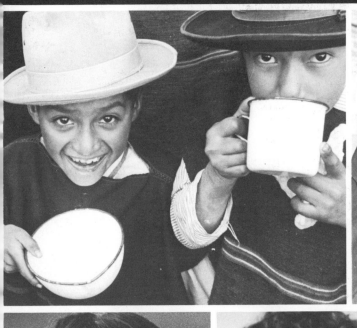
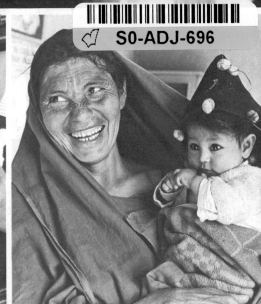
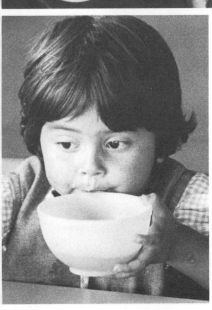
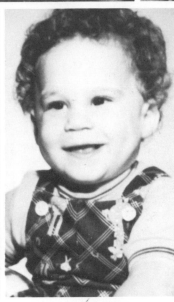
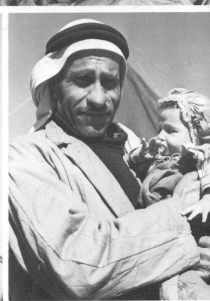
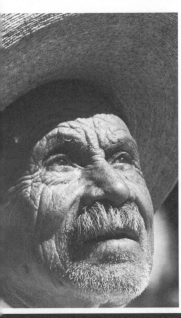
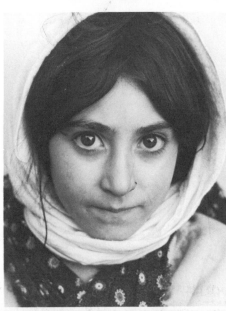
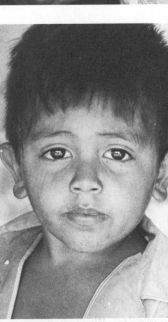

NUTRITION AND PREVENTIVE HEALTH CARE

NUTRITION AND PREVENTIVE HEALTH CARE

Mary Alice Caliendo, Ph.D.

University of Maryland

Macmillan Publishing Co., Inc.
New York
Collier Macmillan Publishers
London

Picture editor: Enid Klass

Endpaper credits: United Nations photos. Top row, left to
right: photo by J. Corash; FAO photo by F. Botts; photo by
Kay Muldoon; United Nations photo; photo by Kay Muldoon.
Second row, left to right: second photo by J. Littlewood;
third, by Nagata; fourth: WFP/FAO photo by Peyton Johnson;
sixth photo: UNATIONS. Bottom row, left to right: first,
second, and third, United Nations photos; fourth, FAO photo
by E. Boubat; fifth, FAO photo by F. Botts.

Macmillan Publishing Co., Inc.
866 Third Avenue, New York, New York 10022
Collier Macmillan Canada, Ltd.

Library of Congress Cataloging in Publication Data

Caliendo, Mary Alice.
  Nutrition and preventive health care.

  Bibliography: p.
  Includes index.
  1. Nutrition disorders — United States —
Prevention. 2. Nutritionally induced diseases.
3. Diet — United States. 4. Nutrition policy —
United States. 5. Nutrition — Study and teaching —
United States. I. Title.
RA645.N87C34   613.2   79-16986
ISBN 0-02-318330-6

Printing: 3 4 5 6 7 8   Year: 6

ISBN 0-02-318330-6

To Nat

Preface

The science and the art of nutrition are dynamic and rapidly evolving. Fifteen to twenty years ago, nutritional concerns were largely limited to providing enough food to stave off nutrition deficiencies, or to prescribing modified diets to aid in the treatment of disease. But nutrition is presently gaining stature as a significant influence on the health of the American population; increasingly it is being viewed as a factor in the health care of our nation.

Today there is a growing appreciation of the interrelations between food and health as well as an increasing awareness of social, environmental, and political factors affecting nutrition. It is important that nutrition and health professionals not only be knowledgeable about these issues, but also be able to shape the complex forces which impact on the relationship between nutrition and health.

This book addresses the role of nutrition in preventive health care. The first section examines changing notions in nutrition. The current U.S. system for the delivery of medical care is reviewed, and alternative systems for providing health care are discussed. The integration of nutrition components into the health care delivery system is then explored.

Section Two looks at the current American diet and at the nutritional status of the American population, with particular emphasis on the nutritional problems of groups vulnerable to nutritional deficiencies. Section Three focuses on the relationship between nutrition and the prevention of the so-called "diseases of civilization" such as heart disease, cancer, dental caries, and other disorders related to overconsumption.

Section Four examines the role of nutrition education in health promotion. After an overview of factors affecting the American diet, the section considers definitions and concepts of nutrition education. Current issues in nutrition education, such as the role of the Federal government, nutrition education and the media, nutrition education to combat misinformation, and nutrition in the medical school curriculum are then discussed.

The final section reviews the development of nutrition policies and programs and ways to shape nutrition policy in terms of participating in the legislative and regulatory process. The administrative structure for the delivery of nutrition programs is reviewed and then various nutrition programs such as the Special Supplemental Food Program for Women, Infants and Children; the Child Nutrition Programs; the Food Stamp Program; and the National Nutrition Program for the Elderly are discussed. The final chapter discusses the current state of a national nutrition policy.

The book is intended for upper level undergraduate or graduate students, not only in community nutrition, but also in therapeutic and clinical nutrition. It should also be useful for those engaged in the practice of community nutrition, for nutrition educators, and for those who work in the areas of clinical and therapeutic nutrition. All nutrition professionals must be aware of the impact of nutrition on health promotion. We can no longer limit our concerns to providing modified diets to hospitalized patients, or to teaching the public about planning a balanced diet by using the basic four food groups. Nutrition professionals should be aware of the expanding nature of nutrition, of the impact of multiple forces on nutrition, and how to be influential in affecting nutrition policies and programs. It is to this end that *Nutrition and Preventive Health Care* was written.

Mary Alice Caliendo

Acknowledgments

I am indebted to many friends, colleagues, and students who encouraged me in this effort. I could never properly thank everyone who contributed to or influenced this work, but I would like to acknowledge a few very special people: Diva Sanjur, who first made me aware of the many complex factors affecting diet and nutrition; Victoria Thiele and Jean Bowering, who always seemed to be there when I most needed help and encouragement; Betty Prather, whose unflagging support and confidence buoyed me in moments of uncertainty; and Eleanor Williams and Laura Sims, who provided insightful suggestions and comments as they read successive drafts of the manuscript. Finally, very special thanks go to my parents, Robert and Juanita Herman, whose example and expectations taught me the importance of hard work, patience, and endurance.

Contents

Nutrition and the health care system

Section Objective

This section is designed to review current issues that relate to the promotion of health, with special emphasis on the relationship between nutrition and health.

Section Overview

The state of American health care is a frequently discussed topic today as we begin to recognize that improvements in health may result not so much from an improved medical care delivery system, but from individual and societal efforts to promote health through changes in life-style and in the environment, and in a general focus on health care rather than on medical care.

Nutrition is perhaps the most easily modified environmental factor that can directly contribute to improved health. Accordingly, we must learn to effectively integrate nutrition components into the health care system.

Developing the ideal health care delivery system — effectively incorporating nutrition into this system and determining which nutrition components should be included — is the subject of this section.

1

Introduction – nutrition and health promotion

Reader Objectives

After completing this chapter the reader should be able to
1. Define and describe the costs of poor nutrition in the United States.
2. Describe quantifiable economic benefits from improved nutrition in the United States.
3. List at least six barriers that limit improved nutrition in the United States.
4. Describe four general strategies for increasing the effectiveness of the role of nutrition in preventive health care.

CHANGING NOTIONS OF NUTRITION

Only recently has the idea of a "nutrition policy" stressed ensuring that North Americans drink orange juice for breakfast, eat enough protein, and limit the intake of candy, soda, potato chips, and "empty calorie food" and that the government make some provision of food aid for the needy overseas. Current thinking on nutrition has, however, dramatically shifted from this parochial notion. To understand the basis for present attitudes on this question it is helpful to briefly review the long-term development of views on nutrition at the national level.

During the 1920s and 1930s nutrition policy focused on nutritional deficiencies, especially as they related to vitamins. With World War II, the focus shifted to the improved and more efficient use of food supplies. The United States became the provider of food aid to its Allies, and the government took an active role in domestic nutrition. The U.S. Department of Agriculture provided posters displaying the "eight basic foods." Ration books were issued, and government charts were offered as useful guides for meal planning.

After the war, the emphasis remained on providing food supplies to the needy overseas, particularly those foods rich in protein. The surplus foods produced by the U.S. farmer formed the basis for much of the food aid that was shipped overseas. The food and agricultural industries worked to increase food production in a cost-efficient, profit-reaping way. It was not until the late 1960s that attention was drawn to the existence of domestic hunger and malnutrition. Partly as a result of the Civil Rights movement, and especially because of the influence of Dr. Martin Luther King and the Southern Christian Leadership Conference, North Americans were made to realize that much hunger existed within their own country.

By the 1970s there was mounting concern over the extent of malnutrition in the United States. The Ten-State Survey,[1] followed by the Health and Nutrition Examination Survey (HANES),[2] attempted to assess the prevalence of malnutrition in the United States. Many North Americans were found in these studies to be at nutritional risk.

Malnutrition does not always present itself in the stark conditions that are more frequently found in developing nations. As H. G. Birch notes:

When we think of malnutrition our imaginations conjure up images of the Apocalypse. We have visions of famines in India, of victims of typhoons, and of young Biafrans starved by war. These images reflect only a highly visible tip of an iceberg. Intermittent and marginal incomes as well as technology which is inadequate to support a population result less often in the symptoms characteristic of starvation than in subclinical malnutrition or what Brock has called "dietary subnutrition . . . defined as any impairment of functional efficiency of body systems which can be corrected by better feeding." Such subnutrition when present in populations is reflected in stunting, disproportions in growth, and a variety of anatomic, physiologic, and behavioral abnormalities. Our principal concern in this country is with these chronic or intermittent aspects of nutritional inadequacy.[3]

There is another aspect to malnutrition — problems of "overnutrition" and excess food intake plague a large proportion of the population and have led to obesity as well as to other diseases commonly associated with "civilization."

The overconsumption of fat, in general, and specifically of saturated fat, as well as cholesterol, sugar, salt, and alcohol have been associated with some of the major causes of death and disability in the United States. Many nutrition and health experts have suggested that some simple changes in North American life-style and in the dietary and food habits of North Americans could significantly reduce the incidence and severe effects suffered from leading "killer diseases."[4,5]

These disorders include:

1. Coronary heart disease — associated with excessive intake of cholesterol, saturated fats, and excessive calories — the nation's number one cause of death.

2. High blood pressure — hypertension — associated with dietary salt and excessive calories contributing to obesity — affects 25 million Americans.

3. Diabetes mellitus — associated with excessive caloric intake and obesity — is the number six cause of death.

4. Dental caries — associated with high intake of sugar and sticky-sweet foods — affects 98 per cent of the American population.

5. Liver disease — associated with heavy intake of alcohol — one of the five leading causes of death.

6. Obesity — associated with excess calorie intake — affects 25-45 per cent of the North American population.

These diseases cause untold expense in terms of medical costs and in loss of quality of life and productivity.

In testimony before the Select Committee on Nutrition and Human Needs in July 1976 D. Mark Hegsted noted: "I wish to stress that there is a great deal of evidence and it continues to accumulate, which strongly implicates and, in some instances, proves that the major causes of death and disability in the United States are related to the diet we eat."[6]

Health and medical experts have become increasingly vocal in expressing their concern with current American eating habits:

Rome's revered heart specialist, Professor Vittorio Puddu, calls it "dietary dying"; Chicago's Dr. Jeremiah Stamler uses evangelistic fervor in an attempt to switch Americans from dietary animal fats to the low animal fat–high polyunsaturate diet; New York's Dr. George Christakis is major-domo of an eating club — the "Anti-Coronary Club" — that would make traditional Princetonians blush; . . . Dr. Jean Mayer believes we're in the midst of a "coronary epidemic"; the dean of American heart specialists, Dr. Paul Dudley White, looks at most American eating habits in terms of a suicidal orgy; and the famed Framingham Heart Study documents that most young men are playing "cardiac roulette."[7]

New notions of nutrition have evolved in the last decade. Nutritional concerns are no longer limited to the processes of the ingestion, absorption, transport, utilization, and excretion of nutrients. Nutrition has become a national concern and is now viewed as a social way to attain the goal of meeting the health needs of the public.[8] Current notions of a "nutrition policy" consider the nutritional dimensions of health to range from problems of nutritional deprivation and undernutrition, to excessive nutrient intake (overnutrition), to the safety, quality, and wholesomeness of the food supply, to the relationship between nutritional status and the incidence of certain diseases such as cancer and coronary heart disease, as well as to the various aspects of therapeutic and rehabilitation needs of the ill patient.

COSTS OF POOR NUTRITION

Literature offers much evidence that the diets of a large number of North Americans, regardless of socioeconomic level, are routinely less than optimal. The impact of this on the health of the nation may be seen in greatly increased vulnerability to complications of pregnancy for the undernourished mother and in the increased likelihood that her child may be of low birth weight with the risk of adverse effects on physical or mental growth and development, in the large numbers of both overweight and underweight children and adults, in the poor health and quality of life of the poorly nourished elderly, in widespread dental disease throughout the entire population, and in the increased incidence of chronic and long-term illnesses that necessitate dietary management, evaluation, and follow-up.[9] The results of improper eating habits have been documented in economic as well as in human health terms. Improper eating habits have been implicated as the prevailing factor responsible for as much as one third of the total national health care bill in the United States.[10]

ECONOMIC BENEFITS FROM IMPROVED NUTRITION

B. Popkin developed a model to determine the economic costs of malnutrition in the United States. The application of the model revealed quantifiable economic benefits from improved nutrition in five general areas:[11]

education — $6.4–19.2 billion

physical performance — $6.4–25.8 billion

morbidity — $201–502 million

mortality — $68–157 million

intergenerational effects — $1.3–4.5 billion

Initially the number of malnourished individuals in the United States was determined from a number of sources, including the Office of Economic Opportunity and other agencies, private and public. The estimated number of malnourished Americans was found to be 7.6 million.

The economic effects resulting from the elimination of malnutrition were calculated, and an evaluation was then conducted. Several costs were not accounted for in the model, the most significant of which was the cost of present medical expense for the treatment of the malnourished. However, the analysis underscores the magnitude of the economic cost of malnutrition.

G. Briggs estimated, based on data from the USDA, that improved nutritional status of North Americans might reduce the national health bill by one third. Briggs analyzed the cost of poor nutritional status relative to some of the common diseases in the United States and suggested that savings might be realized by improved nutrition annually, "based on the more conservative end of the range of current scientific opinion."[10] The national annual costs of some common diseases are:

	Dollars (billions)
Dental disease	$ 3
Diabetes	4
Cardiovascular disease	10
Alcoholism	20
Digestive diseases	3
Total	$40

This analysis does not include complications related to poor nutrition from cancer, kidney disease, or maternal malnutrition and low-birth-weight infants.

Other significant savings can be realized from improved nutritional habits. Improved nutrition presents the possibility of alleviating or eliminating much suffering and loss of work and productivity. It can also help tremendous numbers of individuals to enjoy life of greater quality.

The USDA has suggested that significant improvements in health may result from improved nutrition. Table 1-1, pages 8-10, illustrates the magnitude of benefits from nutrition research. [12,13]

Table 1–1.

Magnitude of Benefits From Nutrition Research

Health Problem	Magnitude of Loss		Potential Savings from Improved Diet
	Part A. Nutrition-related Health Problems		
Heart and vasculatory	Over 1,000,000 deaths in 1967		
	Over 5 million people with definite or suspect heart disease in 1960–62.		25 percent reduction.
	$31.6 billion in 1962		20 percent reduction.
Respiratory and infectious	82,000 deaths per year		
	246 million incidents in 1967		20 percent fewer incidents.
	141 million work-days lost in 1965–66		15–20 percent fewer days lost.
	166 million school days lost		Do.
	$5 million in medical and hospital costs		$1 million.
	$1 billion in cold remedies and tissues		$20 million.
Mental health	2.5 percent of population of 5.2 million people are severely or totally disabled. 25 million people have manifest disability.		10 percent fewer disabilities
Infant mortality and reproduction	Infant deaths in 1967 — 79,000		50 percent fewer deaths.
	Infant death rate 22.4 per 1,000		Do.
	Fetal death rate 15.6 per 1,000		Do.
	Maternal death rate 28.0 per 100,000 live births		Do.
	Child death rate (1–4 yrs.) 96.1 per 100,000 in 1964		Reduce rate to 10 per 100,000.
	15 million with congenital birth defects		3 million fewer children with birth defects.
Early aging and lifespan	49.1 percent of population, about 102 million people have one or more chronic impairments.		10 million people without impairments.
	People surviving to age 65:	Percent	
	White males	66	1 percent improvement per year to 90 percent surviving.
	Negro males	50	
	White females	81	
	Negro females	64	
	Life expectancy in years:		
	White males	67.8	Bring Negro expectancy up to White.
	Negro males	61.1	
	White females	75.1	
	Negro females	68.2	
Arthritis	16 million people afflicted		8∿million people without afflictions.
	27 million work days lost		13.5 million work days.
	500,000 people unemployed		125,000 people employed.
	Annual cost $3.6 billion		$900 million per year.

continued

Health Problem	Magnitude of Loss	Potential Savings from Improved Diet
Dental health	44 million with gingivitis; 23 million with advanced periodontal disease; $6.5 billion public and private expenditures on dentists' services in 1967; 22 million endentulous persons (1 in 8) in 1957; ½ of all people over 55 have no teeth.	50 percent reduction in incidence, severity, and expenditures.
Diabetes and carbo-hydrate disorders	3.9 million overt diabetic; 35,000 deaths in 1967; 79 percent of people over 55 with impaired glucose tolerance.	50 percent of cases avoided or improved.
Osteoporosis	4 million severe cases; 25 percent of women over 40	75 percent reduction.
Obesity	3 million adolescents; 30 to 40 percent of adults; 60 to 70 percent over 40 years.	80 percent reduction in incidence.
Anemia and other nutrient deficiencies	See improved work efficiency, growth and development, and learning ability.	
Alcoholism	5 million alcoholics; ½ are addicted	33 percent.
	About 24,500 deaths in 1967 caused by alcohol	Do.
	Annual loss over $2 billion from absenteeism, lowered production and accidents.	Do.
Eyesight	48.1 percent, or 86 million people over 3 years wore corrective lenses in 1966; 81,000 become blind every year; $103 million in welfare.	20 percent fewer people blind or with corrective lenses.
Cosmetic	10 percent of women age 9 or over with vitamin intakes below recommended daily allowances.	
Allergies	32 million people (9 percent) are allergic	20 percent people relieved. .
	16 million with hayfever asthma	
	7–15 million people (3–6 percent) allergic to milk	90 percent people relieved.
	Over 693 thousand persons (1 in 3,000) allergic to gluten.	Do.
Digestive	8,495 thousand work-days lost; 5,013 thousand school-days lost; about 20 million incidents of acute condition annually.	25 percent fewer acute conditions.
	$4.2 billion annual cost; 14 million persons with duodenal ulcers; $5 million annual cost; 4,000 new cases each day.	Over $1 billion in costs.
Kidney and urinary	55,000 deaths from renal failure; 200,000 with kidney stones.	20 percent reduction in deaths and acute conditions.
Muscular disorders	200,000 cases	10 percent reduction in cases.
Cancer	600,000 persons developed cancer in 1968; 320,000 persons died of cancer in 1968.	20 percent reduction in incidence and deaths.

continued

Health Problem	Magnitude of Loss	Potential Savings from Improved Diet
	Part B. Individual Satisfactions Increased	
Improved work efficiency		5 percent increase in on the job productivity.
Improved growth and development	113,000 deaths from accident. 324.5 million work-days lost; 51.8 million people needing medical attention and/or restricted activity.	25 percent fewer deaths and workdays lost.
Improved learning ability	Over 6.5 million mentally retarded persons with I.Q. below 70; 12 percent of school age children need special education.	Raise I.Q. by 10 points for persons with I.Q. 70–80.

Source: C. E. Weir. Benefits from human nutrition research. Washington, D.C.: Science and Education Staff, USDA, 1971.

BARRIERS TO NUTRITION AND HEALTH PROMOTION

Numerous barriers exist to the implementation of preventive strategies of good nutrition in efforts to improve the national health status. Perhaps the most pervasive barrier is that of the "American way of life." The first national comprehensive survey on the health status of the U.S. population noted that, whereas the population was, on the average, healthy, the lifestyle of most Americans was a health hazard. The survey findings indicated that individual action and life-style changes could result in significantly improved health status.[14] As individuals become more affluent there is a gradual shift in their eating patterns and in their general life-styles. There is a tendency to overconsumption, a sedentary life-style, and often, an increased consumption of alcoholic beverages.

Sociocultural, as well as economic and individual factors, contribute to these patterns. As H. Blackburn notes, "the result of affluence also seems to assume new and independent value status which is in turn passed down as conditioned desire and socially acceptable, though risky behavior. These behaviors and excesses eventually become inalienable personal rights, any suggested change of which is regarded as deprivation and a threat to the American Way of Life"[15]

Life-style and behavioral change are essentially the right and the responsibility of the individual. Although the government as well as educational and health institutions can provide information and support to enable the individual to be knowledgeable about the benefits and risks involved in improving life-styles and behavioral patterns, the change should not be forced. Individual rights raise many difficult and complex issues. For example, what are the individual's rights in choosing to participate in governmental programs? Does the pregnant woman have a responsibility to take advantage of a nutrition program for the well-being of her child, if she herself cannot adequately meet her nutritional needs? When does the right of the individual take precedence over the right or good of others in the "system?" Such issues could be debated at length, and illustrate the complexity of governmental efforts to promote health and good nutrition.

Life-styles, however, are in part an illusory issue. The environment (i.e., social, economic, and political factors) in large part determines what life-style must be adopted. Many people, perhaps the majority of Americans, are not free to choose their life-styles, but are forced by economic necessity to adopt the way of life thrust upon them by the environment. Thus, the environment for many is a factor that significantly limits their food availability and restricts improvements in their food habits. This is discussed in greater detail in Chapters 5 and 12. The North American agricultural system and food industry also exert powerful influences on the nutritional status of the U.S. public. The North American agricultural system has, over the years, developed a highly efficient, cost-effective system of producing and processing massive quantities of food and is able to accommodate the North American food needs with huge surpluses available for export. The emphasis of the total agricultural network, including the farms, the marketing, distribution, and processing systems, the regulatory agencies, and the land-grant universities, is designed for maximum productivity, that is, making available a wide variety and tremendous quantity of foods.

In a sense, the system has been almost too successful. Once geared for high levels of production of such foods as dairy, meat, egg products, and highly refined, processed foods, the agrarian and industrial establishment is now reluctant to consider nutritional objectives in the scheme of priority goals. There is a certain conflict between objectives designed to prevent nutritional deficiencies and those designed to protect the population against overnutrition. In a sense, we have been too successful in assuring an adequate diet for North Americans. It is clear that these institutions exert a tremendous effect on nutritional status.

A very real barrier to improving North American food habits relates to the current state of scientific and technical knowledge. Although a significant body of epidemiological evidence attests to the relation between dietary habits and health status, hard laboratory data are limited. Data on current North American eating habits are also limited. Where data on food consumption exist, it is often difficult to correlate food consumption with health because of a lack of sophistication of data, funds, survey structure, timing, and coordination. Many nutritionists and health professionals agree with the critic who suggested that:

> Nutritional science is not significantly advanced beyond the stage of the Ten Commandments. We have a science of nutrition based on the avoidance of deficiencies, of ill health. What we lack, and sorely need, is a science of well-being, of nutritional sufficiency. We have some idea of what deficiencies are most dangerous, particularly in the area of vitamins. We have very little scientific knowledge of the nutritional qualities of a diet that will maximize well-being and healthy growth.[16]

As M. Lalonde notes:

> The spirit of enquiry and skepticism, and particularly the Scientific Method, so essential to research, are, however, a problem . . . science is full of "ifs," "buts," and "maybe's" while messages designed to influence the public must be loud, clear and unequivocal. To quote I Corinthians, Chapter XIV, Verse 8: 'If the trumpet give an uncertain sound, who shall prepare himself to the battle?'[17]

In advocating nutrition as an essential component of a health promotion strategy, we are confronted by a lack of definite causal relationships between the elements of life-style and environment on the one hand, and ill health on the other. It is not difficult to find scientists arguing both sides of questions such as the following:

Does a diet high in cholesterol necessarily increase the likelihood of developing coronary-artery disease? Will a diet designed to reduce serum lipids reduce the probability of mortality caused by coronary heart disease?

Is the lack of dietary fiber necessarily a risk factor in the etiology of various forms of cancer?

Should the average American drastically limit his or her consumption of eggs because of their cholesterol content?

The fact remains, however, that there is sufficient evidence to suggest that many of America's major health problems are somehow linked to dietary factors, even if the evidence is not conclusive. Ideally, the posture to be taken might be patterned after the Chinese expression "Moi Sui" (pronounced *Moo Sue*), which means "to touch, to feel, to grope around," and which suggests a deliberate stance to innovative and novel actions even when hard scientific proof is not available. The research and scientific professions should take a serious look at the relationships between health and nutrition and prevention, and should aim to establish proven principles. But in the meantime the "Moi Sui" principle should be applied to the search and encouragement of health promotion.[17]

Much of the difficulty in relating the current state of scientific knowledge to the development of practical dietary recommendations to the public revolves around the question, "At what point should generally agreed upon scientific opinions be shared with the public and be the basis for the development of dietary recommendations?" A. Gotto suggests that we remember an extremely important point:

> Medical practice often must be based on the best available existing evidence, even though it falls short of final scientific proof. Certainly all of the scientific evidence concerning diet and its relationship to the major killer diseases is not in, but even when much more evidence accumulates from the surveys, epidemiological studies and basic research, there will continue to be honest professional disagreement concerning the basic dietary path to good health.
>
> However, because there already is much evidence which points in a general direction and because health problems in our country are now enormously pressing . . . it is critical to take some action now.[18]

STRATEGIES TO IMPROVE NATIONAL NUTRITIONAL WELL-BEING

Policymakers can pursue various approaches to increase the role of nutrition in preventive health care. First, nutrition can be integrated into existing health services; that is, nutritional care can become an integral component of the continuum of services available to prevent as well as treat illness and rehabilitate the ill. Chapters 2 and 3 discuss this in greater detail.

Second, social intervention programs can directly provide food and nutritional assistance to target groups through programs such as the WIC supplemental feeding program, the Food Stamp Program, and the School Lunch Program. Social intervention programs can also affect nutrition indirectly by assisting target groups to obtain the economic and social resources needed to obtain adequate nutrition. These programs are discussed in Chapter 17.

Third, the government can influence the nature and quality of the food that is available to the American public. This can be done in two ways: (1) regulations can be designed and implemented to control the content, processing, delivery, storage, and packaging of food supplies so that the nutritional value is maximized, and (2) the government can adjust food prices and, in so doing, can affect the demand for food and the supply of food. Governmental regulation of the food supply is discussed in Chapter 12.

Fourth, the emphasis can be placed on providing the public with nutrition education to enable them to make wise food choices and, in so doing, improve their nutritional status and food habits. Chapters 13 and 14 discuss concepts and activities of nutrition education.

All these approaches are currently being used, to some extent, by the government, by health and nutrition educators and professionals, and by other individuals and groups concerned with optimal nutrition. The political arena in large part determines the area of emphasis. For instance, the most cost-effective approach to improve the nutritional status of a population might involve the direct control of the food supply and the diets of all of the population. Obviously this alternative would be unacceptable in terms of sociocultural and political considerations. The appropriate mix and balance of policy options and interventions will depend upon the political process in which general policy objectives are determined and policies are implemented.

If the health of the public is to be improved through strategies of prevention, and if nutrition is to play a prominent role in achieving improved public health, the approach requires joint efforts among health professionals, educators, the health system, namely, factors that influence the food supply, the educators, the government, and the general public. In other words, the approach must involve national as well as community organizations. The aims must include (1) motivating the public to modify those dietary and life-style characteristics associated with disease and (2) modifying the environment to support such changes.

This will require changes in the health and social system, support systems for the modification of behavior, appropriate changes in the food available to the public, a national policy implemented at all levels, and the appropriate administrative and organizational structure to implement such a strategy.

Dietary habits and nutrition behavior are dynamic and constantly changing; with or without supportive environmental modifications and nutrition education, change in food patterns will continue. If we are to provide input into the evolution of policies and programs designed to influence nutrition, we must be aware of what we are doing, of what the issues are, and of the data supporting both sides of various controversies.

Policy and programs will be influenced by the values, attitudes, and beliefs needed to initiate and sustain change. Policy often evolves more from belief than from hard facts and evidence. An important way to influence the formation of values lies in promoting an awareness of nutrition and in stimulating conversation, discussion, and exchange of knowledge and ideas in various levels of society.

By helping to promote such awareness, by creating a forum for discussion and by contributing and guiding the processes whereby the public can participate in the determination of nutritional programs and policies, we can help to promote health through improved nutrition.

SUMMARY

It is clear that the concept of nutrition as a vital component of efforts to promote health involves complexity and controversy. The remaining chapters are designed to clarify some of the issues involved.

REFERENCES

1. U.S. Department of Health, Education, and Welfare. *Ten-State Survey, 1968–1970*, Publ. No. (HSM) 72-8134. Washington, D.C.: Government Printing Office, 1972.
2. National Center for Health Statistics. *Preliminary Findings of the First Health and Nutrition Examination Survey, 1971–72*. Washington, D.C.: Government Printing Office, January 1974.
3. Birch, H. G. Malnutrition, learning, and intelligence. *Am. J. Publ. Health* 62 (1972): 773–784.
4. U.S. Senate Select Committee on Nutrition and Human Needs. *Dietary Goals for the United States*, 2d ed. Washington, D.C.: Government Printing Office, December 1977.
5. Belloc, N. B., and L. Breslow. Relationship of physical health status and health practices. *Prev. Med.* 1 (1972): 409.
6. Hegsted, D. M. Testimony to U.S. Senate Select Committee on Nutrition and Human Needs. Washington, D.C.: Government Printing Office, July 1976.
7. Medcom, Inc. *Three Times a Day*. New York, 1970.
8. Huenemann, R. L., and M. M. Murai. Philosophy and status of an education program for public health nutritionist–dietitians. *J. Am. Diet. Assoc.* 61 (1969): 669.
9. American Dietetic Association. Promoting optimal nutritional health of the population of the United States. *J. Am. Diet. Assoc.* 55 (1969): 452.
10. Briggs, G. In U.S. Senate Select Committee on Nutrition and Human Needs, *Dietary Goals for the United States*, 2d ed. Washington, D.C.: Government Printing Office, December 1977.
11. Popkin, B. Economic benefits from the elimination of hunger in America. *Public Policy* 20 (1972): 133.

12. Weir, C. E. *Benefits from Human Nutrition Research.* Washington, D.C.: U.S. Department of Agriculture, Science and Education Staff, 1971.

13. Winikoff, B. In U.S. Senate Select Committee on Nutrition and Human Needs, *Diet Related to Killer Diseases.* Washington, D.C.: Government Printing Office, July 27–28, 1976.

14. U.S. Department of Health, Education, and Welfare. *Health United States 1975*, Publ. No. (HRA) 76-1232. Rockville, Md.: National Center for Health Statistics, 1976, pp. 152–156.

15. Blackburn, H. Diet and mass hyperlipidemia: Public health considerations, in U.S. Senate Select Committee on Nutrition and Human Needs, *Diet Related to Killer Diseases.* Washington, D.C.: Government Printing Office, 1977.

16. Gross, L. P. Can we influence behavior to promote good nutrition? *Bull. N.Y. Acad. Med.* 44 (1971): 613.

17. LaLonde, M. *A New Perspective on the Health of Canadians.* Ottawa: Information Center, 1975.

18. Gotto, A. In U.S. Senate Select Committee on Nutrition and Human Needs, *Diet Related to Killer Diseases*, Vol. 2. Part I. Washington, D.C.: Government Printing Office, February 1977.

2

Health and the American health care system

17

Reader Objectives

After completing this chapter the reader should be able to
1. Describe general dissatisfaction with the current medical care system in the United States.
2. Distinguish between medical care and health care.
3. Describe the evolution of the American medical care system.
4. List the four components of the health field concept.
5. Define prevention.
6. Classify prevention activities and state which category has met with the most success in the United States.
7. Justify the prevention approach to health care.
8. List three chronological levels of preventive focuses used to categorize intervention measures, and give a food or nutrition example of each.
9. List eight barriers to health promotion strategies.
10. Describe the mandate of the Health Planning and Resources Development Act of 1974.
11. Define the Health Maintenance Organization (HMO); ambulatory care services; Health Promotion Organization (HPO).

The ideal of medicine is the prevention of disease, and the necessity for curative treatment is a tacit admission of its failure.

— *Sir George Newman*

INTRODUCTION

The traditional system of medical care delivery has been only partly successful in the prevention and control of disease. Billions of dollars have been spent in attempts to cure disease. Although this expenditure is important, and must continue, this effort has brought us to the point at which it is becoming more evident that the prevention of disease should be the primary focus of health care efforts.

New models for the delivery of health service are clearly needed. Improved nutrition may be the cornerstone for efforts designed to promote health and to prevent disease. To create new models requires an understanding and examination of the traditional curative model of medical care. This section reviews some of the basic characteristics of the traditional medical model and some of the alternative models suggested as improvements over the traditional model, and then discusses the integration of a nutrition component into the comprehensive health care system.

THE NATIONAL HEALTH BILL

Health care in the United States is big business. In 1975, 4.8 million workers were involved in providing health care, making it the third largest industry after manufacturing and wholesale/retail trade. The United States spent $139.3 billion for health services in the fiscal year ending June 30, 1976. This was 14 per cent more than was spent in the previous fiscal year. The yearly rate of expansion in national health spending exceeded the growth of expenditures for all other types of goods and services.[1] Health care costs are now responsible for 10 per cent of the national production of goods and services. This is double that of the mid-1960s. The total health cost to the United States approached $200 billion in 1978 — this is almost triple the cost in 1970.[2]

Since 1960 the proportion of the Gross National Product (GNP) allocated for health care expenditure increased from 5.2 per cent to approximately 8.6 per cent; the proportion is expected to reach 10 per cent in the early 1980s.[3]

In 1960 health expenditures accounted for 2 per cent of the federal budget; the comparable figure for 1977 was 10 per cent. Projections for 1980 place the figure at 12 per cent if current trends continue. Personal health expenditures have also greatly increased in recent years. Between fiscal years 1960 and 1976 there was more than a tenfold increase — from $10.4 to $120.4 billion.

Joseph Califano, former secretary of Health, Education, and Welfare in the Carter administration, suggested that "spending on health care will, without some kind of restraint, have ballooned to $229 billion — or more than $1,000 for each man, woman and child in America."[4] These trends in expenditures for national health care are illustrated in Figure 2-1. Many factors influence these increased expenditures, including the increased population growth, increased utilization of medical services, higher medical service prices, and inflation in the prices of technological advances.

With this phenomenal pattern of spending for health care, we might expect an excellent national health status; it does not seem unreasonable to expect optimal health returns for huge health expenditures. But a lack of access to quality health care is a reality for many individuals and population subgroups in the United States. There is evidence from a variety of sources that the increased spending for health care has not significantly been translated into improved health status of the population.

HEALTH STATUS, U.S.A.

A substantial portion of the gain in longevity between 1900 and 1973 was made during infancy. About half of the total gain was made during the first five years of life, and almost all the remainder during the years prior to high school. For white males at age 45, the gain in longevity — considering all advances in medical science and levels of living — was less than four years. . . . The relatively small gain after age 45, especially for males, reflects two facts. One is that heart disease and cancer cause death mainly after that age, and progress against these diseases has been slow

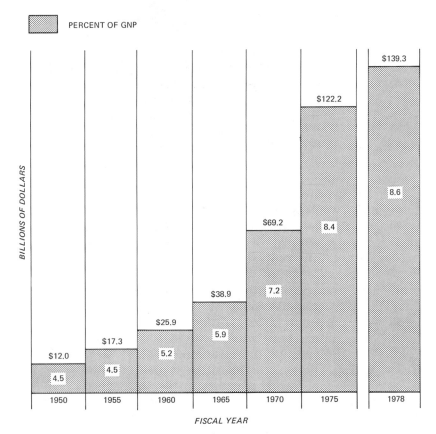

Figure 2-1. Our national health bill: national health expenditures and percent of GNP for selected fiscal years, 1950–1978. (HEW)

. . . the other fact is that certain forms of cancer and heart disease have actually increased substantially since 1900, especially lung cancer and coronary heart disease.[5]

The life span of the average American male is seventeenth among nations in the world when compared with the life spans of males living in other countries. The life span ranking of the American female is twelfth, and the United States ranks thirteenth among nations in infant mortality.[6] These trends are illustrated in Figure 2-2.

Despite the staggering expenditures for health care and the improved availability of medical service, the national health status in the United States relative to illness, disability, and premature death evidences little sign of improvement.

After a 50-year period of decreasing mortality rates, the total death rate in the United States ceased to improve during the 1960s, and between the 1960s and early 1970s the death rate continued to stabilize, ranging from 9.7 to 9.3 per 1,000 population.[7]

The average sickness or injury rate for Americans in 1972 was estimated to be about 450 million — a figure that translates into two episodes per individual. Individuals over the age of 17 missed 5.4 days of work as a

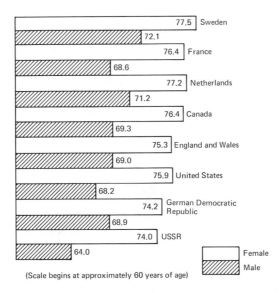

Figure 2-2. Average life spans in different countries. (Department of Health, Education and Welfare: *Health in the United States, 1975,* Publication no. (HRA) 76-1233, p. 45)

result of sickness or injury, and children aged 6 to 16 missed 5.1 days of school.

Few people are satisfied with the tangible returns from the health care dollar; we may have come to the point of diminishing returns on the health care dollar.

How should the health care system contribute to health? A brief look at the evolution of the current health care delivery system will be helpful in suggesting answers to this question.

HISTORICAL PERSPECTIVE ON MEDICAL/HEALTH CARE

Medical care in the United States has always been viewed as a biosocial science and an interpersonal art. The history of medical care is replete with practitioners who recognized the inseparability of health and illness and man's life-style. But the emphasis in delivery of services has focused primarily on treatment and cure rather than on the prevention of disease.

The traditional view of health as the "absence of symptoms" guided the practice of crisis-oriented health care. This traditional concept of health was reflected in medical research, medical care, and social judgments about the levels of well-being the society as a whole was willing to tolerate.

The focal point of the traditional medical care delivery system was the physician. The physician was directly involved in helping the patient gain entry into the system and was directly involved in patient care at every stage of the process, from diagnostic and assessment procedures to therapeutic treatments, evaluations, and follow-ups.

The traditional medical care delivery system has "evolved over the years with little deliberate planning."[8] During the early 1900s the medical care available was rather primitive and centered around the physician. Only ill patients sought any type of medical services. As technology, science, and medical knowledge increased, an expanded array of services was made available to the patient, but the physician remained at the heart of the delivery system.

Medical education has undergone significant changes since the early 1900s, and these changes have affected the practice of medicine and the delivery of health care. More than a century ago, Dr. Edward Jarvis expressed concern for the way medical education ordered its priorities:

> Our education has made our calling exclusively a curative and not a conservative one, and the business of our responsible lives has confined us to it. Our thoughts are devoted to, our interests concerned in, and our employments are connected solely with, sickness, debility or injury — with diminution of life in some of its forms. But with health, with fullness of unalloyed, unimpaired life, we, professionally, have nothing to do.[9]

In 1910 the Flexner report sharply criticized a variety of medical education factors, notably the use of part-time general physicians used as primary faculty — this in turn resulted in various changes in the training of health professionals.[10]

A strong biomedical research base introduced as an integral component of the academic medical school curricula was one of the important results of the Flexner report. This brought special science skills to the treatment of patients, and it influenced the development of a vast number of medical specialists rather than the general practitioner. New drugs, new scientific techniques, and a knowledge explosion characterized the practice of medicine. Focus began to move from the humanistic, patient-centered approach to the technological approach. Although these trends resulted in vastly improved care of the seriously ill and improvements in areas of diagnosis, detection, and follow-up treatment, similar advances were not made in the care of ambulatory patients. It is argued that such increasing specialization and the characteristic geographical maldistribution of health professionals have adversely affected the health care provided for common illness and preventive health supervision.[11]

Summarizing his thoughts on this subject, H. Mahler notes:

> Most of the world's medical schools prepare doctors, not to care for the "health" of the people, but instead for medical practice that is blind to anything but "disease" and the technology for dealing with it; a technology involving astronomical and ever-increasing prices, directed towards fewer and fewer people who often are selected not so much by social class or wealth as by medical technology itself, and frequently focused on persons in the final stages of life. They prepare doctors to deal with rare cases which are hardly ever encountered, rather than with the common health problems of the community; for cure rather than for care. They tend to forget that technical solutions must respond to social goals, not dictate them.[12]

Mahler further asserts that the medical care delivery system at times seems more of a threat than a help to positive health. "The general picture is that of a cost-explosive medical establishment catering not for the promotion of health but for the unlimited application of disease technology to a certain ungenerous proportion of potential beneficiaries and, perhaps, not doing that too well either."[12]

The 1970s ushered in a time of increased concern over the ability of the medical care system to meet the needs of its clients. Medical care had evolved to the point of offering sophisticated diagnostic and treatment services, and it now required the costly teamwork of a variety of medical specialists, elaborate treatment facilities, and expensive equipment. No longer was the system reserved for the very ill; a mix of what S. R. Garfield terms "worried well" and "early sick" also sought the attention of medical experts.

Throughout this evolution, the delivery of health services remained relatively unchanged, "as though oblivious to the great need for new forms of organization equal to the task of applying new techniques and knowledge."[8] But signs of strain and inefficiency began to surface as more people began to demand services and the costs for health care skyrocketed.

Critics have suggested that medical care in the United States is more a collection of fragmented pieces, with much overlapping, alarming gaps in care, inflated costs, and ineffective effort rather than a comprehensive, integrated system in which need and efforts are closely related and benefits are the greatest.

DISSATISFACTION WITH THERAPEUTIC MEDICINE

An extensive review of the weakness of the current system is beyond the scope of the present discussion, but a cursory discussion will provide detail sufficient for understanding the effects of possible modifications of presently existing elements of the health care system.

The existing system is composed of a great number of health care providers who often work independently of other practitioners; the current system lacks coordination, organization, and effective planning; many needed services are not properly integrated into existing services. These characteristics have led to a variety of weaknesses:[13]

1. Duplication of very expensive facilities, resources, and equipment; the brunt of this financial cost must be borne by the consumer of services.

2. Maldistribution of medical and health care services; affluent, often urban, areas enjoy a plethora of services and resources whereas rural and economically poor areas face serious medical service shortages.

3. The piecemeal and fragmented system leads to a lack of continuity in care.

4. Current third-party payment plans, legal restrictions, and professional attitudes limit the development of paramedical personnel who could provide many important services currently provided by the physician, thereby reducing skyrocketing costs and increasing the range of services available to the economically poor.

5. Current third-party payment plans also encourage the consumer to use expensive hospital services; often the medical needs of the client could be met less expensively and equally well through ambulatory care facilities.

6. Payment plans also encourage the service provider to overprescribe services, such as office visits or surgery that may be marginally needed or nonessential.

7. Payment plans often discourage the consumer from taking a preventive strategy to meet his or her own health needs; warning signs of serious illness may be ignored until the illness becomes full blown and requires expensive and prolonged medical care.

8. Formulas for the reimbursement of hospital costs, coupled with the prevalent desire to have hospitals become highly prestigious through the provision of highly expensive, sophisticated equipment, tend to encourage hospitals to acquire costly facilities and equipment; such acquisition is often not proportional to the resulting benefits.

9. The medical profession exerts the predominant influence over operation and regulation of the medical care system. Critics contend that such a monopoly has resulted in a system that is frequently more responsive to the interests of the medical profession than to consumer needs.

Dissatisfaction with the current system also relates to areas beyond these issues and to the high rates of preventable illness and death. Considerable evidence suggests that medical intervention per se cannot satisfactorily contribute to the management of serious disease and sickness. Illustrating this are the growing evidence of patient noncompliance with prescribed therapeutic treatments, the widespread evidence of unneeded surgery, the overprescribing of medication, the growing recognition that technical skills and expertise do not always translate into high-quality human health care, the frequently revealed poor care offered to nursing home patients, the growing public clamor for the appreciation of human treatment for they dying, and an awakened interest in euthanasia.[14]

Many developments in the larger societal context have also contributed to the dissatisfaction with the current system of health care and have stimulated a search for something better. Among these developments are the shifting of societal values toward increased concern with the impoverished and deprived, the environment, and the need for individual and local initiative as a means of stimulating health and development.

All these developments suggest that the public is becoming impatient with crisis-oriented medical intervention, as well as with the sophisticated and inhuman characteristics of advanced medical technology.

The Health Field Concept[15]

One reason for the inadequacy of the current medical health care system appears to be its myopic approach to health care. This reflects a focus on the health care delivery system to the neglect and exclusion of other aspects affecting health status.

The National Health and Welfare Department of Canada developed a broader approach, suggesting that the health field (a general term including all matters related to health) can be divided into four principal elements:

> Human biology
>
> Environment
>
> Life-style
>
> Health care organization

These four elements, which were identified as the etiology of illness and disease, can be briefly described as follows:

1. *Human biology:* "all those aspects of health, both physical and mental, that are developed within the human body as a consequence of the basic biology of man and the organic makeup of the individual." Included in this element are genetic individuality, processes of growth, development, maturation, and aging and the numerous internal body systems such as skeletal, muscular, pulmonary, cardiovascular, endocrine, and digestive.

2. *Environment:* "all those matters related to health that are external to the human body and over which the individual has little or no control." Examples of environmental impacts on health status include the food supply, water supply, and air quality.

3. *Life-style:* "the aggregation of decisions by individuals that affect their health and over which they more or less have control." Life-style variables include traditions, sociocultural practices, recreation activities, eating habits, and exercise patterns.

4. *Health Care Organization:* "the quantity, quality, arrangement, nature, and relationships of people and resources in the provision of health care." Included in this element are hospitals, clinics, medical practice, drugs, community health services, and dental services. Often referred to as the health care system, this has been the focus of most direct efforts to improve health as well as of most health expenditures.

This health field concept suggests that the main causes of ill health are to be found in the first three elements. As M. LaLonde notes, "It is apparent, therefore, that vast sums are being spent treating diseases that could have been prevented in the first place. Greater attention to the first three conceptual elements is needed if we are to continue to reduce disability and early death."[15]

The premise underlying the health field concept is that a holistic approach to improved health status is needed. Such an approach is fundamental to the promotion of health.

It has been estimated that medical care provided by physicians accounts for less than 10 per cent of the difference in health status between any two Americans. An estimated 90 per cent of the variation is the result of factors beyond the control of the physician, such as life-style; personal eating, smoking, and drinking habits; and environmental factors such as air, water, and food supply.[16]

'Twas a dangerous cliff, as they freely confessed.
    Though to walk near its crest was so pleasant;
But over its terrible edge there had slipped
    A duke, and full many a peasant.
The people said something would have to be done,
    But their projects did not at all tally.
Some said, "Put a fence 'round the edge of the cliff;"
    Some, "An ambulance down in the valley."

The lament of the crowd was profound and was loud,
    As their hearts overflowed with their pity;
But the cry for the ambulance carried the day
    As it spread through the neighboring city.
A collection was made, to accumulate aid,
    And the dwellers in highway and alley
Gave dollars or cents — not to furnish a fence —
    But an ambulance down in the valley.

"For the cliff is all right if you're careful," they said;
    "and if folks ever slip and are dropping,
It isn't the slipping that hurts them so much
    As the shock down below — when they're stopping."
So for years (we have heard), as these mishaps occurred
    Quick forth would the rescuers sally,
To pick up the victims who fell from the cliff
    With the ambulance down in the valley.

Said one, to his plea, "It's a marvel to me
    That you'd give so much greater attention
To repairing results than to curing the cause;
    You had much better aim at prevention.
For the mischief, of course, should be stopped at its source,
    Come, neighbors and friends, let us rally.
It is far better sense to rely on a fence
    Than an ambulance down in the valley."

"He is wrong in his head," the majority said;
    "He would end all our earnest endeavor.
He's a man who would shirk this responsible work,
    But we will support it forever.
Aren't we picking up all, just as fast as they fall,
    And giving them care liberally?
A superfluous fence is of no consequence,
    If the ambulance works in the valley."

The story looks queer as we've written it here,
    But things oft occur that are stranger.
More humane, we assert, than to succor the hurt,
    Is the plan of removing the danger.
The best possible course is to safeguard the source;
    Attend to things rationally.
— Yes, build up the fence and let us dispense
    With the ambulance down in the valley.*

*The value of prevention is expressed succinctly in the "Parable of the Dangerous Cliff," author unknown, reprinted from *Farm Safety Review* (May–June, 1966, National Safety Council).

DEFINITION AND TECHNIQUES OF PREVENTION[17]

In general, prevention activities include social factors such as health education, adequate sanitation, good nutrition, and a safe environment. These prevention activities can be categorized in a number of ways:

1. Governmental prevention activities in which the public plays a largely passive role. Examples of this include water supply purification, mandatory immunizations, water supply fluoridation, and safety and sanitation regulations. In these activities, the responsibility belongs to the public sector, whereas the individual remains a largely passive recipient of the benefits obtained.

2. Health professionals involved in health care delivery that offer varying types and degrees of health care of a preventive nature to their clients. Such preventive services include screening for nutritional deficiencies, physical examinations and history, blood pressure measurement, education and counseling about family planning, adequate nutrition, and positive health behavior. In addition, community-wide programs such as chest X rays, diagnostic Pap smears, and immunizations can be included in this category.

3. Preventive programs in which the individual must actively participate and take the responsibility for personal health care. This type of prevention relates not only to the prevention of communicable diseases but also to diseases related to life-style. The individual, in this regard, must learn, become motivated, and implement healthful practices such as employing wise food habits, avoiding smoking and excessive drinking, taking the responsibility to follow prescribed treatment regimes for known and existing diseases, and taking advantage of available educational programs and services that will aid in improving personal health.

Of these three classifications, success has been greatest in the first, in which the individual remains almost a passive recipient of benefits. The second most successful type of program is that in which preventive health services are actually delivered to the individual by the health professional. The least successful category is that in which the individual must take an active role in his or her own personal health care.

THE IMPORTANCE OF HEALTH PROMOTION STRATEGIES

In his volume *Who Shall Live?*, V. R. Fuchs offers support for the notion that "The greatest current potential for improving the health of the American people is to be found in what they do or don't do to and for themselves." Fuchs notes that:

the most important thing to realize about such differences in health levels is that they are usually not related in any important degree to differences in medical care. Over time the introduction of new medical technology has had a significant impact on health, but when we examine differences among populations at a given moment in time, other socioeconomic and cultural variables are now much more important than differences in the quantity or quality of medical care.[18]

The relationship among life-style, individual behavior, environmental conditions, and health status is becoming increasingly evident. The concept of health promotion and preventive health is being seen as a necessary and important response to the major causes of death and disability in the United States today. In view of the condition of the current medical care delivery system, and the resulting costs and dissatisfactions with national health status, the role of prevention cannot be ignored.

Public health efforts are in agreement in fostering the prevention of disease, the prolongation of life, and the promotion of physical and mental health and efficiency through planned, organized efforts. The importance of timing is significant. Health costs and overall social costs are reduced when the community and the individual receives early treatment. Ideally the "treatment" is initiated before the disease processes actually begin. It is clear that community health is best sustained when healthful living styles can be fostered from the very start of the life cycle, or even before, through healthful behavior of the parents.

A number of recent studies suggest strong relationships between good health habits and good health.[19,20] For example, N. Belloc and C. Breslow report on the results of a study of 6,928 Alameda County, California, adults that demonstrated that habits of sleep, meal regularity, physical activity, weight control, and smoking and drinking were related to health; positive practices were associated with improved health, regardless of the influence of sex, socioeconomic status, or age.[20]

A follow-up study by the same authors demonstrated that positive health habits were also related to increased life expectancy.[19]

Fuchs dramatically illustrates the impact of life-styles in his discussion of mortality rates in Utah and Nevada:

> The two states are very much alike with respect to income, schooling, degree of urbanization, climate, and many other variables that are frequently thought to be the cause of variations in mortality. . . . What then explains these huge differences in death rates? The answer almost surely lies in the different lifestyles of the residents of the two states. Utah is inhabited primarily by Mormons, whose influence is strong throughout the state. Devout Mormons do not use tobacco or alcohol and in general lead stable, quiet lives. Nevada, on the other hand, is a state with high rates of cigarette and alcohol consumption and very high indexes of marital and geographical instability. The contrast with Utah in these respects is striking.[18]

The case for prevention has been argued by many health experts. E. J. Pellegrino suggests:

> Disease prevention and health maintenance are inevitably included in any list of medical responsibilities. With equal inevitability, they are among the most neglected sectors of health care. Indeed, at no time and in no country have the available preventive measures been applied vigorously or to a whole population. . . . Were we to make effective use of this (available) information on a wide scale, we could materi-

ally alter mortality, morbidity, and disability. Yet, we do not do so and we are not likely to do so without some major alteration in the organization of health care and the development of the specific functions of prevention . . .[21]

One of the major themes of the activities of the Department of Health, Education, and Welfare is preventive medicine.[22] The long-term goal of health promotion is the maintenance of health and the prevention of disease. The immediate goal is to influence the individual as well as the physical and social environment to promote health and prevent disease.

Activities in this prevention theme include specific measures directed toward individuals (e.g., screening procedures or modification of eating habits), which may be directed by community workers, industry advertising, private physician interest, and other forms of patient education and motivation. Environmental changes, such as changing food supply and improved environmental sanitation, may either aid or deter the consumer from performing protective health activities. Social factors must also be considered; sociocultural values figure prominently in determining behavior and related activity outcomes. Religious custom, ethnic heritage, political leadership, legislation, and group and community activities are all sources influencing social behavior and determining tradition, law, and value systems.

The specific characteristics of any disorder or disease condition, as well as its natural history, will influence the focus and type of preventive action that are most appropriate. The Forward Plan for Health categorization of the health/disease complex is summarized in Table 2-1.

Three chronological levels of "preventive" focuses are used to categorize intervention measures. Primary prevention is the fostering of health and prevention of disease before it begins; this involves the removal of the underlying causes of the disorder, illness, and health problems. For example, food programs to reduce malnutrition would constitute a direct attack on a cause of ill health. Primary prevention may involve a life-style change to improve personal health status, or it may entail the regulation of harmful substances in the environment.

Inherent in the concept of primary care are the following:[23]

First-contact care — primary care is the patient's entry point into the health care system

Outreach and follow-up responsibility for patient and community are assumed

Care is comprehensive and multidisciplinary

Ongoing responsibility for patient in terms of health and sickness are assumed

Responsibility for coordinating the care of all patient's health problems is assumed

Primary care is "personal care in the broadest sense"

Secondary prevention is early intervention into existing illness; it includes early detection of disease and speedy action and intervention to

Table 2-1
Categorization of Health/Illness Complex

Susceptibility to specific disease — understood in terms of a healthy person in "danger of contracting disease upon exposure unless he is immunized." The objective of preventive action here is to provide immunity to particular diseases. This concept may also relate to the prevention of some noninfectious disorders. For example, the modification of inappropriate dietary patterns may help to prevent the incidence of atherosclerotic heart disease in an individual otherwise susceptible to it. Another factor influencing susceptibility to specific disorders relates to an individual's "propensity to seek preventive measures" and treatment early in the development of a disease condition; such action may help to ameliorate the adverse effects of the condition.

Precursors of disease — early detection through screening may alert the individual to certain disease precursors that may lend themselves to early treatment and therapy. For example, obesity (a disease in itself) is often the forerunner of other health disorders such as hypertension, diabetes, and coronary heart disease. An individual with hypertension is at an increased risk of developing heart disease, stroke, and renal disease. If these conditions were detected and treated early, their adverse effects on other illnesses might be prevented.

Presymptomatic disease — the condition of an individual who has a disease but is not yet experiencing symptoms. For example, an individual may have slightly elevated high blood sugar levels but will not be experiencing overt symptoms of diabetes. Detection may involve screening procedures or complete physical and diagnostic workups.

Diagnosed disease — the condition of an individual who presents symptoms indicative of a disease.

Treatment phase of disease — that phase that seeks to prevent further deterioration and disease progression and to help the patient to return to a disease-free state.

Disability Limitation Phase — an advanced progression of the previous phase. Some disorders result in chronic problems and discomfort and morbidity for an extended period of time. Preventive measures involve attempts to shorten this stage and limit the disability, as well as to make the patient as comfortable as possible during convalescence.

Rehabilitation phase — another continuation of the treatment stage involves helping the patient to adjust, physically, psychologically, and socially to what may be a decreased state of functioning and, at the same time, to return the patient to positive health as soon as possible.

Health (Phase Two) — when the ill patient has been returned to the best state of health that is feasible for him or her, after having been ill. The primary objective is to maintain this state of health.

Source: U.S. Department of Health, Education, and Welfare, *Forward Plan for Health, FY 1978–1982*. Washington, D.C., Government Printing Office, 1976.

relieve discomfort, prevent disability and death. An example of secondary prevention is screening for the detection of high blood pressure in apparently healthy individuals with appropriate follow-up action to prevent coronary heart disease.

Tertiary prevention involves encouraging recovery from episodes of sickness; this includes attempts to relieve discomfort, to help people live acceptable lives while suffering from a chronic dysfunction, and to improve health status through a variety of rehabilitative techniques.

Primary prevention demands a deep commitment to community organization and planned change that is traditionally foreign to American ways of life. However, there are promising signs that this approach is becoming increasingly important to people in the United States. Programs such as well-baby clinics and antipoverty programs are evidence of the community's will to prevent disease.

Secondary prevention is also becoming more widespread. A notable example is the high blood pressure detection program in which intervention is founded on a broad community orientation. (See page 371.)

Tertiary prevention is increasingly looking to the community for treatment and care modalities. There is a growing thrust toward offering the elderly an alternative to institutionalization. Intermediate facilities, ambulatory treatment centers, and programs for home care aim to prevent further deterioration without requiring institutionalization. Figure 2-3 illustrates some of the agencies and levels that are involved in the delivery of health care.

Figure 2-3. Some of the agencies involved in the delivery of different levels of health care. (HEW, Public Health Service and Health Resources Administration, *Trends Affecting U.S. Health Care System*, 1976, p. 202)

SPECTRUM OF HEALTH CARE DELIVERY

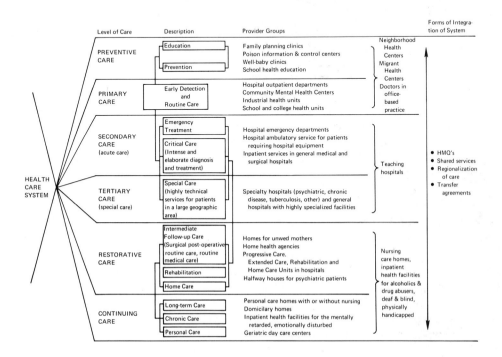

BARRIERS TO HEALTH PROMOTION STRATEGIES[24,25]

The barriers to achieving true health care are numerous.

Health Care as a Political Issue

As previously mentioned, health care has become the nation's third largest "business." Thus the politics of health form a most important barrier to total concern. It is even asserted that "health is not viewed by those who hold the reins of power in terms of the immediate and urgent needs of the citizenry but rather in terms of the benefits to be derived for greater advantage in the political area."[24] Congressmen, national medical organizations, and the insurance industry have vested interests in health concerns beyond human welfare, and all stand to benefit greatly from certain programs. The fact that benefits of health promotion programs are often deferred, that is, long range and appearing in the future, takes political benefits away from these programs. Public officials often allocate fewer dollars for long-range benefits than those that might be allocated to programs that reap more immediate benefits.

A second consideration in this regard is that a real constituency for health promotion has not been developed.

Finally, governmental policies often conflict with policies that are believed to be in the best interests of health. For example, although it is generally agreed that cigarette smoking is hazardous to health, the government continues to pay tobacco growers a price support subsidy. The government spends ten times more to develop a "safe" cigarette than it does in attempts to alleviate smoking. Furthermore, different government agencies oppose one another in their actions.[16]

The Right to Health — Social/Economic Considerations

There is no general agreement about the universal right to health in the United States. Although there is a widely held "right to health" concept, which first appeared in the *Congressional Record* in 1976, there is not yet total agreement that this concept is intended for everyone. The idea has been frequently reiterated since 1944 when President Franklin D. Roosevelt called for the "right to adequate medical care and the opportunity to achieve and enjoy good health." In the current usage, the right to health refers to both curative and preventive medicine for the individual as well as for the community. Although few if any would openly dispute the right to health, there is little effort to stimulate societal conditions that would support and facilitate the realization of this right for all individuals. Conditions of poverty, social deprivation, and adverse environmental conditions negate many efforts of health promotion.

The question — for health care as an individual's right, for health as a state of positive well-being, rather than the concept of medical care as a crisis-oriented, disease-treating service — involves tangible preventive strategies and necessitates the fostering of individual self-responsibility. To plan for health rather than for disease means to foster in individuals a capacity for attending to their own health needs. This is impossible if environmental conditions are hazardous to health and beyond individual control. The important question is, What concept of the right to health shall prevail? Until the nation is fully committed to the concept, optimal health care delivery systems will be limited in quality and accessibility.

Cultural and Behavioral Constraints

The easy, pleasurable, self-indulgent way of life that is advocated for the North American people is contrary to the notion of health promotion. Advertisements promote self-medication to relieve any ache or pain; sedentary activities, spectator sports, and machinery to facilitate the easy life are widely touted.

Programs that attempt to counteract this life-style must recognize what they are up against. These programs must be fully planned with the participation of those who will use and benefit from their services. J. G. Freymann's observation on the health behavior of individuals as far back as the ancient Greeks illustrates the difficulties involved in changing the individual life-styles of a population. According to Freymann, "Greek mythology may contain a clue to the deepest reason of all for this schism (promotion of health, and prevention, vs. cure). Hygeia, the goddess of health, was subservient in the Olympian hierarcy to Aesculapius, the god of healing. Apparently it has always been easier to depend upon healers than living wisely."[26]

Legal/Ethical Concerns

One of the basic individual freedoms is often considered to be the right to self-abuse. The notion is that unless an individual action is harmful to another, it cannot be prohibited. This notion is tempered, however, by the idea that the individual's right to self-abuse must be limited when others suffer from that abuse. For example, whereas the consumption of an inadequate diet may often be harmful only to the individual involved, if that individual happens to be a pregnant mother, the harm will likely extend to the unborn child.

By emphasizing life-style and individual action as being implicated in health status, there is often a tendency to "blame the victim." Although it is logical and sensible to suggest that Americans cut down on smoking and decrease their intake of calories, saturated fats, and highly sweetened foods, these strategies often fail because they do not take into consideration the characteristics, values, cultural traditions, and behavior patterns of individuals. Before we can effectively change individual behavior, society must first correct its own shortcomings. Health professionals and government agencies have traditionally regarded human activity as individual and voluntary; in so doing they have ignored the social preconditions that impinge on individual health and well-being.

Organizational Aspects

The bulk of federal health care expenditures are devoted to medical care activities; less than 2.5 per cent of the yearly health care expenditure in the United States is allocated to activities of prevention. Many health services that are essential to health promotion, such as diagnostic screening, counseling, nutrition education, or screening programs, are not reimbursable by third-party payers, either public (such as Medicare) or private (insurance companies). Such reimbursement is essential to a full commitment to health promotion.

Technology

A grave constraint is the lack of technical knowledge as it relates to physiological/biochemical knowledge of health and nutrition in the individual, and also as it relates to principles of motivation and behavior. For example, we cannot state with certainty what the nutrient requirements of the population are, or the exact effect of a diet that is high in certain elements on health status. We also lack knowledge about the types of strategies and health messages that are most appropriate for reaching population subgroups and the most appropriate ways to induce planned behavior change.

Policymakers are faced with a number of hard questions for which practical answers are needed to base policy. Policymakers are hampered in their efforts by the scientist who responds with the proposal to initiate a methodological study of long-term duration to obtain valid and reliable answers. Although the need for sound, solid basic research cannot be disclaimed, many scientists cannot accept the real need for practical guidelines and direction for policy. As A. Berg has suggested:

> information that today is 80 to 85 per cent accurate is much more useful than 99 per cent accurate information six or eight years from now and is clearly more useful than no information at all. Data for initial planning and policy purposes do not need to be as precise as for the professional journal article. Scientists, in their reluctance to offer what, in their view, are premature judgments, often fail to recognize that in their search for purity, they are losing impact. Moreover, in the process, they are losing a reputation for usefulness.[27]

Resource Allocation

The popular saying, "an ounce of prevention is worth a pound of cure," is not widely accepted by policymakers and planners. In the 45 years between 1929 and 1974 there was a decrease of almost 50 per cent in national health expenditures for public health activities. This is illustrated in Figure 2-4. Spending patterns of this nature surely impose tremendous barriers to the development and effective implementation of a widespread health promotion strategy.

Professional Societies as Restrictive Guilds

As P. B. Cornely asserts, the fragmented health care and the patchwork organization of delivery systems exist, in part, because of traditional professional education and values.[24] Critics contend that there is a sharp stratification of professional and paraprofessional groups, with group identification sometimes being a more unifying concept than client welfare. Each profession sets its own standards, maintains tight reins on entrance to the profession by nonmembers, and subscribes to a certain eliteness for its members. This is certainly an important barrier to a total concern for health care.

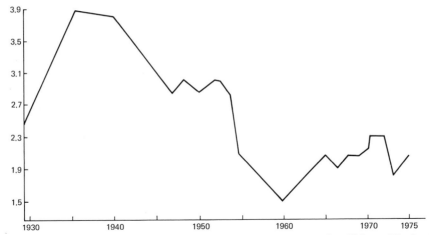

Figure 2-4. Percentage of total national health expenditures for U.S. public health activities, 1929-1974. (*Compendium of National Health Expenditures Data,* **1970,** pp. 20-46; ibid., **1974**)

Lack of Health Education

There is currently only 1 health educator in the schools and medical facilities for every 17,000 people. By contrast, there is 1 physician for every 515 people. Much of the health information that reaches the public is ineffective as education and is often conflicting. Health professionals themselves are rarely trained in nutrition and other preventive health aspects.[16]

FEDERAL INITIATIVE

The federal initiatives and efforts in health-related concerns have expanded considerably in recent years and now recognize the significance of health promotion.[28-30]

Avowing its stance on the health promotion concept, the Congress, in 1976, through the Health Promotion and Disease Prevention Act[28] established an office for the coordination of all health education and health promotion efforts nationwide. The law (P.L. 94-317) notes the importance of controlling current advertising of the "indiscriminate consumption of liquor, food, drugs, or tobacco smoke with little regard for the consequences." The mandate of the Public Law 94-317 provides authority for activities of health promotion and health prevention; its scope encompasses educational and preventive health services.

The National Health Planning and Resources Development Act (P.L. 93-601) of 1974 was enacted to provide a national health planning system and to coordinate state health plans, health facilities expenditures, the development of new institutional health services, and the ongoing review of existing health services.[30] This act is an effort by the Congress to provide equal access to quality health care as a federal priority. The purpose of the act is to facilitate the development of a national health planning policy, to facilitate area-wide and state health planning, and to authorize financial assistance of needed resources to further these ends.

Relevant health agencies and associations and professional societies are invited to actively participate in the health planning process and to communicate recommendations to the secretary of Health, Education, and Welfare (HEW). The act specifically addresses "the promotion of activities for the prevention of disease, including studies of nutritional and environmental factors affecting health and the provision of preventive health care services."

The goals of the act include the provision of equal access to high-quality health care for all individuals; the equitable distribution of health resources, facilities, and personnel; the participation of both providers and consumers in planning, developing, and using health care services; and general public education to promote public awareness of the need for self-responsibility in health care.

The federal agency charged with the responsibility for overseeing the operation of the system is the Health Resources Administration (HRA). The HRA is to advise the secretary of HEW about national health guidelines, the implementation of the regulations of the act, and a new health delivery system.

The act further provides for the United States to be geographically divided into approximately 200 health service areas, each of which is to serve areas of approximately 500,000 to 3 million people except where populations are extremely dense or sparse. A governing body for each area, the Health Systems Agency (HSA), would prepare and implement plans for area-wide health planning. The HSA is comprised of 10 to 30 members, more than half of which must be health consumers, the remainder being health providers (physicians, nurses, representatives of health insurers, HMOs, and the like). Five broad categories of providers are identified, one of them being the "allied health professions."

The HSA is responsible for developing goals for the attainment of long-range objectives. Activities undertaken by the HSA include planning and construction of health facilities, developing health resources, reviewing federal funding applications, and assisting the State Health Planning and Development Agency in its activities.

The responsibilities of the HSAs include the following:[31]

Gathering, analyzing and reporting conclusions from available data, including statistics.

Gathering and analyzing data available from more subjective sources such as people's felt needs, problems, and experiences.

Developing solutions to identified problems and then finding ways of implementing them, in view of legal and financial restraints; determining community reaction to these plans.

Recommending ways to implement identified solutions that are acceptable to the community; incorporating any available resources, including those of the local community.

Increasing the understanding and commitment of the community to obtain maximum long-range involvement in the health care delivery.

The vehicle for carrying out these mandates in each state is the State Health Planning and Development Agency (SA). At the state level, the SA is served by a statewide Health Coordinating Council that coordinates the state's HSA activities. The health planning scheme is intended to provide a mechanism for a logical, organized, and integrated health planning system.

Nutrition is cited among the ten health priorities listed in the preamble to the legislation:

The promotion of activities for the prevention of disease, including studies of nutritional and environmental factors affecting health and the provisions of preventive health services.

The tenth priority, which is less specific but very pertinent to nutrition education and counseling, addresses the need for developing effective methods of educating the general public about suitable personal and preventive health care.

The implementation of these priorities at the local level should be closely monitored. Nutrition advocates, consumers, and professionals should become actively involved in local HSAs and should attempt to make nutritional and other health promotion activities a high priority in the design of services and the allocation of resources.

It is not yet possible to predict the impact that the National Health Planning and Resources Development Act of 1974 will have on the health care delivery system in the United States. Although tangible improvements may be years away, critics suggest that changes in the current health care system are, unfortunately, likely to be minimal.[31-35]

Although the act provides for a much more integrated method of planning and implementing health care delivery services, it also poses many problems for the health care system. Of significant concern is the fact that the act is essentially disease oriented, rather than health oriented. Health status indices are not emphasized; rather, the focus is on treatment for the sick and possibilities for prevention are not stressed.

The implications of this include ignoring the importance of environmental health planning. The act implies an endorsement of the medical care, rather than the health care, model. Thus, concerns about health care must be carefully considered at local, regional, and state levels.

Another important concern involves deciding who will actually be most involved in the planning process at each level. Because the act uses a highly sophisticated approach to planning, members and participants need to be carefully chosen and then provided with some type of training that will enable them to effectively accomplish their task. The act does not specify methods for specifically selecting members from the local community to serve. Unless the appropriate people are appointed, the results of health planning may be contrary to the actual needs of the people whom this planning is intended to benefit.

The involvement of the nutritionist in HSAs can be identified in terms of general program planning. This is discussed in greater detail in Chapter 3. It is important not to underestimate the importance of participating in activities of health planning bodies. Unless the importance of nutritional components is made known to health planners, needed resources will not be allocated to this end and the nutrition components of health planning will be neglected.

The nutritionist must function in close collaboration with health administrators, planners, legislators, economists, and other health professionals so that all may advance the goal of improving the quality of health care delivery.

HEALTH PLANNING WITHIN A NUTRITIONAL CONTEXT — A CASE EXAMPLE[36]

The following is an example of the recognition by a local HSA of the need for more nutritional services in general preventive health care services.

Statement of the Problem

In a northeast rural/urban community with a population of 38,300 people, the HSA has been operating its health services program for more than four years. During this time it has become increasingly apparent that a major gap in the primary care program was the lack of nutritional services. Increasing demands are being placed on present providers, including physicians, midlevel practitioners, and dentists among others to deal with nutritional assessments, problems, and programs. Although no specific data were available, the health professionals believed that, even with the current inadequate systems of identification of nutrition problems, and utilizing busy personnel who were often undertrained in the nutritional sciences, the load was great and the results were discouraging.

To help remedy the situation, the HSA sought temporary assistance from the inservice education program at a local hospital to train some of the HSA program staff on site. A pediatrician was sent to an ADA program on pediatric nutrition problems. Several of the staff, particularly nurse clinicians, attended local continuing educational programs in nutrition.

These measures were, however, deemed inadequate for the long run. With over 50,000 patient visits expected at the two HSA centers per year, and with considerable projected growth in future years, the health planners believed that it was a critical time to begin the development of a nutrition services program. The planners therefore desired to find some way in which to include a nutritional component in the health care centers.

The Community Nutritionist as Health Planner

The HSA health personnel next enlisted the services of a community nutritionist to aid in health planning for the inclusion of a nutritional component in the total HSA health services. She assessed the community, considering various aspects of the community such as those who live in certain areas, and analyzed the community's most important nutritional needs. Through the nutritionist's community assessment, it became even more evident that the community's nutritional needs were not being met.

The nutritionist, in consultation with the other HSA planners, determined that the principal barrier to the inclusion of nutritional services was financial — the HSA did not have sufficient funds to hire a nutritionist to provide needed services.

The consensus was that outside funding should be sought for assistance in including nutritional services in the HSA program. The next step involved the determination of general goals and objectives for planning and developing the nutrition services program. A major effort was to be made to integrate nutrition services with other health support services. General program goals and more specific nutrition service program objectives to aid in accomplishing these goals were developed. These goals are summarized in Table 2-2.

Table 2-2
Goals and Objectives for Nutritional Component of the HSA Program

General: Principal goal is to implement nutrition services as a basic component of a health care delivery system. In the initial planning and implementation stages, a major effort will be made to integrate nutrition services with medical, dental, and other multidisciplinary support services.

Considerations:
1. Establishing measurable objectives and determining priorities in nutrition with the medical and dental staffs.
2. Analyzing the food and nutrition needs of the patient population.
3. Establishing criteria to be used for identifying the "nutritionally vulnerable" who are most likely to need nutrition services.
4. Planning for the most efficient and effective use of nutrition resources, including nutrition and other health personnel.
5. Identifying and establishing referral relationships with available nutrition resources.
6. Integrating nutrition services into the total pattern of health services.
7. Evaluating the efficiency and effectiveness of the nutrition component of health care services.

Objectives:
1. Identifying potential problems and plan for continuing surveillance of care:
   a. screening for nutritional problems.
   b. assessment of food practices and nutritional status.
   c. referral for corroboration.
   d. data input into patient information systems.
2. Preparing and educating patients and their families to assume responsibility for their own nutrition care and to manage early symptoms to prevent complications:
   a. individual patient counseling.
   b. group teaching.
   c. development and/or evaluation of nutrition methods and materials.
   d. training and continuing education for medical, dental, and other professional staff; technical consultation.
   e. training and continuing education for dietetic supportive personnel (nurses, physicians, pharmacists, dentists, and other counselors).

Goals and Objectives for Nutritional Component of the HSA Program (*continued*)

---

    f. referral to, and liaison with, food assistance and other nutrition-related community programs.

    g. leadership in seeking solutions to nutrition problems.

3. Developing and implementing immediate and long-range individualized nutritional care plans for patients:

    a. most of the activities previously described.

    b. ongoing participation in health team planning, direct nutritional assessment and counseling, and evaluation.

    c. health team staff conferences.

    d. initial and follow-up counseling in regard to normal and therapeutic nutritional needs.

    e. input into clinical records.

4. Assisting patients and their families with long-term health problems to attain and maintain adequate diets:

    a. most of the activities previously described.

    b. assistance in adjusting home environment to maximize independent functioning in activities in and outside the home.

    c. liaison with noncontact services or programs helpful in carrying out the nutritional care plan.

Nutritional care activities clearly will overlap and seldom will be restricted to a single phase of operation.

To meet these goals, specific activities were identified and were then broken down into individual tasks required and the time allowance needed to accomplish the tasks. These activities and tasks are summarized in Table 2–3.

With these goals, objectives, and specified activities in mind, the health planners and the nutritionist developed a proposal and submitted it to various agencies. They requested funds for a full-time nutritionist as well as funds to create office space, clerical help, and other needed materials and supplies.

This is an example of how the nutritionist can function in the overall process of health planning, in concert with other health professionals, to improve the effectiveness of health and nutritional service delivery. Appendix III presents an outline of important factors to consider in developing proposals for outside funding, such as the one discussed in this example.

HEALTH PROMOTION IN PRACTICE

Despite public, professional, and political support for the concept of health promotion, the practice has thus far been disappointing. Where the preventive approach exists, it is often in a fragmented and fractionated form as a specific part of therapeutic prescriptions. For example,

Weight reduction may be suggested as a means to improve the health of a diabetic or cardiovascular patient.

Salt reduction may be advised for the hypertensive.

A diet restricted in dietary saturated fat and cholesterol may be prescribed for a patient with elevated blood lipids who is considered to be at risk for the development of atherosclerosis.

The crisis-oriented approach to medical care is supported by the current financial payment system that reimburses physicians for their healing arts, but less frequently reimburses health promotion efforts such as nutritional counseling or physical fitness programs. Similarly, the organization and mandates of federal and state health agencies focus attention on medical, rather than on health care.

A Model Health Promotion Center

One model for implementing the concept of a preventive approach to improve health is being developed by Erling Stordahl, a blind Norwegian visionary. The concept is operationalized through the Beitostolen Health Sports Center, a facility designed to serve a wide variety of handicapped individuals for periods of from 3 to 12 weeks. The facility attempts to alter the life-styles of its clients. Rehabilitation activities are blended with education and counseling to teach skills of diagnosis as well as ways to promote health through positive health habits.

The nutritional component of the center, described in detail by B. Epes, provides individual and group teaching, counseling, therapy, outreach activities, and follow-up nutrition education.[37] The long-term goal is to create a positive and sustained change in life-style and dietary habits and an improvement in health status.

The philosophy behind the center's design, as described by T. Dahl, is based on the notion that each person bears the principal responsibility for improving and maintaining wise health habits. Through an approach that is organized, coordinated, and integrated into other daily life-style habits and that promotes and teaches diagnostic skills, self-care, positive health habits, and sound life-style patterns, the individual is introduced to the concept of health promotion and is helped to an understanding and appreciation for the value of this approach. It is hoped that the individual will be motivated to assume responsibility for his or her own health status.[38]

In the United States there is evidence of a trend to increased health care delivery through the Health Maintenance Organizations and through organized ambulatory care settings.

HEALTH MAINTENANCE ORGANIZATIONS (HMO)

The HMO has been proposed as an alternative to existing systems of medical care. HMOs are organizations "which integrate the provider elements (i.e., practitioners, hospitals, extended-care facilities and perhaps even first-aid stations) necessary to deliver a comprehensive range of services."[39] An HMO is organized health care designed to deliver an agreed upon pack-

Table 2–3
Nutrition Activities and Tasks

Activity	Task	0	2	4	6	8	10	12
Screening for nutritional problems	Develop criteria for screening	———						
	Identify risk factors for poor nutrition	———						
	Staff education and implementation of process		———					
	Develop means of patient referral to RD	———						
	Evaluation of screening activity		———	———	———	———	———	———
Assessment of nutritional status by provider staff	Develop criteria for *clinical assessment* by medical staff, i.e., physical signs of dietary inadequacy, malnutrition, vitamin deficiency, obesity, etc.	———						
	Develop criteria for *biochemical assessment*, i.e., laboratory analysis to determine biochemical signs of dietary deficiencies	———						
	Develop criteria for *dietary assessment*, diet history questionnaire and analysis. Food intake records and analysis	———						
	Develop criteria for *anthropometric assessment*, i.e., measurements of weight, height, head circumference, skinfold thickness	———						
	Staff education	———						
	Evaluation		———	———	———	———	———	———
Dietary counseling	Develop an individual patient counseling service to meet normal and therapeutic needs including follow-up diet counseling for hospital discharged patients	———						
	Develop criteria for follow-up care	———	———					
	Development of a nutritional component in the medical chart	—						
	Establish referral to agencies and community services	———						
	Evaluation		———	———	———	———	———	———
Nutrition education	Develop and implement group teaching programs for weight control	———						

Nutrition Activities and Tasks *(continued)*

Activity	Task	Time Allowance (months)
		0 2 4 6 8 10 12
	maternal nutrition and lactation	——————— (0–6)
	infant and child feeding	——————— (0–6)
	diabetes mellitus	——— (0–2)
	hypertension	————— (0–4)
	cardiovascular disease	——————————— (0–8)
	Develop and/or evaluate nutrition education materials	———————————————— (0–12)
	Training and continuing education for professional staff	——— (0–2)
	Evaluation	———————————————— (0–12)
Evaluation of nutritional services	The goals of the service are defined and problem areas for quality improvement are selected	—— (0–1)
	Standards of criteria for those problem areas are developed	—— (0–1)
	The care provided is completely documented in the patient record	————— (0–4)
	The care provided is reviewed and compared against the standard to identify deficiencies of care	————— (0–4)
	Steps are taken to correct the detected deficiencies for the individual patients whose records were reviewed	——————————— (0–8)
	Development of a cost analysis study to justify the financial advantage of nutritional services	———————————————— (0–12)
Recording pertinent data	Record pertinent data in the patient's problem oriented medical record	——— (0–2)
	Evaluation of records	———————————————— (0–12)

age of comprehensive and organized preventive and treatment services for a voluntarily enrolled group of individuals. The HMO is funded through a prenegotiated payment made by or for each individual enrolled in the plan.

The HMO provides a continuum of health services for individuals. Care is to be comprehensive and organized; continuity of care is inherent in the concept. The ultimate goal is to provide the greatest quality of care for the consumer dollar.[40]

The federal government provides financial support for HMOs. The government also requires that any company providing health benefits to more

than 25 employees must offer HMO coverage as an alternative to traditional health insurance.

Basic to the idea of the successful HMO is care designed to keep individuals healthy, so that more sophisticated and expensive services can be
avoided. A variety of different HMO delivery programs are in operation,
such as the Kaiser Foundation Health Plans in California, the Health Insurance plan of Greater New York, the Group Health Association of Washington, D.C., and the San Joaquin Medical Care Foundation. No matter
how the HMO is organized, it offers the client a combination of outpatient
and hospital services through a single umbrella organization and a single
payment plan.

Prepayment, which is essential to the success of the plan, in effect institutes what might be termed a new "medical economics." This stems from
the fact that the total health care income is received not as a fee for service but as a lump sum. This reverses the typical medical economics in
which physicians are paid more for more services. Under the HMO system,
the doctors are thus better off if the subscribers stay well, and the hospitals are better off if the beds are unfilled. The emphasis is therefore on
prevention. Because the fee is constant and prepaid, people are encouraged to seek care at the early stages of their illness, thus helping to prevent
serious illness and complications.

In the traditional delivery system, the patient more or less decides what
care he or she needs. The patient seeks out a physician and pays for service. The fee regulates the flow of people into the medical care delivery
system. Hoping to save money, the patient is likely to put off visiting a
physician until the patient is acutely ill. This limits the number of well
and "early sick" people who seek the advice of a physician, and it places
the emphasis of the delivery system on the treatment of illness.

It is now recognized that early entry into the delivery system is essential
for early treatment and prevention of major illness. But to eliminate the
fee is equally disastrous for the delivery system. The result is an "uncontrolled flood of well-worried, early-sick and sick people into the . . . doctor's appointment on a first-come, first-served basis that has little relation
to priority of need."[8] This overloads the system and usurps available
physician time that might otherwise be devoted to the care of the sick.

One solution to the problem involves a regulator that is more sensitive
to real medical need than to the ability to pay and can, at the same time,
encourage preventive medicine while setting priorities for the care of the
sick. The system, which is variously termed multiphasic screening, health
evaluation, or health testing, has the potential not only to replace the fee
for service as a regulator of entry into the health care system but can also
become the heart of the health care delivery system.

The ideal health testing component of the health care delivery system
combines a computerized medical history with a comprehensive series of
physiological and biochemical tests administered by paramedical personnel. Figure 2-5 illustrates a proposed place for the health testing system
relative to other components in the total delivery system. The testing
system is easily suited to be a regulator of patient entry into the system;
it can separate the well from the "worried-well" and the "early-sick"

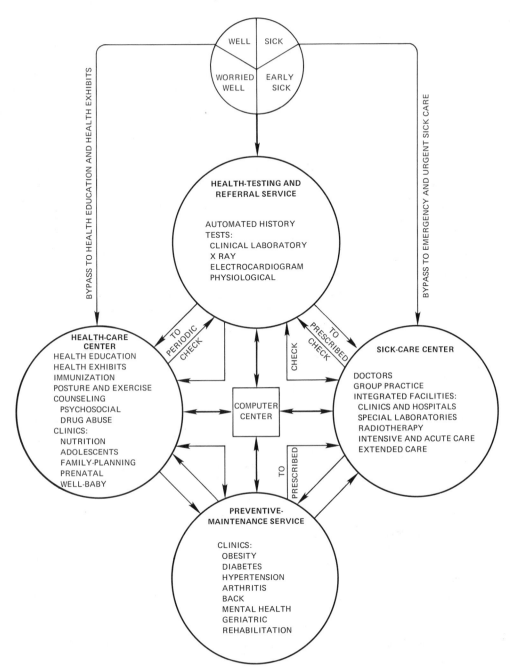

Figure 2-5. Proposed health care delivery system. This system establishes a new method of entry, the health testing service. After testing, the patient can be referred to sick care, health care, or "preventive maintenance." The computer center would regulate patient flow and would be the point of coordination for the system. (S. R. Garfield, The Delivery of Medical Care, *Sci. Am.* **222** (1970) : 15)

from the more acutely or chronically ill. Patients can then be directed toward the type of service that is most fitted to their needs. The computerized profile of each patient can be kept as a record of baseline information, which is useful for future reference. Thus, the physician's time can be saved from routine diagnostic and assessment tasks, and maximum use of paramedical personnel can be made.

With health testing as the heart of the total delivery system, patients can be directed to one of three other main divisions of service: a health care service, a preventive-maintenance service, and a sick care service. The health care division would aim to affect the life-styles of individuals in such a way as to encourage preventive care. Ideally, health care services could channel funds and resources into keeping people healthy. Services would include education and counseling, immunizations, and a variety of "well clinics."

The preventive-maintenance service is geared to accommodate chronic illness that necessitates routine treatment, monitoring, and follow-up. The goal is to maintain patients in a stable condition and prevent further deterioration by disease. In both health care and preventive maintenance, paramedical personnel can function under the supervision of physicians, thus freeing doctor time for the more acutely ill.

The sick care division focuses on returning ill people to health. An organized and comprehensive array of services could concentrate on cures through intensive and intermediate levels of skilled medical care.

According to the proposed system, consumers would be able to choose from among competing HMOs as well as from traditional health providers. Those who opt for the HMO would agree to obtain needed health services on a subscription basis, probably for at least a year. HMOs could be operated through public or private channels and could function in a number of different ways. They could be single, autonomous entities, or they could be part of a state, regional, or national network. Although single or group practice could remain a viable form of health care delivery, it would be subject to the competitive pressure of the HMOs.

One of the underlying assumptions of HMOs is that they would be controlled independently of the health practitioner. The quality of practitioner service could be monitored and evaluated by an objective, outside agency.

It is anticipated that by operationalizing the HMO concept on a large scale, there would be a shift in orientation from crisis-oriented medical care to a preventive, long-term health maintenance approach. Such a system would facilitate continuity of care and the integration of a number of supplemental health services into the HMO operation. Presumably, the economy of health care delivery would be increased. Research has confirmed the savings that can be realized through the operation of HMOs.[22,41]

M. Barthel, for example, reported a study in which HMO enrollment over a 3-year period was compared with traditional health service delivery. Results indicated that an average cost savings of 25 per cent resulted from the HMO as compared with the traditional system. At present there are slightly less than 200 HMOs with approximately 6 million subscribers.[42]

By contrast, in 1964 there were only 18 HMOs; in 1973 there were 42 HMOs serving 4.3 million people.[43] The growth of HMOs is illustrated in Figure 2-6. According to projections of HEW, an estimated 500 new health maintenance organizations will be in the planning or operational stage by 1985. Three hundred of these will be funded by HEW; the private sector is expected to pay for 100, and the remaining 100 would be in the planning stages.[44]

Limitations of HMO

Although the HMO concept clearly offers advantages to the current system of health care delivery, it is not without its limitations. For example, because the HMO concept would replace the fee-for-service barrier to medical care with characteristics of the specific provider, the providers may offer less medical care than that required by the consumer. This allegation can be disputed on the grounds that a new system of health care delivery would be able, through monitoring systems, to protect against such purposeful nondelivery of needed services.

Critics suggest that a loss of consumer confidence in personal privacy, a reduction in confidentiality of client medical records, and a decrease in the freedom to choose one's own physician will result from the HMO. Further, the presumed economy of service delivery may not be realized. Opponents of HMOs also predict that physicians may lose some of the existing financial rewards and become less satisfied with their practice with the result that quality of care will suffer.

Perhaps the more fundamental problem is that the HMO concept relies for its effectiveness upon its ability to identify an enrolled clientele. By paying a set fee for a period of service delivery, the client is able to receive required services. The difficulty concerns the mass of public patients, that is, those who now use the public hospital system and who are characteristically transient in time, locale, need, responsiveness, and eligibility. This clientele is not easily or successfully enrolled in a program of prepayment for services. Thus, from a practical point of view, transient clientele be-

Figure 2-6. Growing number of health maintenance organizations. (HEW)

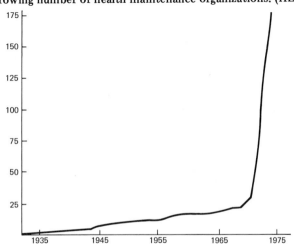

comes excluded from the HMO concept and is relegated to seek other ways of coping with its medical or health needs.

AMBULATORY CARE SERVICES[45]

The movement toward organized ambulatory services (OAS) characterizes much of the health care delivery today and is increasingly recognized as "the only approach to active health care equity in the modern world."[45] The historical origins of primary care extend back to the 1700s. The first American dispensary was organized in Philadelphia in 1786, just 35 years after the first hospital was established in the same city.[46]

The first national Congress of Hospitals and Dispensaries met in Chicago in 1893. A 1916 survey of the Committee on Dispensary Work (American Hospital Association) found 495 hospital outpatients in the United States and 185 independent dispensaries, but by 1918 most of these had been absorbed by hospitals that were the focus for primary health and medical care services.

Specialized clinics to arrest communicable disease sprang up as newer methods of disease detection and treatment were discovered. Charitable clinics designed to aid mothers with infant and child care were initiated for poor and employed mothers in New York in 1893. Public funding for the first governmental division of child hygiene was available through the New York City health department in 1908. Seven years later, 538 infant welfare stations, both publicly and privately supported, were identified in the United States. By 1921, support for the establishment of well-baby clinics to focus on health promotion and the prevention of illness was mandated by the Sheppard-Towner Act. This set the precedent for Title V of the Social Security Act on maternal and child health care.

The development of other types of health clinics and ambulatory care units paralleled these trends. In the early 1900s, the need to arrest communicable disease and to detect disorders that might be responsible for learning impairment stimulated the organization of school health clinics. Other types of clinics include those founded for industrial workers in large factories and governmental services for military veterans, and special populations such as migrants, Indians, farm workers, and others with unique and special needs.

In the 1920s there also emerged a new movement for integrated health centers that was the forerunner of the establishment of health facilities in urban slums to house health department clinics, the Visiting Nurse Association, and similar groups aiming to advance primary health care. Similar centers were constructed as part of the New Deal's Public Works Administration in the 1930s, with support provided by the Hill-Burton Act in the 1940s. By the 1960s, the comprehensive health center idea was translated into reality. Based on the assumption that increased access to primary health services can decrease the utilization of more costly medical services and can improve the health and quality of life for clients, federal, state, and local efforts developed the concept now known as the community health center. In response to the tremendous pressure of rising health problems and of unmet health needs, New York City, in 1961, authorized the Department of Hospitals to transform Gouverneur Hospital into an ambulatory clinic at which 150,000 individuals could obtain health services on a walk-in basis.

In 1965, the federal government established the first neighborhood health center in Boston, providing medical care services to approximately 6,000 inner-city residents. Similar health centers were soon set up in Denver, New York, Chicago, and Los Angeles.

The Office of Economic Opportunity (OEO), established in 1964, administered the early federally funded health centers. These centers were a part of the War On Poverty that tried to deal with the economic, social, and health problems of the poor in this country. The health centers became the focus of many efforts to improve the life and health of those in poverty.

In 1966 the Comprehensive Health Planning and Public Health Services Act was passed, directing that a range of comprehensive health service programs were to be developed in impoverished areas. The programs were to provide an organized system of primary health care services.

By 1975, centers provided for by this act were established in more than 40 states, the District of Columbia, Puerto Rico, and the Virgin Islands, and health care services were made available to approximately 1.6 million individuals.

The initial programs were expanded in the 1970s, when family health centers joined the range of previously existing services. Family health centers provided services for a fixed payment fee basis. Under this plan people enrolled in the program would be eligible to receive as many services as needed and as often as they needed them upon payment of the fixed fee for the specified package of services.

In 1975 the Public Health Service Act mandated the development of specifications for community health centers. A minimum group of services specified were physician services, diagnostic (laboratory and radiologic services) emergency medical services, and preventive medical and dental services, as well as provisions for increasing access to these services.

The Bureau of Community Health Services administers the Community Health Center program that currently includes not only the neighborhood health centers, but family health centers, community health network, and rural health initiatives in accord with the following principles:[47]

Health services must be available to people where they are.

The prevention of conditions that endanger health by assuring comprehensive, continuing care is the best way to ensure a healthy community.

The program must be continually responsive to methods of operating programs frugally by recovering operating costs through Medicare, Medicaid, and insurance companies; by pooling resources within programs so that more people might be served; and by encouraging communities to help themselves.

Table 2-4 compares the program components of some of the various community health centers.

Table 2-4
Community Health Centers Comparison of Program Components

	Neighborhood Health Center (NHC)	Family Health Center (FHC)	Community Health Network (CHN)	Rural Health Initiative (RHI)
Service Mode	Ambulatory Services Health-related supportive services, e.g., home health care and transportation Outreach	Primary Ambulatory services	Ambulatory and inpatient services provided at multiple sites	Primary Ambulatory services provided as part of an integrated health system Outreach Transportation
Principal Locations	Inner-city urban locations	Rural and semi-rural communities	Inner-city Urban location	Rural areas
Target Population	Medically underserved populations	Enrolled families living in medically underserved areas	Enrolled families living in medically underserved areas	Medically underserved populations in critical manpower shortage areas
Financing	Fee-for-service Project grant funds Federal, state, and local funds Third-party payments	Experimental prepaid capitation Individual payment Federal, state, and local funds	Prepaid capitation Project grant funds Federal, state, and local funds Third-party payments	Fee-for-service Third-party payments Project grant funds Local community funds
Consumer Participation	Majority consumer membership on governing board	Majority consumer membership on governing board	Majority consumer membership on governing board	Majority consumer membership on governing board
Operating Status	Average project age — 4½–5 years	First grants — spring 1972 Maximum age of operational projects — 2 years	OEO initiated Transferred to HEW authority — 1973	First grants — spring 1975 All projects operational less than one year

Source: Department of Health, Education, and Welfare. *DHEW — Promoting Community Health* — 1976, Publ. No. (HSA) 77-5000. Washington, D.C., Government Printing Office, 1976.

As should be obvious from this brief review, a variety of modern and distinct types of OAS exist in the United States today. The current definition of an organized ambulatory service (OAS) is "a setting in which several health personnel collaborate and make decisions through some team process (or as part of an organizational framework), and where the services usually (though not always) are financed in a collectivized or shared manner."[45] M. I. Roemer has identified seven types of OAS units: clinics of public health agencies, industrial health units, school health services, private group medical practice, special governmental programs, special voluntary programs, and hospital outpatient departments.

Although a precise figure for the number of individuals served by these health clinics annually is not available, there is little dispute that the figure has been gradually increasing; there has also been a broadening

Table 2-5

Estimated Number of Visits to Different Types of Ambulatory Services, Annually, in the Early 1970s

Type of Service	Number of Visits	Percentage
Hospital outpatient departments	200,000,000	18.2%
Public health clinics	30,000,000	2.7
Industrial health units	40,000,000	3.6
School and college health clinics	55,000,000	5.0
Private group practice	185,000,000	16.8
Special government programs (veterans, military, Indians, migrants, etc.)	25,000,000	2.3
Special voluntary agencies, e.g., cancer, hypertension, alcoholism, family planning	20,000,000	1.8
Private medical practice	545,000,000	49.5

Source: M. I. Roemer. From poor beginnings, the growth of primary care. *Hospitals.* 49 (1 March 1975): 38.

of types of clinics available. Table 2-5 illustrates the estimated number of visits to these different types of ambulatory services annually through the early 1970s.

Roemer has estimated that about half of the ambulatory physician-patient interchanges occurred in organized settings; the other half took place in the private offices of the physician. Although this is necessarily a rough estimate, the proportion of ambulatory services occurring in organized settings outside the private office is increasing.

Ambulatory health centers have provided evidence that access to ambulatory care, especially primary health services, can decrease costs and the use of additional medical services. Many centers have documented the fact that participants' need for hospitalization was reduced. For example, in Rochester, New York, the local center reported a 50 per cent reduction in hospitalization among the enrolled children. Although ambulatory care services are costly, the annual funds per patient served are less than the cost of *one* hospital bed day. Thus, the hospital is beginning to take its rightful place in the health care delivery system — as the point of entry for the acutely ill or for those requiring a particular type of service that is not available at an ambulatory care clinic.

These health care centers have proved so effective that a community health service system, a nationally established and funded system that is locally governed has been suggested as an alternative to the current fragmented system of care delivery. Such a concept would involve government control over most of medical care; it parallels health care delivery systems currently used in countries such as Great Britain. G. E. Pickett justifies this alternative, suggesting that it will eventually "emerge as the only complete way to guarantee the right "of access and contribute to the nation's health. If that is socialized medicine, then we must agree that it is similar to socialized education, and that system has always been accepted as a right."[48]

It is unlikely that the operationalization of the concept on a national scale will occur in the near future. But the notion that providers and consumers must band together to plan, implement, and evaluate health service that is agreeable to both will necessarily improve satisfaction and national health status and the costs for this service will not necessarily be inflated.

HEALTH PROMOTION ORGANIZATIONS (HPO)[49]

In addition to federal efforts, private business has become increasingly cognizant of the importance of health promotion. Many companies now offer innovative health programs, which include such services as primary care clinics located on company premises, health services to all employees, and HMOs for the employees and their families. Some health care agencies have also introduced health promotion innovations. For example, Hawaii's Blue Shield offers health examinations including preventive screening and health promotion services to subscribers. The Rhode Island Blue Cross provides members with a program intended to increase individual responsibility for health care.

Strategies for increasing health promotion must involve cooperation between individual behavior and life-style improvements (i.e., individual actions), corporate efforts at improving the health and physical fitness of employees, the educational system, and the government. A general approach is needed that involves the cooperation of public efforts, the health care delivery system, the health insurance industry, business, and various types of consumer-related enterprises such as recreation, nutrition, and mass media so that the public will have the necessary institutions, incentives, and range of choices to improve its life-style in a manner that is conducive to good health. The federal responsibility in this collaborative enterprise would be to provide needed legislative and economic incentives to create an environment that is supportive of these health promotion efforts.

To accomplish this, K. Lorenz et al. have proposed the establishment of voluntary, community-based health promotion organizations (HPOs). These organizations would reward healthy life-styles and would provide incentives for promotion of health by supporting a close collaborative relationship among sectors of government, private industry, labor, the health care system, the community, and individuals.

All community members would be encouraged to join the local HPO and to solicit other family members and friends to also become involved in health-oriented community service. Such a model would be an incentive to individuals, as well as to community and government interests. In addition, utilizing the tremendous public resources, such as mothers, teachers, and paraprofessionals, would stimulate a type of "grass roots" health promotion effort.

Table 2–6
Premises and Health Goals of the HPO

Premises on Which the HPO Ought to be Based:

1. All people can strive to improve their health, relative to their own individual capacities and restrictions.

2. Achieving physical and mental well-being is a learning process for people. Individuals can develop and maintain behaviors that are consistent with good health if they are given appropriate incentives and rewards and are shown how to do it.

3. Involving and teaching people about self-help and self-control practices in disease prevention and health promotion is possible only if the public and private sectors are willing to make major intermediate and long-range investments in the restructuring of economic and social incentives that will encourage change in the behavior of both consumers and providers.

Health Goals of the HPO Include the Following:

1. It is better to be slim than fat.

2. The excessive use of medication is to be avoided.

3. The fewer the cigarettes smoked, the better it is.

4. Exercise and physical fitness are better than sedentary living and lack of exercise.

5. Alcohol is a danger to health, particularly when driving a car.

6. Mood-modifying drugs are a danger to health, unless properly supervised.

7. Tranquility is better than excess stress.

8. The more responsibility one takes for one's own health, the better it is.

9. The less polluted the environment, the healthier it is.

Source: R. Y. Lorenz, D. L. Davis, and R. W. Manderschied. The Health Promotion Organization: A practical intervention designed to promote healthy living. *Publ. Health Rpts.* 93 (1978): 446–455.

The premises and health goals on which the HPO is based are summarized in Table 2–6. As Lorenz emphasizes, these goals are to be viewed as open-ended and empirical — as additional knowledge becomes available they should evolve and be expanded and changed.

As Lorenz et al. conceive it, the HPO would be structured as a modification of Garfield's model.[8] (See Figure 2–5.) The HPO structure is presented in Figure 2–7. The entry point into the system, evaluation, would consist of three recorded components — the health profile assessment, the health hazard appraisal, and the personal health passport.

The health profile assessment would be based on objective medical criteria and clinical and life-style self-report histories. The health hazard appraisal would include specific importances of adverse health influences such as overeating, alcohol or drug abuse, or occupational exposure. This appraisal would be used to motivate people to modify these behaviors by relating them to reductions in longevity. The health passport would describe an individual's personal health status and health risk status and would serve to inform individuals about their health and to then motivate

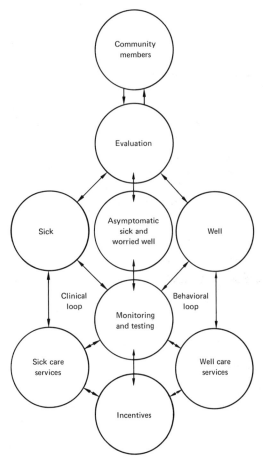

Figure 2-7. Operational components of the health promotion organization. (After Lorenz et al.[49])

them to improve their health. After this evaluation, the members would be directed into one of the categories described by Garfield.[8] (See pages 44–46.

The incentive system, central to the HPO, would support positive health actions at the individual level. Incentives might include educational courses in nutrition or self-care, consumer discounts on material goods, recreational and physical fitness facilities, and economic incentives (e.g., health stamps allowing an individual to "purchase" additional incentives, such as healthy foods, that would in themselves encourage healthy life-styles.) The economic rewards could be provided by local businesses that, in turn, might receive tax benefits for such offerings. Reductions in insurance premiums for those who improve their health status might also be offered. Another incentive might be a sociocultural status symbol, such as media recognition of healthy behavior.

General funding for the HPO might come from the federal government as part of a comprehensive health insurance program, from health insurance companies, or from industry as part of employee fringe benefits.

TOWARD A NATIONAL HEALTH PROGRAM

Although there is general agreement about the need for a national health policy, there is less consensus about what should be included in such a policy. Ideally, a system ensuring continuous, complete, and comprehensive health care should be available and accessible to all.

Comprehensive health care is defined as "planned and supervised flow of services which assures completeness and continuity of care."

Completeness implies that all needed services are available; this includes medical screening, diagnosis, treatment, as well as dental, nursing, nutrition, social services, psychological, audio, and speech, as well as any other services needed to promote health and to prevent illness.

Continuity relates to "the ordered flow of services, including screening assessment of needs (or diagnoses), intervention (or treatment), and follow-up." Continuity also includes activities designed to promote health and to prevent illness, such as ongoing screening, assessment, diagnosis, follow-up, and periodic reassessments.[50]

In effective health care, these components should be carried out simultaneously. There should be no significant delineation between them. For example, in assessment and screening an individual with poor dietary habits may be identified and should then be given counseling; in this case, follow-up and prevention functions are the same.

Continuity also refers to the need to provide a continuum of health care delivery that includes a focus on the home, the neighborhood, and the community. Health care must be coupled with, and integrated into, other aspects of local community development. The American Public Health Association, after considerable deliberation, suggested that any national health program should consider certain elements as mandatory. These are summarized in Table 2-7.[51] Implicit in this design for a national health program are certain basic ingredients. Preventive care, as opposed to crisis-oriented care, must be regarded as the goal.

Realistic and practical health service delivery standards are essential. A national health policy must not generalize about the availability of high-quality care for every citizen, but rather determine realistic goals that can be provided for all. The minimum standards of quality of care must be determined, and must then form the basis for the health care that is available to all. Standards of care should not be fragmented and directed to specific groups, but should be universally applied to everyone.

The most effective approaches to health care should offer mechanisms to give people themselves a share in the responsibility to improve their overall health status. The basic resources must be within the means of the individual family, and must permit personal decisions about the use of these resources to meet varying needs. An important objective of health policy is to include the poor, the minorities, and the disadvantaged in the decision-making process and thus to improve the government's responsiveness to the needs of all.

Table 2-7

American Public Health Association Recommendations for a National Health System

1. Universal coverage — for all civilian residents of the United States.

2. Comprehensive benefits including preventive, diagnostic, therapeutic, health maintenance, and rehabilitative services for all types of illness and health states; provided through primary care, linked with specialty consultative personnel, facilities, and services as needed to meet total health needs; meeting specified quality standards.

3. Financing by a blend of federal social insurance and general tax revenues to provide health care as a social right for all and to assure reasonable equity in funding it.

4. Reform of the health care delivery system to assure equal access for all in an efficient and effective way, and to facilitate interaction between the private and governmental functions.

5. Organization and administration involving federal, state, and local governments with health-oriented direction available at all levels.

6. Public accountability to maximize the responsiveness of the health system to public needs.

7. Economic leverage of public financing on the delivery system, including payment for providers of services, annually negotiated rates for institutional providers and choice of prepayment or fee-for-service payment for professional providers, and incentives for providers to adopt patterns of organization and payment to achieve high quality service.

8. Revamped state programs for licensing of health facilities and personnel to ensure that they meet minimum standards, allow for consumer participation in policy development, and allow for reciprocity of licensure of health professionals from state to state; also important in this regard is periodic inspection and examination of facilities and personnel, the promotion of development to be responsive to social needs and the provision of disciplinary action against those who fail to meet standards.

9. Adequate personnel, service, and facility resources with massive federal support for reorientation and expansion of education programs in health areas; broadened federal support of organized health service, with emphasis on the support of regionalized services, and expanded research in the area of health service delivery.

V. Navarro suggests that a prerequisite for an improved national health status is a more democratized society in which individuals and communities exercise control over health resources and channel them in directions to meet their needs.[52]

All services must be responsive to the real and felt needs of those for whom the services are designed. Citizens are not only to be on the "receiving end" as passive consumers of services but, rather, should be active participants in all phases of health care delivery, from the planning and design stages, through the delivery and evaluation of services. Their interest, knowledge and skill, and desires should become an integral contribution to the entire health care delivery system.

There are a variety of rationales for encouraging consumer participation in one's own health care:[53]

Program acceptance is usually facilitated; involving consumer participation in the planning process has been found to increase consumer attendance, increase active participation of other consumers, and improve informal outside communication.

Opposition to programs is more easily overcome.

Modification of attitudes and behavior is facilitated; consumer participation is positively associated with preventive health behavior attitudes and is also related to increased development of attitudes of self-assertiveness and self-responsibility.

Allows consumer to take an active role in controlling programs that greatly affect one's own life.

Facilitates a closer relationship between consumers and program directors, planners, and officials.

Citizens can also be valuable advocates and supporters of needed services, can be instrumental in sensing the pulse of consumers, and in alleviating many of the primary problems that affect low-income families. For example, citizens can help in organizing support for a Food Stamp Program, in developing the type of total, comprehensive health care program needed in their community, in performing outreach services, and in obtaining needed community support for programs.

Social planning is essential to the implementation of a universal and suitable health care system. All programs should be part of an organized system that is designed to provide equal quality of care and services for all citizens, regardless of their race, nationality, sex, age, or economic, educational, or social background. All programs should have an inherent flexibility that can allow the system to be responsive to the diversities found.

STRATEGIES FOR IMPLEMENTATION OF THE HEALTH PROMOTION CONCEPT IN AMERICA

A forerunner in mapping out a statewide strategy for prevention is the Massachusetts Department of Public Health. A number of approaches have been taken by the department, some of which are summarized below.

1. "Compile and disseminate information demonstrating the favorable ratio of benefits to costs for health promotion programs." Such cost-benefit analysis data for programs such as nutritional counseling and improved nutritional status is necessary to convince the providers, consumers, and public representatives that health promotion should be espoused, not only for the resulting improvements in the quality of human life, but also for purely economic reasons, because of the cost-effectiveness of reduced prevalence of illness and the financial burdens of morbidity and premature mortality.

2. "Develop methods to have insurance premiums reflect self-imposed health risks." An example of the implementation of this notion would be to require higher insurance premiums for obese individuals based on the elevated health risks of obesity. Such legislation would provide incentive for behaviors conducive to good health.

3. "Develop economic incentives for health care institutions to invest in health

promotion." The Health Systems Agency could be charged with the responsibility of providing proper economic incentives to emphasize health promotion.

4. "Encourage the involvement of civic groups and local boards of health in community-based approaches to lifestyle issues." Greater interest on the part of such groups might be encouraged by demonstrating to them the benefits of their work and by providing some funds to match their own resources.

5. "Adopt a taxation policy that provides disincentives for use of harmful products and provides funds to promote their non-use." Such a bill recently introduced into the Massachusetts legislature called for part of the tax revenues on alcohol to be used for detoxification, halfway houses, and other treatment and services for alcoholics.

6. "Institute as part of primary medical practice a clear explanation to patients of the risks associated with their lifestyle." Practitioners might demonstrate to a patient the associated risks of early morbidity, mortality, or of possible life-style changes, such as loss of work and modification in leisure style, that would result from certain illnesses and disorders. By being more informed about the adverse consequences of certain behaviors, for example, habitual excess food consumption, individuals might be more motivated to assume greater responsibility for their own behavior, and in the process, improve their health.

7. "Develop and utilize school health education curricula that permit students, from an early age, to understand the significance of their individual role in keeping health." Although knowledge of healthful practices does not ensure their practice, it is well established that life-long habits and behavior patterns are developed during the early years. In addition to the provision of knowledge, school personnel, as well as others who play a role in influencing the attitudes and behavior of the young, including parents, media advertisers, and health professionals, should work to provide helpful role models and good examples of behavior and life-style that support health promotion.

8. "Make health promotion a high priority in the plans of the Health Systems Agencies and State Health Planning and Development Agencies." This can be accomplished as health planning agencies support and encourage the health promotion efforts of providers, facilities, individuals, and consumer groups. By stating health promotion as an explicit priority, these agencies would also signal public elected officials that their constituency expects, and would support, legislation to the end of health promotion.

9. "Develop partnerships with the media in the promotion of healthful activities." Health promotion advocates could use the media to their advantage, thus making the public more aware of the need for healthy behavior. By joining with interested private interests, by implementing public service campaigns, or otherwise employing the media to advertise health promotion, it is possible to motivate the public to at least look at their behavior as it relates to health, and perhaps make some improvements.[54]

Lessons from the Massachusetts Experience[54]

The Massachusetts experience has indicated the benefits of emphasizing limited numbers of measurable objectives, channeling resources to meet these top priorities, and thus obtaining success in these stated areas. Such visible successes make greater public support for future health promotion programs possible. Another suggested strategy is to develop and distribute lists of resources and of organizations promoting health in given localities. Publishing the names, addresses, phone numbers, and brief descriptions of such resources can be of great help to other interested groups and individuals in developing their own strategies for health promotion. If these approaches are to work effectively, a general change in the health care delivery system must be developed that is supported by legislation and is economically viable.

This emphasis goes far beyond that which appeals to individuals to modify their own life-styles and behavior patterns in the interest of personal health. By acknowledging the important role that the environment plays in determining individual as well as societal health, and by attempting to avoid confrontation with powerful interest groups and commercial concerns whose activities may be harmful to health, the Massachusetts Public Health Department has provided a model from which to build and improve efforts for health promotion.

CONCLUSION

Although many of the approaches discussed in this chapter may be tentative and as yet idealistic, they provide a serious attempt to address the issue of disease prevention. It has been conservatively estimated that the application of prevention measures to diseases of the heart, cancer, stroke, accidents, chronic obstructive lung disease, and cirrhosis of the liver might result in an annual savings of $20 billion and 400,000 lives in the United States.[55] If we are to realize this savings and if we are to achieve true health care rather than medical care, the community as a whole must be the focus of care as well as of education and training. The hospital must be seen as a place where "a certain state of the disease process" can be treated. If the orientation is strictly hospital-focused, it is difficult to train health professionals for real social responsibility. Instead, we need a multifaceted, multiprofessional, team approach to training and to health care. "In short, we need in every respect to adopt an open-door policy."[12]

If we are to achieve true health promotion and preventive health care, rather than medical care, we need to foster a new attitude among Americans. We need to realize the importance of individual and community responsibility for personal health care. We need to recognize that the health care delivery system should be as concerned with keeping individuals healthy as it is with restoring health to the sick. We need to recognize good health as a basic human right and to encourage all segments of society to pursue this right.

REFERENCES

1. U.S. Congress, Congressional Budget Office. *Expenditures for Health Care: Federal Programs and Their Effects.* Washington, D.C.: Government Printing Office, 1977.
2. Shabecoff, P. Soaring price of medical care puts a serious strain on economy. *The New York Times,* May 7, 1978, pp. 1, 69.
3. U.S. Department of Health, Education, and Welfare. *Monthly Vital Statistics Report — Summary Report: Final Morbidity Statistics, 1973.* Rockville, Md.: National Center for Health Statistics, February 10, 1975.

4. Califano, J. A. What's wrong with U.S. health care? *Washington Post,* June 26, 1977.
5. American College of Preventive Medicine and Fogarty International Center of N.I.H. *Appendix of Report.* Bethesda, Md.: National Conference on Preventive Medicine, June 1975.
6. Gray, S. E. *Community Health Today.* New York: Macmillan, 1978.
7. U.S. Department of Health, Education, and Welfare. Administrative confidential draft. I. Preamble, in U.S. Senate Select Committee on Nutrition and Human Needs, *Nutrition and Health.* Washington, D.C.: Government Printing Office, December 1975, p. 243.
8. Garfield, S. R. The delivery of medical care. *Sci. Am.* 222 (1970): 15.
9. Jarvis, E. Communications, quoted in J. E. Fielding, *Am. J. Publ. Health* 67 (1977): 1082.
10. Flexner, A. *Medical Education in the United States and Canada.* New York: Carnegie Foundation, 1910.
11. Aiken, L. H. Primary care: The challenge for nursing. *Am. J. Nurs.* (November 1977): 1828.
12. Mahler, H. Tomorrow's medicine and tomorrow's doctors. *CAJANUS* 10 (1977): 153.
13. U.S. Department of Health, Education, and Welfare. *Towards a Systematic Analysis of Health Care in the United States.* Washington, D.C.: Health Services and Mental Health Association, 1972, pp. 5-8.
14. Fogarty International Center et al. *Preventive Medicine, USA. Health Promotion and Consumer Education.* New York: Prodist, 1976.
15. LaLonde, M. *A New Perspective on the Health of Canadians.* Ottawa: Information Center, 1975, pp. 31-37.
16. Brody, J. Specialists look to preventive medicine to improve the nation's health. *The New York Times,* May 30, 1978, p. B5.
17. Hilbert, M. S. Prevention. *Am. J. Publ. Health* 67 (1977): 353-356.
18. Fuchs, V. R. *Who Shall Live?* New York: Basic Books, 1975, p. 55.
19. Belloc, N. B. Relationship of health practices and mortality. *Prev. Med.* 2 (1973): 67.
20. Belloc, N. B., and L. Breslow. Relationship of physical health status and health practices. *Prev. Med.* 1 (1972): 409.
21. Pellegrino, E. J. Preventive health care and the allied health professions. *Rev. Allied Health Educ.* 1 (1974): 1.
22. U.S. Department of Health, Education, and Welfare. *Forward Plan for Health, FY 1978-1982.* Washington, D.C.: Government Printing Office, August 1976.
23. U.S. Department of Health, Education, and Welfare. *Guide for Developing Nutrition in Community Health Programs.* Rockville, Md., 1978.
24. Cornely, P. B. Community concern for total health care. *J. Am. Diet. Assoc.* 60 (1972): 105.
25. Fielding, J. E., J. H. Hyde, and P. K. Russo. *A Program for Prevention in Massachusetts.* Boston: Massachusetts Department of Public Health, June 1, 1978.
26. Freyman, J. G. Medicine's great schism — prevention versus cure — an historical interpretation. *Med. Care* 13 (1975): 525.
27. Berg, A. A fear of trying. *J. Am. Diet. Assoc.* 68 (1976): 311.
28. U.S. Congress. Health Promotion and Disease Prevention Act of 1976, PL-94-317, June 23, 1976.
29. U.S. Congress. National Disease Prevention and Health Promotion Act of 1978, S.3115, May 19, 1978.

30. U.S. Congress. National Health Planning and Resources Development Act of 1974, PL–93–641, January 7, 1975.
31. Frank, R., and A. Yanochik-Owen. *Nutrition in the Community: The Art of Delivering Services.* St. Louis, Mo.: C. V. Mosby, 1978.
32. Vladeck, B. C. Interest-group representation and the HSAs: Health planning and political theory. *Am. J. Publ. Health* 67 (1977): 23–29.
33. Waters, W. J. State level comprehensive health planning: A retrospect. *Am. J. Publ. Health* 66 (1976): 139–144.
34. Mott, P. D., A. T. Mott, J. M. Rudolph, E. R. Lane, and R. L. Berg. Difficult issues in health planning, development, and review. *Am. J. Publ. Health* 66 (1976): 746.
35. Picket, G. Toward a national health policy — values in conflict. *Am. J. Publ. Health* 65 (1975): 1335.
36. Callie, P., and F. Ganni. Personal communication. Syracuse, N.Y., Summer 1978.
37. Epes, B. The nutrition component of the Vinland National Center, in T. Dahl, ed., *The Vinland National Center — A New Concept in Health.* Minneapolis: Fairview Community Hospitals, 1976.
38. Dahl, T. Economics, management, and public health nutrition. *J. Am. Diet. Assoc.* 70 (1977): 144.
39. Health Services and Mental Health Administration. *Health Maintenance Organizations. The Concept and Structure.* Washington, D.C.: Government Printing Office, 1971.
40. Smith, P. L. Nutrition and the HMO. Unpublished report. Syracuse, N.Y.: Syracuse University, June 1978.
41. U.S. Department of Health, Education, and Welfare. *DHEW — Promoting Community Health — 1976*, Publ. No. (HSA) 77–5000. Washington, D.C.: Public Health Service, 1976.
42. Barthel, M. Washington, D.C. project analyzes medical costs in HMO setting. *Urban Health* 5 (December 1976): 28.
43. Sullivan, R. Health maintenance groups take growing role as resistance eases. *The New York Times*, May 20, 1978, pp. 1, 47.
44. The HMOs. *ADA Courier* 17 (January–February 1978): 3.
45. Roemer, M. I. From poor beginnings, the growth of primary care. *Hospitals* 49 (1 March 1975): 38.
46. Davis, M., and A. Warner. *Dispensaries: Their Management and Developments.* New York: Macmillan, 1918.
47. U.S. Department of Health, Education, and Welfare. *Programs of the Bureau of Community Health Service*, Publ. No. (HSA) 74–5007. Rockville, Md.: Public Health Service, 1973.
48. Pickett, G. E. The basics of health policy: Rights and privileges. *Am. J. Publ. Health* 68 (1978): 236.
49. Lorenz, K. Y., D. L. Davis, and R. W. Manderschied. The Health Promotion Organization: A practical intervention designed to promote healthy living. *Publ. Health Rep.* 93 (1978): 446–455.
50. Hallstrom, B. J., and D. E. Lauber. Multidisciplinary manpower in the nutrition component of comprehensive health care delivery. *J. Am. Diet. Assoc.* 63 (1973): 23.
51. American Public Health Association. Resolutions. *Am. J. Publ. Health* 61 (1971): 186.
52. Navarro, V. *Prevention and Health Promotion: Is It a Viable Alternative?* American Public Health Association Annual Meeting, Washington, D.C., October 1977.

53. Ittig, K. B. *Consumer Participation in Health Planning and Service Delivery: A Selective Review and a Proposed Research Agenda.* Rockville, Md.: National Center for Health Services Research, August 1976.
54. Fielding, J. E. *A Program for Prevention in Massachusetts.* Boston: Massachusetts Department of Public Health, February 24, 1977.
55. Terris, M. *Costs and Benefits of Prevention: The Challenge to National Policy.* Paper presented at the Annual Meeting of the American Public Health Association, Miami, Florida, October 1976.

Nutritional components of the health care system

Reader Objectives

After completing this chapter the reader should be able to
1. State the significance of nutrition in health promotion.
2. State the importance of the team approach in improving nutritional care.
3. List three general benefits from including a nutritional component in a comprehensive health care system.
4. List at least six strategies to be used if the quality of nutritional care is to be significantly improved.
5. List the four elements encompassed by nutritional care.

Nutrition affects health from the time of conception to death. Faulty nutrition leads to increased infant mortality and maternal morbidity; it stunts development, both physically and mentally; and it predisposes to or aggravates a spectrum of disease conditions, diminishing the quality of life, personal productivity and longevity. . . . Sufficient sound information exists with respect to food practices, nutrition, and general health to allow much greater control of health through dietary practices than is now being done. Maximum benefit from existing knowledge will require greater organization of all releveant resources than has been achieved to date. Without such organization and marshalling of resources, much human potential will go unrealized; and, more noticeably, significant relief to the health care system and cost containment will be lost.[1]

The universal significance of nutrition in medicine was recognized early by Hippocrates (460 B.C.) and stated as follows:

> For the art of medicine would not have been invented at first, nor would it have been made a subject of investigation . . . if when men were indisposed, the same food and other articles of regimen which they eat and drink when in good health were proper for them, and if no others were preferable to these. But now necessity itself made medicine to be sought out and discovered by men, since the same things when administered to the sick, neither did nor do agree with them . . .[2]

Nutrition is one of the environmental factors that is most readily subject to human control in the total contribution to individual health. It follows that there is a need to integrate nutritional services into systems that deliver medical and health care.

The significance of nutritional care during illness and rehabilitation is widely accepted. But the role that nutrition might play in promoting health and preventing disease has not been so widely appreciated. There is an increasing recognition that the most practical and effective approach to nutritional care is through a blend of the therapeutic emphasis with that of preventive care. The integration of both orientations into a comprehensive delivery of nutritional care is much needed and is long overdue.

It is becoming apparent that the inclusion of nutrition as a component of health care will greatly reduce the numbers of individuals who need sick care services. Improved nutrition will help to relieve strain on the national health care delivery system, and will result in a reduction in rising health care costs and in an improvement in general physical, psychological, and social well-being of individuals so that they are able to achieve productive lives of high quality.[3]

Nutrition services should thus be included as a component of *all* health and health-related programs. Further, nutrition services should be designed to reach the total population with priority given to those who are nutritionally vulnerable, such as infants, children, pregnant women, and the elderly.[4]

This requires a change in perspective. The preventive approach demands not merely attempting to deal with the consequences of poor nutrition but instead attacking the basic causes at their roots. The causes must be dealt with, rather than the traditional approach of treating the symptoms. It is clear that the traditional approach to nutrition must be broadened to include a responsiveness to community needs. The public's nutritional status must be considered in every phase of the delivery of nutritional services.

This section discusses the integration of a strong and effective nutrition component into existing health care delivery systems.

HISTORICAL PERSPECTIVE

B. S. Kunis has reviewed the highlights of the history of the integration of nutritional services into medical services; her review is summarized here.[5]

The professional nutrition literature, in recent years, has attempted to evolve a practical model for the integration of nutritional care into innovative health care delivery systems. The teaching of nutrition in university teaching hospital clinics was the start of the attempt. Nutrition gradually became a part of many such clinics including prenatal and perinatal, diabetic, hypertension, and other clinics organized to meet specialized population group needs. For the most part, the nutritionists were limited to short-term, rather fragmented sessions with the clinic population referred through the physician. Patient-nutritionist contacts were often sparse and ineffective because of limitations of time, space, or other resources needed to properly incorporate nutritional services into the clinic delivery system.

Limited opportunity for nutritional services to be incorporated into school and industrial clinics was usually dependent upon the "goodwill" toward nutrition of those operating the clinics. As a result nutrition was frequently excluded from the expanding development of ambulatory care systems that were aimed at preventive health care.

Nutrition never gained a foothold as an integral component of private health care that was offered through the private physician. Limited by the lack of recognition of the importance of nutrition in preventive health services, by the physician's lack of nutritional knowledge, as well as the fact that the consumer was rarely willing to pay for new types of services, nutrition was increasingly excluded from systems of health care delivery.

It became increasingly evident that an innovative approach was needed to bring nutritional services into the mainstream of health care delivery. In the early 1960s, an attempt was made to include an integrated normal and therapeutic nutrition education/counseling section into the medical services and preventive health education program of a prepaid health plan.[6,7] The Yale University-based family practice teaching program also provided nutrition as part of the total health care team efforts.[8,9]

Government programs also set the stage for the incorporation of nutrition into program offerings. The Child and Youth Programs (C & Y), Health Maintenance Organizations (HMO), and Family Health Care Centers integrated nutritional care into comprehensive and continuous care delivery.[10-12]

Thus, through a process of slow evolution, the integration of nutrition services into primary care, not only in the hospital but in ambulatory care clinics, became a reality. The nutritionist became a team member, contributing with others from a variety of disciplines to patient health care. Gradually, there was the realization that nutrition should be considered as an important component of all attempts to promote health and to prevent sickness.[3,4,11,13]

A variety of nutritional services have been incorporated into existing community health care programs. Dietary counseling in aspects of consumerism and normal nutrition, therapeutic dietary counseling as ordered by a physician, maternal instruction about infant and toddler diets, aid in obtaining food assistance, referral to the services of a social agency or another health service, and ongoing assessment and surveillance of nutritional status are some of the nutritional services most commonly performed by trained nutritionists. In addition to these examples of nutritional care, comprehensive health care programs ideally should include:[13]

1. Nutrition education for the public, especially in schools and community groups.
2. Dietary counseling for individual health problems, with recognition that telling people the facts about food does not necessarily result in changes of habits; support and reinforcement are needed.
3. Linkages and cooperation among all community health services and community nutrition programs to provide continuity and follow-up.
4. Research to provide knowledge in areas where food and nutrition information is inadequate.
5. Research to establish methods of evaluating programs, educational techniques, and the impact of nutrition services.

All these services should be considered, planned for, combined, and coordinated into the total health care delivery system for comprehensive care. For instance, group feeding programs, such as the School Lunch Program, that concentrate entirely on food service and ignore nutrition education fall short of their potential for improving the health and the nutritional status of the target group. If the program is to be successful and comprehensive, it must be founded upon a sound knowledge of the dietary habits, preferences, and problems of the children being served. Similarly, a meal program for the elderly without nutrition education will not solve the nutrition-related problems of America's older persons. To be comprehensive, services should be designed so that screening includes an assessment of nutritional status that is valid and relevant in relation to significant health risk factors.

Nutritional needs are significant at all levels of service delivery. They must be considered within the framework of the total requirements for alleviating the basic problems of poverty, in dealing with the levels of financial assistance to families (which would affect the quality of their diets), in determining the types of supportive services available to the poor, in designing the programs of employment and manpower opportunities, and in providing home management services to families needing such assistance.

A preventive approach to health care must consider a continuum of services required throughout the life cycle. Beginning with "health promotion" and health education, people must be prepared and counseled to take responsibility for their own health care. The American public has become aware of the relationship between food habits and their health; the media, the medical profession, and the food industry have had an impact. But this groundwork must be built upon by an organized mass nutrition education campaign supported by and carried out by the federal, state, and local levels of government, schools, industry, and medical personnel.

Until such time as comprehensive health care plans are available for all, adequate funding for preventive as well as curative nutritional services should be advocated. This too will be long in coming. Thus, it is important that nutritional services and nutritional care be integrated into existing specialized health care programs and services including services for pregnant women and lactating mothers, infants, and children; programs for the elderly, the poor, migrants, and Indians; school health programs; family planning programs; chronic disease control services; communicable disease control programs; rehabilitation services for alcoholics; prison programs; drug control centers; and group care services such as those provided in hospitals, halfway houses, day care centers, extended care facilities, and residential living centers.[14]

THE NUTRITION COMPONENT OF COMPREHENSIVE HEALTH CARE

Nutritional care has been defined as "the application of nutrition science to the health care of people."[3] The term can be used in reference to individual or community care, but regardless of the frame of reference, nutritional care encompasses the following essential elements that address individual as well as group needs:[15]

1. Assessment of nutritional status; this includes:

    (*a*) information on the availability and acceptability of food.

    (*b*) food consumption data.

(*c*) biochemical measurements of nutrients in body fluid or tissues.

(*d*) clinical and anthropometric measurements.

2. Planning and implementing nutritional counseling and education to meet normal as well as therapeutic needs.

3. Provision of referral to appropriate resources for aid in attaining optimal food and nutrition. Such resources may include food programs (see Chapter 17); nutrition or consumer education; social or economic assistance; and medical/health aid.

4. Program planning, implementation, monitoring, and evaluation, including ongoing, periodic follow-up to determine the effectiveness of nutritional care and to modify the care as appropriate.

These general services encompass a variety of specific nutrition services that should be provided, in the necessary mix, in every operational phase of health care. Examples of the range of nutrition services to be provided in the comprehensive health care delivery system are illustrated in Table 3-1.[16] As the table illustrates, nutritional care should properly be integrated into the continuum of health-sickness states, from preventive, health promotion activities, to diagnostic and assessment, to curative, therapeutic, restorative, and rehabilitative health services.

Table 3-1

Possible Pattern for Nutritional Services in a Comprehensive Health Care Program

Phase of Program Operation	Nutritional Care Goal	Nutritional Care Activities
Public health service and health promotion	To stimulate an awareness, understanding, and appreciation of the relationship between nutrition and health.	Mass public nutrition education, screening, and surveillance.
Health assessment; screening and referral	To identify risks or problems and develop appropriate care plans.	Assessment of food and nutritional status. Referral. Collection of data for patient information systems.
Environmental protection; health promotion; health maintenance	To prepare clients and their families to assume greater responsibility for their own health status. To encourage clients to recognize early warning signals and act appropriately.	Individual or group counseling Planning and implementation of nutrition education materials and evaluation. Development, implementation, and evaluation of nutrition education programs for health professionals, educational professionals. Referral to appropriate food assistance resources or other social, physical, or health resources. Provision of leadership in response to local or state or more global nutritional and health problems.

Possible Pattern for Nutritional Services in a Comprehensive Health Care Program (*continued*)

Phase of Program Operation	Nutritional Care Goal	Nutritional Care Activities
		Provision of consultation to institutions or organizations. Documentation of activities.
Acute and Intensive care	To develop and implement short- and long-term individualized nutritional care plans.	Activities previously listed, plus ongoing participation in health care teams. Planning, development, and implementation and follow-up of food service programs. Initial and follow-up nutrition counseling. Documentation of activities in reports and records.
Restoration and rehabilitation; extended care	To assist individuals and their families with long-term health problems. To help patients attain their maximum potential and improve the quality of their life. To allow individuals to be functioning members of their communities. To prevent unnecessary hospitalization or institutionalization.	Activities previously listed, plus home health care; assistance in helping patient to adjust to difficulties and modified life style; Communication with other health professionals or noncontact programs and services to aid individual in achieving goals set forth in his or her care plan.

Source: Position paper on nutrition services in health maintenance organizations. *J. Am. Diet. Assoc.* 60 (1972): 317.

NUTRITIONAL ASSESSMENT AND EVALUATION

Nutritional assessment is important to determine those individuals who are vulnerable to nutritional problems. It is also helpful in providing information about the general nutritional status (or level of nutriture) of the community; those nutritional problems that are particularly prevalent; the trends and time frame in which nutritional problems appear, are treated, and are alleviated; other environmental factors associated with the development of nutritional difficulties. Nutritional assessment is a mechanism for determining specific individuals who are suffering from malnutrition, so that therapeutic and corrective measures may be undertaken. Nutritional status evaluations also provide helpful data on which to base program objectives, planning, implementation, and evaluation components.

Nutritional status surveys, conducted on the same population at two or more different points in time, using similar survey techniques, can provide helpful information about changing trends in nutritional status. Such an activity has been referred to as monitoring or surveillance. In contrast to a single survey, surveillance implies some type of continuity, of ongoing "watching-over."[17]

A surveillance system can be used in a number of ways, such as the following:[17,18]

1. To identify the extent and type of particular deficiencies or problems in given population groups.

2. To provide mechanisms to identify particularly vulnerable or at-risk populations; as such, surveillance will facilitate the design and implementation of specific interventions.

3. To provide baseline data for comparison with "after-the-intervention" information and, thus, to aid in an evaluation of intervention and preventive programs.

4. To provide data for the setting of priorities for program design, allocation of support, and provision of other resources.

5. To provide data on local situations, so that appropriate targets for public assistance or private aid can be determined.

6. To provide a research base to determine the interaction between various factors that affect nutritional status of individuals or of the community.

7. To enable the selection of appropriate methods for intervention.

Community Assessment of Nutritional Status

A system of delivering nutritional services must recognize that the mustering of health care is intimately related to the structure of the community. A publication entitled *Health Is a Community Affair* (Cambridge, Mass: Harvard University Press, 1967) exemplifies this concept. The general problem of modern public and community health is to find methods of mobilizing the community so that both lay persons and professionals can act together to attack health problems.[19] Prevention must necessarily involve participation of the local community in two basic guises. First, service organization and delivery demands a fundamental knowledge of local health problems, nutritional disorders, and the resources for alleviating health and nutritional disorders. Second, the development of interventions to specific groups demands basic knowledge of the life-styles, habits, dietary practices, beliefs, and motivations of those groups that are at high risk for such problems.

Public health professionals have long held that "the community is the patient," a maxim that suggests that, rather than directing services to individuals, the health professional should first focus on the health of populations considered in their social milieu. This concept of community-as-patient dramatically affords a starting point for community assessment of nutritional status. Such an approach is by no means a simple one, but it can and should guide action. We can never know enough about the complex structure of a community or of a given human subgroup to be confident that we understand patterns of human behavior or that we can effectively work with a local community group to achieve specific change in the intended direction. But a community assessment can provide helpful information and point the health professional in the right direction.

The community can be viewed in a variety of ways, but fundamental to any analysis are the considerations that the community involves complex relationships and that every community is unique. The community must be perceived as a system so that influences of various parts of the community on one another can be assessed. This concept leads to a consideration of such questions as: What are the important political, economic, health, educational, and other institutions, resources, and personnel? Which persons exert the most influence on others in the community? How is the population divided according to demography (age, sex, race, ethnicity, socioeconomic status)? What are the pertinent nutritional or other health needs? What resources are available to attend to these needs? Which population subgroups are particularly in need of nutritional intervention? The answers to these questions can be helpful not only in uncovering needs and setting priorities for action but also in identifying the unique "personality" or style of living that is so intimately related to acceptance of nutritional programs, innovations, and interventions.

Individual Assessment of Nutritional Status

The nutritional surveillance system encompasses a continuum of activities, all of which, in combination, serve to identify existing nutritional problems and needs and suggest possible points of intervention. Screening is one aspect of the assessment process. Basic screening for nutritional problems involves, at a minimum, an evaluation of certain dietary, clinical, biochemical, and anthropometric data to identify the possible existence of a nutritional problem. If an individual does not present a significant indication of a nutritional disorder, based on the data evaluation in the screening process, there is probably no nutritional problem. The individual should be instructed in the preventive aspects of sound dietary practices. The individual need not be scheduled for an immediate follow-up but his or her nutritional status should be reassessed after a period of a year or two, in the event of a change in health status or of the individual's suspicion of a difficulty.

If the data indicate some type of abnormality, the individual should be directed to undergo a further assessment. This may consist of additional laboratory studies, a more sophisticated dietary assessment, roentgenographic studies, or other diagnostic tests to either confirm the disorder or remove the suspicion of a problem. For example, if a dietary history indicates that the individual has very erratic eating patterns or a diet with little variation, an interview and counseling session with a qualified nutritionist should be scheduled. If anthropometric studies indicate a weight for height that is in the range of the 1–5 percentile of accepted standards, further study should be conducted. If the clinical examination suggests that a specific deficiency might be present, this should be further investigated by biochemical tests that are specific for the nutrients in question. If abnormal laboratory values are found, the test should be repeated and the results confirmed. If low values are repeated, further study or treatment is indicated. Figure 3–1 illustrates the components involved in the

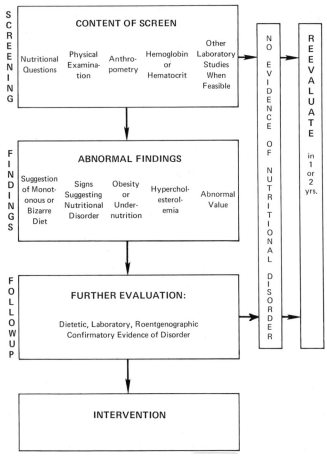

Figure 3-1. Nutritional screening and assessment process. (After Fomon[20])

overall surveillance process.[20] Table 3-2 summarizes criteria for selecting individuals for additional nutritional study.

NUTRITION EDUCATION AND COUNSELING

All primary health care facilities should provide some type of health education to clients. Nutrition should be included in this education either as part of a general health maintenance and preventive program or as a disease-specific education. Health and nutrition education should be provided for and financed as a routine part of client care; it should be an integral and sustained component of all aspects of health care.

As discussed in Chapter 2, the health care system is being challenged to improve its efficiency and effectiveness. One strategy to meet the challenge is the successful use of health and nutrition education. This may not only aid in containing costs but can also help to improve the quality of care and to enhance patient understanding of his or her condition and increase the patient's compliance with prescribed treatments. "Patient edu-

Table 3-2

Criteria for Selecting Individuals for Further Nutritional Assessment

For all individuals	Serum cholesterol concentrations greater than 230 mg/100 ml.
	Dental caries.
	Low hemoglobin concentrations less than 11.0 gm/100 ml for individuals under 10 years of age, or less than 12.0 gm/100 ml for individuals over 10 years of age, except for males over 14 years of age which is less than 13.0 gm/100 ml.
	Diseases or conditions in which nutrition plays a key role — cardiovascular disease, hyperlipidemias, diabetes, gastrointestinal disorders, hypertension, metabolic disorders, physical or mental handicaps affecting feeding, allergies, surgery, burns.
	Weight for height below the 5th percentile or above the 95th.
	Height for age below the 5th percentile (charts are currently available for ages birth to 9 years).
	Inadequate income, food supply, and facilities for food preparation.
	Substance abuse — alcohol, drugs, tobacco.
	Pica.
	Use of oral contraceptives, dilantin, or other drugs or medication affecting nutritional requirements.
For special groups	Any of the above considerations plus:
For pregnant and lactating women	Under 15 years of age; over 35 years.
	Previous unfavorable outcome.
	Short interval between pregnancies.
	Preexisting complications such as cardiovascular disease, renal disease, diabetes.
	Significant deviation in gain in weight.
For infants and children to 18 years of age	Any of items listed for all individuals, plus:
	Low birth weight.
	Failure to thrive.

Source: Department of Health, Education, and Welfare. *Preliminary Guide for Developing Nutrition Services in Health Care Programs.* Rockville, Md., 1976.

cation reinforces the patient's awareness of his responsibility for his own health, and self-responsibility is crucial for the ultimate effectiveness of health care."[21]

Patient health education is multifaceted. It entails the mutual identification of current and projected health care needs by both professional and patient, along with planning the combination of professional and patient responsibilities and roles for meeting needs, disseminating information related to treatment; motivating both patient and professional to perform appropriate roles, and ongoing monitoring of the process of health care. Educational methodologies should be aimed at particular desired behavioral changes and the results of such interventions relative to cost and quality of care should be documented. Program evaluation should be sustained and should provide feedback to help in program revision.

For the most part, nutrition education programs in health care facilities have been crisis-oriented, patchwork, and limited in defined objectives, educational methodologies, and financial resources. Most nutrition education conducted in the hospital or clinic involves individual patient counseling on a specific prescribed diet, or organized group classes for specific types of patients such as the obese or diabetics. Some HMOs and other clinic-based operations offer formal nutrition education programs. Limited numbers of state and local health departments and groups of affiliated hospitals also operate such education programs. Professional groups, such as the American Hospital Association and the American Dietetic Association, have restated their strong positions of approval for hospital health and nutrition education programs.

Diet Counseling

Diet counseling is the provision of individualized professional assistance to help an individual modify his or her food intake in accordance with the individual's health needs.[22] The process of diet counseling entails three separate but related activities: interviewing, counseling, and consulting.[23] The ultimate aim of this counseling is to aid clients in assuming responsibility to improve their own nutritional status.

Interviewing entails a needs assessment; it should identify current dietary habits as well as personal and environmental factors relevant to the improvement of nutritional status. Counseling involves listening, appreciating, understanding, and aiding an individual to understand the relationship between diet and health and, where necessary, to guide the individual to modify the diet in the best interests of good health. The effective nutritional counselor is able to guide, but not manipulate, the client's thinking so that the client is able to take ultimate responsibility for modifying his or her own food habits. Consulting involves the development of a nutritional care plan or a guideline for a client that is based on the client needs.

Counseling should be directed to helping the client learn to acquire a sustained improvement in nutrition behavior. Thus, counseling must involve more than the mere dissemination of information if it is to be effective. Nutrition education is discussed in greater detail in Chapters 13 and 14.

COORDINATION AND REFERRAL SERVICES

To provide the individual with continuity of care, to avoid unnecessary duplication of services, and to make sure that no gap in the provision of service exists, the implementation of nutrition services should be integrated and coordinated with the cooperation of individuals, groups, organizations, and agencies concerned with health care delivery. The following are especially important and should be considered in the development of nutrition programs:[24]

1. Nutrition personnel at the state and local level as well as community individuals working in special projects. By sharing information, resources, ideas, plans, and service standards between health professionals, these personnel can improve the quality of health and nutrition service.

2. Health personnel and nutritionists in nonhealth organizations such as in the education system, the welfare department, cooperative extension, and home economics groups. Such groups are often oriented toward health promotion as they provide health support for families and individuals; a working relationship with these professionals can provide for a comprehensive client referral system.

3. Nutritional personnel in primary care centers and other community health care programs, such as ambulatory care clinics, well-baby clinics, and group care facilities. By maintaining ties with treatment centers, the nutrition service can facilitate continuity or care for the appropriate clients.

4. Other health professionals. If nutritional services are to be maximally used, the importance of the other professionals must be understood and appreciated by nurses, physicians, and other health personnel who are in a position to refer clients to these services.

Referral to other health care services or to welfare, food, food assistance programs, counseling, or education services is basic to a continuity of care as well as to maximizing quality of the services provided. Established procedures, based upon defined criteria and specified standards, should characterize the referral process. A sample nutrition referral form should contain the following information:[24]

Patient's identification (name, address, telephone, Social Security number).

Identification of referring source, address, and telephone.

Reason for referral.

Suggested service to be provided.

Special medical, dietary, or personal factors to be considered.

Patient's physician or other health personnel who have worked with person to whom the follow-up records should be sent.

A sample referral form is included in Appendix II, p. 661.

PLANNING, IMPLEMENTATION, AND EVALUATION OF NUTRITION PROGRAMS

How is an effective nutrition program developed, implemented, and evaluated? Much has been written about the art of program planning and evaluation in relation to nutritional services. Two excellent books[25,26] are *The Dynamics of Clinical Dietetics* by Mason, Wenberg, and Welsch (New York: John Wiley & Sons, 1977), which describes the planning and evaluation of nutrition programs in the clinical setting, and *Nutrition in the Community: The Art of Delivering Services* by Frankle and Yanochik-Owen (St. Louis, Mo.: The C. V. Mosby Co., 1978).

The literature is replete with articles written to acquaint health professionals with the need for organized and systematized approaches to program planning and evaluation. But it is generally agreed that there is a gap between what is suggested in the literature and what is actually practiced. There is a great discrepancy between the concept of planning and evaluation and its implementation.[27]

J. Vermeersch and E. Peck used a system termed POME to study current program planning and evaluation practices of local health department nutritionists and to determine factors associated with planning and evaluation. POME is an acronym for

P — Problem identification

O — Objective statement

M — Method specification

E — Evaluation of results

The POME system assumes that there is an identification of problems based on information that reveals an undesirable situation in a community. The system entails the stating of objectives that are formulated to reduce or eliminate the identified problem, the development of methods to meet objectives, and outcome evaluation — that is, an evaluation designed to determine whether the program effectively met its stated objectives.[27]

The POME process is objective and relies on sound information and data rather than on the subjective approach in which priorities are determined according to "felt need" and evaluation is conducted by counting outcome results, such as the number of clients reached by the program.

Vermeersch and Peck used elements of the POME system to determine the extent to which a national sample of public health department nutritionists were involved in program planning and evaluation. They found that there was a great discrepancy between the concept and the practice of program planning and evaluation. They also found that some nutritionists were involved in program planning to a greater extent than others. They noted that people's inclinations to conduct planning and evaluation were related to individual personality and interests, but that the formal authority of the nutritionists' positions as well as the general organizational environment were the most significant factors influencing general performance.

They suggested that, if planning and evaluation are to become more common, health professionals must have some control over the resources and situations that are related to the development and outcome of programs.[27]

Table 3-3
Guidelines for Program Implementation

1. All those engaged in any aspect of the program planning, implementation, or evaluation or those who are target groups for program benefits should participate and should have a clear understanding of what the project aims to accomplish.

2. Precautions should be taken to compensate for the possible adverse influences of outside factors such as personnel and resources that might conflict with nutrition program objectives.

3. Attempts to broaden the base of support within the sponsoring agency or organization should be made; as much visibility as possible should be given to program activities.

4. Programs should be systematized with a general, broad administrative base and should be integrated into the normal operation of broader programs; they should not be piecemeal appendages to existing programs; they should not be afterthoughts.

5. Promoters of the program should present the program operations in terms that have high priority for the agency or other organization expected to support the program.

6. Those expected to benefit from the program (i.e., clients) should be actively engaged in every step of program planning and implementation; they should aid in identifying possible side effects.

7. A written plan should clearly specify who is responsible for particular program activities.

8. Prior to program implementation, all steps required for each activity should be identified. Time frames for implementing each step should be formulated.

9. Needed resources should be located.

10. Possible program constraints should be identified and addressed.

11. Specified plans for evaluation of program, as well as for the use of evaluative data, should be clearly stated before program implementation.

This book does not intend to describe in detail a method for program planning and evaluation. However, Tables 3-3 and 3-4 and Figure 3-2 summarize some of the important considerations. The components of program planning are presented in Figure 3-2. Guidelines for program implementation are summarized in Table 3-3. Table 3-4 illustrates examples of the nutritional component of comprehensive health care, objectives relating to these components, and possible activities to reach the goal of improved nutritional status of the population.

OPERATIONALIZING THE MODEL FOR INTEGRATION OF NUTRITIONAL CARE — A CASE EXAMPLE

The theory supporting the significance and need for an organized nutritional component of the health care system has evolved, but continuous efforts, testing, refinement, and development are needed before nutrition will be well received in all health care delivery programs.

Table 3–4

Nutritional Components, Objectives, and Activities of Comprehensive Health Programs

Components	Objectives	Activities
Assessment Surveillance Monitoring	To assess nutritional status. To identify strengths in dietary patterns. To identify nutrition status problems. To monitor the progress of those at nutritional risk.	Nutritional assessment program using one or more methods; clinical, dietary, anthropometric, or biochemical.
Referral	To refer those in need to food assistance, other health, social, or educational services.	Develop a manual of food assistance resources for nutritionists and other health professionals. Design and distribute to health professionals a nutrition referral form.
Counseling Education	To solve consumer problems regarding nutrition. To educate consumers and clients about health and nutrition. To educate health providers about health and nutrition.	Design and implement public service announcements on local media with consumer information on nutrition. Design grocery displays to explain nutrition labeling. Conduct nutrition education seminars for health professionals. Assist in developing nutrition curriculum in medical schools.
Program Planning, Development, Implementation, Evaluation	To determine needs for program; set goals and objectives. To identify alternative activities, resources available, and methods for implementation. To determine effectiveness in meeting stated goals. To use evaluation in information to revise and improve program.	Survey needs and available resources. Compare resources with assessed needs. Develop standards of care. Recruit qualified personnel to aid in implementing program activities. Plan for referral and for education. Design tools for program evaluation. Specify methods for use of evaluation data.

One such opportunity for testing and developing the model was reported by B. S. Kunis, from experiences in the Illinois Family Health Centers, Inc. (IFHC). The IFHC, a private corporation of six medical centers and a hospital emergency room, is founded on the premise that comprehensive health services should be available and inclusive at every center. The package of primary care service includes services of a family physician, pediatrician, dentist, nurse-manager, nutritionist, pharmacist, and laboratory. Support services are provided through the disciplines of optometry,

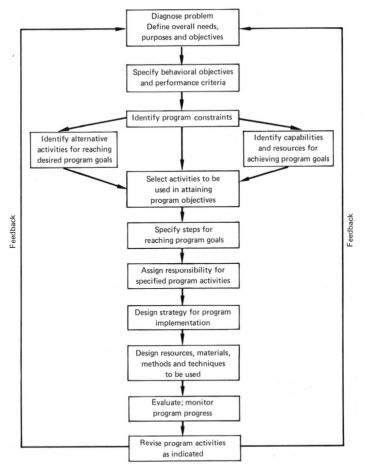

Figure 3-2. Program planning, implementation, and evaluation are continuous and on-going activities.

podiatry, speech therapy, and other medical specialties. The focus is "on continuing health care maintenance through 24-hour availability of medical service, geographic accessibility of medical facilities, and quality care by multidisciplinary professional personnel in identified communities."[5]

Nutrition staff work at permanent locations from one to three days weekly, by appointment. They receive fee-for-service paid to the center and also receive referrals from health professionals and from health consumers. The setting for the delivery of nutrition services is the nutrition office located among the medical examining rooms, an arrangement that provides visibility and accessibility to the health consumers and encourages communication with other team members. The initial patient-nutritionist meeting includes the taking of a nutrition history structured to look for patterns in body weight, food habits, health values, problem-solving techniques, and other important indicators that might contribute to the development of a nutritional-health care plan. Such plans are formulated in consultation with the patient. The aim of the plan is to help the consumer realize and appreciate the need for, and be motivated to follow, a plan designed to maximize his or her dietary and nutritional status. Follow-up appointments are then scheduled as needed.

The philosophy of nutritional care provided in such a framework focuses on the delivery of comprehensive and complete health care services, such as counseling in areas of preventive as well as crisis and remedial areas at reasonable cost levels. The nutritionist offers needed and appropriate levels of nutritional care for all levels of health care, ranging from dietary and consumer difficulties to special therapeutic management. The ultimate objective of this type of approach is to provide the health consumer with guidance, counseling, and education needed in all areas in which food is related to health care.

WHO PROVIDES NUTRITIONAL CARE?

The planning, development, and implementation of the nutrition component of health services is primarily the responsibility of qualified nutrition personnel. Several publications have discussed nutrition services along with the academic, experience, and personal qualifications for nutrition professionals.[14, 24, 28, 29, 30, 31]

The trend away from crisis-oriented medical care to health-oriented services (see Figure 3-3) necessarily involves an alteration in the traditional staffing patterns through which illness-oriented care was provided. Responsibility for service delivery extends from the physician, as primary care provider, to other health professionals. These are the so-called physician extenders who are becoming increasingly important in their own right as providers of health care.

Such trends require a rethinking of traditional roles, functions, and activities that have been delegated to nutrition professionals. Questions about *who* is able and qualified to provide *what* kind of care to *whom* must be examined and answered. This implies a need to reevaluate the education and training through which health professionals are provided with needed knowledge, skills, and expertise to carry out their responsibilities.

If nutritional needs are to be successfully provided, all health professionals must consider nutrition as an integral component of health care. It cannot be assumed that nonnutrition health professionals will automatically understand and appreciate the important relationship between good nutrition and optimal health status. It is important that nutrition professionals establish links for coordination and cooperation among all health professionals involved in health care delivery. One of the most effective ways to achieve this involves the active participation of nutritionists on the health care team.

Team Approach

The health care team concept has received much attention from health planners and health practitioners. Nutrition professionals typically participate in team activities by contributing to team care plans, communicating and sharing knowledge with other professionals, providing unique insights

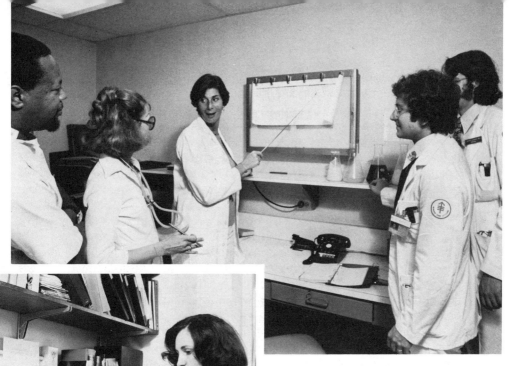

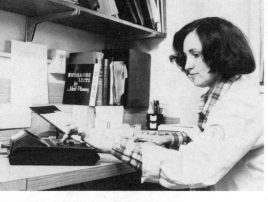

Figure 3-3. Assessment, counseling, and education are important aspects of nutritional care that should be integrated into every aspect of health care. (American Dietetic Association/Doyle Pharmaceutical Company)

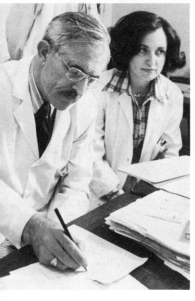

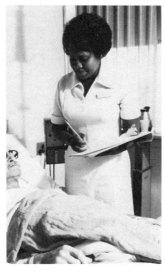

into the nutritional needs of clients, helping other primary care professionals to make sound judgments about patient care, and participating in the evaluation of patient progress. The health care team is a group of health professionals with various backgrounds, skills, and expertise who cooperate and work together to deliver health care services. Each individual team member needs the other team member to provide the best service. Patient problems are so complex that no one individual has all the skills or expertise to meet all needs. Thus, the health care team is able to maximize the skills of each team member.[32]

The health care team has been variously referred to as a comprehensive care, interdisciplinary, or multidisciplinary team. These terms typically refer to a team approach to patient care that is centered around a client's broad health goal (this is more extensive than the traditional medical care goals) and that involves participation by various health professionals in client assessment, design of care plans, implementation, and evaluation of goal-directed activities.

No member of the health care team can ignore the nutritional component of health care. Physicians and nursing personnel can conduct nutritional assessments, provide education and counseling in normal nutrition, make appropriate referrals of clients to nutrition professionals, and support the patient's need to attend to the nutritional advice. Other health professionals such as social workers, physical therapists, occupational therapists, dentists, dental hygienists, speech and hearing specialists, and health educators can assist in the development of referral mechanisms and in counseling clients with nutritional needs.

The approach provides nutrition professionals with the opportunity to integrate nutritional care into all levels of health service. It also offers an effective way to establish and maintain communication among health professionals and patients, thereby promoting an awareness of the significant role of nutrition in health promotion. The team approach can help all health professionals develop and maintain close working relationships that can lead to the attainment of mutual patient care goals and objectives. As nutrition professionals become more involved in the health care team, and as they are able to stimulate an interest, understanding, and appreciation for nutritional care, they will be able to extend and expand the nutrition services available at all levels of health care.

Alternative Staffing Patterns

Flexible use of nonnutrition personnel for activities that are often assumed to be the responsibility of the professional nutrition staff has been needed because of financial and other resource constraints. Such delegation of tasks has been shown to assist a multidisciplinary team in the provision of comprehensive care, and it may be an indication of ways in which nutrition can be made an integral component of the health care delivery system.

Some nutritional care services can be shared among a variety of professionals. Some activities must be independently performed by members of a given profession, whereas other activities may allow for an overlap among two or more disciplines, providing a common base for judgment and collaboration.

Experiences with the C & Y projects formed the basis for the identification of three major areas of commonly shared functioning. The area of *delegated functioning* involves activities variously performed by certain members of the health care team. For example, the referral of children to the nutritionist for nutritional assessment on the basis of overt clinical and/or anthropometric criteria, such as weight for height, allows a variety of health personnel to participate in the delivery of nutritional care.[31]

The second area, that of *collaborative functioning*, involves activities shared by nutrition professionals as well as by other team members. For example, physicians, nurses, and other team members, as well as nutritionists, share responsibility for such activities as collecting health histories and socioeconomic data.

The third area is also one of collaborative functioning, but it relates to a different staff pattern. For example, in matters of family life, meal planning, child care, and home management, nutrition and nursing and social work professionals are apt to collaborate. Many elements in the provision of nutritional care require the unique skills and expertise of nutrition professionals. For example, nutrition personnel usually do not share responsibility with other team members for the activities of nutritional and dietary assessments and for nutritional counseling.

Supportive nutrition personnel, such as the dietetic technician, the nutrition aide, and the dietetic assistant, also provide, under the supervision of the nutrition professional, various aspects of nutritional care.[33] M. A. Scialabba identified 68 role functions for nutritional care dietitians and for dietetic technicians who practice in ambulatory care settings. The functions were categorized under the primary headings of manager, consultant, educator, diet therapist-counselor, and advocate. These functions are listed in Table 3-5.[34] Community nutrition aides can extend the service provided by the nutrition profession. Aides such as Expanded Food and Nutrition Education Program workers are indigenous to the community and assist the community with food supplies as well as nutrition and consumer education.

Table 3–5

Functions Identified as Appropriate for the Dietitian and/or Dietetic Technician

Function	Dietitian	Dietetic Technician
Manager		
1. Identify need for nutritional services in the population served	X	
2. Set priority of need for nutritional services	X	
3. Develop nutritional programs according to priority of needs	X	
4. Write proposals for nutritional programs	X	
5. Set guidelines, standards, policies, and staffing pattern for the nutritional care unit	X	
6. Develop criteria for client referral to nutritional services	X	
7. Recruit and hire nutritional care personnel	X	
8. Prepare budget for nutritional care unit	X	

Table 3–5

Functions Identified as Appropriate for the Dietitian and/or Dietetic Technician *(continued)*

Function	Dietitian	Dietetic Technician
9. Determine appropriate personnel to provide various nutritional services	X	
10. Monitor nutritional care provided by other personnel	X	
11. Delegate tasks appropriately	X	
12. Develop system of records for nutritional programs and services	X	
13. Supervise staff and technical dietetic personnel	X	
14. Represent nutritional staff and program at administrative meetings, giving them visibility and status	X	
15. Write periodic and annual reports	X	
16. Develop program evaluation procedures	X	
17. Periodically review nutritional program in relationship to goals and effectiveness	X	
18. Coordinate nutritional services with affiliated hospitals and community agencies to provide for continuity of care	X	
19. Formulate long- and short-range goals for nutritional programs	X	
20. Interpret and sell nutritional programs to administration, staff and clients	X	X
21. Keep records of nutritional services.	X	X
22. Channel communication up and down organization structure	X	X
23. Organize space and equipment of nutrition office	X	X
24. Channel communication to and from the community and other community agencies	X	X
25. Identify and interpret own role within the immediate organizational structure	X	X
Consultant		
26. Serve as resource person to other professionals for nutritional information and availability of community nutritional resources	X	
27. Up-date other professional staff members on relevant nutrition-related research and literature	X	
28. Contribute to and criticize hypotheses and research designs from point of view of dietary habits	X	
29. Provide information to program planners in the setting and in the community on availability of funds for nutrition-related activities and programs	X	
30. Serve as resource person to program planners on questions of nutritional needs	X	
31. Provide information on foodservice aspects of projected programs	X	
32. Interpret nutritional research reports for staff in relation to food and eating behavior	X	
33. Up-date other staff on new food products and food production trends	X	X

Table 3–5

Functions Identified as Appropriate for the Dietitian and/or Dietetic Technician *(continued)*

Function	Dietitian	Dietetic Technician
Educator		
34. Plan in-service nutrition educational programs for all appropriate professional and non-professional staff	X	
35. Present in-service educational programs for staff	X	
36. Evaluate acceptance and effectiveness of educational programs relative to actual learning or behavior change	X	
37. Write columns or reports providing nutrition education for agency newsletter or bulletin	X	
38. Develop informational literature on aspects of nutritional care as required, i.e., food values, economics, and preparation; special dietary needs; special programs, such as supplemental food programs	X	
39. Service an an authority on questions of food, diet, and eating behavior	X	
40. Respond to claims of food faddists and others with objectivity, stating what is known as fact and what is yet to be learned or proved	X	
41. Plan group instruction for clients relative to nutritional needs in the agency and in the community	X	X
42. Present group instructional programs for clients in the agency and in the community	X	X
43. Develop training programs for lay auxiliary workers around appropriate nutritional topics	X	X
Diet therapist — counselor		
44. Assess nutritional status of clients, utilizing data from dietary history, medical history, and laboratory studies	X	
45. Lead group counseling sessions	X	
46. Prescribe appropriate specific dietary regimen based on physicians' diagnosis and general orders	X	
47. Participate in diagnostic decisions	X	
48. Interview clients to determine dietary status	X	X
49. Assess dietary status of clients	X	X
50. Plan nutritional care programs with clients on an individualized basis	X	X
51. Implement and adapt care plan on follow-up visits	X	X
52. Instruct clients on normal and modified diets as required	X	X
53. Record pertinent information on clients' records	X	X
54. Communicate with and refer clients to other nutritional care resources in the community	X	X
55. Participate in staff conferences and case presentations regarding nutrition	X	X
56. Evaluate clients' progress	X	X
57. Evaluate self in role effectiveness	X	X

Table 3-5

Functions Identified as Appropriate for the Dietitian and/or Dietetic Technician *(continued)*

Function	Dietitian	Dietetic Technician
58. Keep records of services rendered	X	X
59. Write reports of nutritional care activities	X	X
60. Communicate with other professionals as appropriate regarding clients' nutritional needs and progress	X	X
61. Calculate nutrient value of diets as required for the client, for adding to the dietary data in the clinic, and as required for research purposes	X	X
62. Follow up with home visits as required	X	X
Advocate		
63. Serve as spokesman in the agency for the inclusion of nutritional programs to meet established eeds	X	
64. Sell need for nutritional services to appropriate legislative, political, and community leaders and other health professionas	X	
65. Work for representation of nutritional services' interests on planning agencies, boards and committees, with primary focus on requirements for optimal patient care	X	
66. Engage in community outreach activities	X	X
67. Work actively in support of legislation relative to health in general and food and nutrition specifically	X	X
68. Attend meetings of community organizations as participant and as nutrition advocate	X	X

Source: Scialabba, M. A. Functions of dietetic personnel in ambulatory care. *J. Am. Diet. Assoc.* 67 (1975) : 545.

It is evident that all those who provide nutritional care must be ready to meet a variety of challenges. They must demonstrate competencies, not only in the area of planning to meet nutritional needs of clients but also in fiscal planning; implementation and evaluation of programs; coordination and integration within the health care team; successful communication with various health professionals, clients, and public and private concerns; and "most important — showing their effect on the outcome of patient care, not simply their activity based on number of persons seen." As Scialabba emphasized, this necessitates skill in the art and the science of nutrition, as well as professional self-confidence, assertiveness, communication skills, and expertise in the planning, implementation, and evaluation of programs.

How well these nutrition-related responsibilities are performed by those trained to provide nutritional care will, in large part, determine the place of nutrition in comprehensive health care delivery systems. Administrative and planning personnel are more likely to support nutrition personnel in the system if they view them as offering a useful, effective, and unique contribution to health care.

BENEFITS FROM INCLUDING A NUTRITIONAL COMPONENT
IN A COMPREHENSIVE HEALTH CARE SYSTEM

The numerous advantages to providing nutritional care in a comprehensive health care system may be summarized as follows:[13]

1. Evaluation of dietary status and consideration of nutritional needs, whether preventive or restorative, can serve as a positive reinforcement of appropriate habits and can direct early intervention when indicated.

2. Dietary modification is a major factor in recovery from certain illnesses and in lessening the impact of some factors that contribute to long-term health problems. In some diseases such as diabetes, nutritional management is basic to treatment.

3. A health care team in a comprehensive care plan, which seriously attends to nutritional needs, can demonstrate smooth working relationships among professionals, reduced patient visits to the physician, decrease hospitalization, and increase patient care satisfaction.

These benefits can be accounted for in terms of financial savings. Documentation is available that supports the financial savings resulting from the inclusion of nutritional services in comprehensive health care programs. T. Dahl has reported the results of an analysis of the efficiency of comprehensive health care delivery in which the presence of a nutritional functional area in programs designed for children and youth had reduced the average yearly registrant cost. Dahl suggested that "an increase in the allocation of funds to the nutritional functional area by 1 percentage point would be likely to reduce total cost per registrant per year by about 1/11 of a percentage point." These percentage points, translated into dollar amounts, demonstrate that the average yearly registrant cost of $271.52 was actually $27.30 lower than it would have been if the nutritional component were absent.[35]

In a similar study, Dahl demonstrated that the principal source of nutritional services, in which there was no nutritional functional area, was through medical personnel. This analysis indicated that by increasing the cost of the nutritional component by one percentage point, the medical functional area cost was reduced by about one sixth of a percentage point. The total dollar savings in medical costs was as high as $14.62 per registrant annually, whereas the added cost for the nutrition area ranged from only $1.81 to $2.66 per registrant annually.[36]

Although some have questioned the data on which Dahl based his calculations, his model serves to illustrate the cost effectiveness of including a nutritional component in a comprehensive health care service deserves consideration.

Legislation authorizing comprehensive health care programs has acknowledged that nutritional care should be considered as a therapeutic functional area in the same way as medical, social, dental, nursing, psychologic, and similar services are. Thus, where nutritional functional areas were not included in a program, the service had to be delivered by an allied health or medical area at an increased cost. It is clear that the inclusion of nutritional functional areas in health care delivery programs is a cost-effective measure.[37]

BARRIERS TO THE INCLUSION OF NUTRITION IN COMPREHENSIVE HEALTH CARE

Recognition of the significance of nutrition in total health care does not easily translate into common practice. The following are some of the barriers to carrying out the full potential of nutritional care:[13]

1. Limited public appreciation for the importance of nutrition education in health promotion and maintenance, and of nutritional care in health care programs.

2. Inadequate support for nutritional services and the organizational structure within which nutritional care can be provided. This is especially true for providing nutritional care and counseling in ambulatory clinics.

3. A lack of public recognition of the importance of ongoing research support in nutrition and nutritional care delivery.

4. A lack of basic and continuing education in nutrition in medical, dental, and other professional staff curricula.

5. A lack of acceptance or expansion of the role of the nutrition professional in planning and implementing care.

6. A lack of inclusion of nutritional status measures of biochemical, clinical, anthropometrical, or dietary assessments in routine screening procedures; where they are included, they often do not stimulate indicated nutritional referrals.

7. Nutritional services are seldom reimbursable in health insurance plans or by third-party payers.

8. Nutritional services are more accessible to those of higher socioeconomic status and to the indigent who qualify for welfare or public health programs. The working poor and middle-income people have only limited access to nutritional services except on a crisis-initiated basis.

In view of the importance of nutrition in health promotion, nutritional concerns should be reflected in national policy and public or private health programs.

RECOGNITION AT THE NATIONAL LEVEL

The federal government has become increasingly aware of the need to incorporate nutritional care components into existing health care delivery systems. According to the mandate of the National Health Planning and

Resources Development Act, (see pp. 35–36) the Department of Health, Education, and Welfare is to issue, on a periodic and ongoing basis, guidelines for national health planning and policy.[38] Topics to be included in these guidelines are standards for health resources and national health planning goals. To date, three guidelines have been issued under the title Forward Plan for Health; the most recent was issued for the fiscal years 1978–1982.[39] These guidelines are designed to be blueprints for health decision making at the national level.

Several sections of the second plan, Forward Plan for Health, FY 1977–1981, were devoted to nutrition. The Plan appendix recognized nutrition as a preventive health discipline and outlined a comprehensive "nutrition plan." The emphasis on nutritional care laid the groundwork for legislation and regulations that will enhance future opportunities to incorporate nutritional care into the health care delivery system. The part of the plan that concerns nutrition and prevention is especially significant:[40]

Health Maintenance — Make nutrition concerns a mandatory component of all DHEW activities. Include nutrition and health concerns in the policy development processes of all DHEW agencies and of other federal agencies. Strengthen monitoring activities to establish nutritional status, eating habits, and relationship of consumption to various health states.[1]

In Appendix II of the plan there is an equally important statement:

Nutritional care, including dietary counselling, should be integrated into the preventive, diagnostic and restorative health services of all the PHS programs for all family members. However, it is especially important that nutrition services for the subsets of the population with high vulnerability to malnutrition and with special nutritional requirements . . . have priority in efforts to reduce morbidity and mortality rates.[1]

In its third *Forward Plan, FY 1978–1982*, the Deparment of Health, Education, and Welfare, in recognition of the value of proper nutrition, advocated a three-pronged approach to meet the nutritional needs of clients.[39]

1. Identification and monitoring of nutritional needs and problems; the responsibility for this phase falls primarily to the Center for Disease Control and the National Center for Health Statistics. Guidelines and technical assistance are needed to aid in obtaining of accurate and reliable nutrition information. A nutrition education program designed to prepare health personnel to obtain and evaluate nutritional status information must also be developed.

2. Improvement of organization and delivery of nutrition services; this strategy will be implemented through improved planning, guidelines, standards, and criteria for the nutrition-related components of the health care delivery system. Improved coordination and exchange of knowledge, technical assistance, and information among various federal agencies involved with nutrition should receive top priority.

3. Quality assurance; this will be implemented through the development

of standards of nutritional care services and requires increased technical assistance to the providers of health and nutritional care.

The importance of preventive health services, including nutritional services to health promotion, has been recognized, and the significance of the nutritional component has been established at the federal level. To succeed, these approaches must have the enthusiastic support of the medical profession, the medical insurance industry, and the public.

RECOMMENDED STRATEGIES

If nutrition advocates and professionals are to significantly improve the quality of nutritional care, a number of priorities deserve attention.[40–42]

Planning, Organization, and Implementation of Nutritional Care Programs

Nutrition should be mandated as a required component of comprehensive health care. Legislation addressing preventive health care should specifically include the nutritional care component. The type and quality of nutritional care should be specifically covered by written guidelines. Policies should be developed to consider flexible plans allowing nutritional services to meet varying human needs and preferences.

Proponents of nutritional services will have to work within the planning network and will have to join efforts to advocate, promote, and achieve this goal. By supporting legislators, planners, and policymakers who are sympathetic to espoused concerns, by lobbying for the advancement of sound nutrition policies, by being active in promoting effective services at the local level, and by developing support in the public sector and among other health providers, the nutrition advocates can best advance the delivery of sound nutritional services.

Nutritionists need to be knowledgeable about the workings and operation of health planning bodies, they need a commitment from their constituents, and they need a source of data or information on a county and a metropolitan area level. Nutritionists must be able to assist health planners in compiling data on local nutrition problems and on resources that are available and that are needed. Nutrition assessment and surveillance programs, as well as studies designed to meet the local assessment and diagnostic needs, are important to indicate the needs of the community and to demonstrate the impact of nutrition services. If nutrition services are to become an integral component of existing health service delivery programs, they must be appreciated as essential and important not only by nutritionists but by other health professionals and by health consumers as well. There is a need to demonstrate the importance of including nutritional services and to educate planners, health professionals, and the public to this need.

Provision of Nutritional Care

Nutritionists must be knowledgeable and skilled in the provision of nutrition care. This requires a general background in health education, including the methodology of planning, implementation, and evaluation of programs, as well as specialized education in dietetics. To follow up college-level education, there is a need for continuing education to improve skills in the speciality area of nutrition, as well as to improve skills in communication and related areas.

Reimbursement

Reimbursement for nutrition services is important if there is to be a continuing growth of nutrition components of existing health care delivery systems. A variety of options are available. A fee-for-service payment, reimbursement by public or private third parties, or the reallocation of existing resources to pay for nutrition services are three possible ways to provide reimbursement for nutrition care. Legislation mandating health care services should provide for suitable financial incentives to implement nutritional services. The issue of reimbursement for nutrition services underscores the importance of developing methodologies for the documentation of contributions that nutrition care can make to health and well-being.

Continuing Competence and Accountability

The Department of Health, Education, and Welfare in its 1977 report, *Credentialing Health Manpower*, cited a variety of problems in the delivery of health care services, one of which is the problem of equating continuing education with continued competence. The report suggests that professionals should demonstrate continued competence in their fields of expertise as a requirement for continued practice. The report supports the development of sophisticated approaches to continued competence, some of which may include peer review through Professional Standards Review Organizations, reexamination, self-assessment techniques, and supervisory assessment. Continued education is still needed, but it is no longer regarded as a valid indicator of competence. The development of national standards for giving health credentials are suggested as a way to assure continued competence.[40]

To this end, a National Commission for Health Certifying Agencies has been developed to set standards for groups that provide health credentials. This group has as a stated objective "to establish standards for certifying bodies that attest to the competency of individuals that participate in the health care system."[40]

Standards of Care

The development and implementation of standards of care at the local, state, and national level, as well as the design of guidelines for the provision of nutrition care, is crucial. As various interest groups in the health care field become more powerful in competing for scarce health resources, nutritionists must become increasingly skilled in mounting programs to gain national and state support. Basic to gathering such support is the development of guidelines for nutrition services and standards for nutrition manpower. Some states, such as Oregon, have already developed standards for nutrition services. These guidelines might serve as an example to other state nutrition professionals.[41]

SUMMARY AND CONCLUSION

The factors that are essential to an effective nutrition service are summarized in Table 3-6. Because of the long neglect of nutrition, as well as preventive approaches in the United States medical care system, organizations and individuals advocating the role of sound nutrition in health promotion must use their influence to ensure that they share a part of the allocation of health resources.

If nutrition advocates do not play a leading role in shaping health and nutrition policy and implementation, then some other vested interest group is bound to advance their concerns and nutrition may continue to be bypassed.

Table 3-6

Factors Essential to an Effective Nutrition Service

1. Provision of adequate support for screening and monitoring; existing needs of client, felt needs of clients, and factors related to the causes, significance, and modification of existing problems are identified through the nutrition service.

2. Adequate coordination; the nutrition service should be coordinated with other existing health services as well as with other available nutrition services. Such coordination is basic to the continuity of care, to ensure no unnecessary duplication of services, and to avoid gaps in the services available to the client.

3. Operational referral system; criteria should be established for the referral of clients to other services, such as medical or welfare services or nutrition counseling.

4. Systematic planning efforts; there should be a recorded procedure for designing, implementing, and evaluating nutrition services.

5. Adequate resources for achieving nutrition objectives; this includes nutrition personnel, financial support, supplies, facilities, and identified and operational links with other community resources.

5. An evaluation component based on measurable stated objectives. Basic to this is accurate recordkeeping and documentation to report service delivery and progress of the system, as well as individual client progress. There should also be a feedback effort to report evaluation results to clients, administrators, and personnel.

6. Nutritional quality standards; stated standards are essential in screening, monitoring nutritional progress, and in diagnosing nutritional disorders.

REFERENCES

1. U.S. Department of Health, Education, and Welfare. *Forward Plan for Health, 1977–81.* Washington, D.C.: Government Printing Office, August 1975.
2. Hippocrates, in F. Adams, trans., *The Genuine Works of Hippocrates.* London: The New Sydenham Society, 1849.
3. American Dietetic Association. Position paper on the nutrition component of health services delivery systems. *J. Am. Diet. Assoc.* 58 (1971): 538.
4. American Dietetic Association. Promoting optimal nutritional health of the population of the United States. *J. Am. Diet. Assoc.* 55 (1969): 452.

5. Kunis, B. S. Family nutritionist on the primary health care team. *J. Nutr. Educ.* 8 (1976): 77.
6. Katz, M. The role of the nutritionist in a prepaid medical care program. *Am. J. Clin. Nutr.* 13 (1963): 259.
7. Katz, M. *Model of a Nutrition Program and Other Unpublished Documents from the Nutrition Division of Health Insurance Plan.* New York, 1974.
8. Beloff, J., and E. R. Weinerman. Yale studies in family health care. I. Planning any pilot test of a new program. *J.A.M.A.* 199 (1967): 383.
9. Beloff, J., P. S. Snoke, and E. R. Weinerman. Yale studies in family health care. II. Organization of a family health care program. *J.A.M.A.* 204 (1968): 355.
10. Egan, M. C. Building nutrition services in comprehensive health centers. *J. Am. Diet. Assoc.* 61 (1972): 491.
11. Egan, M. C. Nutrition services in child health programs. *J. Am. Diet. Assoc.* 59 (1971): 555.
12. Batchelor, T. M., A. McNowell, and M. G. Wagner. A comprehensive health care program in the community. *J. Am. Diet. Assoc.* 60 (1972): 112.
13. American Dietetic Association. The dietitian in primary health care. *J. Am. Diet. Assoc.* 70 (1977): 587.
14. American Dietetic Association. Position paper on recommended salaries and employment practices for members of the American Dietetic Association. *J. Am. Diet. Assoc.* 58 (1971): 41–42.
15. U.S. Senate Select Committee on Nutrition and Human Needs, Subpanel of Health Care Systems. *Implementation and Delivery of Nutritional Care Services in the Health Care Systems.* Washington, D.C.: Government Printing Office, June 1974.
16. American Dietetic Association. Position paper on nutrition services in health maintenance organizations. *J. Am. Diet. Assoc.* 60 (1972): 317.
17. Nichaman, M. A. Developing a nutritional surveillance system. *J. Am. Diet. Assoc.* 65 (1974): 15.
18. Habicht, J. P., J. M. Lane, and A. J. McDowell. National nutrition surveillance. *Fed. Proc.* 37 (1978): 1181.
19. Wilson, R. *The Sociology of Health: An Introduction.* New York: Random House, 1970.
20. Foman, S. *Nutritional Disorders of Children*, Publ. No. (HSA) 77-5104. Rockville, Maryland: U.S. Department of Health, Education, and Welfare, Public Health Service, 1976.
21. Blue Cross Association White Paper: Patient health education, in Fogarty International Center et al., *Preventive Medicine, U.S.A., Health Promotion and Consumer Education, Appendix K.* New York: Prodist, 1976.
22. American Dietetic Association, Joint Committee on Community Nutrition and Diet Therapy Sections. Guidelines for developing dietary counseling services in the community. *J. Am. Diet. Assoc.* 55 (1969): 343.
23. American Dietetic Association, Diet Therapy Section Committee. Guidelines for diet counseling. *J. Am. Diet. Assoc.* 66 (1975): 571.
24. U.S. Department of Health, Education, and Welfare. *Preliminary Guide for Developing Nutrition Services in Health Care Programs.* Rockville, Md.: Public Health Service, 1976.
25. Mason, M., B. G. Wenberg, and P. K. Welsch. *The Dynamics of Clinical Dietetics.* New York: John Wiley, 1977.
26. Frankle, R., and A. Yanochik-Owen. *Nutrition in the Community: The Art of Delivering Services.* St. Louis, Mo.: C. V. Mosby, 1978.
27. Vermeersch, J. A., and E. B. Peck. Program planning and evaluation practices of local health department nutritionists. *Publ. Health Rep.* 92 (1977): 466.

28. Barney, H., and M. C. Egan. Home economists as members of health teams. *J. Home Econ.* 60 (1968): 427.

29. Phillips, M. G. Nutrition opportunities in specialized health areas. *J. Am. Diet. Assoc.* 55 (1969): 348.

30. U.S. Department of Health, Education, and Welfare. *Guide Class Specifications for Nutritionist Positions in State and Local Public Health Programs.* Washington, D.C.: Government Printing Office, 1971.

31. Hallstrom, B. J., and D. E. Lauber. Multidisciplinary manpower in the nutrition component of comprehensive health care delivery. *J. Am. Diet. Assoc.* 63 (1973): 23.

32. Siegel, B. Organization of the primary care team. *Pediatr. Clin. N. Am.* 21 (1974): 341.

33. American Dietetic Association. Position paper on the dietetic technician and the dietetic assistant. *J. Am. Diet. Assoc.* 67 (1975): 246.

34. Scialabba, M. A. Functions of dietetic personnel in ambulatory care. *J. Am. Diet. Assoc.* 67 (1975): 545.

35. Dahl, T. Estimating the efficiency of comprehensive health care delivery. Paper presented at the 101st annual meeting of the American Public Health Association, San Francisco, 1973.

36. Dahl, T. *The Medical Functional Area in Comprehensive Health Care Delivery for Children: An Economic Analysis*, Study Ser. No. 3-2 (20). Minneapolis: Minnesota Systems Research, 1973.

37. Dahl, T. Economics, management, and public health nutrition. *J. Am. Diet. Assoc.* 70 (1977): 144.

38. U.S. Congress. The National Health Planning and Resources Development Act of 1974, PL-93-641. January 7, 1975.

39. U.S. Department of Health, Education, and Welfare. *Forward Plan for Health, FY 1978–1982.* Washington, D.C.: Government Printing Office, August 1976.

40. Department of Health, Education, and Welfare. Credentialing health manpower: Is continuing education enough? *ADA Courier* 17 (1978): 1.

41. East, D., and V. F. Harger. Oregon dietitians respond to call for health care planning data. *J. Am. Diet. Assoc.* 69 (1976): 400.

42. McCarthy, M. C. *Some Nutrition Issues in National Health Planning.* Washington, D.C.: American Dietetic Association Legislative Workshop, 1976.

section one
END OF SECTION ACTIVITIES

1. With a view toward the future, health planners have proposed various models for organizing medical manpower in different types of ambulatory care centers. Three such models and the minimum population bases needed to support them are listed below. Review these models. Are there any examples in your community where these ideas are implemented? Discuss the models with health professionals and review their ideas about the practicality of implementing them. How would nutritional services be affected by these various models?

Three Models for Organizing Medical Manpower in Ambulatory Care Centers

Comprehensive Ambulatory Care Center

This model is staffed by a multispecialty group of 9–12 physicians. Typically, this model uses general and family practitioners to provide primary care and is supported by all the primary care specialties (pediatrics, obstetrics-gynecology and internal medicine). Physicians from other medical and surgical specialties (e.g., orthopedics, otolaryngology-ENT) might also be affiliated with the center. This center would generally serve 25,000–35,000 people.

Primary Care Center

This model is staffed by 3–6 primary care physicians. For example, such a center might be staffed by two general or family practitioners, one pediatrician and one obstetrician-gynecologist. A primary care center with three physicians would serve approximately 8,500 people; a center with six physicians would serve approximately 17,000 people.

Practitioner/Satellite

This model might be staffed by one or two general practitioner(s) supported by physician extenders, nurses and other health personnel. In areas where it has not been possible to attract a physician a satellite could be developed. The satellite would be staffed by two physician assistants or nurse clinicians supervised by a primary care physician on a part-time basis. The practitioner/satellite with one physician or with one half-time physician and two physician assistants or nurse clinicians would serve approximately 2,700 people. A practitioner/satellite with two physicians would serve approximately 5,400 people. Linkage with other primary care providers is inherent in this model since ALPHA's standards state that the solo practitioners should maintain definite arrangements for referring their patients to specialists.

Source: ALPHA. *Planning for Ambulatory Care: Guidelines for Future Development* (Syracuse, N.Y.: Areawide and Local Planning for Health Action, Inc. 1974) p. 85. Taken from F. F. Yanni: Primary care: future direction or return to basics? *Family and Community Health* 1 (1978): 31.

2. The following table suggests the forces shaping future local health care in the U.S. On the basis of this outline, discuss the possible integration of nutrition services. Develop possible models for health care delivery in the late twentieth century. Compare your ideas with those in B. L. Green. Rural health delivery systems of the 1980s, *Family and Community Health 1* (1978): 95–108. Pay particular attention to the integration of nutrition services into the health care system in the models you design.

Forces Shaping Health Delivery Systems of the 1980s

Force	Strength of Force			Resulting Adjustment in Health Delivery System
	Weak	*Medium*	*Strong*	
Population Location				
Increasing population in nonmetro areas, especially in the West and the South			X	Scarce primary care resources will have large increases in effective demand. Major concern in West with communities whose economic base is mainly energy, and the South where price increases

Forces Shaping Health Delivery Systems of the 1980s (*continued*)

Force	Strength of Force			Resulting Adjustments Delivery System
	Weak	Medium	Strong	
				could reduce access by black Americans
Stable or decreasing population in large metro areas		X		Relatively large stock of health care resources will have shorter queues
Population Profile				
Low, stable birth rates	X			Gradual conversion of obstetrics to other uses
Some postponement of births		X		More impaired infants, and increased use of complex facilities in tertiary hospitals
Increase in proportion of elders			X	Gradual expansion of geriatrics facilities, especially cardiac care units
Economic Condition				
Moderate annual inflation and unemployment	X			Gradual shift toward group practices, and hospital outpatient departments
Education				
Broadening of base of concern about quality of life			X	Reduced tolerance for "gaps" and inadequacies in health care system, and increased interest in modifying lifestyles to achieve better health (health education)
Rapid increase in educational levels of farmers	X			
Medical Technology			X	Unless counterforce emerges, medical goods and services will be additions to existing supply, and will be more suited for metropolitan, tertiary care sector. They will tend to cause costs and prices to increase
Institutional Factors				
Consumers share power in health planning process			X	Increased interest in (1) deployment of mid-level practitioners (midwives, physician assistants and nurse practitioners) and (2) speeding the process of ambulatory care facilities
National Health Insurance		X		Since Medicare-Medicaid is quasi-national health insurance, the major increase in effective demand has already occurred (1965 to 1970). However, regions such as the South with large strata of minorities will experience a large increase in the effective demand for primary care, especially MDs and non-physician providers.

3. Why is such a small percentage of the total federal outlay for health and medical care devoted to public health and health promotion activities? What barriers face a national health promotion strategy? What actions must be taken to overcome these barriers?

4. What various prevention-oriented activities are undertaken in your community? How effective are these activities in promoting health? Are nutrition components part of these activities? Should they be? How might you stimulate action to have nutrition components included in these activities?

5. Investigate the workings of the local HSA in your area. What action has the local HSA undertaken? Who composes the HSA? What is the general stance of the HSA to nutrition and health promotion? Investigate the possibility of becoming actively involved in HSA activities. What strategies might you take to increase the visibility and importance of nutrition activities?

6. Is there an HMO in your area? How does it operate? Is nutrition an important part of HMO activities? How does the structure of the HMO relate to the health care model proposed by Garfield?

7. Justify the presence of a nutrition care component as integral to health care. Survey an ambulatory care clinic in your area. Is nutrition included in the care provided? If not, talk to the director about its absence. Why is nutrition not included? What strategy is needed to make nutrition part of the total health care offered?

8. Use the Nutritional Care Community Agency Report and the Continuing Patient Care Form, pages 98–102 as samples in the following activity.

Mrs. Elsie Watson lives alone in a small rural farm town. She is 87 years old and has three children, but they all live out of state and she rarely sees them. Mrs. Watson does not drive but has been able to walk to the corner grocery store to purchase essential food. However, her arthritis is becoming increasingly painful and her mobility is gradually decreasing.

Mrs. Watson, a mature onset diabetic, is on a 1200-calorie diet. She is 5'4" and weighs 170 pounds.

Mrs. Watson's income is limited — her average food budget is about $10 weekly. She attends a meal program for the elderly, to which she walks two to three times weekly. However, the meals are served in a church basement five blocks away and the walk is becoming increasingly difficult for her.

Assume that you are the public health nutritionist responsible for nutrition needs of the county in which Mrs. Watson lives. You have been asked to interview Mrs. Watson and prepare a community agency report as a baseline care plan for her. Include in your report: (a) nutritional assessment; (b) problems; (c) nutritional care plan; and (d) referral recommendations — for recommended referrals, prepare a nutritional continuing patient care form.

If you were to see Mrs. Watson in person, or have access to her medical records, what information would you like in addition to information of the sort given here?

Nutritional Care Community Agency Report

Date 3-2-77

To: Joan Brown   R.D.

      Dietary Department South   Hospital

      Address:

From: M. Elizabeth Vaughn   R.D.

      Nutrition Department
      Visiting Nurse Association of Metropolitan Detroit
      4421 Woodward Avenue, Détroit 48201
      Phone:

Patient's Name: Ann Wood

      Address:

Note: Pt. re-hospitalized with fracture. On discharge will continue with
supervision and reinforcement of diet.

                                                    12/10/76*
Consultation [X]   12/10/76   Direct Service [X]   2/8/77

Nutritional Assessment
   Sister preparing all food and "weighs meat and measures other food
most of the time." Pt. admits she snitches just a little during night. Following discharge from hospital on 1/20/77 — diet order changed to 1800
cal. 2 gm. Na and 20 gm. Pro. Sister secured special baking mix for Lo-
Pro bread.

Problems Identified
   Need for accurate measurement of all foods. Too much talking — not
enough listening. Lack of understanding of relationship of diet to illness.
Pt. depends entirely on sister for care — needs motivation to participate
in meal preparation.

Nutritional Care Plan
   Replan of diet according to new prescription. Use of single instruction
sheet — simplifying instruction. Change of milk to coffee rich — for coffee
and with cereal. Instruct to use no more than 2 slices regular bread per
day — all other Lo Pro.

   *On former admission to VNA service, Nutrition Consultant made home visit and
attempted to simplify diet for pt. and sister. Pt. re-hospitalized before mission
accomplished.

   Source: E. Peck, ed. Leadership and quality assurance in ambulatory health care. *Proc.
Nat'l Publ. Health Nutrition Workshop*, Chicago, Ill., May 1977.

Nutritional Care Community Agency Report

Date   3-11-77

To: Mary Coy   R.D.

Dietary Department North   Hospital

Address:

From: Elizabeth Vaughn   R.D.

Nutrition Department
Visiting Nurse Association of Metropolitan Detroit
4421 Woodward Avenue, Detroit 48201

Patient's Name: Mildred Clark

Address:

Progress to date: weight loss — 22 lbs. Motivated to lose to 145 lbs. Improved attitude. Allowed increased activity. Interested in maintenance diet when desired weight level achieved.

Consultation ☐   Direct Service ☒   12/29/76
                                                    1/21/76

Nutritional Assessment
    Past eating patterns poor — no breakfast — no lunch or possibly a bologna sandwich. Large portions of meat, potatoes at dinner. Dislikes skim milk and most vegetables. Will eat fruit — loves Pepsi's; used to drink several quarts per day.

Problems Identified
    Limited income for size of family (6). Children age 4, 11, 18 and 23. Gas Co. threatening shut-off. Difficult to make ends meet. Depressed and unable to cope with diet or financial problems. Resisting limited activity. Homemaker presently in home and assisting with shopping and meal preparation.

Nutritional Care Plan
    Diet replan. Encourage increase in total fruits and vegetables. Guidance re: food buying to keep within amount of money available for food. Discuss food preparation. Refer to VNA social worker re: possible eligibility for food stamp participation and T-19.

Nutritional Continuing Patient Care Form

Date 1-20-77

To: Nutrition Department
      Visiting Nurse Association of Metropolitan Detroit
      4421 Woodward Avenue — Detroit 48201

From: South   Hospital

Patient: Ann Wood   Sex F   Age 70

Patient's Address: Phone

Physician: George White   Phone

Diagnosis: Diabetes, Hepatitis, ascites

Modified Diet Prescription: 1500 cal, 40 gm. Protein, 2 gm.

  Na

Meal Plan For Day

Breakfast		*Lunch*		*Dinner*	
Fruit	1	Meat	1	Meat	1
Meat	—	Veg.	2gm. Pro	Veg.	2gm. Pro
Bread	2	Bread	3	Bread	3
Fat	3	Fat	3	Fat	3
Milk	1/4	Fruit	1	Fruit	--
		Milk	1/4	Milk	—

                              N.S. 1 Low Pro Bread
                                    2 fats
                                    1 Fruit
                    Other Feedings (specify)

Patient Counseled   Yes (X)   No ( )

Family Member Counseled   Yes (X)   No ( ) Sister

Group Instruction Program   Yes (X)   No ( ) Diabetic Classes

Problems Identified

Confused re: purpose of diet in relation to diagnoses
Sister — responsible for food preparation asks many questions — but
   doesn't listen to answers

Recommended Nutritional Care Plan
Careful review of diet with patient and sister
Recommend accurate measurement of food — weighing of meat
Encourage self-reliance in relation to meal planning & food preparation.
(Sister often calls dietitian right at meal time.)

Signature   Joan Brown, R.D.

Therapeutic Dietitian

Phone:

Ext:

Nutritional Continuing Patient Care Form

Date   12-18-76

To: Nutrition Department
    Visiting Nurse Association of Metropolitan Detroit
    4421 Woodward Avenue — Detroit 48201

From: North   Hospital

Patient: Mildred Clark   Sex   F   Age 42

Patient's Address: Phone

Ht. — 5'
Wt. — 192 2/3 lbs.

Physician: Thomas   Phone

Diagnosis: MI, Obesity, Hyper-triglyceridemia

Modified Diet Prescription 800 calories

Meal Plan For Day

Breakfast	*Lunch*	*Dinner*
Fruit 1	Meat 2 (Lean)	Meat 3 (Lean)
Meat	Veg. 1	Veg. 2
Bread 1	Bread 1/2	Bread 1/2
Fat 1	Fat 1	Fat 1
Milk 1/2	Fruit 1	Fruit 1
	Milk	Milk

Note: Patient dislikes milk

Other Feedings (specify)

Patient Counseled   Yes (x)   No ( )

Family Member Counseled   Yes ( )   No (X)

Group Instruction Program   Yes ( )   No (X)

Problems Identified
Very difficult to communicate with patient — hates the word "diet" and doesn't want to talk about it.

Recommended Nutritional Care Plan
Anything you can do to encourage adherence to diet.

Signature   Mary Coy

Therapeutic Dietician

Phone:

Ext:

Nutritional status, U.S.A.

Section Objective

This section is designed to describe the dietary and nutritional status of the American population and takes a look at population subgroups particularly vulnerable to dietary deprivation, undernutrition, or malnutrition.

Section Overview

In recognition of the relationship between nutrition and health, and of the importance of optimal nutrition for health promotion, health professionals must concern themselves with the question, What is the nutritional status of the American population? What are Americans eating? How have typical eating patterns changed during the twentieth century? The nutritional status of groups that are particularly vulnerable to malnutrition must also be studied. Of specific interest are those groups that are vulnerable to nutritional problems because of their stage in the life span, such as pregnant women, infants and children, and the elderly. Others are at high risk of developing nutritional disorders because their socioeconomic status restricts their access to adequate food supplies. The poor, with reference to Indians, ethnic subgroups, and migrant workers, will be considered in this context.

4

Dietary and nutritional status of the general United States population

Reader Objectives

After completing this chapter, the reader should be able to
1. Outline general changes in the North American diet since the early 1900s.
2. Describe general findings of the 1965 USDA National Food Consumption Survey.
3. Review types of data collected and results of the Ten-State and HANES surveys.
4. State current national nutrition surveillance activities.

If you want to know where you are going, you must first know where you are.

Abraham Lincoln

FOOD CONSUMPTION IN THE UNITED STATES — OVERVIEW

Since the turn of the century, there have been dramatic changes in food consumption by the North American public. The composition of the average American diet has changed from one in which the mainstay of the diet included fruit, vegetables, and grain products, to one in which these products now often play a much smaller role.[1] Simultaneously, the intake of fat and refined sugar has greatly increased to the point that these two food components now account for approximately 60 per cent of the average American daily energy intake; the comparable figure for the early 1900s was 50 per cent.[2] These changes have stimulated increasing concern among many that the current American diet is excessive in calories, fat, cholesterol, refined sugar, and salt and is deficient in dietary fiber. This chapter focuses on the dietary and the nutritional status of the American population.

WHAT ARE AMERICANS EATING?

The U.S. Department of Agriculture provides annual estimates of food consumption in the United States by examining the types of foods that compose the national food supply and then by calculating the amounts of nutrients available from these foods. To accomplish this, estimates of food consumption are obtained by food balance sheets. Estimates are made by taking annual total national food production, plus imports, minus exports (i.e., the total food supply available), divided by the population, giving food available per person for consumption. A type of disappearance data is derived, indicating the amounts of food that "disappear" into food consumption channels. This food then becomes food consumed or "used up" in the economic sense. The interpretation of such data has certain limitations. Obvious limitations include the fact that such broad data do not indicate individual food consumption or shed light upon how individual consumption varies over time. Furthermore, no account is taken of food wasted and never consumed. However, the data indicate broad trends in consumption that are helpful in providing a base from which to consider the relationship between food and health.

The average per capita food consumption of calories and protein has not changed significantly since the turn of the century, but the types of food consumed have undergone great changes. Although animal products represent a greater proportion of the average diet today than in the early 1900s, there have been few changes in these proportions since the 1960s. A comparison of weight of products consumed now, versus that consumed in earlier years, indicates a slight reduction. Much of this reduction, however, may be attributed to the fact that more foods are now in processed rather than in fresh form so that, bulk weight is reduced.

Food consumption varies greatly according to variability in food supply, as well as in consumer food preferences. For example, severe drought as well as reduced income accounted for a reduced consumption of red meat during the Depression. Poultry consumption has significantly increased with improvements in production processes, which resulted in increased supplies at lower costs. Egg and dairy product consumption peaked around 1950 and then dropped off so that it is currently little different from that in the early 1900s. Tables 4-1 and 4-2 and Figures 4-1 and 4-2 illustrate these trends in food consumption.[2]

Table 4-1

Food Energy and Energy-Yielding Nutrients Available Per Capita Per Day

	1909-1913	1965	1970	1975	1978*
Food energy (calories)	3,480	3,140	3,300	3,210	3,290
Protein (gm)	102	96	100	99	102
Fat (gm)	125	144	156	152	157
Carbohydrate (gm)	492	372	379	370	376

*Preliminary

Figure 4-1. Per capita consumption of food energy, protein, fat, and carbohydrate in the United States, as percentage of 1909-1913 average. (USDA)

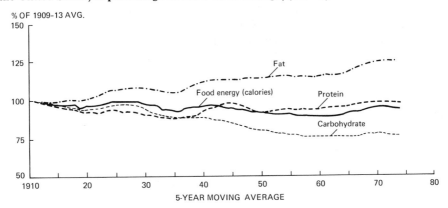

Table 4-2

Trends in U.S. Food Consumption

	1910	*1930*	*1945*	*1960*	*1975*
Animal products (pounds)	576	585	691	633	613
Crop products (pounds) ·	1,013	955	960	795	796
Total all foods (pounds)	1,589	1,540	1,651	1,428	1,409
Meat	139	123	141	147	158
Poultry, fish	31	30	37	48	65
Eggs	37	40	48	42	35
Dairy (including butter)	337	360	440	376	344
Fats/oils	42	49	42	49	57
Fruits, melons	170	180	206	170	161
All vegetables	203	227	268	211	216
Potatoes, sweet potatoes	221	145	136	98	84
Flour, cereal	295	228	201	147	139
Sugar, sweeteners	88	126	93	109	121

Sources: U.S. Department of Agriculture, ERS. *Agricultural Economic Report 138.* Washington, D.C.: Government Printing Office, July 1968; U.S. Department of Agriculture. *Agricultural Statistics.* Washington, D.C.: Government Printing Office, 1977.

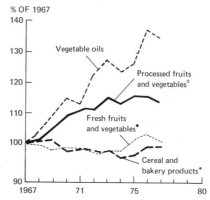

Figure 4-2. Per capita consumption of selected crop products in the United States, as a percentage of 1967 amounts. °includes potatoes and sweet potatoes. ·excludes melons. *grain components only. (USDA)

As the tables and figures illustrate, important changes in national intake have occurred. Protein availability remained stable, but the ratio of animal-to-vegetable protein has almost doubled. The availability of carbohydrates has decreased by 21 per cent, and the level of dietary fiber has decreased by 30 per cent since 1909 and by 47 per cent since 1880. The percentage of calories from fat increased by 31 per cent since 1910.[2]

FAT CONSUMPTION

Between 1900 and 1973, the fat available per person on a daily basis increased from 125 to 156 gm, an increase equal to about 2.5 tbs of butter or margarine; this amounts to approximately 24 lb of nutrient fat per year.[3]

In 1976 saturated fat provided about 16 per cent of "total" dietary calories; polyunsaturated fat provided about 7 per cent and monounsaturated fat provided about 19 per cent of total dietary calories. This is compared with the 10 per cent of total calories recommended for saturated fat content by the Inter-Society Commission for Heart Disease Resources, a group responsible for coordinating the guidelines for care for heart disease patients. The commission suggests that 10 per cent of total calories should come from polyunsaturated and 10 per cent from monounsaturated fats.[4]

The polyunsaturated/saturated ratio (P/S) rose from 0.21 in 1909 to 0.43 in 1974. The availability of cholesterol has not changed drastically, but it has increased from 509 mg per person in 1909 to 556 mg per person in 1970.[5]

Various foods have accounted for the increased fat consumption throughout the twentieth century; however, salad and cooking oils were the principal sources of fat for most of this period. Dairy products and shortening were important during the first 15 years, and margarine, shortening, and meat were next in importance during the later 40 years.[3] Today vegetable oils account for approximately 80 per cent of the total fat intake in American diets.

CARBOHYDRATE CONSUMPTION

Complex carbohydrate foods are no longer the predominant food in the American diet. Until recent years, the primary source of calories was carbohydrate energy that was derived principally from starch. In the 1909–1913 period, for example, starches were the source of 68 per cent of dietary carbohydrates, whereas sugars were the source of only 32 per cent. However, since World War II there has been a decrease in the consumption of complex carbohydrates and an increase in the consumption of simple sugar carbohydrate foods. In 1976, 53 per cent of dietary carbohydrates came from sugars and 47 per cent came from starches. Since 1910 complex carbohydrate consumption has dropped from 37 per cent of total calories to 21 per cent.[6]

The proportion of total carbohydrates in the typical North American diet provided by sugars (carbohydrates in milk, fruit, and sweeteners) has increased since the beginning of the twentieth century, even though per capita sugar consumption has only recently surpassed the levels of the 1920s.[7]

As Figure 4–3 illustrates, sugar consumption accounted for approximately 32 per cent of the total carbohydrates consumed during the years from 1909 to 1913. By 1976, however, sugars had replaced many complex carbohydrate foods and represented the primary carbohydrate sources.

In this same period, there has been an increase in per capita refined sugar and other sweetener consumption from approximately 87 lb to 120 lb annually, or from 12 per cent to 18 per cent of total calories.[6] This is thought to be even higher in specific age and sex groups in the United

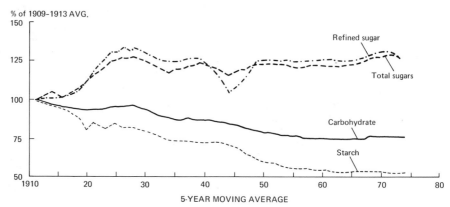

Figure 4-3. Per capita consumption of sugar, carbohydrate, and starch in the United States, as percentage of 1901-1913 average. (USDA)

States.[7] Experts estimate that sugar consumption by those aged 6 to 20 probably ranges from 140 to 150 lb annually.[8]

Table 4-3 and Figure 4-4 illustrate the type of refined sugar used per person per day in the United States. In the time period from 1909 to 1913, refined sugar accounted for approximately 32 per cent of total carbohydrate calories, but by 1976 sugar was the primary source of carbo-

Table 4-3.

Refined Sugar, Estimated Per Capita Consumption by Type of Use, Selected Periods, 1909-13 to 1971[1]

(in pounds)

Type of use	1909-13	1925-29	1935-39	1947-49	1957-59	1965	1971 (preliminary)
In processed foods:							
Cereal and bakery products	4.5	7.7	9.7	12.9	15.4	15.6	17.6
Confectionery products	6.5	8.0	8.2	9.8	9.6	10.4	11.0
Processed fruits and vegetables[2]	3.0	4.6	4.4	9.0	9.8	9.5	10.4
Dairy products	1.5	2.3	2.4	4.6	4.9	5.3	5.8
Other food products[3]	.3	.7	1.2	1.5	1.7	2.5	2.6
Total food products	15.8	23.4	25.9	37.8	41.4	43.4	47.4
Beverages (largely in soft drinks)	3.5	5.0	5.2	10.6	12.6	16.9	22.8
Total processed food and beverages	19.3	28.4	31.1	48.4	54.0	60.2	70.2
Other food uses:							
Eating and drinking places[4]	4.5	5.7	6.3	7.7	7.3	6.2	5.5
Household use[5]	52.1	65.0	58.8	37.4	33.1	28.2	24.7
Institutional and other use[6]	.5	.9	.9	1.3	1.0	1.4	1.1
Total	57.1	71.6	66.0	46.4	41.4	35.8	31.3
Total food use	76.4	100.0	97.1	94.8	95.4	96.0	101.5
Nonfood use[7]	.3	.4	.4	.4	.7	.6	.9
Total consumption	76.7	100.4	97.5	95.2	96.1	96.6	102.4

[1] Prepared by Food Consumption Section, Economic Research Service, U.S. Department of Agriculture.
[2] Canned, bottled, and frozen foods (processed fruit and vegetable products); jams, jellies, and preserves.
[3] Includes miscellaneous food uses such as meat curing, and syrup blending.
[4] Includes hotels, motels, restaurants, cafeterias, and other eating and drinking establishments.
[5] Household use assumed synonymous with deliveries in consumer-sized packages (less than 50 lb).
[6] Largely for military use.
[7] Includes use in pharmaceuticals, tobacco, and other nonfood use.
Source: "Sugars in Nutrition," Levels of Uses of Sugar in the United States, L. Page, B. Friend, 1974.

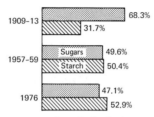

Figure 4-4. Sugar and starch as sources of carbohydrate, per capita per day in the U.S. (USDA)

hydrate calories. One of the major concerns is the fact that much of the sugar consumed is the result of sugar that has been added. L. Page and B. Friend note that the use of sugar in highly processed foods and drink has almost tripled, rising from 20 lb to 70 lb yearly, although the direct purchase by households of refined sugar has decreased from 50 lb to 25 lb yearly. Most of the refined sugar consumption can be attributed to processed food and beverage consumption. Beverages, now the largest single food industry user of sugar, account for about 23 lb of sugar consumption yearly, an amount representing a sevenfold increase since the early 1900s.[7]

OTHER CHANGES IN DIETARY PATTERNS[6]

Other general changes have occurred in the American diet since the turn of the century. Some of the most significant of these changes include:

1. Increased consumption of marketed fruits and vegetables; the largest increase is in canned or frozen, not fresh produce.

2. Reduced egg consumption; current egg consumption is one third less than that at the peak of egg consumption in 1945.

3. Disappearance of regional food patterns.

4. Less seasonal variation in food consumption.

5. More snacking than in previous years, along with an increased consumption of snack foods such as potato chips, pretzels, sweets, candy, and soft drinks.

6. Increased consumption of alcohol; Americans consumed an average of 2.69 gallons of alcohol per person in 1975.

CHEMICALLY DEFINED, HIGHLY PROCESSED FOODS

One of the most significant changes to occur in the eating patterns in the United States during the twentieth century involves the great reliance on chemically defined fabricated foods and additives. Whether such foods were developed for nutrition-related health reasons, that is, foods such as egg substitutes, high polyunsaturated nondairy creamers and margarine, meat replacers, and the like, or for taste preferences, such as soft drinks and snack foods, they all replace natural food components of the diet. Although there may be some benefit to these trends, the important and as yet unanswered question is, What is the impact of these chemically processed foods on the health status of the North American population?

Consumption of processed foods has greatly increased during recent decades. These changes can be illustrated by considering the number of processed food products that are available on the retail market. In 1940 there were about 1,000 different products available in North America; the figure for 1965 was somewhere around 6,000; the figure for 1975 reached 12,000.[9]

Advances in food processing and product development have resulted not only in an increased consumption of processed foods but also in the reduced consumption of unprocessed farm produce. For example, in 1929, Americans consumed less than 100 lb of processed produce and more than 400 lb of fruits and vegetables yearly per capita. By 1971 the consumption of processed foods had risen to 300 lb, whereas consumption of fruits and vegetables fell to about 250 lb per person.[10] Nutrition experts are concerned that in future times we may be unable to hold to the axiom that a varied diet can provide all essential nutrients needed for good health. As the notion of what constitutes a varied diet changes and becomes more difficult for a large number of people to obtain, the concept of a diversified diet and its health relationship is curtailed. As W. Mertz phrased it:

> Regardless of how one evaluates the present nutritional status of people in highly developed societies, it can be stated with certainty that a continuation of the present trend toward consumption of more partitioned, refined, and fabricated food must eventually lead to a point where the rest of the diet cannot meet the requirements for all essential nutrients any more.[11]

There is currently much concern over the lack of dietary fiber in many American diets. Crude fiber intake in the United States averages two-five gm, as compared with the mean level of eighteen gm in the diets of more primitive populations.[12]

HEALTH FOODS AND FAST FOODS

Two other trends in North American eating habits deserve mention, the health foods industry and the fast-food industry. There is no consensus on a definition of health foods. The term may refer to fresh produce or to food supplements such as vitamins and minerals. So-called "health foods" may be a part of religious tradition, such as the special foods used by Seventh-Day Adventists and Buddhists, part of ethnic tradition, trappings of the counterculture, or part of a special modified diet. Health foods may also result from organic production. In 1976 according to the National Nutritional Food Association, there were 750 health food manufacturers in the United States as compared with only 575 in 1972. It has been estimated that the sales of health foods may reach $3 billion by 1980, or a projected 1 per cent of the total national grocery bill. It is clear that the movement to "natural" is making its mark on the mass food market.[13]

Fast-food enterprises continue to consume increasing percentages of the North American food budget. Fast-food restaurants receive approximately $.40 from every dollar spent on food eaten away from home, and they reaped an estimated $20 billion in 1977, the same year McDonald's sold its 23 billionth hamburger.[14]

Some fast-food facts and figures are presented in Table 4-4. These trends in American eating patterns have been identified through very gross estimates. A more refined study of the dietary and nutritional status of Americans has resulted from national surveys.

Table 4-4
Fast Food Facts and Figures

The advent of fast food restaurants has had a great impact on the American diet. McDonald's (the largest fast food chain) sales increased more than twentyfold from $129,600,000 in 1964 to $2,730,000,000 in 1976. The effect of this growth on our diets is reflected in the following statistics:

Ice milk consumption grew *from* 1.2 pounds per person in 1950, *to* 4.5 pounds per person in 1960, *to* 7.4 pounds per person in 1976.
Ice milk, in soft form, is used in cones and shakes at fast food shops.

Frozen potato use climbed *from* 6.6 pounds per person in 1960, *to* 36.8 pounds per person in 1976.
Our use of frozen potatoes is keeping the total potato figure from plummeting. Seven-eighths of all frozen potatoes were sold as French fries in 1976 — three-quarters of them to restaurants and institutional kitchens.

Fresh and frozen fish consumption was up *from* 3.8 pounds per person in 1960, *to* 5.5 pounds per person in 1976.

Chicken consumption rose *from* 27.8 pounds per person in 1960, *to* 43.3 pounds per person in 1976.
Kentucky Fried Chicken outlets serve 2.3 billion pieces of chicken per year — enough to serve 10 pieces to each and every American!

Beef consumption went *from* 64.3 pounds per person in 1960, *to* 95.4 pounds per person in 1976.
McDonald's alone sells a billion hamburgers every 5 months. That equals 6.6 million per day or 11 hamburgers per person per year.

Hard cheese consumption rose *from* 8.3 pounds per person in 1960, *to* 15.9 pounds per person in 1976.
The 92 per cent increase in hard cheese consumption was spurred by our increasing use of mozzarella — "the pizza cheese."

And we are not eating our hamburgers and French fries plain — chili sauce, and tomato catsup, paste, and sauce consumption jumped *from* 7.6 pounds per person in 1960, *to* 13.3 pounds per person in 1976. Meanwhile, pickle consumption grew *from* 4.5 pounds per person in 1960, *to* 8.4 pounds per person in 1976.

And don't forget the drinks we wash our food down with — soft drink consumption rose *from* 192 8-ounce servings per year in 1960, *to* 493 8-ounce servings per person in 1976.

Source: L. Brewster and M. F. Jacobson. *The Changing American Diet.* Washington, D.C.: Center for Science in The Public Interest, 1978.

USDA FOOD CONSUMPTION SURVEYS[15]

The U.S. Department of Agriculture is responsible for studying national food consumption. Surveys by the USDA were conducted in 1935–36, 1942, 1948, 1955, and 1965–66. Data from these surveys provide the basis for developing national food and nutrition policy and for designing other food and nutrition programs. In the spring of 1965, the USDA surveyed the food intake and assessed the nutritive value of diets of men, women, and children in the United States. Information was obtained on the food intake of a 24-hour period for individuals in those households surveyed. This represented the first time that estimates of a one-day's food consumption of a national sample of individuals were studied. Key objectives of the study included:

1. To obtain information on the types and amounts of foods eaten at home, as well as away from home on the days studied; to determine the nutritive contribution of these foods to the daily diet.

2. To determine comparisons of food intake for one sex-age group with others.

3. To determine the frequency and time periods of individuals' food consumption or beverage consumption.

4. To determine the extent and use of vitamin and mineral supplements.

5. To determine the nutritive value of dietary intake of individuals at different phases of the life cycle.

The study obtained food intake reports from 14,519 individuals. Significant results of the 1965 food survey are summarized in Table 4–5. The 1965 survey found that 50 per cent of the households surveyed either met or exceeded the USDA definition of a good diet. In contrast to this, the previous survey (1955) found that 60 per cent of the diets studied were rated as good — thus there was a 10 per cent drop in the diets rated as "good" from the 1955 to the 1965 survey. Diets were rated good if the household food supply met the 1963 Recommended Dietary Allowances (RDA) of the Food and Nutrition Board, National Research Council for

Table 4–5

Significant Results of the 1965 USDA Food Survey

---

1. Quantities of food consumed by males (men and boys) both at home and away from home were greater than those eaten by females of the same age groups, with the following exceptions: tomatoes, citrus fruits, dark-green and deep-yellow vegetables, and other vegetables (not potatoes) and fruit.
2. Consumption of most foods was greatest for males during the late teen and early adult years. Age group differences in intake were less for women than for men.
3. Approximately 40 per cent of surveyed individuals reported eating some food away from home; most food away from home was reported by males aged 12 to 34 and females 12 to 19. For individuals aged 18–19, foods eaten away from home accounted for about 20 per cent of the total daily food intake.
4. For the following nutrients, most age-sex groups consumed 90–100 per cent of the RDAs set in 1968: calories, protein, vitamin A value, thiamine, riboflavin,

Significant Results of the 1965 USDA Food Survey (*continued*)

and ascorbic acid; the nutrients most frequently limited in diets were calcium and iron.

5. For adult males (aged 20 to 64) approximately 45 per cent of calories were derived from high fat foods; for infants the figure was 39 per cent. Mean protein contribution was 15-17 per cent of total calories; all groups averaged protein intakes above the 1968 RDAs—range of protein calories was from 107 per cent to 259 per cent of the RDAs.

6. For many groups, especially females, the intake of calcium and iron was more than 30 per cent below the RDAs; for infants and children under the age of 3 years, iron intake was 50 per cent below recommended levels. For infants less than 2 months of age the ascorbic acid intake was less than that recommended.*

7. Diets of males more frequently met RDA allowances than did diets of females. Diets for children under the age of 9 years were satisfactory except for iron; adolescent and adult females were below the RDAs for calcium, iron, and thiamine. Some age groups were also deficient in vitamin A value and riboflavin; older age groups were also low in dietary calcium, vitamin A value, riboflavin, and ascorbic acid.*

8. For low-income individuals and those living in rural areas and in the South, nutrients often found to be less than the RDAs included ascorbic acid, vitamin A value, calcium, and iron.*

9. Pregnant women averaged dietary intakes of 90-100 per cent of the RDAs for protein and ascorbic acid; they consumed 29-47 per cent less than the RDA for calcium, 19-36 per cent less than the RDA for iron, 22-36 per cent less than the RDA for iron, and 22-35 per cent less than the RDA for vitamin A value. Only the pregnant women aged 20 to 34 consumed below the recommended levels of thiamine and riboflavin.*

10. Estimated intakes of vitamin B_6 and magnesium were considerably less than the recommended levels for many groups, especially for females over age 9 and males over age 55; all males had diets limited in magnesium. Except for women 65 years and older, diets met the RDAs for vitamin B_{12}.*

11. Vitamin and mineral supplements were used by 12 per cent of those females aged 15 to 17 and by males aged 15 to 34. The supplements were consumed by 34 per cent of individuals aged 75 and older; 55 per cent of infants and 43 per cent of children aged 1 to 2 consumed vitamin and/or mineral supplements.

12. Approximately 32 per cent of the sample reported that they ate or drank three to four times daily and 15 per cent of those aged 20 to 34 ate or drank six or more times daily. More than 90 per cent of the individuals in most age groups consumed some food or drink between 5 A.M. and 10 A.M.

U.S. Department of Agriculture. *Food and Nutrient Intake of Individuals in the United States. Household Food Consumption Survey, 1963-66*, Rept. No. 11. Washington, D.C.: Government Printing Office, January 1972.

*Data such as these are frequently misinterpreted to indicate substantial malnutrition in the United States. It is important to remember that intakes of nutrients below the RDAs do not necessarily indicate malnutrition. The RDAs are based on the concept that an individual consuming a diet that provides the recommended amounts of all nutrients would be unlikely to suffer nutritional inadequacy. Thus, the RDAs are estimates of acceptable daily nutrient intakes in the sense that, although the needs of the majority of people will be less than the standards, there may be some who require more. Thus, even if a person has a diet that frequently contains less than the recommended amounts of certain nutrients, that person's diet is not necessarily inadequate for those nutrients.

seven nutrients (protein, calcium, iron, vitamin A value, thiamine, ribo-flavin, and vitamin C).

Further, the percentage of families with "poor" diets was also greater in 1965 — 21 per cent compared with only 15 per cent in 1955. Diets were rated as poor if they contained less than two thirds of the RDA for one or more of the seven nutrients. It is important to note that the results of the study did not mean that the one fifth of the population with "poor" diets were hungry or suffering from malnutrition. Inadequate diets over time often lead to poor nutrition, but there is no way to relate the findings of the USDA study directly to the health of the population studied. Physical examinations and biochemical tests would have been needed to do this.

In both the 1955 and 1965 studies, the nutrients that were most often below the RDAs for households were calcium, vitamin A, and vitamin C. More households were limited in these nutrients in 1965 than in 1955. One possible reason may be the reduced use of dairy products (good sources of calcium) and of fresh fruits and vegetables (sources of vitamins A and C). Results of the study suggested that the reduced milk consumption was related to the increased use of sweetened soft drinks and beverages.

The 1965 study found little evidence of a lack of protein in the average North American diet; only one in every 100 households studied consumed less than two thirds of the Recommended Dietary Allowance for protein. This does not, however, mean that individual groups did not consume diets that were deficient in protein, because average values often tend to conceal the great differences in the amounts and types of food used by individuals in each household and also by different households.

The sixth USDA nationwide food consumption survey began in April 1977. The survey is scheduled to take three years for data collection and analysis will cost an estimated $3 million. The survey sample included 15,000 households. The survey design called for a study of household and individual food consumption; in addition, two supplemental data collections were planned to study food consumption data collected in Alaska, Hawaii, and Puerto Rico and 5,000 households in which elderly individuals resided.[16]

Data on the food consumption patterns of Americans have been available for some time. However, it has only been since the late 1950s that regional or national population samples have been assessed with biochemical, anthropometric, and dietary methods to evaluate nutritional status. In the late 1950s, the Interagency Committee on Nutrition and National Defense (ICNND) studied the nutritional status of populations in about 37 foreign countries. By the mid-1960s, when this study had been completed, we had learned much about nutritional status and problems in developing areas, but little of the nutritional status of the U.S. population.

TEN-STATE NUTRITION SURVEY

Although the previous USDA surveys studied dietary patterns, they did not analyze parameters that would allow a determination of nutritional status. The Partnership for Health Amendment of 1967 instructed the secretary of Health, Education, and Welfare to conduct a comprehensive survey to identify and determine the prevalence of malnutrition among low-income populations in the United States. The bill was signed December 5, 1967. In February 1968 the Nutrition Program of the Health Services and Mental Health Administration (originally called the Interdepartmental Committee on Nutrition for National Defense) was directed to organize and conduct the National Nutrition Survey.

Although the survey was not actually a national survey, ten states were selected to provide broad geographical representation of various areas of the country and to reflect the various economic, ethnic, and sociocultural populations. The survey attempted to assess the nutritional status of high-risk, nutritionally vulnerable groups, such as migrant farm workers, to sample geographical areas where maternal and infant mortality rates were especially high and other areas where participation in federal assistance programs was reputed to be poor. The ten states selected were Texas, South Carolina, Louisiana, West Virginia, Kentucky, New York, Massachusetts, Michigan, Washington, and California.

The sampling procedures and methodology are explained in detail in an HEW publication.[17] The final sample included 24,000 families containing 86,000 individuals. Five general types of data were obtained:

General socioeconomic, demographic, and health data.

Clinical and dental examinations.

Anthropometric measurements.

Biochemical analysis of blood and urine: this type of data was collected to identify the nutritional status of those presumed to be at high nutrition risk; 40,847 individuals, of whom 7,800 were preschool children, were included.

Dietary status information collected through the use of a 24-hour recall.

Not all this data were obtained on all individuals. Specifically, some data, such as dietary information and general socioeconomic, demographic, and health data were collected on households. Other data, such as the biochemical information, were collected on individuals particularly at "high risk," such as pregnant and lactating women, preschool children, and the elderly. Although the information obtained was biased as a result of the sample methods and cannot be generalized to the entire U.S. population, the data were thought to be representative of the population groups sampled and thus enable the prediction of expected problems in groups with similar characteristics. Figure 4–5 summarizes important nutritional problems revealed by the survey.

Biochemical and Dietary Data[17]

Standards for evaluating the biochemical and dietary data were based on ICNND (1963) guidelines that were modified for the Ten-State Survey.[18] The incidence of individuals classified as anemic on the basis of hemoglobin levels varied from state to state; in Louisiana and South Carolina approximately 40 per cent of the individuals studied were found to have

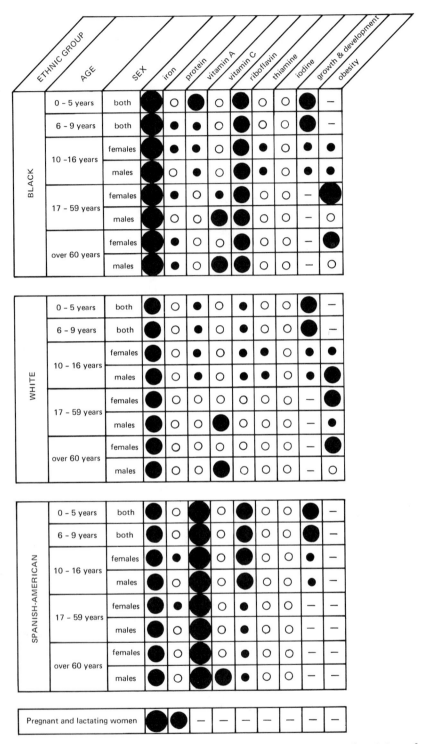

Figure 4-5. Relative importance of nutritional problems in low income ratio states of Kentucky, Louisiana, South Carolina, Texas, and West Virginia (above); and high income ratio states of California, Massachusetts, Michigan, New York, and Washington, (facing page). (HEW)

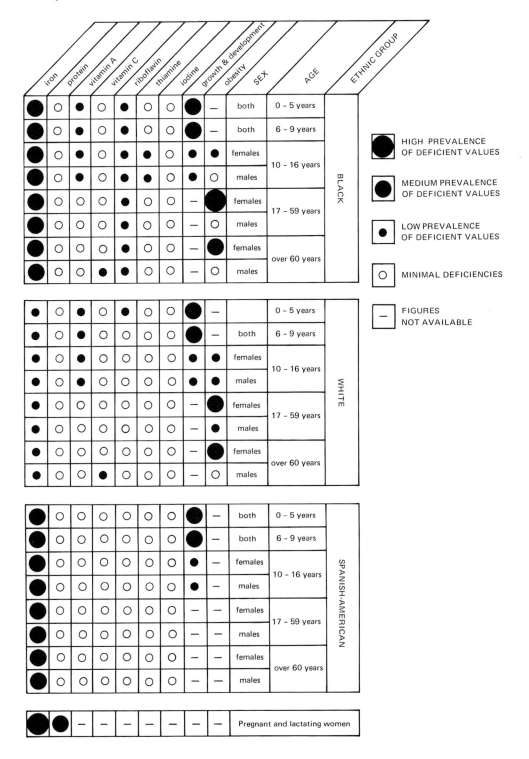

"unacceptable" hemoglobin values, whereas the figure for Washington, California, Massachusetts, and New York was 10 per cent.

Iron

Because anemia can result from various deficiency and illness states, special studies were conducted on samples identified as "unacceptable" to determine levels of serum iron, iron-binding capacity, transferrin saturation index, serum folic acid, and red blood cell folates. These studies found that the major cause of anemia was iron deficiency but was often complicated by low folate levels.

Surprisingly, the study indicated iron and folate deficiency problems in males as well as females. Because males do not suffer the normal blood loss that females do, it had been traditionally assumed that males required less iron. Standards for male hemoglobin levels defined "low" to be less than 14 gm, whereas for females the comparable figure was 12 gm. Thus, with the finding that both males and females had high incidence of iron and folic acid deficiency, the question of appropriate standards was raised.

The incidence of anemia was correlated with low income and with race; black population groups, regardless of their residence, evidenced significantly higher incidence of anemia than did white populations. Different standards of hemoglobin levels should be used for blacks and whites, as blacks tend to have lower hemoglobin levels normally.

Dietary data confirmed the problem of iron status. In populations of all income levels, a high percentage of infants, teenagers, and pregnant women consumed diets containing less than two thirds of the RDA standards for iron.

Vitamin A

Another nutrient of particular concern, as evidenced by the Ten-State data, was vitamin A; a high incidence of "unacceptable serum vitamin A levels" was noted, particularly among children aged 0–16. Although no severe physical lesions associated with vitamin A deficiency were noted, lesions such as follicular hyperkeratosis and Bitot's spots were found. Again, dietary data confirmed the low intake of vitamin A in the diets of many of the individuals studied.

Vitamin C

Ascorbic acid status of individuals varied from state to state; in five states (Texas, Louisiana, Kentucky, West Virginia, and Massachusetts), 6–14 per cent of the sample were found to have "unacceptable serum vitamin C values," whereas in the other states the prevalence was 3 per cent or less. Dietary intakes of ascorbic acid paralleled the biochemical findings.

Riboflavin

Based on urinary riboflavin values, 10 per cent or more of the sampled populations of seven states had "unacceptable values"; dietary data indicated that between 10 per cent and 30 per cent of the sample consumed less than two thirds of the recommended level of riboflavin.

Serum Albumin

In general, dietary data suggested that protein intakes were more often acceptable than were intakes of most other nutrients, but unacceptable intakes were found. Unacceptable serum albumin levels were highest in Texas and Louisiana. The elderly were particularly vulnerable and evidenced highest rates for low serum albumin values.

Clinical Findings[17]

Overt physical evidences of malnutrition were rare, but some cases were found. Marasmus, kwashiorkor, rickets, follicular hyperkeratosis, Bitot's spots (symptoms of vitamin A deficiency), cheilosis, and tongue lesions (symptoms of B-complex deficiency) were noted.* (See Figure 4-6).

Anthropometric Findings (Data Compiled on 62,532 Individuals)

Height and weight data were evaluated by comparison to the Stuart-Meredith growth standards. Growth retardation as evidenced by height retardation was found among all ethnic and income groups. However, income was related to height retardation; often children from higher-income families were found to be advanced by as much as a year over the children from low-income families. For children aged 2, 4, and 6, between 22 per cent and 35 per cent were below the 15th percentile for weight, depending upon sex and ethnicity. The highest prevalence of weight retardation was found in Spanish-American children.

Obesity was common. For adolescents, the mean percentage of obesity (based on the Seltzer-Mayer minimum triceps fat-fold thickness) was 18.3 per cent for white males and 10.0 per cent for white females. The highest prevalence of obesity was found among black women; more than 50 per cent of black females aged 45 to 55 were obese whereas the figure for white women of the same age group was 40 per cent.

HEALTH AND NUTRITION EXAMINATION SURVEY (HANES)

The HANES program was undertaken by the National Center for Health Statistics to establish a continuing national nutrition surveillance system, the purpose being to measure nutritional status of the U.S. population and to monitor changes in status over time. HANES should permit the use of health data as an objective test of programs to improve nutritional status, and it should provide an improved basis for the allocation of scarce program resources.

HANES is the first program to collect measures of nutritional status for a scientifically designed sample representative of the U.S. civilian, noninstitutionalized population in broad age ranges. The probability sample design permits estimates to be made for the total population while at the same time permitting a more detailed analysis of data for certain groups at high risk.

*See Glossary, pages 679-692, for the definition of these terms.

The first data collection for HANES was begun in 1971. Four types of data were collected in the study:[19-21]

1. Dietary information on individual food intake (type, amount, and nutritional quality) obtained by use of a 24-hour recall method (data were analyzed for calories, protein, calcium, iron, vitamin A, ascorbic acid, thiamine, riboflavin, and niacin).

2. Biochemical tests made on blood and urine samples to determine hematocrit, hemoglobin, red and white cell count, serum vitamin A and ascorbic acid, iron, total iron-binding capacity, folate, protein, albumin, magnesium, and cholesterol.

3. Clinical examinations by physicians and dentists to identify physical signs of malnutrition or nutrition-related problems.

4. Anthropometric measurements to determine abnormal body growth and obesity.

Dietary Data

Dietary intake was obtained for 10,126 individuals. The sample was divided according to age groups (1-5, 6-11, 12-17, 18-44, 45-59, and 60 and older), race, and income levels. The data were analyzed and food intakes were compared with recommended daily allowances from the World Health Organization, the Interdepartmental Committee on Nutrition for National Defense Manual, the Recommended Dietary Allowances, and standards used in the Ten-State Nutrition Survey. Results indicated that some nutrients, in particular riboflavin and thiamine, demonstrated adequate or above adequate mean intake for all subgroups sampled in terms of levels of poverty, race, sex, and age.[19,20]

Other nutrients, such as protein, calcium, and vitamins A and C, showed that some (but not most) of the population subgroups had lower mean intakes than the recommended dietary allowance. Mean calcium dietary intakes were lower than the recommended dietary allowance for white adolescents and for young adult females in low-income groups and for adolescent black females in all income groups.

Mean protein intakes were also less than those recommended for many adolescents, adult females, and older males in the low-income groups, for adult black females and older black men, as well as for older white females in the upper-income levels.

Calories were less than the recommended amounts for most of the groups that were surveyed. For all groups except the young children, calorie intakes were below the recommended allowances. Iron intakes were also frequently below the recommended dietary allowance for adult females and for children aged 1-5, adolescent males and adults over 60.

HANES also pointed up a number of current trends in food consumption in the United States. Some of the most interesting include the following:[22]

Meat Consumption — About 83 per cent of the population ate meat at least once a day; another 15 per cent ate meat one to six times a week. Less than 1 per cent of those surveyed said they rarely or never ate meat.

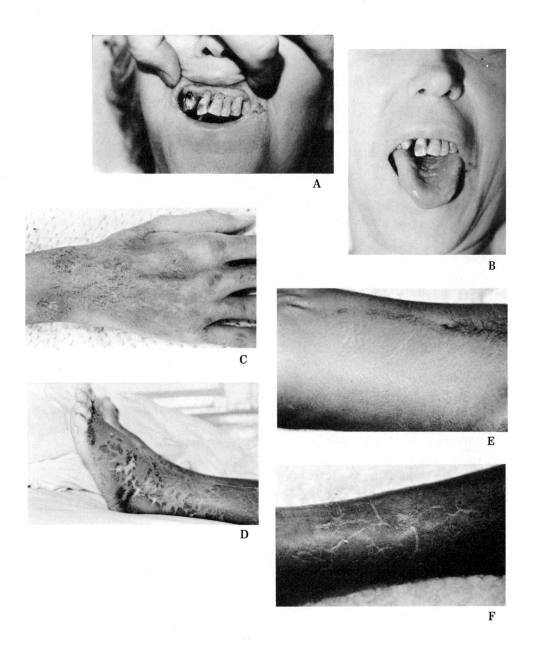

Figure 4-6. A, B Teeth and gums of a patient with multiple vitamin and iron deficiencies, showing cheilosis, glossitis, scorbutic gums, and periodontal disease.
C, D Skin conditions caused by pellagra.
E, F Flaky-paint dermatosis caused by protein and calorie malnutrition.

Milk Consumption — Over half the population drank milk at least once a day, whereas 20 per cent rarely or never drank milk. Milk consumption declined with age; one third of those over the age of 45 reported rarely or never drinking milk.

Fish and Egg Consumption — About half the population seldom or never ate fish, and 18 per cent reported that they seldom or never ate eggs. For those who rarely ate eggs, 67 per cent reported eating them less than once a day, but at least one to six times a week.

Fruit and Vegetable Consumption — Some 68 per cent consumed fruits and vegetables at least once a day; only 4 per cent ate these foods four times a day.

Breakfast Cereal Consumption — Of the total surveyed, 17 per cent ate breakfast cereal once or more a day; 39 per cent seldom or never ate this food.

Desserts — More than 40 per cent of the population ate desserts daily.[22]

Salty Snacks — Only 11 per cent of the population reported eating salty snacks daily, but more than 50 per cent ate them at least once a week.

Biochemical Data

Low hemoglobin and hematocrit values were highest among black adults aged 60 and over in the lowest-income group. Adults in all age groups, regardless of age and income, had more than a 10 per cent incidence of low hematocrits. Black children aged 6 to 11 and 12 to 17 had four times the incidence of low hemoglobins than did white children in each income level.

The greatest incidence of low percentage transferrin saturation values was found in children aged 1–5, 6–11, and 12–17. Black children aged 1–5 had the highest prevalence of low serum vitamin A values. Serum albumin values were adequate in all groups of children, although whites demonstrated a higher prevalence of low serum protein values for all age and income groups.

Clinical Findings and Anthropometric Data[21]

The HANES survey found a low prevalence of clinical signs of malnutrition. The following summarizes some of the clinical evidence related to specific nutrients:

Protein — Clinical evidence of protein deficiency was rare; the only evidence with a prevalence greater than 1 per cent was hepatomegaly and pot belly. Both of these signs were more prevalent in black than in white children.

Vitamin B Complex — Some evidence of deficiency especially in older individuals and in blacks was found. Moderate risk signs evidencing signs of deficiencies of thiamine, riboflavin, or niacin included absent knee and ankle jerks, magenta tongue, angular lesions of the lips, cheilosis and nasolabial seborrhea, and filiform atrophy of the tongue.*

*See Glossary, pages 679–692 for the definition of these terms.

Vitamin C — Some evidence, which was also more common in older individuals and blacks, was found to suggest a deficiency of vitamin C. The lack of vitamin C may have been responsible for swollen, bleeding gums in adolescents.

Vitamin A — Follicular hyperkeratosis of the upper arms existed to some extent among premenopausal females and young children, especially among blacks.

Vitamin D — Disturbing prevalence of bowed legs and knock-knees was found in certain sex-race-income groups. Blacks typically evidenced a higher prevalence of lack of vitamin D than did whites.

Iodine — Goiter was infrequently found in most groups with the exception of young black females and adolescent blacks in the above-poverty income groups, where the prevalence was greater than 10 per cent.

Calcium-Phosphorous — Chvostek's sign, a moderate-risk sign associated with a calcium-phosphorous imbalance, was more prevalent among blacks; prevalence was lower in the older adults of all subgroups.

Black men tended to be leaner than white, whereas obesity was most prevalent among adult females, in particular black females. White men, especially older men, tended to be more obese than black men. Men of higher-income groups were more obese, whereas women of higher-income groups were less obese than their counterparts in lower-income groups.

HANES II

HANES II was begun in 1976, collecting data from 1976 to 1978, and will provide, for the first time, a look at changes in nutritional status over time. The program design was carefully planned around the findings and the experience of the HANES I survey.

We now have much data that broadly defines American nutritional status. Numerous nutritional problems are evident. However, broad-based data is of little use in actually intervening to improve nutritional status.

IMPORTANCE OF IMPROVED NUTRITIONAL SURVEILLANCE

Improved methods of nutritional surveillance (see pages 69–70 for discussion of surveillance) are absolutely essential to improve the nutritional status of Americans. This fact has been emphasized and reiterated by a number of nutrition experts. As. A. Altschul suggests, "a policy of surveillance and monitoring may well be the cornerstone of a National Nutrition Policy, and might well be the structure upon which to build a coordinated nutrition policy."[23]

The Panel on Nutrition and Government of the Senate Select Committee on Nutrition and Human Needs stated the issue in this way:

A primary deficiency in the development of both policy and programs is the lack of information — the kind of information which would be supplied by a surveillance and monitoring system . . . we have scattered bits of information but these do not tell us what we need to know.[24]

There are great limitations to the data currently available. None of the currently existing survey data includes information relating food price changes to food consumption or nutrient intake. Current data allow only very broad conclusions about the nutritional status of the American people. Much additional data are needed to describe the changing nature of the food supply and its effects on eating habits and nutritional status and on the way nutritional status and dietary habits are related to health, especially atherosclerotic heart disease, certain types of cancer, hypertension, and diabetes. Such information is needed to support the design, development, and implementation of corrective measures including educational programs.

We still lack an operational definition of dietary sufficiency, a term that needs to be clarified if real problems are to be solved. It is unrealistic to expect that a single "ideal" standard can meet the needs of people involved in various occupations and activities and of varying levels of health.

These problems of nutritional surveillance were described by the White House Conference on Food and Nutrition in 1969. Since that time, the problems remain with us:

> Many of the methods currently being employed are insufficiently sensitive, cumbersome, tedious and expensive. Micro and automated methods are needed. Methods and standards for the evaluation of nutritional status with regard to some nutrients which may well be of public health importance in the U.S. population are simply inadequate. These include nutrients such as vitamin B_6 and folic acid for which we have inconclusive evidence of the extent or seriousness of the deficiencies in the United States. Finally, there are other nutrients such as some of the trace minerals, which are thought by some to be of health significance in the United States for which data are so fragmentary that no real evaluation can be made.[25]

To remedy this situation, the Senate Select Committee on Nutrition and Human Needs, Panel on Nutrition and Government, suggested that the ideal approach to the development of a nutritional surveillance system ideally would encompass four phases:[26]

1. The identification of goals and objectives of a national nutrition policy.

2. The determination of the types of information essential to achieving policy goals and objectives. For example, if the goal is to reduce the level of saturated fats in the average American diet, it is important to know how much saturated fat is contained in the typical diet.

3. The translation of these basic types of information into indicators that could aid in answering important questions. Using the previous example, we might determine annual sales of foods high in saturated fat, and the incidence of diseases associated with high intakes of saturated fat as possible indicators of national status, relative to saturated fat consumption.

4. A plan to gather information. The plan should indicate information

needed, indicators to be used, who would be responsible for data collection, and how the gathered information would be disseminated to appropriate organizations. Each step in this total process should be included.

Once the goals have been clarified, steps and activities to reach these goals should be decided upon and clearly stated. These steps must then be integrated into an ongoing planning process.

The Food and Agriculture Act of 1977 mandated a proposal for a comprehensive nutritional status monitoring system.[27] Such a system would include assessment, the determination of risk of nutrition-related health problems, the study of various factors causing such nutrition-related problems, an ongoing surveillance system, and program evaluations to determine the effects, adequacy, and efficiency of nutrition-related programs.

In 1972 the Center for Disease Control (CDC) of the Department of Health, Education, and Welfare developed a system to aid states and local governments to monitor specified nutritional status indicators. The program is operated on a voluntary basis. Fourteen states and three metropolitan areas are currently providing information collected by their health clinics on indicators of anemia, obesity, and retarded growth in children from low-income families.

Each month participating states and metropolitan areas receive reports on the results of patients' tests and suggest which of the patients deviate greatly from standard norms. Summary data for all states are also prepared. The Center for Disease Control summarizes all data and publishes a report entitled "Nutrition Surveillance" quarterly. Thus far the data has been used to justify health and nutrition programs, to monitor the effectiveness of interventions, to evaluate programs such as the USDA Special Supplemental Food Program for Women, Infants, and Children (WIC), and to aid program planning and resource allocation.

In response to the nutritional surveillance mandate of the Food and Agriculture Act of 1977, the U.S. Department of Agriculture and the Department of Health, Education, and Welfare formulated a joint proposal for a comprehensive Nutritional Status Monitoring System (NSMS). The proposal, which was submitted to Congress in May 1978, is based on four interrelated elements: nutritional and dietary status, nutritional quality of food, dietary practices and knowledge, and the effects of nutrition intervention programs. Activities suggested to carry out the surveillance include:

1. A decennial, collaborative survey with the Health and Nutrition Examination Survey (HANES) and the National Food Consumption Survey (NFCS).

2. An additional NFCS to be conducted between the decennial surveys — physiological examinations may be added to these surveys.

3. Special surveys of high-risk populations.

4. Expansion of the Center for Disease Control Screening activities to more states, with a broader scope of coverage.

5. Collection of nutrition screening information from programs such as Early Periodic Screening, Detection, and Treatment Program.

6. Evaluation studies of nutrition intervention programs.

The total estimated funding requirement to implement the first year's proposed activities was set at $20 million.

A number of weaknesses have been identified in the proposed surveillance system. Areas of major concern include:[28]

1. Lack of specificity and agreement between the departments of Agriculture and Health, Education, and Welfare. Lack of agreement was noted in several areas: the extent to which the five-year NFCS will collect physiological data, the extent of coordinated research efforts on dietary and physiological assessment of nutritional status, and the nature of the decennial survey.

2. The specific role of the system in program evaluation. The proposal lacked definition of methodologies that would result in meaningful response rates to surveys designed to evaluate programs such as the Food Stamp Program or that could fully evaluate the nutritional impact of such programs on participants.

3. Inadequacy of coordination mechanisms. There was no defined procedure for settling disagreements between the USDA and the HEW relative to responsibilities and work on the surveillance system.

The U.S. General Accounting Office (GAO) made several recommendations as first steps toward implementing the proposed surveillance system. GAO suggested that appropriate congressional committees review the proposed system after a given period of time and, if necessary, designate either USDA or HEW as the agency with primary responsibility for system implementation. Other recommendations included a joint pilot study during the next NFCS to determine the feasibility of combining the NFCS and HANES, and the funding of an independent peer review of the proposal by an outside group.

It is obvious that both HEW and USDA have seriously attempted to improve nutritional surveillance activities. Studies presently in progress will determine the shape that future national nutritional surveillance systems will take.

Nutritional assessment programs are also a part of other programs designed to improve nutritional status. In addition to the nutritional status screening components of the WIC and Headstart programs, the Early Periodic Screening, Detection, and Treatment Program (EPSDT) (sometimes referred to as Child Health Assessment Program, CHAP) also provides for the collection of data that may indicate nutritional problems. EPSDT, under an amendment to Title XIX of the Social Security Act, is designed to make comprehensive health services available to individuals under 21 years of age who are eligible for Medicaid.

The screening component is to include a health history, a physical examination, a review of immunization status, and other selected tests, some of which are intended to identify malnutrition. The screening is then to provide a basis for further referrals as needed.

Other assessment programs are also operating to identify and then follow up nutritional problems. A program managed by the state of California is the Child Health and Disability Prevention Program. The primary goal of the program is "a reduction in the incidence of preventable illness and disability, and a promotion of a positive health status among children in California." The program is geared to approximately 1,128,034 individuals under 21 years of age who qualify for Medicaid as well as the children who entered the first grade in the fall of 1975. Those who provide screening services to eligible children can be reimbursed for their expenses. The program is intended to be a periodic screening program; assessment is conducted at periodic intervals to provide ongoing surveillance of health status.[29]

Tests performed as part of the program include a health history; a physical examination; hearing, vision, and tuberculin tests; biochemical blood and urine tests; and assessment of nutritional, dental, and developmental condition. Part of the program is referral to additional needed services. Immunizations are provided where indicated and follow-up is conducted for those who need additional services.[29]

SUMMARY

Drastic changes in the eating habits of Americans have occurred during the twentieth century. The effects of these changes have been related to American health status. Overconsumption of fat, especially saturated fatty acids, cholesterol, sugar, and salt have been related to the increased prevalence of six of the current ten major "killer diseases" in America: As M. Hegsted noted:

> I wish to stress that there is a great deal of evidence and it continues to accumulate, which strongly implicates and, in some instances, proves that the major cause of death and disability in the United States are related to the diet we eat. I include coronary artery disease which accounts for nearly half of the deaths in the United States, several of the most important forms of cancer, hypertension, diabetes and obesity as well as other chronic diseases.[1]

On the other hand, these dietary trends may be contributing to undernutrition in some segments of the population. Diets composed largely of fat and sugar often tend to contain inadequate amounts of vitamins and essential minerals and, hence, may result in vitamin or mineral deficiencies. The problem is particularly prevalent among low-income groups, who are often easily victimized by advertisements and inducements to eat foods that are high in "empty calories." Resulting effects of the changing North American diet, both in terms of undernutrition and overnutrition, are discussed in the following pages.

REFERENCES

1. Hegsted, M. In U.S. Senate Select Committee on Nutrition and Human Needs, *Dietary Goals for the United States*, 2d ed. Washington, D.C.: Government Printing Office, December 1977.
2. U.S. Department of Agriculture. *1977 Handbook of Agricultural Charts. Agr. Handbook No. 524.* Washington, D.C., November 1977.
3. U.S. Department of Agriculture. *Fat in Today's Food Supply — Level of Use and Sources.* Washington, D.C., 1974.
4. U.S. Senate Select Committee on Nutrition and Human Needs. *Dietary Goals for the United States*, 2d ed. Washington, D.C.: Government Printing Office, December 1977.
5. Stamler, J. In U.S. Senate Select Committee on Nutrition and Human Needs, *Diet Related to Killer Diseases*. II. Washington, D.C.: Government Printing Office, February 1-2, 1977, p. 289.
6. Brewster, L., and M. F. Jacobson. *The Changing American Diet.* Washington, D.C.: Center for Science in the Public Interest, 1978.
7. Page, L., and B. Friend. Level of use of sugars in the United States, in H. L. Sipple and K. W. McNutt, eds., *Sugars in Nutrition.* New York: Academic Press, 1974, pp. 93-107.
8. U.S. Senate Select Committee on Nutrition and Human Needs, Hearings before the Select Committee on Nutrition and Human Needs, Part 2. *Sugar in Diet, Diabetes, and Heart Diseases.* Washington, D.C.: Government Printing Office, 1973, p. 147.
9. Lee, P. R. Nutrition policy — from neglect and uncertainty to debate and action. *J. Am. Diet. Assoc.* 72 (1978): 581.
10. Winicoff, B. Changing public diet. *Human Nature* 1 (January 1978): 60.
11. Mertz, W. Dietary changes pose unknown health danger. *CNI Week. Rept.* 7 (19 November 1977): 4-5.
12. Bickel, J. H., and T. M. C. Urban. Fiber content of the American diet and the diet of the Tarshumara Indian. Unpublished calculations. 1975.
13. U.S. Department of Agriculture. *National Food Situation*, Publ. No. NFS-161. Washington, D.C., September 1977.
14. Gray, P. Want food fast? Here's fast food. *Time*, July 4, 1977, p. 46.
15. U.S. Department of Agriculture. *Food and Nutrient Intake of Individuals in the United States. Household Food Consumption Survey, 1965-66*, Rept. No. 11. Washington, D.C., January 1972.
16. American Dietitians Association. Food consumption survey. *J. Am. Diet. Assoc.* 70 (1977): 303.
17. U.S. Department of Health, Education, and Welfare. *Ten-State Nutrition Survey, 1968-1970*, Publ. No. (HSM) 72-8134. Washington, D.C.: Government Printing Office, 1977.
18. Interdepartmental Committee on Nutrition for National Defense. *Manual for Nutrition Surveys*, 2d ed. Washington, D.C.: Government Printing Office, 1963.
19. National Center for Health Statistics. *Preliminary Findings of the First Health and Nutrition Examination Survey, U.S., 1971-72.* January 1974.
20. U.S. Department of Health, Education, and Welfare. *Dietary Intake of Persons 1 to 74 Years of Age in the United States. Advanced Data. Vital and Health Statistics of the National Center for Health Statistics*, Rept. No. 6. Washington, D.C.: Government Printing Office, March 30, 1977.
21. Lowenstein, F. W. Preliminary clinical and anthropometric findings from

the *First Health and Nutrition Survey, U.S., 1971–72. Am. J. Clin. Nutr.* 29 (1976): 918.

22. *The Nation's Health*, September 1978, p. 2.
23. Altschul, A. In U.S. Senate Select Committee on Nutrition and Human Needs, *National Nutrition Policy Study Hearings*, Vol. 7–A. Washington, D.C.: Government Printing Office, June 21, 1974.
24. U.S. Senate Select Committee on Nutrition and Human Needs. *Report of the Panel on Nutrition and Government, op. cit.*
25. White House Conference on Food, Nutrition, and Health. *Comprehensive Report.* Washington, D.C.: Government Printing Office, December 1970.
26. U.S. Senate Select Committee on Nutrition and Human Needs. *Towards a National Nutrition Policy. Nutrition and Government.* Washington, D.C.: Government Printing Office, May 1975.
27. U.S. Congress. Food and Agricultural Act of 1977, PL–95–113. September 29, 1977.
28. U.S. General Accounting Office. *Future of the National Nutrition Intelligence System*, Rept. No. CED–79–5. Washington, D.C., November 7, 1978.
29. California State Department of Health, Family Health Services Section, Children and Youth Unit. *California's Child Health and Disability Prevention Program Fact Sheet.* April 1975.

5

Poverty and nutrition problems of economically disadvantaged groups

Reader Objectives

After completing this chapter, the reader should be able to
1. Define poverty.
2. State the procedure for determining the poverty level.
3. State the relationship between income and diets.
4. State the general nutritional problems of
   - American Indians and Alaskan Natives.
   - Spanish-speaking immigrants to the United States.
   - Migrant laborers.
5. State recommendations for improving the nutritional status of these vulnerable groups.
6. Describe three general strategies for dealing with poverty.

PERSPECTIVES ON POVERTY

Economic poverty significantly limits man's food choices and, in so doing, makes it difficult for the impoverished to be adequately nourished. Poverty and nutritional deprivation continue in the United States despite large-scale efforts to end them. The War on Poverty, the programs of the Great Society, welfare, food stamps, school lunches, job training, Upward Bound, and Operation Headstart all attempted to alleviate poverty in North America, but the problems continue and, according to some estimates, are worsening.[1]

The alleviation of hunger and malnutrition must be considered in the context of eliminating poverty. Hunger usually results from a lack of resources to procure an adequate diet, and in the long run it cannot be ended without the elimination of poverty. (See Figure 5-1.)

POVERTY — DEFINITIONS AND CHARACTERISTICS

Poverty is not homogeneous. The poverty suffered by what Oscar Lewis has termed the "culture of poverty" is certainly of a much different nature than that suffered by graduate students on limited incomes. Lewis suggested a basic difference between internal and external poverty.[2]

Internal poverty represents the culture of poverty into which an individual is born and is (according to this theory) rarely able to escape. Such poverty is characterized by many distinct factors. For example, the individual in the "culture of poverty" often experiences lack of power, helplessness, lack of self-worth, inability to provide for needs of self and

Figure 5-1. Many population subgroups in America are at high risk of nutritional problems because of economic factors. (Left column, from top: United Nations/John Littlewood; FAO photo by Emmet Bright. Center column: WFP/FAO photo by J. Ciganovic; UN photo; FAO photo by F. Botts. Right column: United Nations/Ray Witlin; FAO photo by J. Ciganovic; UN photo.)

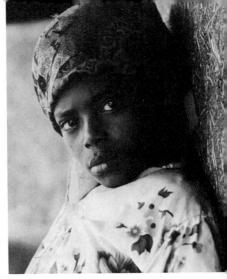
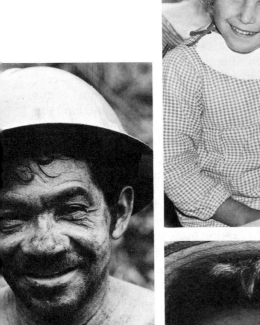
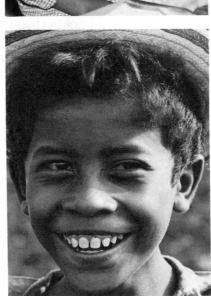
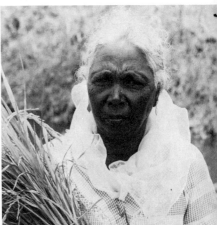
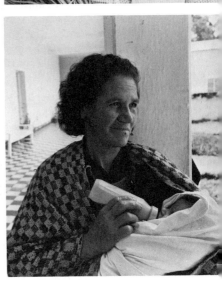
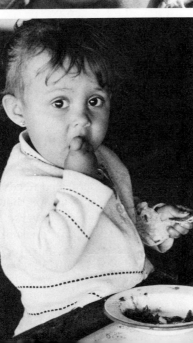

family, disregard for traditional values of the middle and upper class, and different attitudes toward highly regarded middle-class opportunities such as education. The individual born into the culture of poverty faces a spiral of adverse environmental pressures operating to "keep him in his place." For example, poor education, lack of income, and lack of steady employment may result in poor environmental and living conditions, poor sanitary conditions, and reduced access to social services, such as health care. Such factors then lead to poor health status and poor nutritional status, which in turn result in diminished responsiveness to environmental stimuli, loss of time spent in school, lack of attention, and hence diminished learning. These factors in turn lead to a repetition of the cycle. In addition, intergenerational effects (deprivation and the consequences suffered by one generation) result in adverse effects on another generation. Clearly those born into such poverty have a very difficult time overcoming adverse factors and breaking out of the culture of poverty.

External poverty, on the other hand, is usually more transitory: a middle-class family whose head temporarily loses his or her job or the family of a graduate student pursuing an education but temporarily earning no income exhibit external poverty. Although the individuals are forced to reduce the demand for material items and to adjust their lifestyle to reduced income, they do not modify their values, attitudes, self-image, and social relationships and are able to readjust to increased income when economic conditions improve.

Before poverty can be alleviated, however, we must be aware of who is to be considered poor and who is not. The issue of defining poverty is a complex one:

> It might appear a simple matter to define and measure poverty. After all, it is easy to describe a hypothetical situation with terms so harsh and stringent that most persons will agree they denote poverty. But agreement that all persons at and below some level are poor does not constitute agreement that persons above it are not poor. Poverty is not an "either-or" state or condition; it is also a matter of degree.
>
> . . . Policy issues and causality often get mixed up with the definition of poverty. Many people believe that poor people are people who deserve something, sympathy only perhaps, but possibly some kind of assistance. Thus, when it is said that persons of a given type are not poor, what may be meant is that they do not deserve help or sympathy. And, when it is said that somebody is not "that poor," what may be meant is that someone does not deserve "that" much help. The feeling that poor people necessarily deserve help inevitably leads to definitions of poverty which reflect programmatic and policy issues. The definition of poverty is easily confounded by instilling into it a concern about the incentive effects of some program presumed to relieve poverty.[3]

The term *poverty* connotes broad environmental, economic, social, and psychological conditions. An individual who does not command resources sufficient to meet his or her own perceived needs might generally be considered poor. But beyond this basic concept there are various views and perceptions of what constitutes poverty. Poverty definitions are essential for public policy purposes; they allow decision makers and program planners to identify individuals who are "eligible" for public services, and they are necessary for an evaluation of antipoverty programs.

Some social scientists advocate the use of general "social indicators" to measure poverty. By indicating ways in which the "poor" differ from the others in society, these scientists believe that they can focus on such factors as quality of life and social health. Indicators used in this connection include infant, child, or adult mortality; morbidity; nutritional and health status statistics; level of education; housing indices; and neighborhood crime rates. However, the absence of these negative social indicators or an adequate income does not ensure that all other "quality" aspects of life are obtained. It is possible that economically well-off individuals might be considered "poor" if certain social indicators are used.

Poverty in the economic sense can be defined in two ways. *Relative* poverty is determined in terms of what the general population has. Examples of relative poverty include:

a fixed percentage of the population to be defined as "poor," or

defining poverty as those whose incomes fall below 50 per cent of the median income.

Absolute poverty is poverty in terms of an individual's ability to buy a specified set of goods and services. For example, the cost of a basic diet might be objectively determined, and poverty would be defined in terms of those who could not afford to purchase this. Such absolute definitions are valid only when they are used in a specific time period and place.

DETERMINING THE POVERTY LEVEL

There is much controversy over appropriate ways to determine poverty levels. A century ago poverty in the United States might have been defined in terms of survival. But as the average standard of living rose, people began to look at poverty in relative terms. Although most Americans would probably agree that a poverty definition should consider resources sufficient to meet minimum standards of living as well as "fair" levels of resources to provide for human growth and development, there is much debate over the actual level at which the dividing line should be fixed.

The current measure of poverty used in the allocation of federal program benefits was developed in 1964, and, after minor revisions, it was adopted by the Office of Management and Budget in 1969 as the federal government's official statistical poverty measure.

Food, a basic human need, is the cornerstone of the currently used poverty index. Standards of need are based on the NAS-NRC recommended dietary allowances as they are reflected in USDA food plans. These food plans are developed on the premise that a large variety of foods, available at widely varying costs, can provide a nutritionally sound diet. Thus, diets at different cost levels have been developed and serve as the basis for determining the poverty index. Food plans incorporate not only the cost differentials but also consider actual food consumption of households in the United States as determined by USDA Household Food Consumption surveys.

Four food plans are currently in use: the thrifty plan (which replaced the previous economy food plan) and the low-cost, the moderate-cost, and the liberal food plans. The USDA estimates the food cost (prepared and eaten at home) on a monthly basis for the four food plans for 12 different age-sex combinations and also for pregnant women and lactating mothers.

The USDA thrifty food plan is designed to be reasonably tasty and contains certain preferred foods. Waste and the money spent for nonnutritious foods are allowed for in the food plans. Expensive foods such as costly meats and convenience foods are limited whereas lower-cost food items such as whole grain and enriched breads and cereals are allowed in greater quantities.

The cost of the thrifty food plan is low, relative to the food cost reported by households surveyed in the 1965–1966 Household Food Consumption Survey. Approximately 10 per cent of the families surveyed spent less than the thrifty food plan cost in purchasing their food.

The current poverty threshold is determined by presuming that the suitable ratio of nonfood item expenditures to food expenditures would be that of the average in the United States. On the average, food expenditures account for one third of total family income after taxes. Thus, cost of the thrifty food plan is multiplied by three to determine the poverty threshold. The poverty threshold for one- and two-member families is determined by a slightly modified version of this process. Although the validity and appropriateness of this way of determining a poverty threshold is widely debated, it forms the basis for many program and policy decisions.

The standards are modified according to the number in the family and the composition of family. These standards are updated monthly by the Bureau of Labor Statistics according to increases in food prices. There are other statistical measures for poverty such as dollar cutoffs unadjusted for family size, percentiles of the income distribution, and percentages of median family income. All these measures have advantages and limitations that vary depending upon the purposes for which they are intended. Each measure also has a certain degree of subjectivity and limitation related to poor data bases and conceptual difficulties.

U.S. POVERTY STATISTICS

According to official poverty levels, 24.7 million Americans were classified as poor in 1977. Of these, the following pinpoint the poor in terms of population subgroups:[4]

Group	Percentage of Group Classified As Poor
All Americans	11.6%
Whites	8.9
Blacks	31.3
Hispanic	22.4

Group	Percentage of Group Classified As Poor
Aged 65 or older	14.1
Central city residents	15.4
People living on farms	17.1

A committee print from the select Committee on Nutrition and Human Needs, "Hunger 1973 and Press Reaction," summed up the state of poverty in the inner cities:

> They are places in which one family in four is poor, half the unrelated elderly and the youth are poor; where the cost of living is 12 percent higher than the national average, but the full-time wages of one in 14 workers is not sufficient to keep a family of four above the poverty line. The cost of food alone is 13 percent higher in the cities. . . .[5]

Rural poverty is being increasingly recognized as the cause of many heretofore ignored health and education problems. There are approximately 10.5 million people in rural areas in the United States whose incomes fall below federal poverty lines; indeed, the rural poor constitute 41 per cent of the nation's poor. They are usually older, more disabled, and less well educated than the urban poor.[6]

Illiteracy is closely associated with the rural poverty. Among rural poor, the rate of functional illiteracy is almost 60 per cent. One of every four individuals residing in rural areas is poor and 70 per cent of these poor live on less than $2,000 annually. Among the rural poor, there is a disparity in illiteracy rates associated with race; in rural agricultural areas, white illiteracy rates are 2.2 per cent, black rates are 15.2 per cent, and Puerto Rican illiteracy approaches 17.7 per cent. Income levels parallel these differences in literacy; the per capita income of white rural residents is considerably higher than is that of nonwhite rural residents.[7]

The rural poor have other problems and they are at a unique disadvantage. Their needs are very great, but they are not as visible as other disadvantaged segments of the population, and hence their needs are easily ignored or forgotten. Thus, little note has been paid to meeting their needs through public assistance programs.

POVERTY AND PURCHASING POWER

Poverty, considered in terms of lack of command over goods and services sufficient to meet basic needs, is mainly a function of the lack of purchasing power. Purchasing power depends upon three factors:

1. Income
2. The relative prices of needed goods and services
3. The cost of all additional demands made upon income

Incomes and prices directly affect the ability to purchase nutritious food. Other financial expenditures such as clothing, housing, education, and health needs indirectly affect the amount of money available to purchase food.

RELATIONSHIP BETWEEN INCOME AND DIETS

Income is a very important determinant of diet and nutritional status. Three trends are relevant to the relationship between income and diet. The first, which was initially noted by a German, Engel in the nineteenth century and is termed Engel's law, is that as incomes increase, the proportion of total income spent for food decreases, but the absolute expenditures for food rise. There is, however, an exception to this trend in that for the lowest-income groups the absolute expenditures are initially so low that initial income increments may result in a higher percentage of income being spent for food.

A second trend is that the proportion of money spent for different groups of foods varies as income increases. Those with very low incomes usually purchase more carbohydrate foods. As incomes increase, the calories obtained from carbohydrate foods decrease and more calories are obtained from costlier animal and vegetable products. The impact of economic development often results in an increased consumption of fat and protein with a reduction in the quantity and quality of carbohydrate foods consumed. Although low-income people tend to consume larger amounts of complex carbohydrates than do people with higher incomes, many health and nutrition experts now call for an increased consumption of complex carbohydrates. The relationship between the consumption of animal and vegetable protein and income is so well known as to be almost axiomatic: animal protein consumption rises at the expense of vegetable protein as incomes rise. (However, among many people in the United States, this trend has been somewhat reversed with the "back to nature movement.")

A third trend is that as incomes rise there is a shift toward the more refined, processed, and convenience foods within food groups. For example, fiber-depleted foods often replace traditional plant foods.

FOOD PRICES

One of the most important consumer problems relative to food is the very high and rising retail cost of food. Of the various priorities suggested by the Consumer Task Force of the White House Conference, the very first that was singled out for special emphasis was the lowering of food prices.[8] Recent and rising inflation has been devastating to both low- and middle-income households. In many inner-city areas, families are forced to spend a proportion of their income for food that is greater than the proportions spent by many in developing nations. Increasing food prices and resulting limited diets and poor quality of foods have been implicated, not only in poor nutritional status but also in the riots and discontent of the 1960s and 1970s.

DO THE POOR PAY MORE?

The poor have been adversely affected by the inflationary increases in food prices to a greater degree than have other economic classes. One reason for this is that the poor spend a larger part of their incomes on food than do their nonpoor counterparts. According to a Consumer Expenditure Interview Survey, families with incomes below $3,000 spent 46 per cent of their incomes for food in 1973; in contrast to this, families earning $12,000 to $14,999 spent only 12 per cent of their incomes for food. Table 5–1 illustrates the percentage of money income spent for food for the years 1972 and 1973 for families of different income levels.[9] The table also indicates that food expenditures rose faster than income for the poor, and that the proportion of income spent for food increased most for families whose incomes were less than $3,000 annually.[9]

Another reason that the poor are harder hit by inflationary food prices relates to their food-spending patterns. During periods of inflation, the middle and upper class are able to alter their spending patterns and "spend down" by buying less expensive items. For example, if very expensive animal products are too costly, those who are used to such foods can "spend down" by buying the less expensive cuts of meat and thus miss the food-price squeeze.

The poor, who are already buying the lower-cost foods, cannot "spend down" to avoid the inflationary prices. No food items are available that

Table 5–1

Percent of Money Income (Before Taxes) Spent for Food at Home and Away: All Families and Single Persons, Consumer Expenditure Interview Survey, 1972 and 1973

Income and Area	1972	1973	1973 as a Percentage of 1972
Under $3,000	38%	46%	123
3,000–3,999	28	28	100
4,000–4,999	23	24	104
5,000–5,999	21	21	101
6,000–6,999	18	18	99
7,000–7,999	17	18	104
6,000–8,999	15	16	106
10,000–11,999	15	15	101
12,000–14,999	13	13	103
15,000–19,999	12	12	105
20,000–24,999	10	11	105
25,000 and over	6	7	114
All families	14	14	101

Source: A. Manchester and L. Brown. Do the poor pay more? *National Food Situation* 160 (June 1977): 27.

can be used to replace the already relatively inexpensive food. In addition, because of the increased demand for less expensive food items, the prices of these items begin to rise. Thus, the poor are hardest hit by inflation as the food items they routinely purchase sometimes rise in price faster than do the foods typically consumed by the nonpoor. This concept is sometimes referred to as the "inflation tax."

Some studies have developed market baskets of foods eaten by the poor and have then compared these food prices with the Consumer Price Index for food. This index provides an indication of the relative rise in food prices for high-priced and low-priced foods. A USDA study treated meat, poultry, and fish as one category. Within this category, low-priced foods were those with a retail price of less than $1 per pound in 1970. The other food groups were similarly divided.

Results of the analysis indicated that the prices of low-priced foods rose approximately 1 per cent more between 1967 and 1970 than did the prices of the more expensive food items. However, the price movements were divergent. For example, in 1975 and 1976, high-priced foods increased in price more rapidly than did the low-priced foods, but, for price movements over the years from 1967 to 1976, the low-priced foods were 83 per cent higher whereas the high-priced foods were 79 per cent higher.[10]

Table 5–2 illustrates the divergent price movements during the years 1967 to 1976. It is thus difficult to generalize about comparative inflation rates of lower-priced and more expensive foods.

The phrase "The poor pay more" is especially applicable to problems of poor rural and urban shoppers. Low-income people in both areas often do not have the choice of shopping at large, more efficient retail markets, but instead are forced to shop at smaller, less efficient stores that charge higher prices and offer less variety.

Low-income people lack three basic qualities that are important for participation in the free market.[11] First, they are often unable to do comparison shopping; they may have limited transportation and credit and be forced to shop in the corner grocery store where prices are very high. They may be limited by their knowledge and hence unable to make wise

Table 5–2
Inflation Rates of Low- and High-Priced Foods

Year	Relatively Low-Priced Foods	Relatively High-Priced Foods
1967	100.0	100.0
1970	113.5	112.1
1971	115.0	117.6
1972	119.9	122.5
1973	144.6	136.4
1974	169.3	158.2
1975	180.3	174.1
1976	182.9	179.1

Source: A. Manchester and L. Brown. Do the poor pay more? *National Food Situation* 160 (June 1977): 27.

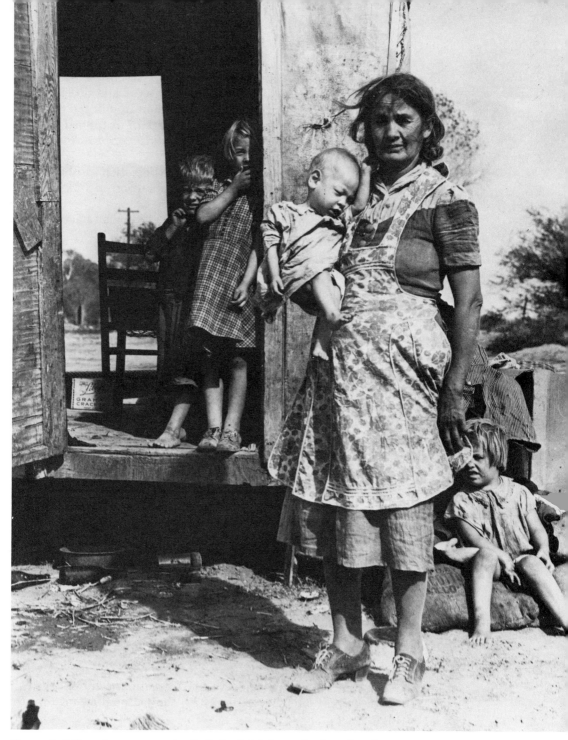

Figure 5-2. Poverty can severely limit food intake and adversely affect nutritional status. (National Archives)

consumer food choices. Second, they are often victimized by crooked business practices that deliberately take advantage of and deceive them. Third, the low-income individual is often least able to enforce consumer rights and privileges. If he or she is taken advantage of or robbed, the low-income person is often unable to obtain legal counsel or professional help to set straight the wrong he or she has suffered.

Low-income consumers face many other barriers that prohibit them from obtaining equality in the marketplace. Such barriers include:

1. Lack of education needed to understand the manufacturer's or advertiser's claims.

2. Language barriers that hinder foreign-born individuals from understanding product claims or from understanding how to shop comparatively for the best buys.

3. Pride that may lead to poor consumer judgment because of an unwillingness to question or to admit confusion about a product.

In addition to these problems, some population subgroups in America face additional compounding difficulties. The following sections review special problems facing the American Indians, low-income Spanish-speaking Americans, and the migrant workers. The effect of economic deprivation on nutritional status is also reviewed.

AMERICAN INDIANS AND ALASKAN NATIVES

The American Indian population is among the poorest and most malnourished ethnic groups in America.[12-25] According to census data, there are 827,108 American Indians and Alaskan Natives, 543,000 of whom live on or near reservations.[12] The impoverished conditions of the American Indians are graphically described by the following statistics:[13-19]

1. Annual family income is the lowest of any ethnic group in the United States — $1,900.

2. Forty per cent of Indians who live on reservations are classified as below the federal poverty line; this is compared with a national average of 4.3 per cent.

3. Forty per cent of Indians who live on reservations who are aged sixteen or over were unemployed in 1970; the national average for this statistic is 4.3 per cent.

4. The average reservation Indian must pay 28 per cent more for food than does his or her urban counterpart.

5. Since over 50 per cent of the Indian population are under 20 years of age, the population is more vulnerable to malnutrition and other disease conditions that may impair physical and emotional health.

6. Maternal mortality rates average two to three times higher than the rates for the overall U.S. population.

7. Infant mortality is 22.4 per cent higher than the national average.

8. Postnatal Indian deaths account for half of infant deaths; the Indian rate of 11.2 per 1,000 is compared with 4.9 per 1,000 in the general U.S. population; leading causes of infant death among Indians include influenza, pneumonia, and diarrheal disease.

9. High incidences of many nutrition-related diseases have been reported: the Indian death rate from cirrhosis of the liver is 38.9 per 100,000 compared with 14.4 per 100,000 for the general population.

10. High rates of anemia exist (one study found that the incidence of anemia among Indians was triple that of the national rate.)

11. Large proportions of Indian children have low hemoglobin, plasma iron, vitamin A, and vitamin C.

12. Obesity has been noted to occur among some Indian tribes at rates of 60 to 90 per cent.

13. High prevalence and mortality caused by diabetes mellitus is 19.4 per 100,000 compared with 17.3 per 100,000 for the American white population.

Nutrition Surveys[25]

A number of surveys of the nutritional status of Indians and Alaska Natives have demonstrated mild to marked deficiencies of specific nutrients.[20-31] Van Duzen et al. in a five-year study of 4,355 patient admissions to the Indian Health Service Hospital in Tuba City, Arizona, found 616 diagnosed cases of child malnutrition. Fifteen of these presented kwashiorkor, and 29 had marasmus. Van Duzen also found that approximately 15 per cent of the children admitted who were under the age of 5 had some type of associated malnutrition.[20]

J. G. French noted vitamin A, C, and other nutrient deficiencies in a study of Navajo infants less than 2 years of age. Twelve of 139 infants had been hospitalized for malnutrition, and ten were hospitalized for anemia.[21] Other studies of native Americans reported that the mean intake of calories, calcium, riboflavin and iron, and vitamins A and C were less than the recommended allowances.[22-25]

These studies also noted growth rates that were well below the standards reported in the Iowa and Boston standards. In the survey of 167 Navajo children studied by W. Carlile et al., almost one third of the children fell below the third percentile in weight.[23] K. Reisinger's group found 73–83 per cent of the Navajo children that they studied were less than the fifty-ninth percentile in weight and height.[24] G. Owen et al., in studying Apache children, found that 38 per cent of the children were less than the tenth percentile in height and 18 per cent were less than the tenth percentile in weight.[22]

Relatively few nutritional surveys and studies of the nutritional status of Indians have been conducted. Data are thus incomplete, and the picture is changing relative to the Indian health status, as well as to the relationship between Indians and their non-Indian counterparts. Some of the results of

existing studies are summarized in Table 5–3. The following conclusions
and summary were suggested on the basis of existing information:[23]

1. Socioeconomic and dietary information suggest that the average reservation Indian family's diet is frequently marginal and in need of supplementation. Deficiencies in diet include those of animal protein,
   milk, fresh fruits, and vegetables. Such deficiencies add to "hidden
   hunger," which in turn results in poor health status of many Indian
   children.

   Food recently "imported" to the reservations is often of a high sim-

Table 5–3

Nutritional Status of the American Indian: Selected Survey

Reference	Population	Major Findings
(26)	645 Navajo subjects at Ganado; 595 subjects at Pinon	Diet had previously consisted mainly of corn, wild game, goat or mutton, and wild plants. Food grown included beans, squash, melons, pumpkins, and potatoes.
		With the introduction of trading posts, this traditional pattern changed; wheat flour replaced corn; herb beverages were replaced by coffee, tea, and soft drinks.
		The typical meal pattern included three meals daily; diets tended to be monotonous with little variation.
		Basic food items were mutton (roasted, fried or stewed), onion, potatoes, bread, coffee, and tea.
(27)	966 Navajos in Greasewood Chapter	Study demonstrated need for increased dietary iron, protein, and vitamin C for adults; more calories for children and elderly.
		More than half of households studied received USDA commodity foods; only 21 per cent had running water; 23 per cent had electricity; 23 per cent had refrigeration; 75 per cent of households stored meat outside; 69 per cent used wood as cooking fuel.
		Main staples were sheep and corn; visceral meats were eaten.
(20)	4,355 children admitted to Hospital in Tuba City	616 of children were malnourished; 15 had kwashiorkor; 29 had marasmus; approximately 15 per cent of children admitted to hospital had some type of malnutrition.
		Growth curves of children were well below standards for American children.
(21)	Western Navajo Indians	Diets of children were low in calories and protein; often were low in vitamins A and C and other nutrients.

Nutritional Status of the American Indian: Selected Survey *(continued)*

Reference	Population	Major Findings
		Infectious diseases were causes of high mortality rates; single most important cause was gastroenteritis; foods most commonly used were potatoes, meat, bread, and cereal.
(28)	49 nutrition aids working on Navajo reservation collected dietary information	Of 281 households receiving USDA commodity foods, 47 per cent used some types of native foods; primary native foods were corn mash and blue corn bread.
		Meal patterns similar to those reported by Darby in 1956.
(29)	67 Head Start Chippewa children in Northern Wisconsin	5–8 per cent were under height for age, 28 per cent were overweight, and 25 per cent had less than acceptable hemoglobin levels.
		Iron intake was the lowest of all nutrients studied.
		No clinical signs of malnutrition were evident.
(30)	Navajo Indian Reservation, Arizona	Comparison of patients admitted with kwashiorkor, marasmus, or weight deficits to Public Health Service Indian Hospital in Tuba City in period 1969–1973.
		The number of patients below the age of 5 years fell between two time periods; there was a 39 per cent decrease in the number of patients admitted for weight deficits; marasmus was found in only two cases after 1969; the incidence of kwashiorkor decreased by 50 per cent.
		Study concluded that infant and child feeding programs contributed to improved health.
(31)	94 females responsible for family food preparation on Standing Rock Reservation	Relative to RDAs, mean nutritional intakes were Kcal, 75 per cent; vitamin A, 93 per cent; niacin, 96 per cent; riboflavin, 73 per cent; thiamine, 90 per cent; vitamin C, 89 per cent; calcium, 51 per cent.
		Iron was satisfactory for women aged 55–75 but not for younger women.
		No typical daily menu; meals lacked variety.
		Commonly used foods included dry bread, potatoes, meat, bologna sandwiches, potato chips, soda, and coffee.
		Most women were overweight; few were aware of basic nutritional facts; only 19 could define "calorie."
		74 per cent of families used government commodity foods.

ple carbohydrate nature and may contribute to high incidence of dental caries.

2. Nutritional surveys have found widespread deficiencies of vitamins A and C, calcium, and iron, and frequent low protein intakes.

3. Although biochemical studies of nutritional status among Indian children are few, the available data suggest that a common finding is low hemoglobin levels from iron deficiency anemia.

4. Anthropometric information demonstrates that the average Indian preschool child lags behind his non-Indian counterpart in growth, height, and weight.

5. Severe malnutrition is rare, occurring primarily in association with child neglect, which is infrequently found.

6. Indian children suffer high infant mortality and morbidity, primarily from respiratory and digestive diseases. The poor nutritional status of the children is likely a contributing factor.

Barriers to Adequate Nutrition

There are numerous reasons for the nutritional problems experienced by native Americans. Logistical difficulties are often involved in obtaining food or in securing food assistance. For example, food stamp offices and suitable retail outlets may be 100 miles away, necessitating travel over poor roads. In addition, language, cultural barriers, racism, and discrimination may also hinder the Indian from access to an adequate food supply. Other barriers to adequate nutrition faced by native Americans include:[13]

1. Cultural disruption resulting in dramatic and often detrimental changes in dietary patterns.

2. Loss of productive lands, water, and traditional rights of hunting, fishing, and agriculture.

3. Poverty, unemployment, isolation, and inadequate housing.

4. Inadequate funding, sensitivity, and understanding of Indian problems in legislated programs.

5. Political impotence resulting from isolation, absence of direct represen tation, poverty, and scattered, small populations.

6. Confusion of federal/state authority and responsibility and failure of the federal government to honor treaty, executive promises, and commitments.

7. Gross inflation of particularly low-cost staple foods.

8. Inadequate knowledge of nutritional status and problems of food availability of Indians by administrators dealing directly with Indian health care.

9. Inadequate knowledge by Indians of proper food choices for nutritional needs.

In 1977 the Food Research and Action Center (FRAC) surveyed Indian reservations to determine the current situation regarding food issues affecting the Indian population. The final report reviewed several important factors limiting Indian participation in federal food assistance programs. Barriers to participation included Indian inability to pay the purchase price for food stamps and antagonistic state or county program workers. Many of the barriers were direct functions of the distant geographical locations of the reservations.[32-33] For example, the survey found that some Indians lived as far as 350 miles (round-trip distance) from the food stamp certification centers and the food stamp issuance center and as far as 400 miles from food stores. Outreach to inform Indians about the existing and available federal food and nutrition programs was extremely limited. Table 5-4[32-33] summarizes some of the survey results.

Recommendations for Improving Nutritional Status on the Reservations

Central to all recommendations is the concept that the native Americans should be involved in every aspect of planning, policy and decision making, implementation, and evaluation of all issues related to nutrition and health in their populations.

At the Conference on Nutrition, Growth, and Development of North American Indian Children, tribal representatives recommended that colleges and universities in various areas of the country become more closely involved in the problems and needs of Indian communities. They also recommended that the federal government provide financial support for this collaboration. A major goal of all Indian improvement activities should be the training and hiring of native Americans in all program efforts.

Further research into the determination of specific nutritional problems in different areas of the country and the effects of such problems on the growth, health, and development of Indian children is needed. Findings from such research should then be translated into educational programs or into intervention efforts designed to improve the health and nutritional status of the Indian people. Sensitivity, appreciation, and consideration should be given to the unique social and cultural traditions of the Indian people.

Most of the recommendations developed as a result of the conference were formalized in the recommendations of the Panel on American

Table 5-4

Accessibility of Food Stamp Program on Surveyed Indian Reservations (Number of Reservations Surveyed Was 62)

Distance (miles)	Number of Reservations with Approximate Round-trip Distances from Farthest Home to		
	Certification Centers	Issuance Centers	Food Stores
0–30	13	12	12
31–80	19	19	15
81–160	16	18	8
161–300	6	5	1
300 plus	1	1	1

Indians and Alaska Natives of the White House Conference on Food, Nutrition and Health. Important focuses included the following:[34]

1. Improvement of the quality and quantity of food; this could be accomplished through federal food assistance programs. Enrichment or fortification of frequently used foods was suggested as a possibility for improving nutritional status. Meat, poultry, and dairy product quality and safety should be improved through the establishment and enforcement of improved grading and inspection regulations.

2. Protection and safety of indigenous foods; this could be accomplished through legal or programmatic approaches. Hunting and fishing sites should be defended, protected, and restocked as needed.

3. Identification and surveillance of nutritional status through comprehensive nutritional surveillance programs. Longitudinal studies of the growth and development of Indian children is needed. Federal financial support should be provided to assist these efforts.

4. Prevention of disease; programs to improve the health of native Americans should be developed and adequately funded.

5. Nutrition education; a comprehensive program should include a combination of professional and paraprofessional nutritionists; native Americans should be trained and used where possible. Education in food and nutrition should be mandated as part of school curricula at all levels; sociocultural beliefs and traditions should be incorporated into the education.

6. Indians should be encouraged to pursue careers in health and nutrition. Such education efforts should be integrated into school food programs.

In February 1977, the USDA sponsored a national workshop on "Food Issues Affecting the Indian Population." The purpose of the workshop was to discuss problems related to Indian participation in federal food assistance programs and to explore alternative methods to deliver needed services. Among the recommendations were the following:[35]

1. Continue the Food Distribution Program in areas where the Food Stamp Program is not meeting adequate food needs.

2. Allow tribal governments the right to administer the Food Stamp Program (such a right is currently granted to some tribes).

3. Provide 100 per cent federal funding of food assistance where tribes are incapable of raising necessary funds.

4. Test the feasibility of using mobile stores or food cooperatives to provide for food needs of reservations; investigate reservation food prices and accessibility of retail food stores.

5. Establish an Indian Advisory Committe within USDA to allow for broader Indian participation.

6. Allow reservations to be designated as food stamp project areas.

7. Provide a food package reflecting nutritional needs as well as sociocultural preferences of Indian populations.

8. Increase outreach activities in native Indian tongues.

9. Ensure that eligibility requirements are translated into native language when necessary.

10. Improve existing data collection methods to obtain more usable statistics on Indians.

The intent of these recommendations remains to be translated into reality.

SPANISH-SPEAKING IMMIGRANTS

Low-income Spanish, Puerto Rican, and Mexican-Americans comprise another U.S. subgroup with a high prevalence of nutritional problems. Since the 1940s there has been an increase in both legal and illegal migration to the United States from Mexico.[36] The "Mexican" immigrant may thus be a native to the area where he or she resides, may be a Mexican national, and may have come legally (*bracero* or "green card" holder) into the country or illegally (wetback) to find work and take up residence.

Spanish-speaking immigrants differ greatly in terms of culture, religion, social practices, language, life-styles, and experience. However, in many cases they are poorly educated and without specialized skills. Folklore, tradition, and social/cultural customs are especially important to immigrants because many of the elders of the people were illiterate and tradition was passed down through the generations. Another difference between Spanish-Americans and those of other ethnic minorities is the fact that, because their homeland is often very accessible to them and they are able to move back and forth from Mexico or Puerto Rico to the United States, they have the opportunity to renew their homeland traditions and practices.

P. Acosta and R. Aranda have described four groups of Californian-Mexicans in different stages of acculturation.[37]

1. Middle-class Mexican-Americans, often the descendants of many California-born generations, tend to display characteristics of the general middle-class culture.

2. The second and third generation of Mexican-Americans at different stages of acculturation still hold to certain of the cultural practices and traditions of their ancestors.

3. The first generation or Mexican nationals are well versed in all the cultural practices of their native homeland and cling to these beliefs and traditions; they often express the desire to return home.

4. Migrant farm workers may come from any of these groups but, because of the demands of the migratory life-style, are often unable to adopt middle-class customs and habits.

Cultural attitudes toward food often integrate the ideology of Greek humoral pathology manifested in the "hot-cold" dichotomy. G. N. Foster summarized the basic characteristics of this belief as follows:

Foods, herbs, illnesses and bodily states (such as sleeping and pregnancy) are characterized by degrees of "hot" and "cold"; sometimes actual temperature is involved, as when a person becomes overheated by the sun or wet from contact with cold water, but more often the putative degrees of heat and cold are innate characteristics, or properties, or substances. "Hot" illnesses or bodily states are treated with "cold" remedies. (And vice versa.) [38]

These ideas are often found, in variations, among Spanish-American populations. The ideas affect food intake, especially in times of illness or during pregnancy and lactation, infancy, and childhood. High-protein foods are often restricted during such periods.

As immigrants move to border areas, there is frequently a decline in breast-feeding with a concomitant rise in prolonged bottle-feeding. Although various foods are offered to the infant before the age of six months, meat is often withheld, possibly because of the idea that meat may be irritating to the infant.

Acosta reviewed the cultural determinants of food habits in young children of Mexican descent in various areas of California. Her findings included the following: In the East Los Angeles area, more mothers breast-fed their infants than did mothers in the border areas. Strained foods, with the exception of meat and eggs, were often added to the infants' diet by the age of 3 months. Mothers continued to believe that certain foods, often high-protein foods, should be restricted from the diets of young children, and of pregnant women and nursing mothers. It was suggested that such beliefs may be related to the factors of the "culture of poverty" influences where the people lived. [37]

Mothers living in Sal si Puedes continued to believe in the "hot" and "cold" theory of health and illness and modified their diets accordingly. Mothers in Hanford, California, said they were not familiar with this ideology, but their diets exemplified a number of factors that fit in with the "hot" and "cold" classification of food.

Factors that may have limited communication of these immigrants with other population subgroups included low educational levels; large families; illiteracy; inability to speak English; social, class, or racial discrimination; and poor socioeconomic conditions. By occasionally returning to their native Mexico to visit, beliefs were reinforced, and this may have helped to perpetuate the native ethnic traditions and ideology that influenced diets and nutritional status. [37]

Nutritional status surveys of Mexican-Americans have revealed significant problems, such as vitamin/mineral deficiency, low height for age, anemia, overnutrition, overweight, and elevated serum cholesterol.

Screening of 2,241 children in the 2- to 5-year-old age bracket indicated that the Arizona Mexican-American population had a high prevalence of short stature children. The low-weight-for-height condition did not appear to be a problem in the 2- to 5-year-old age groups. In fact, 13.3 per cent of the Mexican-American children were overweight. About 20 per cent of the 2- to 5-year-olds had hemoglobin readings below 11 gm/100 ml. Of the 294 Mexican-American children whose serum cholesterol levels were tested, 56.1 per cent had a reading greater than 160 mg. [39] Other studies have reported similar nutritional problems. [40]

MIGRANT LABORERS

It is not to die of hunger that makes a man wretched; many men have died. . . . But it is to live miserable [and] not know why; to work sore and yet gain nothing; to be heart-worn, weary, yet isolated, unrelated . . .

— Thomas Carlyle

In a real sense the migrant farmers form a "subculture" in this Nation. They live apart from the rest of us in a regular number of ways. By definition they are on the move, regularly or irregularly, living each year in several states and in the process usually managing to lose the many advantages of a permanent residence in any one of them.

— Coles, 1969

The traditional life-style of migrant families has hindered them from obtaining many of the basic comforts that are common to the majority of Americans. The migrant farm workers have been excluded from protective labor legislation, from educational opportunities, and from participation in many federal programs designed to improve the lives of needy Americans. (See Figure 5-3.)

Migrants face many serious problems related to obtaining needed social, educational, health, and nutritional services. It has been charged that the migrant farm work force actually subsidized agricultural policies through low wages, poor working conditions, and unsanitary, low-quality living conditions.[41] Federal, state, and local governments have been charged with institutionalizing the deprivation and poverty of the migrant people. The migrant worker has traditionally been excluded from protective labor legislation; where such legislation is applied to the migrant,[42] lack of enforcement often makes its effects meaningless.

Because the migrant is by definition transitory, the migrant's family is denied many social and educational opportunities that most Americans take for granted. The Report and Recommendation of the Panel on Nutrition and Special Groups charged that:

> Simply stated, the migrant has been maintained as a separate class — the poorest of the working poor — through deliberate societal policy. Because of their poverty and life style, migrants are economically eligible for most of the so-called benefit programs. Yet although their eligibility is dictated by social and economic policies which keep them poor, there has been an outright refusal to establish or administer benefit programs in such a way that they can meet migrant needs.[43]

Socioeconomic Conditions Experienced by Migrant Workers

In 1975 the USDA conducted a survey to determine the extent of USDA program services to migrant farm workers and the living conditions of migrants, to identify difficulties in obtaining nutrition benefits, and to suggest strategies for necessary improvement.

The study found that many of migrant workers' problems are directly related to their work. For example, the harvesting of food crops requires large numbers of workers at certain times of the year, but these times are often short and infrequent. Thus, the migrant farm worker must shift his or her life, family, and belongings according to climate shifts and the developing crops.

It is difficult to obtain an accurate count of migrant farm workers. The U.S. Department of Labor places the number at 208,000. Program managers of migrant assistance agencies set the figure at 500,000. At the opposite end of the spectrum, the figure used by organizations advocating the use of migrant workers, such as the United Farmworkers and the Teamsters, is 750,000. Accurate counts are complicated by the changes in residency and the difficulty in locating the migrants.[44] Most of the migrant workers are concentrated in ten states: Texas, California, Florida, Michigan, Arizona, Oregon, Ohio, Washington, New Mexico, and New York. Table 5–5 lists the breakdown of migrant workers' homes as obtained in the USDA survey.

According to the Economic Research Service's Hired Farming Working Force of 1974, the average income of migrants is $3,097, but this figure is deceiving. The gross income of the migrant worker is reduced by a variety of factors such as transportation, food, and housing, as well as by payoffs demanded by crew leaders, the withholding of income by farm managers, or the inability to collect promised cash bonuses.[45]

The USDA summed up the living conditions of the migrants as follows:

> Migrants, in most cases, are poor, minority, have a fourth grade education, possess few or no marketable skills, do not know how to avail themselves of public or private services, receive little information on programs designed to assist them, live a day to day existence, have an immediate need for income that deters them from enrolling in programs that may provide them with skills for other employment, have an average age range between 18 and 30 and a family size averaging five members.[44]

Table 5–5
Migrant Populations of Surveyed States

Area	Percentage of Migrants
Arizona	4%
Southern California	20
Central California	4
Florida	10
Mississippi	5
Oklahoma	3
South Carolina	5
Texas	42
Puerto Rico	5
Other	2

Source: U.S. Department of Agriculture, Office of Equal Opportunity, Compliance Enforcement Division. *USDA Reports on the Migrant Farm Worker.* Washington, D.C.: Government Printing Office, March 1976.

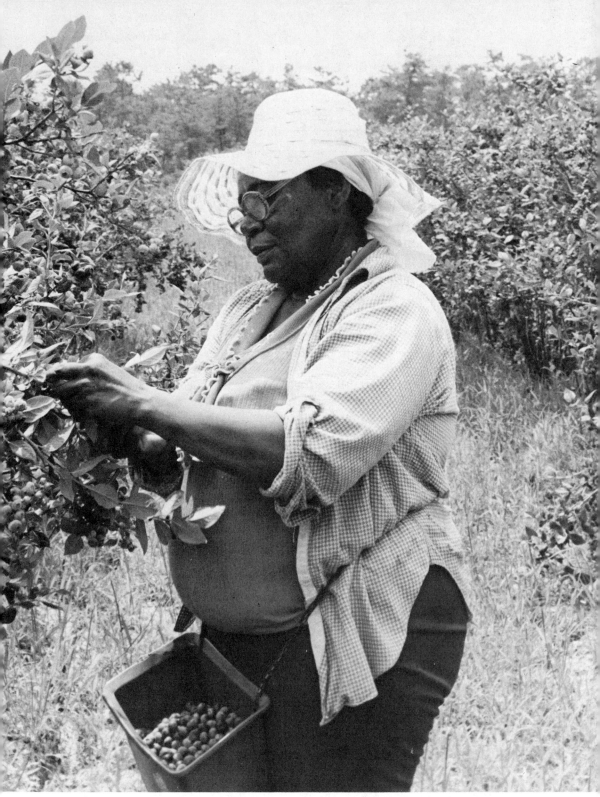

Figure 5–3. Migrant laborers are often the victims of an insidious exploitation that takes a devastating toll on their health and nutritional status. John Ripton photo, copyright 1978 by Food Monitor magazine. Reprinted by permission.

Further illustrating the tremendous living problems among migrants are the following:[46]

1. Anemia is common as are parasitic disorders that are found in almost 80 per cent of the migrant population.

2. The postnatal death rate per 1,000 live births in California is about 4.5 per cent above that of other occupational groups.

3. The average migrant family is composed of at least seven persons, with no fewer than five children in each family.

4. Deteriorated and substandard housing and poor sanitation conditions are other major problems of the migrant worker.

5. More than 800,000 migrant children work beside their parents as farm laborers; they thus miss out on formal education. Some 300,000 travel constantly with their families, attending two to three schools a year.

Nutrition Problems of Migrants

Describing their nutrition problems one observer noted: "stores were furnished to just half of the migrant employees, cooking utensils and dishes to only one-tenth, refrigeration was available to 9%; 3% had running water in their quarters, and 22% had running water outside."[47] Many migrants had to rely on drawing water from a well as their only source of water. If a company store was provided, the prices were always inflated, but, when there was no store run by the farmer, the migrants often had worse food problems because they had no transportation to go elsewhere to purchase food.

In *The Slaves We Rent*, T. Moore suggested: "A poor diet condemns the child from the start." He cited a case of 28 babies dying in a migrant camp in the San Joaquin Valley as a result of dehydration and malnutrition. "A report on a camp in Mathis, Texas, showed that 96 per cent of the children had no milk in six months. Their diet consisted mainly of cornmeal and rice. A doctor commenting on the report said there was evidence of "ordinary starvation." The migrant children were often noted to have scurvy, rickets, and kwashiorkor.[48]

W. Heaps, in *Wandering Workers*, discussed many case studies of migrant families. In response to his question, "Tell me about your food . . . ," one migrant mother replied that their meals consisted of fried pork, oxtails, pigs' feet, and beef bones, tomatoes (they picked these), chitlings when in the South, rice, grits, cornmeal, and yams. "Salads and desserts, never! Of course, we eat the fruits and vegetables we pick (the bad ones they give us free)." The mother reported using flour for biscuits and gravies. Butter was never used as it did not keep and there were no refrigerators. Food items were purchased daily at the company store and charged; they were paid for at the end of the migrants' stay. Heaps noted that, "Vitamin deficiencies are common and excessive intake of starches and fats causes a dietary imbalance which affects their general health." Migrant mothers are often very concerned about the diets of their children, but do not know how to improve them.[49]

The results of a nutritional survey of Florida seasonal farm workers provides a perspective on the life-style and nutritional status of farm worker families.[50] Many farm worker families seem to live from day to day with little interest or ability in planning for the future. Often dependent upon public assistance for resources to obtain their food, these families tended to eat better at the beginning of the month. Children were taught to become independent at a very young age, as reflected by their dietary patterns. Children were often responsible for preparing their own meals or for buying snacks to stave off hunger. Many schoolchildren received free or reduced-price meals, which provided a large part of their nutrition.

Rarely did families eat the evening meal together. In many cases, there were not enough chairs or space in the home to allow the family to sit down together. Individual family members frequently ate what they wanted, when they wanted. Diets tended to lack variety, and new foods were seldom introduced. Although generalizations may obscure the individual family differences, the following provide some insight into "typical" meal patterns and dietary habits of subgroups of farm workers.[50]

Spanish-Americans often ate refried beans (pinto, navy, or chick peas) with fried rice at many meals. A large pot of rice, to which was added pieces of sausage, peppers, tomatoes, or potatoes was often boiled in the morning and provided food throughout the day. Puerto Ricans followed a similar pattern, boiling a pot of salted codfish, yams, yautias (similar to white potatoes), and plantains.

Black families observed "boiling" or "frying" days. On a weekly basis, families boiled a large pot of greens with lard, salt pork, bacon, neck bones, or ham hocks. Dried beans and blackeyed peas were also prepared. Other popular foods included fried cornbread, biscuits, and gravy. Both Spanish-Americans and blacks liked fried chicken and fish and fresh fruit.

A survey of the nutritional status of the workers suggested that the most serious problem was iron deficiency anemia. Other problems included folacin deficiency, retarded growth of the children, and obesity among the adults.[50]

In an attempt to address these problems and to improve the dietary and nutritional status of the population, an intensive nutrition education program was implemented. The project included community health workers who provided a great service by making health information relevant, understandable, and available to their peers. As intermediaries between the professionals and the client group, their aid was considered indispensable. Resurveys of nutritional status after the three-month education program indicated slight improvements.

Knowledge of the nutritional status of various migrant groups is very limited. Those migrants who have been studied seem to be fairly consistent with those reported by Kaufman.[50] Results of selected other studies of Mexican-Americans or migrants and their nutritional status are presented in Table 5–6.

Nutrition Programs for Migrants

A number of programs have been designed to improve the health and nutritional status of migrant workers and their families. USDA programs

Table 5-6
Nutritional Status Survey of Mexican Americans or Migrant Workers

Reference	*Population*	*Major Findings*
(56)	149 Mexican American families studied over 3 years in Lower Rio Grande Valley, Texas	Vit. A intake compared favorably with RDA. Vit. D intake generaly deficient. Consumption of fruits, vegetable and milk products was low. Iron intake low, protein intake adequate. Biochemical and clinical evidence of Vit. A deficiency. Low height and weight of children was common.
(52)	65 Mexican migrant families in California	Families shopped once a week, spending an average of $40 at markets chosen for low prices. Demonstrated food habits reflecting poverty: high consumption of beans, white bread or tortillas. Ethnic backgrounds reflected in food preferred and frequency of consumption, in folklore about menstruation, in knowledge of other peoples' foods.
(53)	175 preschoolers of Mexican descent evaluated on basis of data from physical, dietary, biochemical, dental and medical history evaluations	One third were 1 or more S.D. below mean of Iowa growth standards for height. One fourth were below 16th percentile for weight. Most children met 2/3 RDA for protein. 12% didn't meet 2/3 of 1968 RDAs for energy; for other nutrients, the following % didn't meet 2/3 RDA: % nutrient 11 calcium 44 iron 13 thiamine 23 preformed niacin 7 Vit. A 29 Vit. C More than 50% were iron deficient; 1% had low plasma Vit. A; 9% had low plasma Vit. C.

available to the migrant include the school lunch, school breakfast, special food service programs for children, special milk program, nonfood assistance program, food stamps, the WIC programs, and the Nutrition Program for the elderly (however, there are usually few elderly among the migrants).

Migrant health programs offered through the Department of Labor provide preventive health services, including services designed to prevent malnutrition, prenatal, and postpartum services, ongoing periodic screening for young children, and health education.[54]

According to the Migrant Health Center Act, P.L. 94-673, primary health services, which all grant recipients must provide, are preventive health services, which include medical, social, nutritional assessment and referral, preventive health education, family planning, immunizations, and prenatal and postpartum care, and well-child care (including periodic screening).[54]

In addition, supplementary health services, which are not required but may be provided by a migrant health center, include nutrition education. Other programs for migrants that provide nutrition assistance include those sponsored by the Migrant Ministry of the National Council of Churches and special programs for migrant workers and their families through Community Action Programs.

In addition, some local migrant centers and programs are designed to meet the health, educational, and nutritional needs of the migrants. In one such program in Colorado, an effort is made to enroll students in free and reduced-price school lunch and special summer food programs. There is also an attempt to get the children to accept new foods and to include ethnic foods in the menu. Techniques used in this program include tasting parties designed to introduce unfamiliar foods to the children, providing nutrition and food-related information in cafeterias in Spanish, and hiring local migrants to work as cafeteria aides and cooks.[55]

Another successful project is the Migrant Nutrition Education Project located in Hidalgo County in Texas.[56] The project provides nutritional assessments of Mexican-American migrant farm workers' children, followed by nutrition education and increased enrollment in food assistance programs. Bilingual Mexican-American mothers from the target population, hired and trained as nutrition aides, work primarily on a one-to-one home visit basis with migrant homemakers. Those migrant farmers who worked with the aides made more progress than did others, suggesting that the use of additional homemakers as aides was desirable.[56]

Recommendations for Improving the Nutritional Status of the Migrants

Any recommendations designed to improve the nutritional and health status of the migrant worker must consider the migrants' unique situations, which are very different from those of many other impoverished groups. The Panel on Nutrition and Special Groups suggested that basic improvements should include the provision of an adequate income for all individuals.[13] But beyond this, the panel suggested that USDA create an Indian and Migrant Program Division to attend to the unique needs of these two vulnerable groups. Existing food programs should have provisions for the participation of migrant laborers. For example, centralized administrative control and decentralization of program operations for migrants would allow them to have continuous, rather than "hit or miss" opportunities to participate.

Other recommendations included:

1. The creation of a national food and nutrition program for the migrant farm worker, centralized in a single office.

2. The creation of grants and contracts with private organizations and community groups to develop new techniques for delivering food and nutritional services to migrants.

3. The funding for development of cooperatives and other food-purchasing ventures.

4. Expanded and improved outreach to familiarize the migrant with available assistance.

5. Programs to be systematically organized and provided in a bilingual manner.

Conclusions — Solutions to Poverty[1]

Basic to the alleviation of economic-related malnutrition is the elimination of economic poverty. There are two general strategies for alleviating poverty.[1]

1. The universal services approach — this involves the creation of free or reduced-price services available to all on an equal basis, without consideration of income.

2. The selective programs approach — various target groups are selected to receive specified program services; goals of programs are tailored to the perceived needs of the clients.

The universal services approach is evidenced by the American system of free public education through high school or protective services such as police and firemen. In many European nations, this concept of universal services has been extended to include programs of free health and dental care, job training with pay, public housing, and low-cost day care centers.

There are many reasons for the lack of success of the selective programs approach. Such programs have been defined and described in terms as "programs for the poor are poor programs." Limitations of such programs that are directed only at the poor include the following:

1. Benefits are maintained at a low level to discourage workers from stopping work to participate and to encourage participants to look for work.

2. Poverty programs tend to enjoy limited political support. The middle class, which usually bears the burden of supporting such programs, has the attitude, "Why should I work hard to support those who don't work? Why should my hard-earned dollars be spent on the poor who are too lazy to work?"

3. Thus, there is a social stigma surrounding the operation of these programs. Many eligible poor decline to participate because of the loss of respect entailed.

4. Such programs may blame the victims; those who are poor, not through their own fault, are blamed for their situation; the social system, which in reality is also responsible, is not blamed.

5. The underlying assumption of all such poverty programs is that, by helping the poor to reenter the market system, they will function adequately on their own; such is not necessarily the case as was pointed out in preceding paragraphs.

By contrast, the universal services strategy does not have many of these drawbacks. Some advantages of universal services programs are the following:

1. Because all participants benefit, the programs usually enjoy strong political support. An example is that of the school lunch program whose benefits extend to all children attending schools where the programs operate. Such programs are more successful than most federal food programs.

2. Because benefits are available to all, there is no need to keep them unreasonably low as a disincentive.

3. Because all are able to participate, there is no social stigma.

4. Universal services programs engender cooperation and union among the poor and the middle class (the nonrich) instead of placing them at odds.

In the long run, the nutritional status of the poor in the United States can be best improved by increasing the social circumstances of the disadvantaged. In other words, nutrition and health can be improved by allowing the underdog a chance to enjoy a life of better quality, one that is more likely to enable him or her to improve his or her dietary patterns. Inherent in such a process is the fostering of a different system of values and attitudes toward the poor.

But such a goal will take a tremendous period of time to be realized. Given human nature and the American societal and political structure, this goal may never be achieved. An alternative suggestion is to switch from the selective programs approach to a universal services approach. It is clear that the political ramifications of such an approach would be tremendous; but it is, according to some, the only feasible way to improve the health and nutritional status of the poor.[1]

Beyond such approaches, other strategies have been suggested to improve the health and nutritional status of low-income groups. The following provide a basis for developing comprehensive programs to this end:[50]

1. Nutritional surveillance should be available to all; it should be ongoing and integrated into other health care services. It should serve as a guide to referral and follow-up care and for the design of nutrition education programs. It should be integrated into school physical examinations for schoolchildren, into baby clinics for infants, and into other health care services available to the population. The surveillance should be followed up with referrals as needed, dietary evaluation, education, and counseling.

2. Nutrition education and counseling should be integrated into the

school curricula, into family health programs, and into programs geared to the pregnant woman and lactating mother, infant, and young child. Such education should be comprehensive, long-term, and provided as part of a total community, health, education, and welfare effort.

3. Existing food assistance programs, such as the school lunch and breakfast program, the WIC Program, and the Food Stamp Program, should be strengthened and expanded and should include the development of effective nutrition education efforts.

Food Cooperatives[57]

Food cooperatives have been suggested as another strategy for helping the low-income poor to improve their diets through food production and distribution. Food cooperatives offer a mechanism whereby the poor can work together to advance their own interests and can help themselves to better diets by participating in the food distribution system. Food cooperatives, if properly managed and supported (through human, financial, and technological resources), can offer people an alternative access to the food supply.

Food cooperatives may take a variety of forms:

1. Buying Clubs — associations of families who join efforts to buy food from wholesale dealers. If labor is shared among members, the savings in food costs can be substantial. In some areas, coalitions of individual buying clubs join efforts and improve the effectiveness of the cooperatives.

2. Cooperative Stores — more formal than buying clubs, these formed when individuals organize and start their own food stores.

3. Direct Charge Outlets — defined as "amalgams" of the cooperative store and food buying club, such outlets entail the establishment of a warehouse facility that displays food without promotional materials. Participants are charged a wholesale rate plus a small fee per week.

Food cooperatives are usually established to provide open membership to interested individuals who desire similar services. Each member has one vote in determining cooperative operation. There is a restricted return on the capital invested in the cooperative, and surplus is refunded to members. In other words, cooperatives operate on a cash basis, but not for profit. There is frequently an effort to provide ongoing education of members. There are numerous advantages and benefits to food cooperatives, but there are also many limitations. The Panel on Nutrition and Special Groups reviewed the subject of food cooperatives and listed advantages as well as restraints. These are presented in Tables 5–7 and 5–8.[43]

Although the limitations of food cooperatives are considerable, the benefits are strong enough to conclude that cooperatives do offer a significant and workable alternative for groups who desire to work together to improve nutrition by surmounting some economic difficulties.

Table 5-7
Food Cooperatives — Benefits

1. Cooperatives are by their very structure and nature democratic-egalitarian institutions, based on equality of participation rather than the predetermined privileges of accumulated wealth. Co-ops allow people to participate in a cohesive effort on an equal basis with one man-one voice-one vote.

2. Cooperatives can, through astute purchasing, careful management, and membership loyalty, reduce the cost of food purchases to consumers. These savings can be realized immediately or accumulated as a surplus and invested for longer term benefits from the enterprise.

3. Cooperatives can provide some employment to a limited number of low income people connected with their development and operation.

4. Through purchasing from a cooperative, members with no investment can earn equity through the "patronage principle" of returning surplus margins to members according to use of the co-op. Thus, poor people with large families, who do all their purchasing through the co-op, will earn a proportionately high share of refunds which can be converted to equity ownership or withdrawn as savings.

5. The development and ownership of a cooperative enterprise can instill a sense of pride and accomplishment in poor people. The dignity and responsibility of owning their own enterprise is a less tangible but perhaps more significant result of economic cooperation among the poor.

6. Consumer cooperatives, with an interest in the health and welfare of their members, can often put emphasis on sales of higher quality and more nutritions products than other more competitive outlets. Cooperatives can and do provide members more education on nutrition and the proper balance of foods to buy and eat.

7. A strong urban consumer's movement among the poor could stimulate more contacts, linkages and markets for producer cooperatives of small family farmers in rural areas. This linkage between consumer and producer interests could produce real economic benefits and savings for both groups.

Source: U.S. Senate Select Committee on Nutrition and Human Needs, Panel on Nutrition and Special Groups. *The Development of Poor People's Food Cooperatives. National Policy Study, Part 3.* Washington, D.C.: Government Printing Office, 1974.

Table 5-8
Food Cooperatives — Limitations

1. The inability of isolated, small, consumer cooperative outlets to compete in their purchasing, pricing, and public relations, with large national and multinational food chains. The economics of scale, vertical integration of products, managerial expertise, and system of suppliers, developed by these food system giants is difficult for a small community-based group to overcome. Only through a large, unified, integrated effort of consumer cooperatives, acting in concert, could any countervailing pressure or alternative be built to the present oligarchial control of the food processing and distribution industry.

2. Consumer cooperatives among the poor suffer from a deficiency of trained and dedicated managerial personnel. More training programs are needed to prepare managers for entreprenurial positions like that of community co-op store managers. Black colleges and other educational institutions, in their present effort to develop

Food Cooperatives — Limitations (*continued*)

programs of community responsibility and involvement, ought to take note of the need for more trained managers for small businesses and adjust their curricula accordingly.

3. Consumer cooperatives, as other ventures among the poor and minority people, are usually under-capitalized at the outset, which contributes to stifling growth and frustrating the fulfillment of their basic promises. More flexible sources of credit, at more concessionary interest rates and terms, must be found to support consumer cooperatives and other community development enterprises.

4. More membership education and understanding is needed to undergird poor peoples' organizations from within. More funds, time and technical people need to be made available for this training task.

Source: U.S. Senate Select Committee on Nutrition and Human Needs, Panel on Nutrition and Special Groups. *The Development of Poor People's Food Cooperatives. National Policy Study, Part 3.* Washington, D.C.: Government Printing Office, 1974.

SUMMARY

Most of the current approaches to the alleviation of poverty attempt to meet the short-term needs and problems of the poor by improving existing programs. Increased funding, personnel and outreach efforts, improved organization and administration, and better public support are all aimed at increasing the effectiveness of existing antipoverty programs.

However, there is scant evidence of improvement in the lives of the poor or in reducing the numbers afflicted by poverty. Some even contend that "systemic social forces prevent the success of such programs and are creating hunger and poverty faster than programs can be enacted."[1]

Basic to alleviating poverty and the resulting malnutrition is a diligent attempt to understand the real nature and the causes (including the social systems and institutions) of poverty. When these factors have been discovered and carefully defined, attempts can be made to design new programs in line with new goals.

REFERENCES

1. Moyer, W. A strategy for ending domestic hunger. *Church and Society* (November–December 1975): 37.
2. Lewis, O. *The Children of Sanchez: An Autobiography of a Mexican Family.* New York: Random House, 1961.
3. U.S. Department of Health, Education, and Welfare. *The Measure of Poverty: A Report to Congress as Mandated by the Education Amendments of 1974.* Washington, D.C.: Government Printing Office, April 1976.
4. In the race between income and inflation. *U.S. News and World Report,* August 21, 1978, p. 76.
5. U.S. Senate Select Committee on Nutrition and Human Needs. *Hunger 1973 and Press Reaction.* Washington, D.C.: Government Printing Office, 1973.

6. Brown, W. Rural poor shortchanged on public aid, report says. *Washington Post*, February 28, 1979, p. A3.

7. Gardner, N. The plight of rural women in upstate New York. *Conference Proceedings*, Syracuse University, Syracuse, N.Y., April 2, 1976.

8. White House Conference on Food, Nutrition, and Health. *Report of the Consumer Task Force*. Washington, D.C.: U.S. Government Printing Office, 1969.

9. U.S. Department of Agriculture, Consumer Expenditure Survey. *National Food Situation*, Publ. No. NFS-152. Washington, D.C., May 1975.

10. Manchester, A., and L. Brown. Do the poor pay more? *National Food Situation*, Publ. No. NFS-160. Washington, D.C.: U.S. Department of Agriculture, June 1977, p. 27.

11. Schnapper, D. Comment. *Yale Law J.* 76 (1967): 745.

12. U.S. Department of Commerce, Bureau of Census. *Statistical Abstract of the United States*. Washington, D.C.: Government Printing Office, 1975.

13. U.S. Senate Select Committee on Nutrition and Human Needs. *National Nutrition Policy Study. Part 3. Nutrition and Special Groups*. Washington, D.C.: Government Printing Office, June 19, 1974.

14. Taylor, T. V. *The States and Their Indian Citizens*. Washington, D.C.: U.S. Department of the Interior, Bureau of Indian Affairs, 1972.

15. U.S. Department of Commerce, Economic Development Administration. *Helping Them to Help Themselves*. Washington, D.C.: Government Printing Office, May 1972.

16. U.S. Department of Health, Education, and Welfare. *Health of the American Indian*. Washington, D.C.: Government Printing Office, April 1973.

17. U.S. Department of Health, Education, and Welfare, Office of Program Statistics. *Indian Health Trends and Services*, 1974 ed. Washington, D.C.: Government Printing Office, 1974.

18. Farris, C. Indian children: The struggle for survival. *Social Work* 21 (1976): 386–389.

19. Kunitz, S. J., J. E. Levy, C. L. Odoroff, and J. Bollinger. The epidemiology of alcoholic cirrhosis in two southwestern Indian tribes. *Q. J. Stud. on Alc.* 32 (1971): 706.

20. Van Duzen, J., J. P. Carter, J. Secondi, and C. Federspiel. Protein and calorie malnutrition among preschool Navajo Indian children. *Am. J. Clin. Nutr.* 22 (1969): 1362.

21. French, J. G. Relationship of morbidity to the feeding patterns of Navajo children from birth through twenty-four months. *Am. J. Clin. Nutr.* 20 (1967): 375.

22. Owen, G. M., C. Nelson, K. Kram, and P. Garry. Nutrition survey of White Mountain Apache preschool children, in *Nutrition, Growth, and Development of North American Indian Children*, Publ. No. (NIH) 72–26. Washington, D.C.: U.S. Department of Health, Education, and Welfare, 1969.

23. Carlile, W. K., H. G. Olson, J. Gorman, C. McCracken, R. VanderWagen, and H. Connor. Contemporary nutritional status of North American Indian children, in *Nutrition, Growth, and Development of North American Indian Children, op. cit.*

24. Reisinger, K., K. Rogers, and A. Johnson. Nutrition survey of lower Greasewood, Arizona Navajo, *ibid.*

25. Moore, W. M., M. Silverberg, and M. S. Read, eds. *Nutrition, Growth, and Development of North American Indian Children*, Publ. No. (NIH) 72-26. Based on a conference cosponsored by the National Institute of Child Health and Human Development, Indian Health Service, and American Academy of Pediatrics Committee on Indian Health. Washington, D.C.: U.S. Department of Health, Education, and Welfare, 1972.

26. Darby, W. J., C. G. Salsbury, W. J. McGanity, H. F. Johnson, E. B. Bridgforth, and H. Sanstead. Study of the dietary background and nutriture of the Navajo Indian. *J. Nutr.* 60 (1956): Suppl. 2, 3–85.

27. University of Pittsburgh. *Nutrition Survey of the Lower Greasewood Chapter Navajo Tribe, 1968–1969.*

28. Nance, E. B. Food consumption of 200 Navajo adults receiving USDA-donated foods. Unpublished Master's thesis. Denton, Texas. Texas Woman's University, 1972.

29. Horner, M. G., C. M. Olson, and D. J. Pringle. Nutritional status of Chippewa Head Start children in Wisconsin. *Am. J. Publ. Health* 67 (1977): 185.

30. Van Duzen, J., J. P. Carter, and R. Vander Zwick. Protein and calorie malnutrition among preschool Navajo Indian children. A follow-up. *Am. J. Clin. Nutr.* 29 (1976): 657.

31. Bass, M. A., and L. M. Wakefield. Nutrient intake and food patterns of Indians on Standing Rock Reservation. *J. Am. Diet. Assoc.* 64 (1974): 36.

32. Carmody, T. In Testimony before the U.S. Senate Select Committee on Nutrition and Human Needs. Washington, D.C.: Government Printing Office, March 25, 1977.

33. U.S. Senate Select Committee on Nutrition and Human Needs. *Recommendations for Improved Food Programs on Indian Reservations.* Washington, D.C.: Government Printing Office, April 1977.

34. White House Conference on Food, Nutrition, and Health. *Report of the Subpanel on American Indians and Alaska Natives: Eskimos, Indians, and Aleuts. Final Report.* Washington, D.C.: Government Printing Office, 1970, pp. 82–88.

35. U.S. Department of Agriculture. *Food Issues Affecting the Indian Population.* Washington, D.C., 1977.

36. Burma, J. H. *Spanish-speaking Groups in the United States.* Durham, N.C.: Duke University Press, 1954.

37. Acosta, P. B., and R. B. Arand. Mexican-American low-income groups, in *Practices of Low-income Families in Feeding Infants and Small Children with Particular Attention to Cultural Subgroups. Proceedings of a National Workshop.* Rockville, Md.: U.S. Department of Health, Education, and Welfare, 1972.

38. Foster, G. N. International conference on prevention of malnutrition in the preschool child. Social anthropology and nutrition of the preschool child, especially as related to Latin America, in *Preschool Child Malnutrition: Primary Deterrent to Human Progress.* Washington, D.C.: National Academy of Sciences, National Research Council, 1966.

39. Yanochik-Owen, A., and M. White. Nutrition surveillance in Arizona: Selected anthropometric and laboratory observations among Mexican children. *Am. J. Publ. Health* 67 (1977): 151–154.

40. Jacob, M., I. F. Hunt, O. Dirige, and M. E. Swendseid. Biochemical assessment of the nutritional status of low-income pregnant women of Mexican descent. *Am. J. Clin. Nutr.* 29 (1976): 650.

41. U.S. House Subcommittee on Agricultural Labor of the House Committee on Education and Labor. Seminar on Farm Labor Problems. Washington, D.C., June 2–3, and 10, 1971.

42. U.S. Congress. The National Labor Relations Act, 29, U.S.C. Sections 207 (3), 207 (c)-(d).

43. U.S. Senate Select Committee on Nutrition and Human Needs, Panel on Nutrition and Special Groups. *Nutrition and Migrant Laborers, Part 4.* Washington, D.C.: Government Printing Office, June 1974.

44. U.S. Department of Agriculture, Office of Equal Opportunity. *USDA Reports on the Migrant Farm Worker.* Washington, D.C.: Government Printing Office, March 1976.

45. U.S. Department of Agriculture. *Income of Farm Wageworker Households in 1971*, Rept. No. 251. Washington, D.C., 1974, p. vii.

46. Fuentes, J. A. The need for effective and comprehensive planning for migrant workers. *Am. J. Publ. Health* 64 (1974): 2–10.

47. Brooks, M. S. *The Social Problems of Migrant Farm Laborers.* Carbondale, Ill.: Southern Illinois University, Department of Sociology, 1960, pp. 82–83.

48. Moore, T. *The Slaves We Rent.* New York: Random House, 1965, p. 57.

49. Heaps, W. A. *Wandering Workers.* New York: Crown Publishers, 1968, pp. 29–30, 71, 138–147.

50. Kaufman, M., E. Lewis, A. Hardy, and J. Proulx. Florida seasonal farm workers. Follow-up and intervention following a nutrition survey. *J. Am. Diet. Assoc.* 66 (1975): 605.

51. Larson, L. B., J. M. Dodds, D. M. Massoth, and H. P. Chase. Nutritional status of children of Mexican-American migrant families. *J. Am. Diet. Assoc.* 64 (1974): 29.

52. Bruhn, C. M., and R. M. Pangborn. Comparisons between Mexican-Americans and "Anglos." Food habits of migrant farm workers in California. *J. Am. Diet. Assoc.* 59 (1971): 347–355.

53. Acosta, P. B., R. G. Arand, J. V. Lewis, and M. Read. Nutritional status of Mexican-American preschool children in a border town. *Am. J. Clin. Nutr.* 27 (1974): 1359.

54. Legislative highlights. *J. Am. Diet. Assoc.* 65 (1974): 570.

55. Reaching the migrant child. *Food and Nutr.* 4 (February 1974): 10–11.

56. Larson, L. B., D. M. Massoth, and H. B. Chase. A potpourri of nutrition education methods. *J. Nutr. Ed.* 6 (1974): 20–21.

57. U.S. Senate Select Committee on Nutrition and Human Needs, Panel on Nutrition and Special Groups. *The Development of Poor People's Food Cooperatives. National Policy Study, Part 3.* Washington, D.C.: Government Printing Office, 1974.

6

Nutritional status of vulnerable groups throughout the lifespan

Reader Objectives

After completing this chapter, the reader should be able to
1. Define the "at-risk" concept.
2. State the reasons why the following might be considered at risk for developing nutritional problems:
   — Pregnant women and lactating mothers.
   — Infants and children.
   — Adolescents.
   — The elderly.
3. Describe the use of the "at-risk" concept for the planning of intervention programs.

OVERVIEW — PERSPECTIVES ON THE AT-RISK CONCEPT

This chapter reviews population subgroups who are "at-risk" relative to optimal nutritional status. The at-risk concept has recently been given a scientific definition and increased attention as a tool in nutritional assessment and surveillance. The concept has been defined in terms of the health and nutrition of young children as follows:

> a major, identifiable biological or environmental circumstance or event, affecting women in child bearing years, especially during pregnancy and lactation, or infants and young children, which increases the risk of severe illness, especially malnutrition . . . and therefore suggests the need for prevention, and special care and attention.[1]

At-risk factors have been variously categorized as environmental, biological, or social factors and may be identified at the level of the community, the family, or the individual. As an example, various at-risk indicators of malnutrition that may be identified in industrial nations are illustrated in Figure 6–1. Many of the economics-related risk factors have been discussed in greater detail in Chapter 5.

Use of the At-risk Concept for the Planning of Interventions

The at-risk factors should be viewed as dynamic and constantly changing, rather than as static. Once data have been collected on the prevalence and incidence of risk factors, analysis would include the frequency with which given risk factors were associated with undesirable outcomes. As an example, is it a biological risk factor? What percentage of the cases evidence the factor?

When problem identification has been accomplished, the problems should be rated according to priority for action; the priority can be assigned in view of the following considerations:[1]

1. Ranking associated factors in an agreed-upon order.

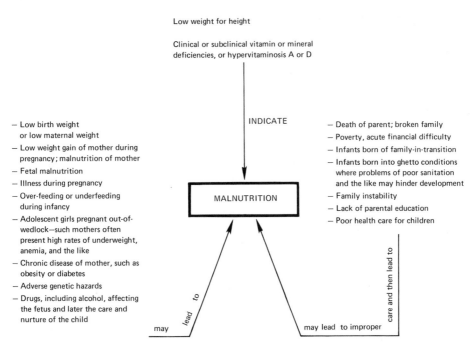

Figure 6-1. At-risk indicators of malnutrition in industrialized nations. (Adapted from IUNS, 1977)

2. Examination of the factors to identify interrelationship or interactions. For example, the combined effects or the synergistic effects of two or more factors may be greater than the total of the individual effects.

3. If available resources allow, and if program needs indicate, more sophisticated statistical analysis may be undertaken. Such techniques as correlations, multiple regression analysis, or path analysis may disclose helpful results.

4. The first result should be a guide that can be easily and practically applied to problems at the community, family, or individual level. The main objective is to identify from "an as yet unaffected population on the basis of at-risk factors, these individuals most likely to develop the undesirable outcome," and from this information to devise and implement appropriate intervention actions.

Information derived from the at-risk concept can be used not only to identify possible intervention points but also to improve the economy of health care delivery services, which can be achieved in a number of ways:

1. To identify the population most at risk.

2. To identify the point at which intervention actions are likely to be most successful.

3. To identify changing trends in a given situation; such information can serve to warn policymakers and planners about the need to develop appropriate actions before there is a severe crisis.

4. To evaluate the effect of the program as a whole, rather than to look at individual performance.

In sum, the at-risk concept is a helpful tool in the planning and implementation of programs. There is need, however, to broaden an awareness of the usefulness and applicability of the approach and to increase research into various ways in which the concept can be expanded and its operationalization increased. This chapter focuses on groups throughout the life span who are frequently at risk of developing nutritional problems. The groups discussed are pregnant and lactating women (at risk because of their increased nutrient needs and because of the nutrient needs of their offspring), infants, children and adolescents (at risk because their rapid growth demands high-quality diets), and the elderly (at risk because of various social, physiological, and economic problems that may prevent their obtaining adequate nutrition).

NUTRITIONALLY VULNERABLE MOTHERS AND CHILDREN

Pregnant women and lactating mothers and very young children are especially vulnerable to malnutrition. Lack of adequate nutrition during pregnancy or during the child's early years may restrict nutrients that are needed for proper physical and mental growth and development.

PREGNANCY

The object of maternity care is to ensure that every expectant and nursing mother maintains good health, learns . . . child care, has a normal delivery, and bears healthy children. Maternity care in the narrower sense consists in the care of the pregnant woman, her safe delivery, her postnatal care and examination, the care of her newly born infant, and the maintenance of lactation. In the wider sense, it begins much earlier in measures aimed to promote the health and well-being of the young people who are potential parents, and to help them to develop the right approach to family life and to the place of the family in the community. It should also include guidance in parentcraft and in problems associated with infertility and family planning.[2]

Despite its wealth and vast technological advancement, the United States does not have an impressive record of favorable pregnancy outcomes. Infant, neonatal, and maternal death rates as well as percentage of low-birth-weight infants in the United States are much higher than they should be. Table 6-1 summarizes some of these statistics.[3]

No one factor is responsible for these poor pregnancy outcomes. A combination of limited health care and poor economic circumstances is probably the underlying cause of many maternal or neonatal difficulties. Increasing attention is also being paid to the quality of the pregnant mother's diet as being significantly associated with maternal and infant health and welfare.[4-5]

Table 6-1
Statistics Indicating Health Risks Affecting U.S. Mothers and Infants

Percentage of U.S. Infants with Low Birth Weight (less than 2,500 gm)	
1960	7.7%
1965	8.3
1970	7.9
1975	7.4

Infant and Neonatal* Mortality Rates per 1,000 Live Births		
	During First Year of Life	*During First 28 Day of Life*
1960	26.0	18.7
1965	24.7	17.7
1970	20.0	15.1
1973	17.7	13.0
1975	16.1	11.6

Maternal Deaths Resulting from Complications of Pregnancy, Childbirth, and Puerperium** per 100,000 Live Births	
1960	37.1
1965	31.6
1970	21.5
1973	15.2
1975	12.8

*Neonatal — during first months of life.
**Puerperium — period during and immediately after childbirth.
Source: C. Olson and M. Mapes: Nutrition, growth and reproduction. Reducing the risks for mothers and infants. Ithaca, N.Y.: Cornell University, May, 1977.

It has been estimated that between 10 per cent and 20 per cent of low-birth-weight babies born yearly, or 120,000 babies, in the United States have suffered malnutrition before their birth. Malnutrition *in utero* can be the result of many factors such as inhibited nutrient transfer across the placenta — it does not necessarily reflect maternal lack of adequate nutrients. We do not know how many of these infants were born to malnourished mothers.[6]

Nutrition and Pregnancy

We cannot yet precisely define the role of nutrition in determining pregnancy outcome, but increasing evidence indicates that malnutrition of the mother is associated with low birth weight, stillbirth, neonatal mortality, and birth defects. Research is continuing to investigate the relationship between maternal malnutrition and brain development and the later mental and physical performance of offspring.

The most important factor in infant mortality rates is that of low-birth-weight babies, those who weigh 2,500 gm or less at birth.[7] Other abnormalities associated with low birth weight include congenital anomalies of the central nervous system, such as cerebral palsy and mental retardation, deafness, and blindness.[8]

Before looking more closely at the relationship between maternal nutrition and low-birth-weight babies, it is important that we distinguish between two different classes of low-birth-weight babies. One class is composed of babies of normal weight for gestation, but who are delivered before term. These infants are called "premature." The other classification, often called small-for-gestational-age infants, or small-for-date infants (SFDI), are delivered at full term but are underweight.

The SFDI have been termed "undernourished term infants."[9] They are believed to be underdeveloped *in utero* as the result of intrauterine growth retardation or fetal malnutrition. This group is the concern of the following paragraphs.[10] It has been estimated that as many as 50 per cent of the infants born among populations living in poverty are SFDI.[11] Several factors contribute to the condition: maternal preeclampsia, cigarette smoking by the mother after 20 weeks gestation, and small maternal size (i.e., small height for weight indicating possible maternal malnutrition earlier in life) have been associated with SFDI.[8]

R. Williams studied 84.1 per cent of the live babies born in California between 1966 and 1970. A total of 1,424,637 infants were categorized by birth weight, gestational age, and race, and intrauterine growth curves (i.e., curves relating mean birth weight to completed gestation time) were constructed for different ethnic groups. Up to the gestational time of 36 weeks, the growth curves of whites (non-Spanish), Spanish, blacks, and Orientals were similar; beyond 36 weeks the growth curves of the black and Spanish infants were lower than the other two groups, a factor that neither race nor environment could account for. When race was held constant, the effect of the environment on intrauterine growth was demonstrated. Although environmental factors such as medical care, housing, sanitation, and other living conditions were not studied, the author concluded that "the mother's nutritional status during the third trimester of pregnancy is far the most likely single cause for prenatal growth retardation." [12]

The effect of maternal malnutrition on fetal growth is not fully known. It is very difficult to define a direct cause-and-effect relationship between the nutritional status of the mother and the pregnancy outcome, in part because nutrition is associated with so many socioeconomic variables and exerts its influence in concert with many other factors. Most researchers believe that a prolonged lack of an adequate diet during pregnancy can be harmful to either mother or to offspring. Although fetal nutrition is not always related to maternal diets, there is evidence to suggest that severe food restriction in late pregnancy can result in a low-birth-weight infant.[13]

Animal Studies

The notion that maternal malnutrition might be related to fetal or pregnancy anomalies was studied through animal studies as early as 1935. In the 1940s, J. Warkany showed that pregnant animals severely deprived of adequate diets produced offspring suffering from various kinds of abnormalities. These studies demonstrated that the fetus was not always a parasite, able to satisfy needs at maternal expense.[14]

Pregnancy outcome depends upon the timing of the dietary restriction, the severity, and the duration. B. Chow and C. Lee found that a reduction in food by as little as 25 per cent of total calories without qualitatively affecting the diet can result in increased stillbirths, neonatal mortality, and morbidity.[15]

In general, from existing data on animal experiments, we can conclude that maternal malnutrition is one of a host of factors that can interfere with normal fetal growth and development. A variety of ill effects caused by prolonged and severe maternal malnutrition during pregnancy include reduced size and number of brain cells, organs, and placenta as well as changes in normal physiological functioning and cell constituents.

Human Supplementation Studies

Paralleling these animal experiments, researchers found that reproductive risk appeared to be associated with dietary intake, often as a function of poverty. B. Burke et al. addressed the question of the effect of maternal diets on pregnancy outcome by studying 216 diet histories of pregnant women and relating the rated histories (rated good, fair, or poor on the basis of the RDAs) to outcome of pregnancy. Results showed a significant tendency for ratings of diets and ratings of offspring of mothers to correspond. Mothers whose diets were rated good were more likely to give birth to an infant in optimal condition. Other supplementation programs for the poor in developing countries, or in populations presumably at risk of malnutrition, have been shown to increase the birth weights of the infants.[16]

Although these sources of evidence seem to confirm what many believed was common sense, the studies have been criticized on various counts. One fault related to the fact that dietary intake by itself could not be taken as a valid, conclusive measure of nutritional status. Very few of the early studies even considered the past nutritional status of the mother. Sampling procedures as well as supplementation procedures were criticized as being unscientific.

Studies of Human Organ Systems[6]

Other studies have tried to associate the weight of fetal organs and cells with maternal health and nutritional status. R. Naeye et al. studied the organs of 252 infants in the United States who were stillborn or died during the first two days after birth. Infants were grouped according to socioeconomic status of the family. Infants from poor families tended to have diminished mass and size of fat cells as well as smaller livers, adrenals, thymuses, and spleens relative to the infants from nonpoor families. Naeye suggested that undernutrition may have been responsible for the growth retardation in the low-income group.

In another investigation, Naeye studied 1,044 stillbirths and neonatal deaths. Medical records were reviewed to determine maternal prepregnancy weights and heights and weight gain during pregnancy. These variables were studied in relation to weights of the infants and weights of internal organs of the infants. Although no significant relationships were found for infants who died before 33 weeks gestation, Naeye found that overweight mothers with a high pregnancy weight gain as well as underweight mothers with a low pregnancy weight gain had infants with reduced-size livers and adrenal glands. Mothers who had been restricted to 1,000–1,500 calories during their pregnancy bore infants with smaller overall and organ size than mothers who were not so restricted. The correlations remained when variables of race, marital status, employment status, and interval since last pregnancy were controlled for.[17,18]

Data from Populations Subjected to Famines[6]

Experiences of different population groups that were subjected to wartime famines also demonstrated that maternal diet was related to reproductive capacity. Studies in Holland[19] and in Leningrad[20] suggested that malnutrition could result in low-birth-weight infants, with greatest maternal deprivation being related to the greatest reduction in the size of the offspring. These studies also found that many women under conditions of semistarvation experienced amenorrhea (cessation of menstruation) and thus failed to conceive.

Nutritional Status of Pregnant Women in the United States

Relatively few published studies relate maternal nutritional status to infant health status in the United States. Most of these studies focused on the poor in developing nations. One study done among low-income Americans was reported by N. Springer et al.[21−22] They evaluated personal, medical, and dietary information of 198 pregnant women who attended a maternity and infant care project in Detroit. All the women were from the low socioeconomic level; the mean age was 20.5 years with an age range of 13–40 years. Of the 198 women, 193 were black, 4 were white, and 1 was a native American. The average educational level of the women was 11 years.

About one third of the women in the study were 20 per cent or more above the standard weight for their height. Dietary modifications had been prescribed by physicians for 40 per cent of the patients. One fourth were on 1,800 kcal with no added salt diets, 13 were limited to 1,800 kcal, 6 were on no added salt; 1 was on a bland diet limited to 1800 kcal; and 3 were diabetics on calorie- and carbohydrate-modified diets. Although most of the women were eligible to participate in the food program offered by the project or in federal food programs, only one third of them actually did take advantage of these programs.

The average dietary intakes of the women in the study included the following number of servings per day:*

meat	1.5	legumes	0.8
milk	1.6	vegetables	1.0

*It is interesting to compare these servings with those recommended for pregnant woman by the four basic food groups in which the suggested number of servings for the various groups are meat, two servings; milk, four servings; fruit and vegetables, four servings; and bread and cereals, four servings.

eggs	0.5	fruit	1.3
	cereal	4.4	

This suggests that women's diets were inadequate in milk, vegetables, and fruit; the mean dietary score was 8.3 as compared with the recommended 13.0. Prenatal supplements (vitamins and minerals) were prescribed for all of the mothers, which possibly offset adverse effects from their inadequate diets.

However, these group findings obscure the fact that a high percentage of the women did not consume any eggs; approximately one third to one half consumed no vegetables or fruits on the day of the 24-hour recall. Their mean heights and prepregnancy weights were within normal ranges, and their mean hemoglobin and hematocrit levels also tended to be in the normal ranges.

The study also assessed the dietary and nutritional status of the infants born to these mothers at the time of the first postpartum (after birth) clinic visit. The mean protein intake was 32 gm, was considerably higher than the recommended 18 gm. Fewer than 25 per cent of the infants received a nonfortified formula; none of the mothers nursed her infant. The mean height and weight of the male infants were above the tenth percentile of the standards — the mean height and weight of the female infants were below the tenth percentile. Mean hemoglobin levels of the infants were better than the normal acceptable levels.

Maternal weight gain was shown to be an important index influencing the infant's birth weight, height, and head circumference. Although these findings cannot be extrapolated to all pregnant women throughout the United States, they suggest a cause for concern relative to nutritional status.[21,22]

Summary on Nutrition and Pregnancy

One of the best summaries of the result from epidemiological, animal, and clinical studies on diet, nutrition, and pregnancy was presented by M. Winick during hearings before the U.S. Senate Select Committee on Nutrition and Human Needs. His conclusions were:[23]

1. An association exists between the amount of weight gained during pregnancy and birth weight in all types of populations.

2. An association exists between maternal nutritional status prior to pregnancy and birth weight in poor populations.

3. The difference in birth weight between rich and poor accounts for the difference in mortality between rich and poor.

4. The larger the number of smaller infants in a population, the greater the chance of mental retardation.

5. Malnutrition retards infant growth thereby producing smaller infants with reduced organ growth and smaller brains.

6. Feeding a better diet during pregnancy increases maternal weight gain,

birth weight, and, therefore, should decrease mortality and the incidence of retardation.

Implications

There is a need for additional study of normal physiological adjustments
that occur during pregnancy and for epidemiological studies to help in
understanding the effects of various environmental, health, sociocultural,
economic, dietary, and educational variables on pregnancy outcome.

Although much research remains to be done, the available evidence provides significant bases for public health implications and recommendations.
However, maternal diets can vary greatly without evidence of harm to
either fetus or mother. The classical results of maternal malnutrition are
evidenced as the result of severe and prolonged dietary deficiencies.

Maternal Weight Gain

The exact relationship between maternal weight gain and infant birth
weight remains to be determined. However, there is generally a positive
association between maternal weight gain during pregnancy and birth
weight of the offspring. In other words, increased maternal weight gain is
associated with increased infant birth weight. Previous maternal weight
is also associated with infant birth weight; in general, the variables of
maternal weight gain and maternal prepregnancy weight gain have the
greatest effect on infant birth weight. However, maternal weight gain
cannot be used to definitely indicate infant birth weight; the quality of
the maternal diet as well as the components of weight gain, life-style,
medical care, and general health status are also important determinants
of fetal growth and development.[24]

Past nutritional experiences of the mother may be equally important in
determining the pregnancy outcome.[25] As H. G. Birch noted:

> The available data therefore suggest that women who are not well-grown have char-
> acteristics which negatively affect them as childbearers. In particular, short stature
> is associated with pregnancy and delivery complications and with prematurity.
> Since growth achievement within ethnic groups is a function of health history and
> in particular nutrition, it is clear that the mother's antecedent nutritional history
> when she herself was a child can and does significantly influence intrauterine
> growth, development and vitality of her child. Moreover, an inadequate nutritional
> background in the mother places this child at elevated risk for damage at delivery.[26]

Although a knowledge of the effects of individual nutrients on pregnancy is not complete, there is a general consensus that an average
pregnancy weight gain of 24 lb (between 20 lb and 25 lb) will support the
most favorable pregnancy outcome. This weight gain would be achieved
through a gain of up to 3.0 lb during the first trimester and about 0.8 lb
per week during the second and third trimesters. This pattern of weight
gain is important and is more related to a favorable pregnancy outcome
than the sum amount of weight gain.

Special consideration should be given to the pregnant adolescent and to
women who become pregnant while in a poor nutritional state. The Com-

mittee on Maternal Nutrition suggested that the restriction of salt during pregnancy is of "doubtful value . . . and is potentially dangerous." Vitamin and mineral supplements are not recommended as substitutes for a nutritionally adequate and varied diet, but iron (30–60 mg daily during the second and third trimesters) and folic acid (0.2–0.4 mg daily) supplements are recommended, as preventive measures. In areas in which soil and water are deficient in iodine, the committee encouraged the use of iodized salt.[24,25] The recommended dietary allowances for pregnant and lactating women over and above the general population, are presented in Table 6-2.[27]

Although maternal nutrition during pregnancy is important, a lifelong history of adequate nutrition is the best preparation for a successful pregnancy. To this end, policies dealing with food availability and affordability, public health and nutrition education programs, and nutritional surveillance of women of childbearing age can be important in ensuring adequate nutrition and a favorable pregnancy outcome. These policies, if implemented at the federal, state, and local levels of government, may figure prominently in reducing current infant mortality rates in the United States.

The Committee on Maternal Nutrition has set forth other general recommendations that are particularly relevant for promoting the health and the nutritional status of the pregnant woman and her child:[25]

1. Standard, high-quality levels of maternal health and nutritional care should be provided and made available to all pregnant mothers.

2. Nutritional needs of pregnant or lactating mothers, the infant, and the young child should receive top priority in the allocation of nutrition services and in the implementation of food programs.

3. Medical school curricula should prepare physicians to recognize and promote the important relation between health and maternal nutrition.

4. A committee on nutrition should be established by the American College of Obstetrics and Gynecology; questions on the relation between nutrition and pregnancy outcome should be part of qualifying exams for gynecologists and obstetricians.

5. Public health officials and personnel with special skills in the areas of pregnancy should be increased in number in order that counseling and health services may be made available for all individuals. Subjects particularly relevant to nutritional counseling include food budgeting, purchasing, preparation, menu planning, and meal service, as well as child care and family living.

6. Sound nutrition education should be a part of the curricula of elementary and secondary education so that children may learn early in life of the importance of good nutritional habits.

7. Public health organizations and health professionals should assume the responsibility of providing sound nutrition information to the public. This is especially important in the face of the plethora of food faddists and quacks.

Table 6-2

Food and Nutrition Board, National Academy of Sciences-National Research Council Recommended Daily Dietary Allowances[1] for Pregnant and Lactating Women, Over and Above Requirements for General Population

	Pregnant	*Lactating*
Protein (grams)	+30	+20
Fat-Soluble Vitamins		
Vitamin A (μg R.E.[2])	+200	+400
Vitamin C (μg)[3]	+5	+5
Vitamin E (mg α T.E.)[4]	+2	+3
Water-Soluble Vitamins		
Vitamin C (mg)	+20	+40
Thiamin (mg)	+0.4	+0.5
Riboflavin (mg)	+0.3	+0.5
Niacin (mg N.E.)[5]	+2	+5
Vitamin B_6 (mg)	+0.6	+0.5
Folacin[6] (μg)	+400	+100
Vitamin B_{12} (μg)	+1.0	+1.0
Minerals		
Calcium (mg)	+400	+400
Phosphorus (mg)	+400	+400
Magnesium (mg)	+150	+150
Iron (mg)	7	7
Zinc (mg)	+5	+10
Iodine (μg)	+25	+50

[1] The allowances are intended to provide for individual variations among most normal persons as they live in the United States under usual environmental stresses. Diets should be based on a variety of common foods in order to provide other nutrients for which human requirements have been less well defined.

[2] Retinol equivalents. 1 Retinol equivalent = 1 μg retinol or 6 μg β-carotene.

[3] As cholecalciferol. 10 μg cholecalciferol = 400 I.U. vitamin D.

[4] α tocopherol equivalents: 1 mg d-α-tocopherol = 1 α T.E.

[5] 1 NE (niacin equivalent) is equal to 1 mg of niacin or 60 mg of dietary tryptophan.

[6] The folacin allowances refer to dietary sources as determined by *Lactobacillus casei* assay after treatment with enzymes ("conjugases") to make polyglutamyl forms of the vitamin available to the test organism.

[7] The increased requirement during pregnancy cannot be met by the iron content of habitual American diets nor by the existing iron stores of many women; therefore the use of 30-60 mg of supplemental iron is recommended. Iron needs during lactation are not substantially different from those of nonpregnant women, but continued supplementation of the mother for 2-3 months after parturition is advisable in order to replenish stores depleted by pregnancy.

Reproduced from Recommended Dietary Allowances, Ninth Edition (1979) with the permission of the National Academy of Sciences, Washington, D.C.

8. The team approach to health care is recognized as being valuable, but a person with special skills in dealing with the pregnant mother, especially the pregnant adolescent, should be available and consulted when high-risk patients are involved.

9. Prenatal care and family-planning advice should be made available to

all. Barriers limiting accessibility to such services should be identified and eliminated.

10. School personnel should be assisted with their attempts to relate school health facilities to community maternity care programs and resources.

11. Pregnant adolescents should be helped to continue with their education and should receive counseling and guidance in subjects of health, child care, nutrition, and other subjects that are essential to help them provide their families with the best health, personal, and nutrition care.

Pregnant Adolescents

Pregnant women of any age are vulnerable to nutritional problems, but the risk of the pregnant adolescent is especially great. The National Research Council summarized the particularly vulnerable status of the pregnant adolescent relative to malnutrition:[2]

> The problems of pregnant adolescents are of particular importance because of the trend in the United States toward marriage at earlier ages and increases in the proportion of infants born to young mothers. . . . Girls are at biological risk if pregnancy occurs before cessation of growth. In the United States, the average age at menarche is 12.5 to 13 years. About four years later, or at about 17 years of age, the great majority of girls have completed linear growth and have achieved gynecologic maturity. Pregnancy after this age should not present special biological hazards.[27]

The number of pregnant teenage girls, particularly those under the age of 17, continues to rise. Births to adolescent mothers accounted for 19 per cent of all births in 1975, compared with 17 per cent in 1966.[28]

A variety of less fortunate circumstances are associated with a teenage pregnancy. The births are frequently illegitimate; in 1975, there were approximately 222,500 illegitimate births to teenagers aged 15 to 19. Young mothers are also less likely than older mothers to have adequate prenatal health care. An estimated 40 per cent of 15-year-old mothers receive prenatal care during the first trimester of pregnancy, compared with 61 per cent of 19-year-olds.[28] Further, studies have demonstrated that teenagers often have poor dietary patterns; babies of young mothers are more often small for date and experience a greater incidence of birth defects than those of older women.[28]

Nutritional studies of pregnant adolescents are limited. Two extensive bibliographic reviews of research on maternal nutrition into the 1970s included only two published reports in this area.[29-31] A more recent review noted that many reports on the nutritional status of pregnant adolescents found suboptimal nutrient consumption relative to the recommended dietary allowances.[31] The studies[32-42] reviewed by E. S. Weigley[31] support the findings of the Ten-State Nutrition Survey that adolescents aged 10 to 16 had the most unsatisfactory nutritional status of any age group.[43] Results of some of these studies are summarized in Table 6-3.[31] These reports indicate that inadequacies in calcium, iron, vitamin A, and calories are not infrequent.

Table 6-3

Surveys on Nutritional Status in Pregnancy and Adolescence

Researchers	Summary Findings
Kaminetsky 1973[32]	Studied 13 to 17 year old girls in Newark, N.J. Maternal and Infant Care Project. Used dietary and biochemical methods of assessment; 35% of sample had engaged in pica; about half did not improve their diets even with counseling. Vitamin supplements were beneficial in terms of folic acid and thiamine blood levels but had minimal effect on other vitamin values; substantial evidence of nutritional deficiency in population studied.
King et al., 1972.[33]	Studied at two San Francisco hospitals; three-day food records 7th and 9th months plus biochemical assessment used to determine nutritional status; least adequate nutrients were calcium, iron, vitamin A and energy.
Osofsky et al., 1971[34]	Studied pregnant 11 to 18 year olds in Syracuse New York with three day food records. Lunch was provided as part of the project. About 95% were below 1968 RDAs for iron and calcium, 90% for vitamin A and 50% for protein.
Seiler and Fox, 1973[35]	Used three-day record to study pregnant and non-pregnant Nebraska girls aged 16 and younger. Based on RDAs, diets of pregnant girls were poorer than those of nonpregnant; dietary supplements were beneficial in some, but use was erratic. The non-pregnant group scored better on a nutrition knowledge test and seemed to be better psychologically adjusted.
Thompson et al., 1973[36]	Studied diets of pregnant women taking dietary supplements. The women aged 14 to 17 evidenced greatest need for iron and calcium supplements.
Dawson and McGanity, 1970[37]	Studied gestational changes in certain plasma free amino acids in pregnant adolescents. Plasma levels of leucine, isoleucine and valine declined during 2nd and 3rd trimesters; methionine, alanine and glutamic acid similarly declined.
Dickens et al., 1973[38]	Of pregnant adolescents studied 25% had anemia although iron and vitamin supplements were advised and provided.
Cohenour and Calloway 1972[39]	Studied panthothenic acid intake of pregnant girls aged 14 to 18; intakes were below accepted standards for non-pregnant adults.
Daniel et al., 1971[40]	Studied folic acid intakes of 114 pregnant girls aged 12 to 15; more than 97% failed to achieve the RDAs; blood folate levels were also low.
Van de Mark and Wright 1972[41]	Studied 3-day intakes of pregnant and non-pregnant 12 to 16 year olds and compared this with their hemoglobin and whole blood folate levels. Dietary and blood values were low.
Ancri et al., 1971[42]	Studied factors determining pregnancy outcome in 98 women aged 12-32, divided into 4 age groups. A significantly higher weight gain noted for youngest; lowest weight gain in oldest group. Weight gain not associated with caloric intake; no correlations between maternal caloric or protein intake and infant's birth weight. Mean caloric intakes were below but protein was above the 1974 RDA's. 10% of infants weighed less than 2500 gm. at birth; birth weight correlated with mother's age and length of pregnancy.

Programs to Help Pregnant Adolescents

In the past two decades, a variety of multidisciplinary programs have been implemented to help the pregnant adolescent. Within recent years, more than 100 communities in the United States have developed interdisciplinary programs to aid pregnant teenagers who live at home. These programs are often the result of several different community organizations, including the school system, who work together in a cooperative service effort. The girls are afforded the opportunity for continuing education in a classroom setting, as well as ongoing prenatal health care and counseling.[44]

Various authors have written about the design, implementation, and evaluation and effectiveness of multidisciplinary programs to aid pregnant adolescents. Some of these programs are reviewed in Table 6–4. Common to most comprehensive programs are elements of health care, social services, and some type of education in parenthood, child care, a vocational skill, or a career.[54]

Table 6–4

Programs Designed to Assist the Pregnant Teenager

Researchers	Programs
Anderson, 1973[45]	Moorhead Area Learning Center, Moorhead, Minnesota; enrolls pregnant girls aged 14 to 18, or grades 9 to 12. The Center offers instruction in business, English and home economics; counseling is available; credits earned at the center can be transferred to the high school. There is also instruction in prenatal care, infant and child development, foods and consumerism.
Backalinick, 1974[46]	Center for Interim Education, Bridgeport, Connecticut. The Center includes academic education, individual and group counseling, natural childbirth training, dental and medical care, tours of the labor and delivery room. Nutrition is offered as part of a "Preparation for Childbirth" course.
Badger, 1976[47]	Cincinnati, Ohio General Hospital. Participants attend weekly classes held in a pediatric clinic until infants are six months of age. Medical attention, health, nutrition and infant stimulation are concerns of the program.
Goldstein, 1973[48]	San Francisco General Hospital; comprehensive maternity program provides vocational education, parent skills, general guidance and the chance to achieve a high school diploma; counseling and prenatal care also offered.
Hansen, 1976[49]	Family Learning Center, New Brunswick, New Jersey; operated by the New Brunswick Board of Education for pregnant teens; offers academic work, as well as instruction in health, nutrition and child care.
James, 1973[50]	Meharry Medical College, Nashville, Tenessee, Outreach provides hospital-based outpatient services; the program is interdisciplinary, with a team including physician, nurse, social worker, medical student, obstetrical fellow and nutritionist; psychiatrist and minister also available.
McAnarney, 1975[51]	Rochester Adolescent Maternity Project (RAMP) of the University of Rochester, New York, School of Medicine and Dentis-

Programs Designed to Assist the Pregnant Teenager *(continued)*

Researchers	Programs
	try; provides total care in a central setting; services offered include comprehensive medical, psychological and social care.
Milk, 1973[52]	Maternal Child Health Program, East Carroll and Ouachita Parishes, Louisiana. Provides prenatal care, diet management, counseling by a medical social worker, and the provision for continuing education. The program features the health care team approach using the service of a nurse, social worker, nutritionist and physician. Cooperative Extension Service also involved.
Osofsky et al., 1970[53]	The Young Mothers Educational Development Program (YMED), Syracuse and Onondaga County, New York. Sponsored by the State University of New York, Upstate Medical Center, Syracuse Board of Education, and Onondaga Department of Health. Provides intensive medical, educational, social and psychological services for low-income pregnant adolescents. Headquartered in a school near the center, YMED offers multidisciplinary, comprehensive care.

Wallace et al., surveyed available help for pregnant teenagers in 130 cities throughout the United States. Eighty-five of the cities offered some type of nutrition program. Unmet needs mentioned by various cities included nutritional services for mothers, nutrition education and food supplements, maternal education on infant feeding, and the provision of food for pregnant teenagers.[55]

IMPORTANCE OF ADEQUATE NUTRITION IN LACTATION

The importance of optimal nutrition for successful lactation experiences has been documented. Breast-feeding has been found to offer physiological, immunological, nutritional, and psychological advantages to the infant and psychological and physiological benefits to the mother.

Lactation does, however, exert significant physiological and nutritional demands on the mother. A mother whose nutrition is inadequate may often deplete her reserves to provide needed extra energy for lactation. The calorie and protein content of milk from undernourished mothers may not significantly vary from that of well-nourished mothers, but the quantity is often reduced.[56] The fatty acid pattern may be changed, and the content of water-soluble vitamins and possibly some trace elements may be reduced in the milk of the undernourished mother. The fat-soluble vitamin content (vitamins A, D, E,) as well as calcium, iron, copper, and fluorine appear to be relatively independent of the mother's diet.[57,58]

Nutritional requirements are higher for the lactating mother. Lactation requires significant increases in energy intake, vitamin E, protein, pyridoxine, vitamin A, folacin, calcium, and iodine. According to the Committee on Recommended Dietary Allowance of the Food and Nutrition Board, intakes of all nutrients except vitamin D should be increased during lactation.[27] The Recommended Dietary Allowances for lactating women are included in Table 6-2.

In spite of these known increased nutritional needs of the lactating mother, there is considerable confusion regarding specific recommendations for dietary patterns during lactation. Few studies are available that assess either quantitative dietary needs or the nutritional status of the nursing mother. To illustrate the conflicting advice offered to the lactating mother, Sims summarized advice on nutrition and diet that are commonly offered in lay publications. This is illustrated in Table 6-5.[59] L. Sims studied the dietary habits of 61 lactating women. Three one-day food records and dietary questionnaires were collected. The sample was largely composed of white, middle-class, highly educated young women who were nursing their first babies. Most were highly motivated, wished to have a successful lactation experience, and were eager to consume a well-balanced, adequate diet.

Eighty per cent of the subjects took vitamin/mineral supplements. Those who did take these supplements, as well as those who did not, consumed approximately 2,100 kcal daily and approximately 90 gm of protein. The mean daily intake was 84.4 per cent of the RDAs for energy. Whereas all women consumed diets described as "fairly generous in terms of meeting the recommended allowances," the women who took supplements had better intakes from food alone. The only nutrient that was not consumed in excess of the allowances from food alone was iron; the non-supplemented group consumed less than 100 per cent of the RDAs for calcium, iron, and niacin.[59]

Implications for assessing the dietary and nutritional status of other groups, particularly those from lower socioeconomic backgrounds, are obvious. Those with lower incomes and less education may be less able to learn about, or purchase, adequate diets. More information on the nutritional status of lactating mothers is clearly needed.[59]

NUTRITIONAL STATUS OF INFANTS AND CHILDREN

Many changes in infant feeding practices have signaled concern among nutritionists. The decline in breast-feeding, with the rise in artificial feeding, as well as the trend toward earlier introduction of solid foods, may adversely affect health in later years.

Considerations in pediatric nutrition related to the development of cardiovascular disease are discussed more fully on pages 267-270, and considerations related to obesity are reviewed on pages 309-310.

S. J. Fomon, in his classic volume *Infant Nutrition*, suggested that the following are important nutritional principles for infants and children:[60]

1. The diet should be adequate but should not contain excessive amounts of water, calories, and essential nutrients.

2. An appropriate distribution of calories should come from protein, fat, and carbohydrates.

Table 6-5

Advice on Diet during Lactation Given in Commonly Used Lay Publications

Reference	Milk	Meat	Eggs	Recommendations for Daily Intake Fruit	Vegetables	Bread and Cereal	Other
Spock and Lowenberg	at least 1 qt	4–6 oz (+ liver, "if you can manage it")	2	3 servings, 2 of which should be citrus	3 or 4 servings + 1 dark green or deep yellow	3 servings + "extra serving or two"	Prenatal vitamins recommended by physician
Spock	1½ qt	1 generous portion, preferably 2; liver valuable — include occasionally	1	6 servings, including 2 raw; 2 of oranges, grapefruit, tomatoes, raw cabbage, or berries; 1 dark green leafy or deep yellow vegetable; potatoes		3 servings, whole or enriched	Butter or margarine; vitamin D preparations
National Dairy Council	4 c. or more	3 "generous" servings	1	3 or 4 servings; 1 should be citrus, melon, berries, or tomatoes	3 or 4 servings, including one potato + raw and dark green or deep yellow, frequently	4 servings, whole or enriched	

Mead Johnson Co.							
Pryor	No diet recommended; suggests avoiding chocolate, cabbage, onions, and garlic to prevent "fussiness or refusal to nurse," because these are greatest offenders in affecting milk and displeasing infants. No specific diet or foods recommended; urges mother to consume "plenty of high protein foods (meat, cheese, eggs, etc.), whole grain cereals and breads, fruit and fruit juices to give quick energy."						
La Leche League	No special diet — just "variety of foods," "natural foods"; avoid: "lots of refined sugar in foods, highly refined grains and cereals; watch liquids — water, juice, milk 50%; tea, coffee 50% is o.k."						Brewer's yeast for energy if needed; vitamin/mineral supplement only if prescribed by physician
Davis	1½ qt	2 servings lean; liver several times a week	1 or 2	3 or 4 servings; at least 1 citrus a day	at least 2 servings a day, including a green, leafy	at least 2 servings whole wheat or whole grain	Wheat germ; yeast; supplements of vitamins, A, D, B-complex, ascorbic acid, and E, + calcium, magnesium, minerals
Eiger and Olds	1 qt	3 or more servings; liver or heart often for iron	1	6 servings, including 1 good vitamin A source; 1 good ascorbic acid source; 2 fair ascorbic acid sources; 2 other fruits and vegetables, including potatoes		3 or 4 servings whole grain or enriched	Vitamins as prescribed by physician

Source: L. Sims. Dietary states of lactating women. I. Nutrient intake from food and from supplements. *J. Am. Diet. Assoc.* 73 (1978): 139.

3. The diet, and the way in which it is fed, should stimulate the development of sound nutritional habits.

4. The diet should be easily digestible.

Recommended dietary allowances for infants and for children are presented in Tables 6-6 and 6-7.

Considerable evidence suggests that children may be at nutritional risk on a number of counts. The Ten-State Survey found evidence of retarded heights and weights, especially among children from low-income families. The prevalence of retarded growth progressively decreased as family income increased.[43] Diets of children, especially those from low-income families, were often limited. Iron intakes were frequently deficient in the children studied. A high prevalence of iron deficiency anemia was found in children of all ages, from infancy to adolescent years. Among preschoolers, 70 per cent of the black southern and 30 per cent of the white northern children had hemoglobin levels less than 12.0 gm/100 ml. Low-income adolescent males had a higher prevalence of anemia than did females of the same economic level. Obesity was widespread and seemed also to be related to income.

Many other studies have found high prevalences of nutrition-related

Table 6-6.

Recommended Dietary Allowances for Infants[1]

	Age: birth to 6 months	*six months to 1 year*
Weight: kilograms	6	9
pounds	13	20
Height: centimeters	60	71
inches	24	28
Protein (g)	kg × 2.2	kg × 2.0
Fat-Soluble Vitamins		
Vitamin A (μg R.E.)[2]	420	400
Vitamin D (μg)[3]	10	10
Vitamin E (mg α T.E.)[4]	3	4
Water-Soluble Vitamins		
Vitamin C (mg)	35	35
Thiamin (mg)	0.3	0.5
Riboflavin (mg)	0.4	0.6
Niacin (mg N.E.)[5]	6	8
Vitamin B_6 (mg)	0.3	0.6
Folacin[6] (μg)	30	45
Vitamin B_{12} (μg)	0.5[7]	1.5
Minerals		
Calcium (mg)	360	540
Phosphorus (mg)	240	360
Magnesium (mg)	50	70
Iron (mg)	10	15
Zinc (mg)	3	5
Iodine (μg)	40	50

Table 6-6 continued

Estimated Safe and Adequate Daily Dietary Intakes of Additional Selected Vitamins and Minerals[7] for Infants

	Age: birth to 6 months	*6 months to 1 year*
Vitamin K (μg)	12	10–20
Biotin (μg)	35	50
Pantothenic Acid (mg)	2	3
Trace Elements[8]		
Copper (mg)	0.5–0.7	0.7–1.0
Manganese (mg)	0.5–0.7	0.7–1.0
Fluoride (mg)	0.1–0.5	0.2–1.0
Chromium (mg)	0.01–0.04	0.02–0.06
Selenium (mg)	0.01–0.04	0.02–0.06
Molybdenum (mg)	0.03–0.06	0.04–0.08
Electrolytes		
Sodium (mg)	115–350	250–750
Potassium (mg)	350–925	425–1275
Chloride (mg)	275–700	400–1200

[1] The allowances are intended to provide for individual variations among most normal persons as they live in the United States under usual environmental stresses. Diets should be based on a variety of common foods in order to provide other nutrients for which human requirements have been less well defined.

[2] Retinol equivalents. 1 Retinol equivalent = 1 μg retinol or 6 μg β-carotene.

[3] As cholecalciferol. 10 μg cholecalciferol = 400 I.U. vitamin D.

[4] α tocopherol equivalents. 1 mg d-α-tocopherol = 1 α T.E.

[5] 1 NE (niacin equivalent) is equal to 1 mg of niacin or 60 mg of dietary tryptophan.

[6] The folacin allowances refer to dietary sources as determined by *Lactobacillus casei* assay after treatment with enzymes ("conjugases") to make polyglutamyl forms of the vitamin available to the test organism.

[7] Because there is less information on which to base allowances, these figures are not given in the main table of the RDA and are provided here in the form of ranges of recommended intakes.

[8] Since the toxic levels for many trace elements may be only several times usual intakes, the upper levels for the trace elements given in this table should not be habitually exceeded.

Reproduced from Recommended Dietary Allowances, Ninth Edition (1979) with the permission of the National Academy of Sciences, Washington, D.C.

disorders in children in the United States. The National Preschool Nutrition survey reported a 7 per cent prevalence of anemia among children aged 1–6. Nutritional risk was most common among the poor; black children were taller and heavier than white, but white children were more likely to be overweight. Children from low-income families were more likely to suffer from inadequate amounts of food, rather than from poor quality of food. Dental problems were most common among poor, black children.[61]

The Health and Nutrition Examination Survey (HANES) found black children to be taller, heavier, but less fat than white children. Socioeconomic status was not related to weight-for-height indices or to the prevalence of thin children. Caloric intakes were lowest for poor children, and

Table 6-7.
Recommended Dietary Allowances for Children[1]

	Age (years)		
	1-3	*4-6*	*7-10*
Weight: kilograms	13	20	28
pounds	29	44	62
Height: centimeters	90	112	132
inches	35	44	52
Protein (g)	23	30	34
Fat-Soluble vitamins			
Vitamin A (μg R.E.)[2]	400	500	700
Vitamin D (μg)[3]	10	10	10
Vitamin E (mg α T.E.)[4]	5	6	7
Water-Soluble Vitamins			
Vitamin C (mg)	45	45	45
Thiamin (mg)	0.7	0.9	1.2
Riboflavin (mg)	0.8	1.0	1.4
Niacin (mg N.E.)[5]	9	11	16
Vitamin B_6 (mg)	0.9	1.3	1.6
Folacin (μg)[6]	100	200	300
Vitamin B_{12}	2.0	2.5	3.0
Minerals			
Calcium (mg)	800	800	800
Phosphorus (mg)	800	800	800
Magnesium (mg)	150	200	250
Iron (mg)	15	10	10
Zinc (mg)	10	10	10
Iodine (μg)	70	90	120

[1] The allowances are intended to provide for individual variations among most normal persons as they live in the United States under usual environmental stresses. Diets should be based on a variety of common foods in order to provide other nutrients for which human requirements have been less well defined.

[2] Retinol equivalents. 1 Retinol equivalent = 1 μg retinol or 6 μg β-carotene.

[3] As cholecalciferol. 10 μg cholecalciferol = 400 I.U. vitamin D.

[4] α tocopherol equivalents. 1 mg d-α-tocopherol = 1 α T.E.

[5] 1 NE (niacin equivalent) is equal to 1 mg of niacin or 60 mg of dietary tryptophan.

[6] The folacin allowances refer to dietary sources as determined by *Lactobacillus casei* assay after treatment with enzymes ("conjugases") to make polyglutamyl forms of the vitamin available to the test organism.

[7] Because there is less information on which to base allowances, these figures are not given in the main table of the RDA and are provided here in the form of ranges of recommended intakes.

[8] Since the toxic levels for many trace elements may be only several times usual intakes, the upper levels for the trace elements given in this table should not be habitually exceeded.

Reproduced from: Recommended Dietary Allowances, Ninth Edition (1979) with the permission of the National Academy of Sciences, Washington, D.C.

Table 6–7 continued

Estimated Safe and Adequate Daily Dietary Intakes of Additional Selected Vitamins and Minerals[7]

	Age (years)		
	1–3	*4–6*	*7–10*
Vitamin K (μg)	15–30	20–40	30–60
Biotin (μg)	65	85	120
Pantothenic Acid (mg)	3	3–4	4–5
Trace Elements[8]			
Copper (mg)	1.0–1.5	1.5–2.0	2.0–2.5
Manganese (mg)	1.0–1.5	1.5–2.0	2.0–3.0
Fluoride (mg)	0.5–1.5	1.0–2.5	1.5–2.5
Chromium (mg)	0.02–0.08	0.03–0.12	0.05–0.2
Selenium (mg)	0.02–0.08	0.03–0.12	0.05–0.2
Molybdenum (mg)	0.05–0.1	0.06–0.15	0.1–0.3
Electrolytes			
Sodium (mg)	325–975	450–1350	600–1800
Potassium (mg)	550–1650	775–2325	1000–3000
Chloride (mg)	500–1500	700–2100	925–2775

iron intakes were lowest for black children, presumably because they consumed less food. The lowest hemoglobin and hematocrit values were found among low-income and black children.[62]

The Center for Disease Control's Nutrition Surveillance Program, in surveying poor children, found about twice the expected rate of children who were underheight for their age. Being overweight was more commonly found than being underweight.[63] Iron deficiency anemia generally is considered to be the most prevalent disorder among American infants and children.[64] Infants and young children, because of their rapid growth, have high dietary iron requirements and collectively as a group are at the highest risk for the development of iron deficiency.[65] The highest prevalence of low hemoglobins in the United States is seen among infants of low birth weight, infants aged 6 to 24 months, and children and adolescents, especially those from low-income families.[64]

Infants and young children are highly vulnerable to potential iron deficiency. The Preschool Nutrition Survey considered a hemoglobin level less than 10 gm/100 ml or a hematocrit less than 31 per cent to be low for children aged 1 to 2 years, and a hemoglobin less than 11 gm per 100 ml or a hematocrit less than 33 per cent for children aged 2 to 6 to be indicative of anemia. About 5 per cent of preschool children surveyed were anemic according to these criteria. Almost half of the population surveyed were deficient in iron on the basis of iron-binding capacity.[61]

Other studies have found greater prevalences of anemia among North American children. It is unfortunate that most data on the incidence of iron deficiency and anemia are based on hemoglobin and hematocrit values as the criteria for the absence of, or presence of, iron deficiency. This is neither adequate nor specific for determining iron deficiency;

rather it is merely an indication of whether or not the individuals sampled did or did not have anemia, of which there are a variety of causes.*

However, the data are sufficient to raise questions about the nutritional status of many American children. Additional, properly designed and executed studies should be undertaken to determine the true magnitude of the problem of iron deficiency in the American population, as well as possible strategies to resolve the problem.

Numerous data indicate that the prevalence of low hemoglobin is related to income levels. The Preschool Nutrition Survey, for example found that 9 per cent of those aged 2 to 6 in the lowest-income group were anemic, but only 4 per cent of those not in low-income groups were anemic.[61] The HANES[66] found that of those aged 1–5 from low-income families 13.8 per cent had hemoglobin levels below 11.0 gm/100 ml. In contrast, only 6.5 per cent of those from families living above poverty level evidenced these low hemoglobin levels. The Ten-State Survey noted that the prevalence of low hemoglobins was greater among low-than higher-income groups, and among blacks than among white children.[43]

T. Haddy et al. studied the iron status of 109 infants and children from low-income families. The ages of the sample ranged from 4 months to 5 years. Evidence of iron deficiency was found as measured by transferrin saturation that was not always confirmed by standard anemic criteria. These researchers suggested that iron deficiency may exist in many individuals who were not diagnosed to be anemic.[67]

Another interesting report by Haddy was the relationship between dietary intake of certain nutrients and anemia. When protein and calories were adequate, according to RDA standards, iron intake at 57 per cent of the RDAs was not correlated with anemia, whereas iron intake at 40 per cent of the RDAs was correlated with anemia. Moreover, R. C. Theurer, in a comprehensive literature review of iron nutriture and status in infants, concluded that iron deficiency anemia very likely occurs in as many as 60 per cent of infants in the United States.[68]

These studies frequently surveyed the easier-to-reach children in an area — those who attended a health clinic or those enrolled in school. The highest-risk populations were probably not seen or evaluated. Thus, the overall picture of the state of nutritional problems among North American children is probably not accurate. But even these data illustrate that malnutrition does exist among North American children. Results of some of the studies on the nutritional status of children in the United States are summarized in Table 6–8.

---

*Although they are not commonly used in nutritional status surveys, three practical tests can be used to determine whether anemia is the result of dietary iron deficiency. These are: (1) the response of low hemoglobin concentration to administration of iron; (2) saturation of transferrin less than 16 to 17 per cent; and (3) a ratio of free erythrocyte porphyrins (FEP) to hemoglobin greater than 5 μg/g when lead concentration in the blood is less than 40 μg/100 ml.

When there is not enough iron for the synthesis of heme, the FEP concentration increases; thus, an excess of "free" protoporphyrin will accumulate in the red blood cells. Excess lead in the body will also interfere with the incorporation of iron into heme and might, therefore, cause an elevated FEP-to-hemoglobin ratio. However, concentrations of lead in the blood less than 40 μg/100 ml will rarely result in increased FEP concentration.[64]

Table 6-8

Dietary and Nutritional Status Surveys of Children in the United States

Reference	Population	Some Major Findings from the Study
Futrell et al., 1971[69]	139 Negro preschoolers in Mississippi	56% of the children had head circumferences below the 50th percentile. Most limiting nutrients were calories, ascorbic acid; both were related to educational levels of parents. Calcium was also limiting.
Futrell et al., 1975[70]	247 black preschoolers in Mississippi	Nutrient intakes related to mother's educational, but not income levels. Nutrients associated with mother's education were iron, calories and vitamin A. At all income levels there were children whose nutrient intakes were low in energy, iron, calcium, vitamin A and ascorbic acid; more than 50% of boys and 67% of girls were below 50th percentile of Boston height standards.
Fryer et al., 1971[71]	3444 preschool children in North Central Region	About 2/3 of children received RDAs for calories; most diets were adequate in protein. Boys had higher intakes than girls in same age groups.
Fox et al., 1971[72]	3444 preschoolers in North Cen. Region	Diets were adequate in calcium and phosphorous but low in iron, relative to 1968 RDAs.
Frank et al., 1977[73]	68 rural school children	Iron, calcium and vitamin A intakes were low for most children; thiamine and niacin intakes were lower for girls than for boys; riboflavin and niacin were generally adequate; high animal fat intakes resulted in a low P/S ratio.
Caliendo et al., 1977[74]	113 preschoolers in Ithaca, New York	22% of children aged 1–4 were anemic (hematocrit less than 34%); 12% of children's heights and 8% of weights were below 5th percentile while 8% of heights and 4% of weights were above 95th percentile for Boston Standards. 21% of children ate no fruit, 13% no vegetable, 55% no food rich in vitamin A or C during day of 24-hour recall.
Margo et al., 1977[75]	344 children aged 1–16 living in poor urban area	Iron deficiency anemia was found in 23% of 1 year olds; 53% of these children evidenced biochemical signs of iron deficiency; anemia decreased with age.
Johnson et al., 1974[78]	150 black preschoolers in Mississ.	74% of children consumed less than 8 mg. of iron daily; more than 99% consumed less than half the RDA for folic acid. 8.7 percent were anemic (hgb less than 10 g/100 ml) transferrin saturation was low in 26.7% of children.
Sturgeon, 1959[77]	term infants to age 1	7% developed anemia, (hgb less than 10G/100 ml).

Dietary and Nutritional Status Surveys of Children in the United States *(continued)*

Reference	Population	Some Major Findings from the Study
Haughton, 1963[78]	underprivileged in New York City	At age 1, 41.3% were anemic. Of those under age 3, 27.3% were anemic (hgb less than 10g/100 ml).
Danneker 1966[79]	364 children aged 6–36 months in child health conference in Allegheny, Penn.	16.4% were anemic (hgb less than 10 g/100 ml).
Kravitz et al., 1966[80]	Chicago preschool children in Operation Head Start	8% were anemic as measured by hematocrit values.
Dwyer et al., 1978[81]	119 vegetarian preschoolers	More of children evidenced length and weight measurements that were below the Harvard 50th percentiles than were expected after, but not before the age of 6 months. The children were also leaner after six months of age than was to be expected from Tanner-Whitehouse standards. All children had normal head circumferences.
Hutcheson 1960[82]	white and black children in rural Tennessee	20.9% of children up to age 6 had hematocrits of 31% or less; Children aged 1 year had higher incidence: 27.4% of whites, 40% of nonwhites had hematocrits less than or equal to 31%.
Gutelius 1969[83]	Negro children at health center, Wash., D.C.	Iron deficiency anemia identified in 28.9% of sample; children aged 12–17 months evidenced 65% prevalence of anemia.
Bryan and Anderson 1965[84]	low income handicapped children in rural N. Carolina	An estimated 71% of black and 35% of white children had inadequate diets; 90% of these resulted from an inadequate family diet.
Child Development Group of Miss. 1967[85]	Mississippi low income children and families	47% of 118 families surveyed never served milk; only 18% served fruit or juice to children.
Owen and Kram 1969[86]	Mississippi preschoolers	On the average, poorer children were smaller and at greater nutritional risk than more affluent; Nutrients most often limiting were vitamin C, calcium, riboflavin and calories.
Kerry et al., 1968; Crispin et al, 1968[87,88]	40 preschool children aged 3½ to 5½ in Lincoln, Neb. children divided into 2 groups: L = lower income, H = higher income	Mean caloric intake for both groups was lower than allowance; Mean intake for all nutrients but iron also met RDAs for both groups, but some children within groups consumed inadequate diets low in iron calcium, and vitamin C. 10% had low hemoglobin values; anthropometric values indicated better nutritional status for those in H group than in L group.

Dietary and Nutritional Status Surveys of Children in the United States *(continued)*

Reference	Population	Some Major Findings from the Study
Cook et al., 1976[89]	compared nutritional status of 18 Head Start and 17 nursery school participants in Maine in Spring and Fall.	Iron intakes were low; — 35.3% of Head Start children consumed inadequate amounts of vitamin C in fall, but only 7.1% were low in spring; Evidence of low vitamin A and niacin intakes found among nursery school children in fall, and in Headstart children in spring.
Lieberman et al., 1976[90]	581 school children attending 2 ghetto schools, predominantly black and low income, in L.A. California	Dietary intake tended to be close to RDAs for most nutrients. 86 children were below 16th percentile for height (Iowa stds.) Weights of 90 were above 84th percentile.

NUTRITIONAL STATUS OF ADOLESCENTS

Nutritional needs of children reach a maximum during the preadolescent and adolescent years; only in pregnancy and lactation are female requirements greater than they are during adolescence. Table 6-9 illustrates the nutritional needs of adolescents.

Adolescents are also very vulnerable to nutritional problems. Their rapid rate of growth (requiring high-quality diets), coupled with their desire for independence, the peer pressure, and social needs for acceptance may contribute to the poor dietary habits of adolescents. *Nutritional Status USA*, a study that looked at the nutritional needs and status of the United States during the 1940s and 1950s, reported that teenage girls evidenced the poorest diets relative to their high needs of any group studied.[91]

Few existing studies of adolescents assess nutritional status in terms of clinical, biochemical, anthropometric, and dietary analysis. The HANES, the only study that is nationally representative, found that mean energy intake was low for both black and white males and females in income groups that were below as well as above poverty level. Other findings from the HANES relative to adolescent nutritional status include:[66]

Nutrient	Finding
Protein	Adequate for all ages, sexes, incomes, and races with the exception of black females aged 18–44
Iron	Low for 12–17-year-olds; low for both black and white females in both income groups in the age range 18 and over; above standards for males
Vitamin A	Above standard for all with exception of blacks aged 12–17
Vitamin C	Adequate for all groups

Table 6-9.

Recommended Daily Dietary Allowances for Males and Females Ages 11-22[1]

	Age 11-14		Age 15-18		Age 19-22	
	Males	*Females*	*Males*	*Females*	*Males*	*Females*
Weight: kilograms	45	46	66	55	70	55
pounds	99	101	145	120	154	120
Height: centimeters	157	157	176	163	177	163
inches	62	62	69	64	70	64
Protein (g)	45	46	56	46	56	44
Fat-soluble Vitamins						
Vitamin A (μg R.E.)[2]	1000	800	1000	800	1000	800
Vitamin D (μg)[3]	10	10	10	10	7.5	7.5
Vitamin E (mg α T.E.)[4]	8	8	10	8	10	8
Water-Soluble Vitamins						
Vitamin C (mg)	50	50	60	60	60	60
Thiamin (mg)	1.4	1.1	1.4	1.1	1.5	1.1
Riboflavin (mg)	1.6	1.3	1.7	1.3	1.7	1.3
Niacin (mg N.E.)[5]	18	15	18	14	19	14
Vitamin B_6 (mg)	1.8	1.8	2.0	2.0	2.2	2.0
Folacin (μg)[6]	400	400	400	400	400	400
Vitamin B_{12} (μg)	3.0	3.0	3.0	3.0	3.0	3.0
Minerals						
Calcium (mg)	1200	1200	1200	1200	800	800
Phosphorus (mg)	1200	1200	1200	1200	800	800
Magnesium (mg)	350	300	400	300	350	300
Iron (mg)	18	18	18	18	10	18
Zinc (mg)	15	15	15	15	15	15
Iodine (μg)	150	150	150	150	150	150

[1] The allowances are intended to provide for individual variations among most normal persons as they live in the United States under usual environmental stresses. Diets should be based on a variety of common foods in order to provide other nutrients for which human requirements have been less well defined.

[2] Retinol equivalents. 1 Retinol equivalent = 1 μg retinol or 6 μg β-carotene.

[3] As cholecalciferol. 10 μg cholecalciferol = 400 I.U. vitamin D.

[4] α tocopherol equivalents. 1 mg d-α-tocopherol = 1 α T.E.

[5] 1 NE (niacin equivalent) is equal to 1 mg of niacin or 60 mg of dietary tryptophan.

[6] The folacin allowances refer to dietary sources as determined by *Lactobacillus casei* assay after treatment with enzymes ("conjugases") to make polyglutamyl forms of the vitamin available to the test organism.

[7] Because there is less information on which to base allowances, these figures are not given in the main table of the RDA and are provided here in the form of ranges of recommended intakes.

[8] Since the toxic levels for many trace elements may be only several times usual intakes, the upper levels for the trace elements given in this table should not be habitually exceeded.

Reproduced from: Recommended Dietary Allowances, Ninth Edition (1979) with the permission of the National Academy of Sciences, Washington, D.C.

Table 6-9 continued

Estimated Safe and Adequate Daily Dietary Intakes of Additional Selected vitamins and Minerals for Adolescents over 11 years of Age.[7]

Vitamin K (µg)	50–100
Biotin (µg)	100–200
Pantothenic Acid (mg)	4–7
Trace Elements[8]	
Copper (mg)	2–3
Manganese (mg)	2.5–5.0
Fluoride (mg)	1.5–2.5
Chromium (mg)	0.05–0.2
Selenium (mg)	0.05–0.2
Molybdenum (mg)	0.15–0.5
Electrolytes	
Sodium (mg)	900–2700
Potassium (mg)	1525–4575
Chloride (mg)	1400–4200

The Ten-State Survey found that significant numbers of 10–16-year-olds consumed energy levels below the standards. Other findings from the Ten-State survey include:[43]

Nutrient	Finding
Protein	Exceeded dietary standards
Calcium	Higher for males than females; increased with age in males; decreased for females; white adolescents had highest mean intake; 20–54 per cent of adolescents consumed less than standard (650 mg)
Iron	Lower than for any other nutrient; black and white females in low-income ratio states evidenced better intakes; more than 80 per cent of adolescent females consumed less than 18 mg
Vitamin A	Exceeded standards for most groups; blacks tended to have higher intakes than whites or Spanish-Americans; intakes higher for males than for females
Thiamine	All groups exceeded standards
Riboflavin	All groups exceeded standards
Vitamin C	All groups consumed intakes higher than standard

R. Huenemann reviewed adolescent nutritional problems and reported that major difficulties were dental caries, obesity, and anemia in females as well as in males. Other problems were low intakes of vitamin A and C.[92] Results of other studies that examined food habits and the nutritional status of adolescents are presented in Table 6-10.

NUTRITIONAL STATUS OF THE ELDERLY

The number of elderly in the United States is increasing at a more rapid rate than is the number of those under 65 years of age. The median age in

Table 6-10
Nutritional Status of U.S. Teenagers

Reference	Population	Major Findings
1965 Household Food Consumption[93]	1400 boys and girls aged 12-19	mean caloric intake for boys was highest for those aged 18-19; girls aged 12-14 consumed most calories; boys' intakes slightly exceeded RDA; girls' mean iron intake (11 mg) was less than the RDA; girls diets also tended to be limited in vitamin A and thiamine.
Hodges and Krehl, 1965[94]	Iowa children, grades 9-12	mean nutrient intakes and biochemical measurements tended to be adequate but a small proportion were low in hemoglobin, vitamin A and C blood levels.
Hampton et al., 1967[95]	127 teenagers in Berkeley, Cal.	mean intakes for nutrients except iron and calcium were adequate; 15% of girls did not meet 2/3 of RDA for vitamin A and C; 10% of boys did not meet 2/3 of RDA for vitamin A and 30% failed to meet RDA for vitamin C; approximately 50% of girls were low in calcium and iron; 10% of all teens consumed less than 2/3 of calorie allowance; obesity was not uncommon.
Wharton, 1964[96]	Illinois teens	noted nutrient intakes were generally lower than those reported by Hampton; a greater percentage of his sample than Hampton's failed to achieve 2/3 of RDA.
Dibble et al., 1959[97]	Junior High School adolescents in Onondaga County, New York — one predominantly black, one white school studied	41% came to school without breakfast in Negro school; in white school only 4-7% missed breakfast.
Huenemann et al, 1968[98]	High School students in Berkeley, Calif.	Black children had poorer intakes than whites; 90% of black children had irregular eating habits.
Christakis, 1968[99]	School children in Manhattan, New York	71% of sample consumed "poor" diets; less than 7% had excellent diets.
Myers et al., 1968[100]	332 4th, 5th and 6th grade students in Roxbury, Mass.	55% of sample consumed "unsatisfactory" breakfast; 60% unsatisfactory lunches; 64% had less than 2 glasses of milk daily; 132 children ate no citrus fruit; 37% of Black, 45% of White children had unsatisfactory intakes of protein rich foods.

1970 was 27.9 years; in 1975 it was 28.8 years; and in 1976 it rose to 29.0 years. There were 23 million Americans over the age of 65 in 1977 and more than 32 million over the age of 60. It has been estimated that by the year 2000, there may be 29–33 million Americans over the age of 65. These figures translate into 1.25 million people who reach the age of 65 every 50 weeks; one in eight Americans is older than sixty-five years. By the year 2000, this figure may be one in five.[101]

It is generally agreed that numerous mechanisms influence the aging process. Many researchers believe that aging is manifested through factors that cause cell destruction or limit cell regeneration. Other factors thought to be associated with the aging process include reduced efficiency of DNA repair mechanisms, flaws in the synthesis of protein, impaired enzyme functioning, deterioration of immunologic processes, actions of free radicals, and the cross linkage of proteins.[102]

The relationships of nutrition to the aging processes are not well understood. Nutrition is known to be a factor in the development of diseases that are associated with old age. Nutrition may be effective in "reducing the burdens that the elderly must bear and curtailing the processes that . . . lead to the physiological state that we at present define as old age."[103] In other words, nutrition must be studied as a possible way to slow or alter the aging process as well as to improve the environment of the elderly and to provide optimal health and welfare for the older individual.

The nutritional problems of the elderly have gained national attention in recent years. Reports from the White House Conference on Food, Nutrition, and Health,[104] the White House Conference on Aging,[105] and testimony before the U.S. Senate Select Committee on Nutrition and Human Needs have stimulated interest in nutrition and the elderly. It is commonly accepted that a large proportion of senior citizens in the United States have poor food habits and consume diets that are not adequate in essential nutrients. The physiological, social, and economic changes in the lives of older citizens frequently make them vulnerable to nutritional problems. (See Figure 6-2.)

Literature describing the food habits of the elderly and their nutritional status has presented evidence that many elderly are extremely vulnerable to the effects of poor nutrition.[106] The USDA study of 1965 demonstrated that many elderly who appeared outwardly healthy were deficient in certain nutrients, most notably protein, the B vitamins, vitamins A and C, iron, and calcium.[93] Other studies seem to corroborate these findings. M. Dibble et al., for example, found that when diets of the elderly were inadequate, they tended to be low in several nutrients, rather than in a single one.[107]

Factors Influencing Dietary Quality

Older individuals often have poor food habits and hence poor nutritional status because of poor physical health, physical disabilities, limited incomes, lack of mobility needed to purchase food, loneliness and depression that cause decreased interest in preparing and eating food, and reduced appetites that result from other physiological, psychological, or environmental changes. Because of these factors, the elderly are often at high nutritional risk.

Although the effects of such poor eating habits are known, there is relatively little known about the environmental factors that may be causative factors. Poverty is certainly a major determinant. Many older men and women, especially those living alone, pay very little attention to the planning of well-balanced meals. Limited incomes prevent the purchase of an adequate variety and quality of foods, and many older people have limited knowledge of the kinds of foods that can provide them with an economical but healthful meal.

I. Harrill et al. observed the foods consumed by elderly women and found that the diets generally met two thirds of the RDAs but that the intake was not statistically related to selected physical, social, or psychological factors. Intakes generally reflected established food patterns that varied with the individual's background and experience.[108]

E. N. Todhunter et al., in a study of noninstitutional older individuals in Middle Tennessee, found that more than 80 per cent of black males, white females, and white males, but 70 per cent of black females, were meeting two thirds of the RDA for protein. Only 44 per cent of the white and 37 per cent of black women had satisfactory intakes of iron; vitamin A intake was unsatisfactory for more than half the group. The factors deemed important in determining an adequate diet were education and income. On the other hand, age, chewing problems, and individual feelings about personal health did not influence dietary quality.[109]

G. S. Johnson studied 234 adults over the age of 60 in Akron, Ohio, and found that the nutritional value of the diets of more than 75 per cent of the sample were appraised as "fair" or "poor." Income was ranked as having the greatest influence on eating habits, followed by nutrition knowledge, convenience foods, dental health, and eating alone. Most of the subjects were concerned with maintaining good eating habits, but the lack of income prevented full practice. The study indicated that the elderly were in need of nutrition education to ensure the availability of an adequate diet.[110]

Other factors reported to have a significant influence on the dietary intakes of the elderly include:[111,112]

Age — energy intake has been reduced 11–19 per cent during the eighth decade.

Location (urban versus rural) — those living in rural areas are somewhat more protected from this energy intake reduction, perhaps more as a result of increased physical activity than of environmental influences per se.

Degree of social participation — the more socially active elderly tend to have better food habits.

Exposure to media — the elderly have been reported to watch more television than any other age group. Their food habits are influenced both by the advertisements and by the inactivity associated with much television viewing.

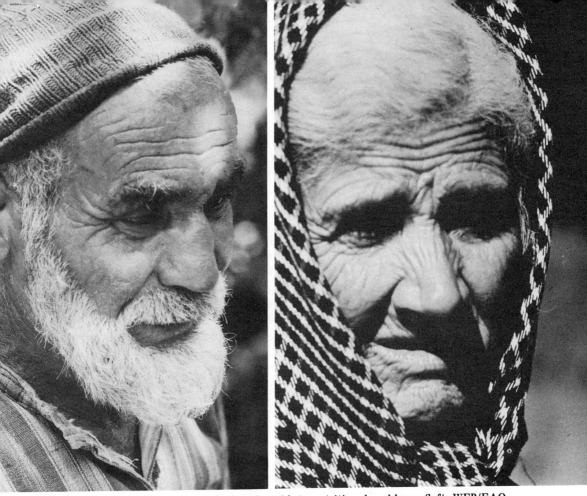

Figure 6-2. Older citizens are increasingly vulnerable to nutritional problems. (left: WFP/FAO photo by F. Iovino; right: UN photo by A. Jongen)

Health Status Related to Nutrition and Food Intake

Physical problems of dentition and gastrointestinal diseases, such as peptic ulcer, gall bladder disease, and pancreatitis, may cause the elderly to reduce their food and nutrient intake. Declining taste and smell sensitivity, which are frequent among the elderly, may also cause a reduced appetite. The health status of the elderly in terms of previously prescribed modified diets, the belief that certain foods are not well tolerated, and the preference for presumed (sometimes falsely) "healthy" foods prohibit consumption of certain foods.

Disabilities and restricted physical activity resulting from accidents and chronic diseases, which commonly affect the elderly, may also limit their food choice and consumption. Some of these conditions influence the need for nutrients. For example, a prolonged confinement in bed may result in significant losses of calcium or nitrogen. Other difficulties may arise when modified diet prescriptions result in appetite failure or limit the intake of preferred foods. Drugs used to treat diseases may also affect nutritional status. For example, digitalis may cause nausea and vomiting; diuretics may result in a loss of potassium.

A number of studies of eating patterns of the elderly have reported relationships between health or dentition problems and food intake. One survey of 283 households reported that 80 per cent of the sample had some type of diet limitation that was linked to health, 30 per cent had a health problem requiring dietary modification, and 30 per cent had a lack of appetite for food, attempts to control weight, and chewing difficulties.[113]

Various physiological and metabolic changes may also affect the nutritional status of the elderly. Table 6–11 summarizes some of these changes. Particular nutrient considerations for the elderly are summarized in Table 6–12.[114–118]

A significant problem among the elderly is osteoporosis, a disorder in which the bone's chemical makeup remains normal but minerals and the supporting matrix of the bone are lost. Bones thus become thinner, lighter, and more porous. Osteoporosis should not be confused with osteomalacia, a disease caused by a deficiency of vitamin D in the elderly, similar to rickets in children. Dietary osteomalacia is rare in the United States, but it may be found, most frequently in patients recovering from gastric surgery.

Osteoporosis occurs in an estimated one third of women over the age of 60; it can also be observed in men and women under the age of 60. The incidence of the disease in the United States has been variously estimated by different researchers. Some estimate that half of postmenopausal women have osteoporosis,[119] and others estimate that at least a tenth of all individuals over the age of 55 suffer from the disease.[120]

The cause of osteoporosis is not yet clear. It is frequently related to a diet that is deficient in calcium. With an insufficient blood calcium supply, bone calcium is resorbed to maintain serum calcium levels. It has thus been suggested that "chronic dietary deficiency of calcium and chronic dietary excess of phosphorous results in bone demineralization."[121] Factors related to this include vitamin D deficiency, vitamin C deficiency, protein deficiency, fluoride, and an imbalance in the calcium/phosphorous ratio, which in bone is 2 to 1. For this reason, it is often considered that

Table 6–11
Physiological Changes Affecting Nutritional Status of the Elderly

General Changes

lean muscle replaced by fat;
reduced calories needs
specific nutrient needs not reduced; therefore, quality of food consumed must be
   maximized;
changes in enzyme activity and secretion of gastric components may occur in elderly;
activity of salivary amylase often decreases with age; proteolytic activity of the enzymes may also decrease;
activity of pancreatic amylase and lipase may decrease;
chlorhydria may increase with age;
glucose tolerance tends to diminish with age;
changes in renal function include reduced rental blood flow and glomerular filtration
   rate;
reduced ability to form either a concentrated or dilute urine.

Table 6-12

Summary of Particular Nutrient Considerations for the Elderly

Vitamins

Absorption may be reduced by disease.

B vitamin deficiency often responsible for mental confusion.

Supplements may be recommended with reduced food intake.

Deficiency of fat soluble vitamins A, D, and E may result from reduced fat in the diet, and from impaired absorption resulting from intake of laxatives or mineral oil.

Minerals

iron — iron deficiency anemia common in elderly; deficiency may result from reduced absorption due to achlorhydria or gastrointestinal malfunction, as well as from reduced intake.

magnesium — deficiency may manifest itself in malabsorption syndromes, with loss of body fluid and cirrhosis of the liver; symptoms include muscular weakness, vertigo, mental changes and tumors, all of which may be easily confused with other disorders of the elderly.

calcium — evidence of need is controversial — conflicting theories relating role of dietary calcium to bone integrity.

A number of factors common to the elderly affect loss of bone calcium: acid ash diet, reduced dietary calcium, reduced exercise, poor circulation; atrophy of organic bone matrix.

fluorine — possible that life-long consumption may reduce risk of osteoporosis.

potassium — diets may be low in; deficiency may be evidenced in confusion and muscle weakness.

Protein — elderly have similar or greater need for essential amino acids, as compared to younger adults; utilization may decrease with age.

Roughage, fiber and water — elderly need sufficient amounts to maintain bowel regularity.

Salt — high intakes should be avoided due to possible relation between intake and congestive heart failure and hypertension.

the appropriate dietary ratio should be similar. However, with the average American diet, the intake of phosphorous is much greater, whereas that of calcium has declined. The ratio of calcium to phosphorous in the typical American diet may now approach 1 to 4.[121] High levels of phosphorous enhance calcium deficiency in animals and perhaps in humans.[122]

It is difficult to determine the degree to which the development of osteoporosis is related to lifelong dietary intakes of calcium and phosphorous. Generally speaking, the prudent diet would include adequate levels of calcium as well as magnesium, other minerals, vitamin D and vitamin C, and protein to protect, to the degree possible, against the development of osteoporosis.

Consumer Buying Practices

The elderly as a group are especially susceptible to fraudulent practices through misrepresentations, health swindles, and faddism. The reasons for this vulnerability include physiological ailments, the desire for quick cures, insufficient information, and the tremendous need for hope that often characterizes the elderly. Minimal research has been devoted to the elderly as consumers.[123] Only recently have the elderly been seen as an important target for advertising. As their numbers increase, however, more interest is being expressed in the elderly by marketers. Many of the elderly are poor, so that they come under the Federal Trade Commission's definition of a "special audience" (one with special needs for information and protection against fraud and deception.)[124]

The shopping process is often a burden to the elderly. Mobility, difficulty in shopping for food buys or walking to the location where prices may be cheaper, limited choice and more expense at the stores frequented by the elderly, food packaging, as well as limited storage facilities — all compound the already difficult task of achieving optimal nutrition for the elderly.

One study conducted to clarify some of the consumer problems of the elderly sampled members of the National Retired Teachers' Association/ American Association of Retired Persons in August and September 1973. The most significant consumer problem reported was food.[125] Respondents were asked what spending areas were reduced in response to inflation. Food away from home was mentioned most often, whereas food eaten at home was the fourth most frequently mentioned item.

The Bureau of Labor Statistics, in its survey of consumer expenses, reported that older families in which the head was between 65 and 74 years of age spent 25.7 per cent of their income for food; families whose head was older than 75 spent 26.7 per cent of their income for food.[126] This leaves little money to cover remaining housing, medical, and other expenses. It is thus clear that the elderly face many problems in attaining optimal nutritional status. Results from studies conducted to determine the dietary habits of the elderly are presented in Table 6–13.[127]

SUMMARY

Describing and interpreting the result of studies on the nutritional status of particular groups is a very complex task. Many uncertainties are involved in ascertaining diets, determining what general indicators of nutritional status actually mean in terms of an individual's nutriture, and identifying causative factors in the development of food habits. Despite the uncertainties, it is clear that many in the United States are not consuming adequate diets. Such poor nutrition will likely translate into health problems. The first step toward the alleviation of nutritional problems is the early identification of factors that predispose an individual to nutritional risk.

CONCLUSION[1]

The subject of this chapter has been the various at-risk populations in the United States. It is useful to consider practical ways for implementing the at-risk concept. If the at-risk factors are to be practically used, it is impor-

Table 6-13
Dietary Status of the Elderly

		Subjects			Recalls	
	Description of Dietary Surveys				*Results of Nutrient Intake Analysis of Dietary Records*	
Reference	Location	No.	Sex	Purpose	Nutrients with Means Less than Standard	Nutrients for Which One-Third Subjects Below Standard
109	Middle Tennessee	343 / 186	F / M	To determine nutritive adequacy of meals and reasons for inadequacies	Not given	Riboflavin, vitamin A, thiamine in both sexes; vitamin C in males; iron in females
128	Luzerne county, Pennsylvania	389 / 184	F / M	To assess impact of congregate meals program for elderly; test validity of 24-hour recall used with elderly persons	Calcium in female nonparticipants	Calories, calcium, vitamin A, thiamine, vitamin C in all subjects; iron in female nonparticipants
66	34 states and District of Columbia	1938	M / F	To measure nutritional status in representative sample of white United States population	Iron in low-income groups; calories in all groups	Calcium, iron, vitamin A, ascorbic acid
129	Rural Pennsylvania	40 / 69	M / F	To evaluate nutritional adequacy of rural citizens	Calcium in females; vitamin A in males and females	Calories, calcium, vitamin A, thiamine, riboflavin, vitamin C
130	Cincinnati, Ohio	135 / 50	F / M	To determine nutritional contribution of meal program to dietary needs of senior citizens	Day including program meal — none below standard; day with no program meal — calories, thiamine in males; calcium in females	Not given
131	Ten provinces, reserves, and crownlands	General Population 926 / 859; Indians 116 / 114; Eskimos 29 / 19	M / F; M / F; M / F	To determine nutritional status of the Canadian population	Not given	*General population:* Iron, vitamin A, calcium, thiamine, riboflavin in both sexes; protein in females only. *Eskimos:* Calcium, vitamin A, vitamin C in both sexes; protein, thiamine, riboflavin in females only. *Indians:* All nutrients except niacin

Dietary Status of the Elderly *(continued)*

| | | Description of Dietary Surveys | | | | Results of Nutrient Intake Analysis of Dietary Records | |
| | | | Subjects | | | Recalls | |
Reference	Location	No.	Sex	Purpose		Nutrients with Means Less than Standard	Nutrients for Which One-Third Subjects Below Standard
43	Ten states	1209 867	F M	To determine magnitude and indication of malnutrition in the United States		Calories in males and females; iron in all black, low-income white, and high-income Spanish-American females; vitamin A in Spanish-Americans; protein in low-income black males and white females, all black females, and high-income Spanish-American females	Calories and eight nutrients except vitamin C intake of high-income black females and calcium intake of white males and high-income Spanish-American males
132	Nationwide	460 624 219 340	M F M F			65–74 years: calories, calcium in both sexes; vitamin A, thiamine, riboflavin in females 75+ years; calories, vitamin C in males; calcium, riboflavin, vitamin A in both sexes	Not given
113	Rochester, New York	179 277	M F	To learn more about dietary problems of the aging		Not given	None
133	Boston, Massachusetts	42 62	M F	To determine relationship of nutrient intake to various social and economic variables		Calories in both sexes	Iron, thiamine, riboflavin
Food Records (one to four days)							
134	Central Missouri	149 317	M F	To evaluate effect of meal program on adequacy of nutrition intake of older Americans		Calories in all groups; calcium in female participants, both nonparticipant groups; niacin in male participants, one nonparticipant group	Not given
135	Indianapolis, Indiana	18 26	M F	To assess adequacy of zinc intake through analysis of hair and determination of taste acuity; to estimate dietary intake of Title VII feeding program participants		Zinc, calcium in both sexes; calories in males	Zinc
136	Berkeley, California	1962 study 98 131 4 study years 68 73	M F M F	To relate nutritional status to mortality rate to determine nutritional status and dietary habits over a 14-year period		1962: calories, niacin in males, calcium, niacin in females	1948, 1952, 1954, 1962: calcium in females; niacin in both sexes

Ref	Location	N	Sex	Purpose		
137	Milwaukee, Wisconsin	23 42	M F	To determine if sufficient food purchased to meet RDA and individual meals of selected patients provide adequate nutrients	Not given	Calories, calcium, vitamin C
				Food Records (over four days)		
138	West Lafayette, Indiana	12 32	M F	To determine differences in status found in elderly ill requiring extended nursing care	Calories, calcium, and niacin in both sexes	Calcium, protein, iron
107	Syracuse, New York	33 67	M F	Information on nutrient intake and status of healthy persons living in own household, either alone or with spouse	Iron, thiamine in females only	Calories in males; vitamin A, vitamin C in both sexes
139	Baltimore, Maryland and Washington, D.C.	252	M	To evaluate effect of age on dietary intake: to estimate energy expenditure and its relation to caloric intake at various ages	Calories in 75–99 years; calcium in 54–64 years	Not given
140	Lincoln, Nebraska	26	F	To determine the intake of nutrients of active, healthy women 65 years or older	Iron	Less than two-thirds RDA: none
133	Boston, Massachusetts	42 62	M F	To determine nutrient intake and its relation to various social and economic variables	Calories: both sexes	Iron, thiamine, riboflavin
				Weighed Intake		
141	Fort Collins and Denver, Colorado	15 45	F F	To compare the nutrient intake of institutionalized and free-living women	Calories, thiamine, calcium in all subjects; iron in 69–75 years group	Less than two-thirds RDA: calcium
140	Lincoln, Nebraska	6	F	To determine intake of nutrients of active healthy women 65 years or older	Iron	Less than two-thirds RDA: none
142	Rhode Island	24 24	M F	To study intake of individuals residing in institution for aged in comparison to RDA and to average portion served in institution	Not given — just range of intake	Protein, iron, niacin, vitamin C
143	Lansing, Michigan	18	F	To determine nitrogen, calcium, and phosphorus retention of older women	Calcium — other results: to maintain equilibrium of protein, calcium, and phosphorus required 1600–1800 calories under 70 years; 1500 calories over 70 years	Not given

Dietary Status of the Elderly (continued)

					Results of Nutrient Intake Analysis of Dietary Records	
	Description of Dietary Surveys				Recalls	
		Subjects				
Reference	Location	No.	Sex	Purpose	Nutrients with Means Less than Standard	Nutrients for Which One-Third Subjects Below Standard
				Dietary Histories		
144	Within 75 miles of Manhattan, Kansas	99 / 98	M and F / M and F	To compare eating behavior of nursing home residents to elderly living in own home	Calcium in both sexes; calories in males	One third had scores of six or lower (less than 67 percent RDA for two or more nutrients)
145	Missouri	45 / 66	M / F	Subgroup of large survey to determine the nutritional status of Missouri residents	Calories	None
146	Boston, Massachusetts	30 / 70	M / F	To study nutritional status of older people living at home	Calories in males; thiamine, iron in females	Less than 75 percent RDA: iron in females; calories in males;
147	Michigan	117	F	To examine relationship between nutritive quality of diets, physical well-being, and body weight	Not given	Less than 80 percent RDA: calories, calcium, iron, vitamin A, vitamin C, thiamine, riboflavin; less than 40 percent RDA: calcium, vitamin A in black women only
				Inventory Method		
137	Milwaukee, Wisconsin	thirteen homes		To determine if sufficient food purchased to meet RDA and if individual meals of selected patients provided adequate nutrients		One home was less than standard in calcium; one home was less than standard in vitamin A; six homes were less than standard in ascorbic acid.

Source: R. O'Hanlon and M. Kohrs. Dietary Studies of Older Americans. *Am. J. Clin. Nutr.* 31 (1978): 1257.

tant that they first be defined through community assessments and epidemiological studies. The factors will vary greatly from one area or situation to another. For example, in a developing country, the single most important factor may be the number of children in the family. In an industrialized nation, the most important factor may be level of income, or it may be the employment status of the mother. After the factors of importance have been identified, their accuracy and predictive value in terms of nutritional status must be assessed. The at-risk factors are dynamic and will change; as one problem is dealt with the importance of other factors will vary.

The concept can be modified so that it can be used by community aides, auxiliaries, or paraprofessionals. Because these individuals are usually of the community and are familiar with the problems there, they can go into the homes for screening as well as for monitoring, intervention, and follow-up. Their work must be supported by strong and effective supervision, and the responsibilities of these workers must be carefully delineated. Some of the simple, practical methods of identification of at-risk populations found useful in different projects include (1) the use of different colored stars on the health records of those at risk, (2) a numerical score, (3) symbols, (4) an "at-risk register," or (5) maps of the district on the wall of the health center with different colored markers indicating the homes of those at risk. As should be clear, it is important that the methods used be of practical value and that they have educational value both for the clients and for the workers or professionals.

Before the at-risk concept can be operationalized in a practical and meaningful way, the given situation must be analyzed and priorities ordered. Criteria to be considered in ordering priorities include:

1. feasibility of management
2. sensibility to change
3. ease of measurement
4. relevance
5. cost
6. interpretation for government
7. production value
8. validity
9. acceptance by population

The evaluation of these at-risk factors may indicate difficulties that are hard to tackle for various economic, sociocultural, or political reasons. However, it is important that the health worker and the planner understand and appreciate the true characteristics of the population, and of the problem as a basis for developing policies and interventions.

If it is to be successfully used, the at-risk concept should be part of a training program for all types of health personnel, including physicians, nurses, nutritionists, and paraprofessional staff. There should also be training in using various mtehods for detecting at-risk factors, such as nutritional anthropometry.

The value of the at-risk concept in identifying and treating nutritional problems has been confirmed in various programs throughout the world. It should become a major influence in the development of programs and of policies designed to alleviate problems of nutrition in the community in the United States, as well. But before this can happen, it is necessary that an awareness of the approach be increased and that health professionals understand and become skilled in the methods for assessing at-risk factors, in setting priorities, and in planning, implementing, and evaluating interventions to alleviate at-risk factors.

REFERENCES

1. International Union of Nutritional Sciences. Guidelines on the at-risk concept and the health and nutrition of young children. *Am. J. Clin. Nutr.* 30 (1977): 242–254.
2. World Health Organization, Organization and Administration of Maternal and Child Health Services. *Fifth Report of the World Health Organization Expert Committee on Maternal and Child Care*, WHO Rept. No. 428. Geneva, 1969.
3. Olson, C., and M. Mapes. *Nutrition, Growth, and Reproduction: Reducing the Risks for Mothers and Infants.* Ithaca, N.Y.: Cornell University, May 1977.
4. Philips, C., and N. E. Johnson. The impact of quality of diet and other factors on birth weight of infants. *Am. J. Clin. Nutr.* 30 (1977): 215.
5. Higgins, A. C. Nutritional status and the outcome of pregnancy. *J. Can. Diet. Assoc.* 37 (1976): 17.
6. Worthington, B. S., J. Vermeersch, and S. R. Williams. *Nutrition in Pregnancy and Lactation.* St. Louis, Mo.: C. V. Mosby, 1977, pp. 10–30.
7. Lowe, C. U. Research in infant nutrition: The untapped well. *Am. J. Clin. Nutr.* 25 (1972): 245–254.
8. McDonald, A. *Children of Very Low Birth Weight.* London: William Heinemann Medical Books, 1967.
9. McBurney, R. D. Undernourished full-term infants: Case report. *West. J. Surg.* 55 (1943): 363.
10. Winick, M., J. Brasel, and E. Velasco. Effects of prenatal nutrition upon pregnancy risk. *Clin. Obstet. Gynecol.* 16 (1973): 184–197.
11. Winick, M. ed. *Nutrition and Fetal Development.* New York: John Wiley, 1974, p. vii.
12. Williams, R. Intrauterine growth curves: Intra- and international comparisons with different ethnic groups in California. *Prev. Med.* 4 (1975): 163–172.
13. Roe, D. A. Concepts of neonatal malnutrition. *N.Y. St. J. Med.* 70 (1970): 420–426.
14. Warkany, J. Experimental studies on nutrition in pregnancy. *Obstet. Gynecol. Surv.* 3 (1948): 693–703.
15. Chow, B. F., and C. Lee. Effect of dietary restriction of pregnant rats on body weight gain of offspring. *J. Nutr.* 26 (1943): 569.
16. Burke, B. S., V. A. Beal, S. B. Kirkwood, and H. C. Stuart. The influence

of nutrition upon the condition of the infant at birth. *J. Nutr.* 26 (1943): 569.

17. Naeye, R. L., M. M. Diener, W. S. Dellinger, et al. Urban poverty: Effects on prenatal nutrition. *Science* 166 (1969): 1026.

18. Naeye, R. L., W. Blanc, and C. Paul. Effects of maternal nutrition on the human fetus. *Pediatrics* 52 (1973): 494.

19. Smith, C. A. Effects of maternal undernutrition upon the newborn infant in Holland. *J. Pediatr.* 30 (1947): 229-243.

20. Antonov, A. N. Children born during the siege of Leningrad. *J. Pediatr.* 30 (1947): 250-259.

21. Springer, N. S., A. M. Byrne, and W. D. Block. Nutritional indexes of clients in a maternity and infant care project. I. The target population. *J. Am. Diet. Assoc.* 71 (1977): 613.

22. Springer, N. S., A. M. Byrne, and W. D. Block. Nutritional indexes of clients in a maternity and infant care project. II. Dietary, anthromopometric, and hematologic indexes of pregnant women and their infants. *J. Am. Diet. Assoc.* 71 (1977): 617.

23. Winick, M. In U.S. Senate Select Committee on Nutrition and Human Needs, *Hearings on Maternal, Fetal, and Infant Nutrition, Part 1.* Washington, D.C.: Government Printing Office, 1973.

24. Committee on Maternal Nutrition, Food and Nutrition Board, National Research Council. Nutritional supplementation and the outcome of pregnancy. *Proceedings of a Workshop,* Sagamore Beach, Mass., November 3-5, 1971. Washington, D.C.: National Academy of Sciences, 1973, pp. 1-153.

25. Committee on Maternal Nutrition, Food and Nutrition Board, National Research Council. *Maternal Malnutrition and the Course of Pregnancy.* Washington, D.C.: National Academy of Sciences, 1970.

26. Birch, H. G. Problems inherent in population of nutrition and mental subnormality, in G. A. Jervis, ed., *Expanding Concepts in Mental Retardation.* Springfield, Ill.: Charles C Thomas, 1968.

27. National Academy of Sciences, National Research Council, Food and Nutrition Board. *Recommended Dietary Allowances,* rev. 1979. Washington, D.C., 1979.

28. U.S. Department of Health, Education, and Welfare, National Center for Health Statistics. *Teenage Childbearing, United States, 1966-75,* Publ. No. (HRA) 77-1120. Washington, D.C., September 8, 1977, vol. 2. (suppl.).

29. Committee on Maternal Nutrition, Food and Nutrition Board. *Annotated Bibliography on Maternal Nutrition.* Washington, D.C.: National Academy of Sciences, 1970.

30. Baizerman, M., C. Sheehan, D. L. Ellison, and E. R. Schlesinger. *Pregnant Adolescents: A Review of Literature with Abstracts, 1960-1970.* Washington, D.C.: Consortium on Early Childbearing and Childrearing, 1971.

31. Weigley, E. S. The pregnant adolescent. *J. Am. Diet. Assoc.* 66 (1975): 588.

32. Kaminetzky, H. A., A. Langer, H. Baker, O. Frank, A. D. Thomson, E. Munves, A. Opper, F. Behrle, and B. Glista. The effect of nutrition in teenage gravidas on pregnancy and the status of the neonate. I. Nutritional profile. *Am. J. Obstet. Gynecol.* 115 (1973): 639.

33. King, J. C., S. Cohenour, D. Calloway, and H. N. Jacobson. Assessment of nutritional status of teenage pregnant girls. I. Nutrient intake and pregnancy. *Am. J. Clin. Nutr.* 25 (1972): 916.

34. Osofsky, H. J., P. Rizk, M. Fox, and J. Mondanaro. Nutritional status of low-income pregnant teenagers. *J. Reprod. Med.* 6 (1971): 29.

35. Seiler, J. A., and F. Fox. Adolescent pregnancy: Association of dietary and obstetric factors. *Home Econ. Res. J.* 1 (1973): 188.

36. Thompson, M. F., E. Morse, and S. Merrow. Nutrient intake of pregnant women receiving vitamin-mineral supplements. *J. Am. Diet. Assoc.* 64 (1974): 382.

37. Dawson, E. B., and W. McGanity. Plasma amino acid alteration during teenage pregnancy. *Am. J. Obstet. Gynecol.* 107 (1970): 585.

38. Dickens, H. O., E. Mudd, C. Garcia, K. Tomar, and D. Wright. One hundred pregnant adolescents: Treatment approaches in a university hospital. *Am. J. Publ. Health* 63 (1973): 794.

39. Cohenour, S. H., and D. Calloway. Blood, urine, and dietary pantothenic acid levels of pregnant teenagers. *Am. J. Clin. Nutr.* 25 (1972): 512.

40. Daniel, W. A., Jr., J. R. Mounger, and J. C. Perkins. Obstetric and fetal complications in folate-deficient adolescent girls. *Am. J. Obstet. Gynecol.* 111 (1971): 233.

41. Van De Mark, M. S., and A. Wright. Hemoglobin and folate levels of pregnant teenagers. *J. Am. Diet. Assoc.* 61 (1972): 511.

42. Ancri, G., E. H. Morse, and R. P. Clarke. Comparison of the nutritional status of pregnant adolescents with adult pregnant women. III. Maternal protein and calorie intake and weight gain in relation to size of infant at birth. *Am. J. Clin. Nutr.* 30 (1977): 568.

43. U.S. Department of Health, Education, and Welfare. *Ten-State Nutrition Survey,* Publ. No. (HSM) 72–8134. Atlanta, Ga., 1972.

44. Howard, M. Multidisciplinary services for school-age pregnant girls. *Am. J. Orthopsych.* 40 (1970): 289.

45. Anderson, R. Meeting the educational needs of the pregnant teenager. III. *Teacher of Home Econ.* 17 (1973): 14.

46. Backalinick, I. A school program designed to help pregnant teenagers. *The New York Times,* June 14, 1974, p. 38.

47. Badger, E., et al. Education for adolescent mothers in a hospital. *Am. J. Publ. Health* 66 (1976): 469.

48. Goldstein, P. J., et al. Vocational education: An unusual approach to adolescent pregnancy. *J. Reprod. Med.* 10 (1973): 77.

49. Hansen, C. M., et al. Effects on pregnant adolescents of attending a special school. *J. Am. Diet. Assoc.* 68 (1976): 538.

50. James, W. F. B. Newer approaches in the management of the pregnant unmarried adolescent. *J. Nat'l Med. Assoc.* 64 (1972): 483.

51. McAnarney, E. R. Provision of maternity and prenatal care to adolescent girls. *Acta Paediatr. Scand.* 236 (1975): 54.

52. Milk, J. C. Adolescent parenthood. *J. Home Econ.* 5 (1973): 31.

53. Osofsky, H. J., R. Rajan, P. W. Wood, and R. Diflorio. An interdisciplinary program for low-income pregnant schoolgirls: A progress report. *J. Reprod. Med.* 5 (1970): 103.

54. Teenage mother and child program. Linkup. N.Y. State Div. for Youth *Newsletter* 4 (1975): 7.

55. Wallace, H. M., E. Gold, H. Goldstein, and A. Oglesby. A study of services and needs of teenage pregnant girls in the large cities of the United States. *Am. J. Publ. Health* 63 (1973): 5.

56. Lindblad, B. S., and R. J. Rahimtolla. A pilot study of the quality of human milk in a lower socioeconomic group in Karachi, Pakistan. *Acta Paediatr. Scand.* 63 (1974): 125.

57. Filer, I. J. Relationship of nutrition to lactation in newborn development, in K. S. Moghissi and T. N. Evans, eds., *Nutritional Impacts on Women —*

Throughout Life with Emphasis on Reproduction. New York: Harper & Row, 1977.

58. Guthrie, H. A. *Introductory Nutrition,* 3d ed. St. Louis, Mo.: C. V. Mosby, 1975.
59. Sims, L. Dietary status of lactating women. I. Nutrient intake from food and from supplements. *J. Am. Diet. Assoc.* 73 (1978): 139.
60. Fomon, S. J. *Infant Nutrition,* 2d ed. Philadelphia: W. B. Saunders, 1974.
61. Owen, G., A. H. Lubin, and P. L. J. Garry. Preschool children in the U.S.: Who has iron deficiency? *J. Pediatr.* 79 (1971): 563.
62. U.S. Department of Health, Education, and Welfare, National Center for Health Statistics. *Preliminary Findings, First Health and Nutrition Examination Survey, United States, 1971–1972. Dietary Intake and Biochemical Findings,* Publ. No. (HRA) 74-1219-1. Rockville, Md., January 1974.
63. Nutrition program evaluated. Report on education research. *Education Daily.* November 30, 1977, p. 4.
64. Fomon, S. J. *Nutritional Disorders of Children. Prevention, Screening, and Follow-up,* Publ. No. (HSA) 77-5104. Rockville, Md.: U.S. Department of Health, Education, and Welfare, 1977 reprint.
65. Hunter, R. E., and N. J. Smith. Hemoglobin and hematocrit values in iron deficiency in infancy. *J. Pediatr.* 81 (1972): 710.
66. Abraham, S., F. W. Lowenstein, and C. J. Johnson. *Preliminary Findings of the First Health and Nutrition Examination Survey, United States, 1971–1972.* Washington, D.C.: Government Printing Office, 1974.
67. Haddy, T. B., C. Jurkowski, H. Brody, D. Kallen, and D. M. Czajka-Narins. Iron deficiency with and without anemia in infants and children. *Am. J. Dis. Child.* 128 (1974): 787.
68. Theuer, R. C. Iron undernutrition in infancy. *Clin. Pediatr.* 13 (1974): 522.
69. Futrell, M. F., L. T. Kilgore, and F. Windham. Nutritional status of Negro preschool children in Mississippi. *J. Am. Diet. Assoc.* 59 (1971): 224.
70. Futrell, M. F., L. T. Kilgore, and F. Windham. Nutritional status of black preschool children in Mississippi. Influence of income, mother's education, and food programs. *J. Am. Diet. Assoc.* 66 (1975): 22.
71. Fryer, B. A., G. Lamkin, V. Vivian, E. Eppright, and H. Fox. Diets of preschool children in the North Central region: Calories, proteins, fats, and carbohydrates. *J. Am. Diet. Assoc.* 59 (1971): 228.
72. Fox, H., B. Fryer, G. Lamkin, V. Vivian, and E. Eppright. Diets of preschool children in the North Central region: Calcium, phosphorous, and iron. *J. Am. Diet. Assoc.* 59 (1971): 233.
73. Frank, G. C., A. W. Voors, B. E. Schilling, and G. S. Berenson. Dietary studies of rural schoolchildren in a cardiovascular survey. *J. Am. Diet. Assoc.* 71 (1977): 31.
74. Caliendo, M. A., D. Sanjur, J. Wright, and G. Cummings. Nutritional status of preschool children. *J. Am. Diet. Assoc.* 71 (1977): 20.
75. Margo, G., Y. Baroni, R. Green, and J. Metz. Anemia in urban underprivileged children. Iron, folate, and vitamin B-12 nutrition. *Am. J. Clin. Nutr.* 30 (1977): 947.
76. Johnson, C. C., and M. F. Futrell. Anemia in black preschool children in Mississippi. *J. Am. Diet. Assoc.* 65 (1974): 539.
77. Sturgeon, P. Studies of iron requirements in infants. *Brit. J. Haematol.* 5 (1959): 45.
78. Haughton, J. Nutritional anemia of infancy and childhood. *Am. J. Publ. Health* 53 (1963): 1121.

79. Danneker, D. *Anemia in Selected Allegheny County Child Health Conference Populations.* Pittsburgh: Allegheny County Health Department, 1966.
80. Kravitz, H. Results of "Operation Head Start" in Chicago. *Illinois Med. J.* 129 (1966): 590.
81. Dwyer, J. T., R. Palombo, H. Thorne, I. Valadian, and R. Reed. Preschoolers on alternate life-style diets. *J. Am. Diet. Assoc.* 72 (1978): 264.
82. Hutcheson, R. H. Iron deficiency anemia in Tennessee among rural poor children. *Publ. Health Rep.* 83 (1968): 939.
83. Gutelius, M. F. The problem of iron deficiency anemia in preschool Negro children. *Am. J. Publ. Health* 59 (1969): 290.
84. Bryan, A. H., and E. L. Anderson. Dietary and nutritional problems of crippled children in five rural counties of North Carolina. *Am. J. Publ. Health* 55 (1965): 1545.
85. Child Development Group of Mississippi, Nutrition Services Division. *Surveys of Family Meal Patterns.* May 17 and July 11, 1967.
86. Owen, G. M., and K. M. Kram. Nutritional status of preschool children in Mississippi: Food sources of nutrients in the diets. *J. Am. Diet. Assoc.* 54 (1969): 490.
87. Kerrey, E., S. Crispin, H. M. Fox, and C. Kies. Nutritional status of preschool children. I. Dietary and biochemical findings. *Am. J. Clin. Nutr.* 21 (1968): 1274.
88. Crispin, S., E. Kerrey, H. M. Fox, and C. Kies. Nutritional status of preschool children. II. Anthropometric measurements and interrelationships. *Am. J. Clin. Nutr.* 21 (1968): 1280.
89. Cook, R. A., S. B. Davis, F. H. Radke, and M. E. Thornbury. Nutritional status of Head Start and nursery school children. *J. Am. Diet. Assoc.* 68 (1976): 120.
90. Lieberman, H. M., I. F. Hunt, A. H. Coulson, V. A. Clark, M. E. Swendseid, and L. Ho. Evaluation of a ghetto school breakfast program. *J. Am. Diet. Assoc.* 68 (1976): 132.
91. Morgan, A. F., ed. *Nutritional Status, U.S.A.,* Bull. 769. Albany, Calif.: California Agricultural Experiment Station, 1959.
92. Huenemann, R. L. A review of teenage nutrition in the United States. *Proceedings of National Nutritional Education Conference,* Misc. Publ. No. 1254. Washington, D.C.: U.S. Department of Agriculture, 1973, pp. 37–41.
93. U.S. Department of Agriculture, Consumer and Food Economics Research Division. *Food Intake and Nutritive Value of Diets of Men, Women, and Children in the U.S., Spring 1965,* Rept. No. 62–18. Washington, D.C.: Agricultural Research Service, 1969.
94. Hodges, R. E., and W. A. Krehl. Nutritional status of teenagers in Iowa. *Am. J. Clin. Nutr.* 17 (1965): 200–210.
95. Hampton, M. C., R. L. Huenemann, L. R. Shapiro, and B. W. Mitchell. Caloric and nutrient intakes of teenagers. *J. Am. Diet. Assoc.* 50 (1967): 385.
96. Wharton, M. A. Nutritive intake of adolescents. *J. Am. Diet. Assoc.* 42 (1964): 306–310.
97. Dibble, M., M. Brin, E. McMullen, A. Peel, and N. Chen. Some preliminary biochemical findings in junior high school children in Syracuse an.¹ Onondaga County, N.Y. *Am. J. Clin. Nutr.* 17 (1965): 218.
98. Huenemann, R. L., L. R. Shapiro, M. C. Hampton, and B. W. Mitchell. Food and eating practices of teenagers. *J. Am. Diet. Assoc.* 53 (1968): 17.

99. Christakis, G., A. Miridjanian, L. Nath, H. Khurana, C. Cowell, M. Archer, O. Frank, H. Ziffer, H. Baker, and G. James. A nutritional epidemiologic investigation of 642 New York City children. *Am. J. Clin. Nutr.* 21 (1968): 107.

100. Myers, M., S. O'Brien, J. Mabel, and F. Stare. A nutrition study of schoolchildren in a depressed urban district. I. Dietary findings. *J. Am. Diet. Assoc.* 53 (1968): 226.

101. Weg, R. B. *Nutrition and the Later Years.* Los Angeles: University of Southern California, Ethel Perry Andrews Gerontology Center, 1978, pp. 1-2.

102. Krehl, W. A. The influences of nutritional environment on aging. *Geriatrics* 29 (1970): 65-76.

103. Winick, M., ed. *Nutrition and Aging.* New York: John Wiley, 1976, p. v.

104. White House Conference on Food, Nutrition, and Health. Washington, D.C.: Government Printing Office, 1969.

105. White House Conference on the Aging. The elderly consumer. *Reports of the Special Sessions on the Elderly Consumer.* Washington, D.C.: Government Printing Office, 1971.

106. Ossofsky, J., and A. Anderson. *A Nutrition Program for the Elderly.* Washington, D.C.: National Council on the Aging, April 1972.

107. Dibble, M. V., M. Brin, V. F. Thiele, A. Peel, N. Chen, and E. McMullen. Evaluation of the nutritional status of elderly subjects with a comparison between fall and spring. *J. Am. Geriat. Soc.* 15 (1967): 1031.

108. Harrill, I., C. Erbes, and C. Schwartz. Observations on food acceptance by elderly women. *The Gerontologist* 16 (August 1976): 349.

109. Todhunter, E. N., F. House, and R. VanderZwaag. *Food Acceptance and Food Attitudes of the Elderly as a Basis for Planning Nutrition Programs.* Nashville, Tennessee: Tennessee Commission on the Aging, 1974.

110. Johnson, G. S. Food intake patterns and the relative positions of factors affecting ingestion of nutrients of selected elderly adults in the Akron, Ohio area. Unpublished Master's thesis. Kent, Ohio: Kent State University, 1971.

111. Clancy, K. L. Preliminary observations on media use and food habits of the elderly. *The Gerontologist* 15 (1975): 529-532.

112. Debry, G., R. Bleyer, and J. M. Martin. Nutrition of the elderly. *J. Human Nutr.* 31 (June 1977): 195.

113. LeBovit, C. The food of older persons living at home. *J. Am. Diet. Assoc.* 46 (1965): 285.

114. Eckerstrom, S. Clinical aspects of metabolism in the elderly. *Geriatrics* 21 (1966): 161-165.

115. Mayer, J. Aging and nutrition. *Geriatrics* 29 (1974): 57-59.

116. Winick, M. Nutrition and aging. *Contemporary Nutr.* 2 (1977); one-page circular.

117. Rao, D. B. Problems of nutrition in the aged. *J. Am. Geriatr. Soc.* 21 (1973): 362-367.

118. Morgan, A. F. Nutrition of the aging. *The Gerontologist* 2 (1962): 77-84.

119. Smith, R. W., and J. Rizek. Epidemiologic studies of osteoporosis in women in Puerto Rico and southeastern Michigan with special reference to age, race, national origin, and to other related or associated findings. *Clin. Ortho. and Related Res.* 45 (1966): 31.

120. Lutwak, L. Osteoporosis: A mineral deficiency disease. *J. Am. Diet. Assoc.* 44 (1964): 173.

121. Lutwak, L. Periodontal disease, in M. Winick, ed., *Nutrition and Aging.* New York: John Wiley, 1976, p. 145.
122. Hegsted, D. M. Major minerals. Section A. Calcium and phosphorous, in R. S. Goodhart and M. E. Shils, eds., *Modern Nutrition in Health and Disease.* Philadelphia: Lea and Febiger, 1973, pp. 268–286.
123. Klippel, R., and T. Swenney. The use of information sources by the aged consumer. *The Gerontologist* 14 (1974): 163–166.
124. Howard, J., and J. Hulbert. *Advertising and the Public Interest. A Staff Report to the Federal Trade Commission.* Chicago: Crain Communications, 1973.
125. Waddell, F. E., ed. *The Elderly Consumer.* Columbia, Md.: Antioch College, Human Ecology Center, 1976.
126. U.S. Bureau of Labor Statistics, Consumer Expenditures and Income. *Urban United States, 1960–61,* Rept. No. 237–38. Washington, D.C.: Government Printing Office, 1964.
127. O'Hanlon, R., and M. Kohrs. Dietary studies of older Americans. *Am. J. Clin. Nutr.* 31 (1978): 1257.
128. Goodman, S. Assessment of nutritional impact of congregate meals program for the elderly. Unpublished Ph.D. thesis. University Park: Pennsylvania State University, 1974.
129. Guthrie, H. A., K. Black, and J. P. Madden. Nutritional practices of elderly citizens in rural Pennsylvania. *Gerontology* 12 (1972): 330.
130. Joering, E. Nutrient contribution of a meals program for senior citizens. *J. Am. Diet. Assoc.* 59 (1971): 129.
131. Nutrition Canada. *Nutrition Canada National Survey, 1970–72.* Ottawa: Information Canada, 1973.
132. U.S. Department of Agriculture, Consumer and Food Economics Research Division. *Food and Nutrient Intake of Individuals in the United States. Spring 1965. USDA Household Food Consumption Survey, 1965–66,* Rept. No. 11. Washington, D.C.: Government Printing Office, 1972.
133. Davidson, C. S., J. Livermore, P. Anderson, and S. Kaufman. The nutrition of a group of apparently healthy aging persons. *Am. J. Clin. Nutr.* 10 (1962): 181.
134. Kohrs, M. B., P. S. O'Hanlon, and D. Eklund. Contribution of the older American's nutrition program to one day's dietary intake. *J. Am. Diet. Assoc.* 72 (1978): 487.
135. Greger, J. L., and B. S. Sciscoe. Zinc nutriture of elderly participants in urban feeding program. *J. Am. Diet. Assoc.* 70 (1977): 37.
136. Steinkamp, R. C., N. L. Cohen, and J. E. Walsh. Re-survey of an aging population — 14-year follow-up. *J. Am. Diet. Assoc.* 46 (1965): 103.
137. Hankin, H. J., and J. C. Antohmattei. Survey of food service practices in nursing homes. *Am. J. Publ. Health* 50 (1960): 1137.
138. Justice, C. V., J. Howe, and H. Clark. Dietary intakes and nutritional status of elderly patients. *J. Am. Diet. Assoc.* 65 (1974): 639.
139. McGandy, R. B., C. H. Barrows, Jr., A. Spanias, A. Meredith, J. L. Stone, and A. H. Norris. Nutrient intakes and energy expenditures in men of different ages. *J. Gerontol.* 21 (1966): 581.
140. Fry, P. C., H. M. Fox, and H. Linkswiler. Nutrient intakes of healthy, older women. *J. Am. Diet. Assoc.* 42 (1963): 218.
141. Harrill, I., C. Erbes, and C. Schwartz. Observations on food acceptance by elderly women. *Gerontology* 16 (1976): 349.
142. Tucker, R., C. Brine, and M. Wallace. Nutritive intake of older institutionalized persons. *J. Am. Diet. Assoc.* 32 (1958): 819.
143. Ohlson, M. A., L. Jackson, J. Boek, D. D. Cederquist, W. D. Brewer, and

E. G. Brown. Nutrition and dietary habits of aging women. *Am. J. Publ. Health* 40 (1950): 101.

144. Clarke, M., and L. Wakefield. Food choice of institutionalized vs. independent-living elderly. *J. Am. Diet. Assoc.* 66 (1975): 600.
145. Kohrs, M. B., R. O'Neal, A. Preston, D. Eklund, and O. Abrahams. Nutritional status of elderly residents in Missouri. *Am. J. Clin. Nutr.* 32 (1978): 2186.
146. Lyons, J. C., and M. F. Trulson. Food practices of older people living at home. *J. Gerontol.* 11 (1956): 66.
147. Kelley, L., M. Ohlson, and L. Harper. Food selection and well-being of aging women. *J. Am. Diet. Assoc.* 33 (1957): 466.

section two
END OF SECTION ACTIVITIES

1. How aware are you of the changes that have taken place in the North American diet during the twentieth century? Take the following quiz and find out.

The Changing American Diet Quiz

1. Of the total vitamin C in the diet of the average North American in 1976, how much came from citrus fruit (processed and fresh; includes orange juice)?

a) 28 per cent   b) 48 per cent   c) 68 per cent

2. How many eight-ounce servings of soft drinks did the average American drink in 1976?

a) 86   b) 367   c) 493

3. In the average North American's diet, how many calories a day come from alcoholic beverages?

a) 90   b) 210   c) 350

4. Was coffee consumption in 1976 higher or lower than it was in 1946? By how much?

a) 62 per cent higher   b) 36 per cent lower   c) 134 per cent higher

5. On the average, how many four-ounce glasses of frozen orange juice did North Americans drink in 1976?

a) 110   b) 240   c) 365

6. Of all the fresh fruit that North Americans bought in 1976, what proportion was bananas?

a) 18 per cent   b) 36 per cent   c) 52 per cent

7. How much cheese (including cottage cheese) did North Americans eat (on the average) in 1976?

a) 20.7 pounds   b) 35.3 pounds   c) 55.5 pounds

8. How much red meat (beef, lamb, pork, and veal) did North Americans consume on the average in 1976?

a) 85.2 pounds   b) 165.2 pounds   c) 242.5 pounds

9. How much of the ice cream and ice milk that North Americans ate in 1976 was vanilla?

      a) 72 per cent   b) 42 per cent   c) 24 per cent

10. What percentage of the daily calorie intake was supplied by added sweeteners (sugar, corn syrup, etc.) in 1976?

      a) 3 per cent   b) 10 per cent   c) 18 per cent

11. By how much is the magnesium content of the 1976 North American diet higher or lower than it was in 1910?

  a) 60 per cent higher   b) 32 per cent higher   c) 16 per cent lower

12. Did North Americans in 1976 get more or fewer of their calories from fat than did those in 1919?

      a) less than 5 per cent more or less   b) 17 per cent more

                    c) 31 per cent more

Answers

1-a, 2-c, 3-b, 4-b, 5-a, 6-b, 7-a, 8-b, 9-b, 10-c, 11-c, 12-c

Source: Center for Science in the Public Interest

2. Nutritional Status, U.S.A.

It is highly possible that hunger and poverty exist in your community. Identify a particular section of your community that is especially vulnerable to nutritional problems. Also identify community groups that work directly with the selected group. Design a plan for identifying nutritional problems suffered by the group. Meet with the identified community group to plan a method to implement your assessment plan.

Use the "at-risk" concept in designing your study. How can the use of this concept and the results of your study be used in planning for interventions into the problems that are uncovered? Could you train paraprofessionals to make use of the "at-risk" concept? What material would you use in such training?

After actual problems have been identified, design an intervention strategy that would enable you to experience a direct relationship with the vulnerable group while attempting to help improve their nutritional status.

If possible, implement the intervention strategy and collect data to evaluate it.

Refer to the Community Study to Identify Nutrition Program Needs" pp. 219–227, for help in your community survey.

3. It is often stated that food habits are very difficult to change. Yet a look at today's food habits, relative to those of 50 years ago, demonstrates great change. What factors influenced these changes? How have the changes influenced the health status of the population in the United States? On balance, have the changes had a negative or positive influence on the health status of the North American public?

4. What is the difference between nutritional assessment and nutritional surveillance? In what instances is each appropriate? Are there any efforts in your community to undertake nutritional surveillance activities? Talk to people in the public health department about this. Do they see a need

(End-of-section activities continue on page 227.)

Community Study to Identify Nutrition Program Needs
_____

To: Nutritionists

Subject: Guide for Use of Community Study to Identify
          Nutrition Program Needs

1. The Community Study to Identify Program Needs is a tool developed to aid in learning about the community influences on nutrition, including key persons and agencies providing nutrition related services or who may influence these programs, results of nutrition status, dietary or other studies and statistical information which provides a basis for better understanding the county and for developing a nutrition program for the community.

2. Some sources of data and information for completing the Community Study include:

1. Most recent edition *Florida Vital Statistics* (also available in county health agencies for information for last complete calendar year)
2. *Florida Education Director*
3. *Directory of State Government* (printed annually)
    Bureau of Economics and Business Research
    College of Business Administration
    University of Florida
4. *Florida Statistical Abstract* (printed annually)
    University of Florida Press
5. Latest Census Report (1970)
6. *New Florida Atlas, Patterns of Sunshine State, 1974*
    Trend Publications

Other printed resources:

1. Directories
    Telephone
    Professional (Dietetic, Nursing Associations, and so
      forth)
    Nutrition Committee
    Community Services
2. Local Newspapers (general information)

Personal and Agency contacts:

1. County Health Department (public health nurses, sanitarians, clerks and other personnel)
2. Other Health Professionals
3. County Courthouse (County Commissioners)
4. Home Economics Extension Agent
5. Schools (School Food Service Director, health coordinator, Home Economics teacher/s, principals)
6. District Division of Family Services office
7. Local Mass Media (food editor or writers, public service directors)

8. Representatives from other community agencies (Red Cross, Voluntary Agencies, and so forth.)
9. Librarians (for miscellaneous county and census data; for aid in locating additional resouces)
10. Chamber of Commerce (local and state — Jacksonville)
11. Area Planning Boards (larger cities, for information on housing)
12. University of Florida Bureau of Economics and Business Research (to request statistical abstracts about age distribution)
13. Florida Department of Commerce, Tallahassee (for employment data)

Public Health Nutritionists should be familiar with and review:

Nutritional Assessment in Health Programs, a November, 1973 *Supplement to the Journal of the American Public Health Association* which includes a thorough description of the assessment of communities to help determine nutritional needs, provides the basis for including different types of information on the community assessment and suggests other resource information.

Information gathered should be reviewed in conjunction with ongoing programs of the county health department, priorities of other disciplines, known interests of other agencies, statistical information and any gaps in service revealed in the assessment. These problems and needs and how they can be resolved should be discussed in space provided.

After completion of the community study, note changes in personnel, programs and additional factors influencing the nutrition program when they occur to save time at a future date and to have the information readily available for yourself and others.

County: _____
Year: _____

Community Study to Identify Nutrition Program Needs

1. Population:
    a. Total _____ White _____ Non-white _____
    b. Age distribution:
        (1) Infants (total resident live births last year)
                          White _____ Non-white _____
        (2) Preschool (8% of total population)_____
        (3) Elementary school age _____
        (4) High school age _____
        (5) Adult population _____
        (6) Estimated population over 65 _____
        (7) Estimated seasonal population _____
                          Migrant_____ Tourist _____
2. County characteristics:
    a. Square miles area _____
    b. Total population _____

Community Study to Identify Nutrition Program Needs *(continued)*

    c. Population density _____

    d. Languages commonly spoken (other than English)

    _____

3. County government:

    a. County Commissioners

        (1) Board Chairman: _____

        (2) Board members: _____

                _____

                _____

                _____

    b. County Health Services

        (1) County Health Officer _____

        (2) County Nursing Director _____

             Number of Nurses _____

             Nurse Specialists_____

             _____

             _____

        (3) County Sanitarian Director _____

             Number of Sanitarians _____

        (4) Other personnel (Dentists, Health Educators, and so forth)

        _____

        _____

    c. County Welfare Director _____

    d. Socio-Economic factors _____

        (1) Range of family incomes _____

            (a) % of population with incomes below current index of

                poverty:

                $ _____% White _____ % Non-white _____

        (2) Rate of unemployment _____

        (3) Major businesses and industries: _____

        _____

        _____

        (4) Number of persons receiving public assistance:

            Aid for dependent children _____

            Supplemental Security Income _____

               for the blind _____ _____

              for the disabled _____

               for the aged _____

            County Welfare _____

        (5) County participation in food assistance programs:

            (a) Food stamp program

                Number participating _____

                Estimated % of eligibles _____

            (b) Supplemental Food Program (W.I.C.)

                Number of participating:

                Women _____Infants _____Children (1–3) _____

        (6) Number of emergency food orders in past year (Welfare

            agency only)_____

(7) Emergency feeding programs for county in cases of disaster

_____

_____

_____

_____

(8) Other sources of emergency food (churches, Salvation Army, and so forth) _____

_____

_____

_____

4. State government:
   a. Area senators: _____

   _____

   b. Area Representatives: _____

   _____

5. Educational facilities:
   a. Universities
      colleges or   Programs in food,
      technical   Estimated   nutrition, home eco-
      schools   enrollment   nomics, etc.

      (1) _____   _____   _____
      (2) _____   _____   _____
      (3) _____   _____   _____
      (4) _____   _____   _____

   b. Schools (total number)_____   Enrollment   Literacy rate

      Public   _____   _____
      Private and/or   Educational
         Parochial   _____   _____   level (Adults)
      Special Schools   _____   _____   _____
      (1) School Board:
          (a) Chairman   _____
          (b) Members_____   _____

          _____   _____

      (2) Supervisory personnel:
          (a) Superintendent of Schools _____
          (b) Supervisor of Instruction _____
          (c) Specialized personnel:
              School Food Service Supervisor _____
              Home Economics Supervisor _____
              Health Coordinator _____
              Other _____
      (3) Special Programs:
          (a) Adult Education _____
          (b) Classes for Young Parents _____
          (c) Preventive Dentistry_____
      (4) Health curriculum includes nutrition _____

Community Study to Identify Nutrition Program Needs *(continued)*

(5) School food service participation
Type A Lunch Breakfast Special Milk
Total No. of
students par-
ticipating _____ _____ _____
No. of students
participating _____ _____ _____
Price range _____ _____ _____
No. served
free _____ _____ _____
No. served at
reduced price _____ _____ _____

6. County and State Institutions (excluding hospitals, schools), (include halfway houses, youth, correctional facilities).

Name Capacity Contact person Phone

_____ _____ _____ _____

_____ _____ _____ _____

_____ _____ _____ _____

_____ _____ _____ _____

_____ _____ _____ _____

7. Community resources:
    a. Hospitals, skilled nursing facilities and nursing homes (use continuation sheet if necessary).

Name # of beds Registered Dietitian Phone FT PT

_____ _____ _____ _____

_____ _____ _____ _____

_____ _____ _____ _____

_____ _____ _____ _____

b. Home Health Care Programs

Name Contact Person Phone

_____ _____ _____

_____ _____ _____

_____ _____ _____

Health and Medical personnel: (number)
(1) Doctors _____
(2) Dentists _____
(3) Midwives _____
(4) RN's _____
(5) PHN's _____
(6) LPN's _____
c. Specialists _____
(7) Registered dietitians _____
(8) Food services supervisors qualitied for HIEFSS _____
(9) Physicians assistants _____
(10) Dietetic technicians _____
(11) Dietetic assistants _____

Community Study to Identify Nutrition Program Needs *(continued)*

d. Health agencies (official, non-official, VNA, Heart Association, and so forth, attach community services guide if available)

_____

_____

_____

_____

e. Home Economics Extension Program:
   Senior or Supervising Home Economics
   Extension Agent_____

   No. of agents _____ No. of program aides _____
   Expanded Nutrition Education Program:
   Total families served_____
   No. of Aides_____

f. Nutrition Committee members and agencies represented (attach directory if available) _____

_____

_____

_____

g. Daytime programs for children: Number _____
      Number of children served _____
      Number serving meals _____
   Headstart Programs: Number _____
      Number of children served _____
      Sponsoring agency _____
      Director _____
   Programs with government reimbursement for meals and snacks:
   Number _____
      Number of children served _____
   Is there a Florida Association of Children Under Six chapter?

   _____

h. Mass media:
   (1) Newspapers   Food Editor or contact person   Phone

   _____   _____   _____

   (2) Radio Sta-   Public Service Director/s   Phone
       tions

   _____   _____   _____

   _____   _____   _____

   _____   _____   _____

   _____   _____   _____

   (3) Television   Public Service
       Stations   Director/s   Phone

   _____   _____   _____

   _____   _____   _____

   _____   _____   _____

Community Study to Identify Nutrition Program Needs *(continued)*

_____   _____   _____
_____   _____   _____

Programs and names where nutrition may be best included:

_____
_____
_____

i. Other pertinent programs, for example, Community Action Programs, Emergency Food and Medical Programs, Home Delivered
Meals, Congregate Dining Programs, Alcohol and Drug Rehabilitation Programs, and so forth (use continuation sheet if necessary).

Name of Program   Contact person   # served   Phone

_____   _____   _____   _____
_____   _____   _____   _____
_____   _____   _____   _____
_____   _____   _____   _____

8. Vital Statistics: (County)
    a. Birth rate 19___ _____
        (1) White   _____
        (2) Non-white   _____
        Actual resident number births _____
        Actual resident number births (W) _____
        Actual resident number births (NW)_____
    b. Death rate 19 ___ _____
        (1) White   _____
        (2) Non-white   _____
        Actual resident number deaths _____
        Actual resident number deaths (W) _____
        Actual resident number deaths (NW) _____
    c. Specific mortality rates (list calendar year)

	(1) *County:*		(2) *State:*	
Maternal:	Total ____ Rate ____		Total ____	Rate ____
# White	____	____	____	____
# Non-white	____	____	____	____
Infant:	Total ____ Rate ____		Total ____	Rate ____
# White	____	____	____	____
# Non-white	____	____	____	____
Neo-natal	Total ____ Rate ____		Total ____	Rate ____
# White	____	____	____	____
# Non-white	____	____	____	____

    d. Deliveries (last calendar year)

	Total	*White*	*Non-white*
(1) # live births	_____	_____	_____
(2) # hospital deliveries	_____	_____	_____
(3) # home deliveries	_____	_____	_____

Community Study to Identify Nutrition Program Needs *(continued)*

       (4) # illegiti-
          mate births   _____   _____   _____
       (5) # births less
          than 5 lbs.,
          8 oz.   _____   _____   _____
       (6) # births to
          mothers under
          18 years   _____   _____   _____

   e. Ten leading causes of death (least calendar year)

       (1) _____   Number _____
       (2) _____   _____
       (3) _____   _____
       (4) _____   _____
       (5) _____   _____
       (6) _____   _____
       (7) _____   _____
       (8) _____   _____
       (9) _____   _____
      (10) _____   _____

9. Food and water supply:
    Extent and type of agricultural production:

    Natural and man induced influences on water and food supply:

    Is water supply fluoridated? _____
    Natural fluoridation? _____

10. Cultural characteristics: (Such as Ethnic Groups, Attitudes, Nutrition, Food and Health Concepts, Opinion Molders, and so forth):

11. Results of any nutrition status or dietary studies done in the county:

12. Potential caseload of high risk groups as found in existing screening programs:

    CVD _____   Diabetes _____   Others _____
    Hypertension _____   Medicaid _____
    List nutrition related problems found in medicaid screening:

Community Study to Identify Nutrition Program Needs *(continued)*

---

13. Results of housing studies or surveys:
    Number of low income public housing units _____
    Total inhabitants _____
    Number of low income public housing units for the elderly _____
    Estimated No. of homes:
       Without electricity _____
       Without any plumbing _____
       Without indoor toilets _____
       Without radios _____
       Without television _____
14. Discussion of food and nutrition problems and needs which can be met through the public health nutrition programs:

Source: E. Peck, ed. *Leadership and Quality Assurance in Ambulatory Health Care. Proceedings of the National Public Health Nutrition Workshop.* Chicago, Illinois, May 1977.

---

for any surveillance activities? What resources are needed to begin such activities? What might be target populations for nutritional surveillance?

5. What are your personal feelings about poverty, hunger, and deprivation? State whether you agree or disagree with the following statements.

a. People who are poor deserve to be so. They usually could find jobs, but don't want to work.

b. My parents worked very hard to be where they are now. Others should do likewise. Welfare should be limited to extreme cases in which physical handicaps hinder an individual's ability to work.

c. I really understand what it is like to be poor.

d. Poverty in the United States is not really related to the way I live.

e. The major problem in the United States is inflation, not poverty.

f. The U.S. government should spend a greater part of its budget to aid the poor and impoverished.

g. Every North American should be guaranteed the right to a nutritious diet; if an individual can't afford it on his or her own, the government has a responsibility to aid in insuring this basic right.

h. The problem of poverty in the United States is so complex that there is really little I personally can do about it.

i. The problems of hunger in the United States are so pressing and urgent that I should take some sort of personal action now; I don't have time to wait until I know all the facts about poverty and nutritional deprivation in this country.

j. Poverty in the United States is in large part the result of monopoly and oligopoly in the North American food industry.

Discuss your responses with those of others. Did you find it easy to respond to these statements? How do responses to statements such as these influence the existence of poverty and malnutrition in the United States? How might certain attitudes be modified?

6. The amount of funds allocated to a given program depends in large part on the priorities of legislators and program planners. There are often many worthy priorities, but, because funds are limited, choices must be made. Use the priorities lists that follow to rank the items in each list, from most to least important, in terms of what you believe is most deserving of attention, concern, and resources. Did you have any difficulty in ranking your priorities? What values were important in your decisions?

Personal priorities

    Many good friends

    A safe, healthful environment

    A satisfying job

    Good grades in school

    Material security, including a home

    A good relationship with family and friends

    A high social and prestige position among your peers

    Much free time to pursue leisure activities

    A college degree

    Good health

National priorities

    A strong national defense

    High-quality health care for all Americans

    Expanded, improved, and reduced-price transportation systems

    Better relationship with Third World countries

    A safe, healthful environment

    Free public education through college

    Universal health insurance

    Elimination of poverty-related hunger in the United States

    Elimination of racial prejudice

    Elimination of sexual prejudice

Nutritional priorities

    Outreach for the Food Stamp Program*

    Increased number of free school lunches*

    Improved nutrition education in the school lunch program*

    Nutrition education for all participants in the WIC* Program

    Increased free food stamps*

*See Chapter 17 for a description of these programs.

Funds for nutrition education through the mass media

Increased number of Meals on Wheels

Increased number of school breakfast programs*

Increased participation in the WIC Program*

Nutrition education in the Nutrition Program for the Elderly*

7. The case history of Mrs. Pamela West illustrates the hardships imposed on many by the current financial crunch and spiraling inflation. These hardships are especially relevant to this section as they relate to the ability of the poor to obtain a nutritious and varied diet.

Mrs. West and her two children are part of America's migrant farmworker class; as such, they are among the poorest and most economically deprived in the United States. Mrs. West's annual earnings are less than $2,000, considerably less than the official poverty level. She has less than $225 available monthly to meet her expenses. She often takes a 20-mile bus trip to the nearest food stamp office, where she can increase her purchasing power with food stamps. The trip is a hardship, not only financially, as it costs her many hours in earnings during planting and harvesting seasons, but it is also a hardship in terms of time away from her children.

Because of her limited income, Mrs. West's family suffers severe consequences related to poor nutritional status and, hence, poor health. Susan, her 10-year-old daughter, has lasting facial marks, the result of early skin disease related to vitamin and mineral deficiency. Joey, the 6-year-old son, also suffers the consequences of poor diet; he frequently falls victim to contagious infections, is anemic, and often suffers from contagious diseases his classmates are able to resist. The eyesight of the children is also impaired, possibly the result of vitamin deficiency.

Mrs. West tries very hard to provide proper sustenance for her children. She is quite concerned about the effects of poor nutrition on her children's health, but also on their education. Because her children are often sick, they frequently miss school. Even when they are in school, their attention is sometimes diverted by hunger pangs. Many days the children go to school without breakfast; the school has a lunch program, but no breakfast program. Federal funds are available for a breakfast program, but local school officials adamantly refuse to have the program in their schools.

Mrs. West dreams that her children will be fortunate enough to graduate from high school, but the statistical odds are against it. Soon the children will be old enough to go out and work daily in the fields. The income they can contribute will help to improve the health and nutritional status of the family, and their education will likely be forgotten.

Many hard choices must be made. You, as a community nutritionist, have been asked to develop a series of plans to help Mrs. West and others in her situation. Outline the steps you would take to identify in greater detail the problems experienced by Mrs. West. What solutions would you propose? Would they be primarily of a nutritional nature? Would they be acceptable to Mrs. West? Would they be acceptable to local health and educational officials? How would you institute needed reforms? How would you evaluate the effectiveness of your actions?

8. The purpose of this exercise is to develop a model for the solution of the problems involved in the case study. The starting point and other considerations include:

a. Identify the problems.

b. Identify the services needed.

c. Identify the resources needed in the solution of problems identified: — consider resources of personnel, money, time, and facilities — who are the most appropriate providers for needed services in terms of cost, availability, accessibility, and acceptability to client group?

d. What is the most appropriate setting for needed services in terms of cost, accessibility, and acceptability?

e. What barriers to needed services exist?

f. How might needed services be linked to existing services?

g. What type of evaluation components might be appropriate?

h. Other considerations?

The following is an article from a local newspaper weekly.

A child born in Cayahoga County, New York, is more likely to die in the first four weeks of life than in any other place in the state. Dr. George Gordon, county health commissioner, described the situation as "abominable." The infant mortality rate in the county is almost 16 children per 1,000 live births; this is compared with a state average of 11 per 1,000. The children who die during their first year in the county number 20 a year, as opposed to a state average of 14.

To correct the problem, a program expected to cost more than $70,000 the first year has been authorized by the county legislature's health and sanitation committee. The program provides for identifying high-risk mothers, determining their nutritional needs, and then providing foods to meet nutritional needs. Administration of the program, the cost of the food, and most expenses are fully reimbursed by the state. However, according to Marilyn Conway, regional public health nutritionist, "we have funds to help a third of the people eligible. What concerns me is the 60 percent that cannot be helped by this program."

According to Conway, the problem in the county is health care, but it is also the diets of pregnant women. Conway stated that "it has long been medical belief that an unborn child will take whatever nutrients it needs from the mother, and it is the mother's health that will suffer. We know now that this is not true. If a pregnant mother does not eat the proper diet, not only is her health but also that of her child likely to suffer."

In an interview, Conway identified some problems created by malnutrition as children who are small for weight at birth, palsied, mentally retarded, or have incomplete digestive systems, kidney problems, or cleft pallets. "Diet is not the only cause of these problems, but in many cases, the problems can be traced directly to the diet of the mother; this is especially true from the fourth to the fourteenth weeks of pregnancy," she said.

9. Review lay publications designed for pregnant or lactating women, such as baby magazines available from hospitals and diaper service. Look at the nutrition information contained in these publications and study it for reliability and validity. What practices are encouraged by these magazines? Is the information supported by scientific nutritional evidence? What advice is given to the mother? For example, is breast-feeding or bottle-feeding advocated? Also evaluate materials hospital- or physician-distributed to new or expectant mothers regarding infant feeding practices. What practices are encouraged by these materials?

10. Susan is a 23-year-old graduate student. She is three months pregnant and has been routinely referred to you, the HMO nutritionist, for nutritional counseling. She is 5'5" tall and weighs 123 lb. She states that her normal weight is 115 lb. Her hematocrit is 31 per cent and her hemoglobin is 10.0 gm.

Susan plans to nurse her baby. She states that she does not now use any drugs, coffee, alcohol, or refined sugars. She is a vegetarian, eating no meat, poultry, or fish. She does eat eggs and dairy products. She buys her food at a local health food store and tries to buy "organically grown" food. She supplements the eggs and dairy products with beans, brown rice, whole grains, fruits, and vegetables. She uses sea salt and rose hips, as well as a daily vitamin E supplement. As a nutritionist, what would you advise Susan about the protein content of her diet? What would you suggest about the iron content? Should she increase her calorie intake? Susan plans to feed her infant a lacto-ovo-vegetarian diet. Would you encourage her in doing this?

11. Jane S. is the wife of a local prominent physician. She has just had her first prenatal visit to the doctor and has been referred to you, the nutritionist, for routine nutritional assessment. Jane is two months pregnant. She is an attorney and has a very demanding work schedule. She is expecting her second child. Jane is 5'4" and weighs 110 lb. During her first pregnancy, Jane limited (with difficulty) her weight gain to 15 lb and was very proud of the fact that she reached her normal weight within 2 weeks of the delivery. She notes with pride that her first child was and is very healthy, well developed, and intelligent. Jane plans to limit her weight gain to 10–15 lb this time also. Because of her demanding work schedule, she frequently does not have time for breakfast. When she does sit down for lunch, she has cottage cheese and fruit. Dinner, preceded by a couple of drinks, is usually limited to 300–400 calories. What suggestions would you have for Jane? What strategies would you use in counseling her about the importance of an adequate diet during her pregnancy?

Overnutrition – the relationship between diet and some of the " diseases of civilization "

Section Objective

The general objective of this section is to consider the current research data and information available on the relationship between diet and the etiology of "diseases of civilization," that is, diseases of wide prevalence among populations in Western, industrialized countries. These disorders include heart disease, cancer, obesity, dental caries, diabetes mellitus, and alcoholism.

Section Overview

In an effort to promote health through diet, many researchers and nutritionists, as well as public policymakers, advocate that specific dietary patterns be recommended for the general public. To this end, the U.S. Senate Select Committee on Nutrition and Human Needs published, and then revised, *Dietary Goals for the United States* in 1977. The aim of these recommended dietary changes is to prevent nutrition-related disorders such as cancer and heart disease. But opponents of this endeavor suggest that we lack evidence to support the theory that modifying the American diet will influence the incidence of these nutrition-related disorders. It is important, therefore, to understand and differentiate between factually based, and theorized, nonsubstantiated nutrition knowledge.

In view of the continuing debate and controversy surrounding the *Dietary Goals*, it is essential that great care be taken to accurately understand and inform the public about the relationship between diet and the so-called "killer diseases" that the goals were designed to prevent. Emotion, misunderstanding, and prejudiced information about nutrition often influence attitudes about what diet can and cannot do to promote health.

This section reviews the current state of research and knowledge relating to diet and the prevention of certain nutrition-related disorders. The conditions reviewed were selected because of their wide prevalence among the American population and because of their hypothesized relation to the American diet and eating patterns.

7

Diet, nutrition, and heart disease

Reader Objectives

After completing this chapter the reader should be able to
1. State the diet-heart hypothesis.
2. Describe the public health significance of heart disease in the United States.
3. List at least ten risk factors associated with coronary heart disease.
4. State the general conclusions of epidemiological studies on the relationships between diet and heart disease.
5. List three types of studies designed to investigate the possibility of preventing atherosclerotic heart disease.
6. State three dietary factors (other than lipids) related to heart disease.
7. Describe three research programs investigating the relationship between diet and heart disease.
8. State general dietary recommendations for the prevention of heart disease.

THE DIET-HEART HYPOTHESIS

Coronary heart disease is now accepted as the "greatest sustained epidemic confronting mankind."[1] Atherosclerosis and coronary heart disease (CHD)* have attracted widespread and appreciable interest in recent decades. However, the disorders remain problematic and poorly defined relative to etiology and physiologic changes. We still lack general consensus about the exact nature of CHD. Various investigators have proposed explanations for the disease process that eventually leads to advanced atherosclerotic heart disease, but none of these explanations has been unequivocally approved.[2-7]

Much current research suggests that the public health problem of atherosclerosis is caused, in large part, by the life-style of modern man. Dietary patterns and food habits figure prominently in the research designed to piece together the parts of the coronary heart disease puzzle.

The U.S. Department of Agriculture estimated that proper diet might reduce cardiovascular disease mortality by 20 per cent to 25 per cent. This has been corroborated by a number of experts on cardiovascular disease and endorsed by the director of the National Heart, Lung, and Blood Institute, R. Levy:

> Let me say that I can think of no subject more worthy of our close attention than the relationship between nutrition and deadly disease as exemplified by the link between diet and cardiovascular illness. . . . the disease problem is massive. A 25 percent reduction in cardiovascular deaths would save over 200,000 lives annually. A 25 percent reduction in the incidence of these diseases would save over $14 billion a year.[2]

---

*Terms used in connection with coronary heart disease are numerous and sometimes confusing. A glossary of commonly used terms can be found at the end of this chapter, pp. 271–272.

PUBLIC HEALTH SIGNIFICANCE OF HEART DISEASE

Cardiovascular disease is the leading cause of death in the United States. Recent estimates suggest that more than 29 million Americans suffer cardiovascular disease that produces significant morbidity. Cardiovascular disease is responsible for more deaths than all other causes combined. Figures 7-1, 7-2, and 7-3 illustrate the magnitude of the problems of cardiovascular disease.

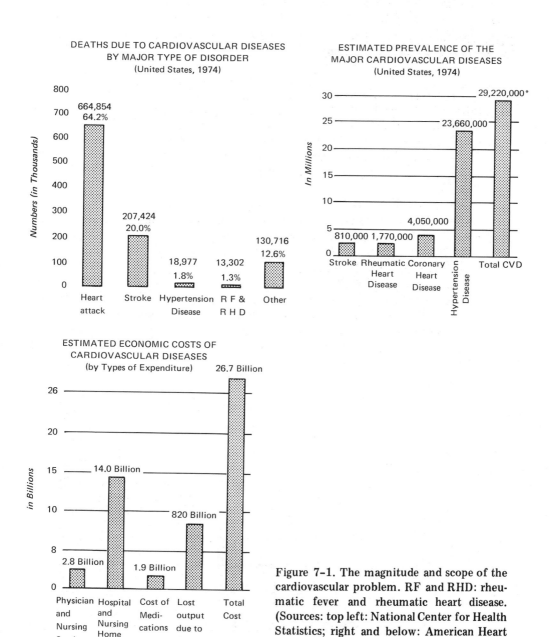

Figure 7-1. The magnitude and scope of the cardiovascular problem. RF and RHD: rheumatic fever and rheumatic heart disease. (Sources: top left: National Center for Health Statistics; right and below: American Heart Association)

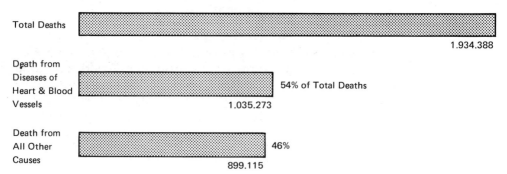

Figure 7-2. Diseases of the heart and blood vessels, the major cause of death in the United States. (American Heart Association)

The average American male has a 33 per cent chance of developing some form of atherosclerotic heart disease before the age of 60; the American female has a 10 per cent chance.[8] Coronary heart disease is the most prominent cause of early disability in the current American work force. About 40 per cent of the more than 350,000 persons who receive Social Security disability allowances each year suffer from some form of atherosclerotic disease.

The economic costs of atherosclerotic heart disease are also high in terms of days of work lost; hospital, diagnostic, surgical, and other medical care; and rehabilitation services. The American Heart Association suggested that annual hospital-related costs were approximately $8 billion in 1976. This figure is drastically higher than a comparable figure ten years ago; the estimated total cost for medical care for the atherosclerotic disorders is thought to be about $10 billion yearly.[8] Although both the direct and indirect costs of heart disease are staggering, they do not tell the whole story. The suffering and agony and pain that one incident of coronary heart disease brings to the victim and to his or her family and life cannot be quantified.

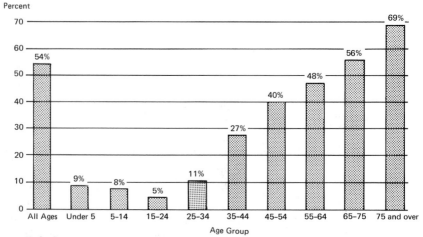

Figure 7-3. Percentage of all deaths caused by cardiovascular disease in the United States by age, 1974. (American Heart Association)

It should also be noted that approximately 70 per cent of all CHD deaths occur suddenly, within minutes from the first appearance of symptoms and before the patient can be treated by medical facilities. About a quarter of these initial heart attacks cause the victim to die within three hours of the onset of symptoms. Another 10 per cent of the victims die within days or weeks of the first attack. For these who survive the initial attack, their chance of dying within the next five years is five times higher than of those who have no history of CHD.[9-11]

A statistical summary of selected cardiovascular disease "facts" is presented in Table 7-1.

The importance of preventing the first attack is thus clear. Current scientific knowledge of the risk factors predisposing an individual to premature CHD suggests that these factors can be modified, controlled, or corrected by changes in the environment or in individual life-styles. In view of these considerations and of the tremendous public health significance of atherosclerotic heart disease, the 1970 Inter-Society Commission for Health Disease Resources report recommended a strategy of primary prevention of premature atherosclerotic diseases. The commission suggested that, to implement this strategy, adequate resources of money and manpower should be devoted to accomplish dietary modification to ameliorate hyperlipidemia, obesity, hypertension, and diabetes.[9]

Recent data suggest that "we seem to have turned the corner in the epidemic of heart disease."[2] Statistics presented at the 1977 annual American Heart Association meeting revealed the following:[12,13]

Since 1968, the mortality rate from heart disease has declined in both sexes, for blacks and for whites.

In 1974 the rates, relative to those of 1968 were down as follows: 15 per cent for white females and 24 per cent for nonwhite females; 14 per cent for white males and 17 per cent for nonwhite males. Such decreased mortality rates continued through the 1977 time period and represent large savings in terms of human life.

The decline in cardiovascular mortality rates since 1960 is almost double that of the drop in other causes of mortality.

In 1975, in spite of an increasingly older and larger population, the number of deaths from cardiovascular disease fell below 1 million for the first time since 1967.

For the age group 65–74, heart disease declined by 30 per cent and mortality rates for stroke dropped 45 per cent.

It appears that we may be on the right track. The task now is to determine the factors involved to accelerate the trend. A number of possible factors have been suggested. For example, between 1963 and 1975, per capita consumption of animal fats and oils dropped 57 per cent, whereas consumption of vegetable fats and oils increased 44 per cent.[14] Some have associated these dietary trends with the decline in mortality rates from cardiovascular disease. Correspondingly, there is evidence that mean serum cholesterol levels of the North American population have recently de-

Table 7–1
Heart Facts Statistical Summary

CVD Cost — $28.5 billion (AHA est.) in 1978.

Prevalence — 29,780,000 Americans have some form of heart and blood vessel disease.
· hypertension — 24,080,000 (one in six adults).
· coronary heart disease — 4,120,000.
· rheumatic heart disease — 1,800,000.
· stroke — 1,840,000.

CVD Mortality — 994,513 in 1975 (53 percent of all deaths). (1978 AHA est.):
1,003,300 (52 percent).
· one-fourth of all persons killed by CVD are under age 65.
· other 1975 mortality: cancer 365,693; accidents 103,030; all others 338,749.

Research — since 1949 nearly $300,000,000 in Heart Association dollars have gone
into research.
· by policy, AHA allocates 57 percent of its national budget to research.
· affiliates allocate about 23 percent of their income to research.

Atherosclerosis — contributed to many of the 836,757 heart attack and stroke deaths
in 1975.

Congenital or Inborn Heart Defects — 35 recognizable types of defects.
· more than 25,000 babies are born every year with heart defects.
· post-natal mortality from heart defects had been reduced to 6,440 in 1975.

Heart Attack — caused 642,719 deaths in 1975.
· 4,120,000 alive today have history of heart attack and/or agina pectoris.
· 350,000 a year die of heart attack before they reach hospital — average victim waits
three hours before decision to seek help.
· About 1,000,000 Americans will have a heart attack this year about about 650,000
of them will die.

Stroke — killed 194,038 in 1975; afflicts 1,840,000.

CCU — most of the 7,000 general hospitals in U.S. have coronary care capability.
· 1,800 have separate CCUs; 3,000 have combined intensive care and coronary care
facilities.
· specialized coronary care for all heart attack victims could save about 50,000 lives
a year; in-hospital deaths could be reduced about 30 percent.

Hypertension (HBP) — 24,080,000 adults.
· of those who do know they have it, many are untreated or inadequately controlled.
· only a minority have it under adequate control.
· for 90 percent of those with high blood pressure science doesn't know the cause; but
it is easily detected and usually controllable.

Rheumatic Heart Disease Prevalence — 100,000 children; 1,700,000 adults.
· killed 12,930 in 1975. Modern antibiotic therapy has sharply reduced mortality in
5-24 age group.

Major Risk Factors
BLOOD PRESSURE — man with systolic pressure over 150 has more than *twice* the
risk of heart attack and nearly *four* times risk of stroke of man with systolic pressure
under 120.
CHOLESTEROL — man with blood cholesterol of 250 or more has about *three*
times the risk of heart attack and stroke of man with cholesterol level below 194.
CIGARETTE SMOKING — man who smokes more than one pack a day has nearly
twice the risk of heart attack.

Am. Heart Association 1978

clined. The lipid research collaborative study under the National Heart, Lung and Blood Institute reported a fall of about 10 per cent in the mid-1970s versus 15 or 20 years ago.[2] Other encouraging trends include the massive public health efforts to detect and treat potentially dangerous high blood pressure (see Chapter 11).

However, experts stress that the problem of heart disease is far from solved. In spite of recent progress, the CHD mortality rate in the United States is one of the highest in the world. There is still much to be done. The current decline in the mortality rate from coronary heart disease may be interpreted as an endorsement of preventive approaches recommended to the North American public during the past years. A continued effort must be made to broaden existing preventive activities. To date, commitment has not been made to mount sufficient large-scale efforts to improve the aspects of life-style that are crucial to improving the picture.

RISK FACTORS ASSOCIATED WITH HEART DISEASE

Current research into the etiology, development, and prevention of coronary heart disease focuses on the study and identification of factors predisposing an individual to a high risk or probability of developing CHD. Risk factors have been defined as "those habits, traits, and abnormalities associated with a sizeable (e.g., 100 per cent or more) increase in susceptibility to the atherosclerotic disease. In particular, they are associated with greater proneness to premature onset of these diseases."[10]

Currently known risk factors appear to account for a large part of the variance in incidence of heart disease either within a given population or between various world populations.[15-17] The ability of individual risk factors to predict individual susceptibility is marred by lack of sophistication of screening and detection of the disease. It is well known that many who do not present clinical evidence of heart disease may in fact have the initial lesions and will eventually succumb to the disorder. Another problem lies with the sensitivity of methods to detect risk measures and to adequately interpret the relation of these factors to the disease process. For example, a one-time identification of risk is not able to account for the effect of risk existing over a period of several years. Nor can it separate out interrelationships between risks, which may be of a synergistic nature.

Although it is impossible to predict on the basis of risk factors the probability that a given individual will succumb to CHD, individuals from areas of low CHD prevalence exhibit, on the average, lower levels of risk factors than those from areas of higher prevalence. Risk factors associated with coronary heart disease are listed in Table 7-2.

Some of these risk factors are of more significance than others. D. Kritchevsky conceptualized the relative importance of various factors by the use of a "pie chart," illustrating the relative size of the different "wedges" or factors that vary for each individual.[16] This demonstrates the notion that each person reacts to different factors differently, and suggests that factors noted to be risk factors for population groups as a whole

Table 7–2
Risk Factors Associated with Coronary Heart Disease

Risk Factors Not Easily Altered:

Heredity: there appears to be an inherited tendency to coronary heart disease for some individuals.

Sex: premenopausal females have a lower mortality rate from heart disease than do men; after menopause, the female mortality rate from heart disease increases, but remains lower than that for males.

Race: black Americans have twice the likelihood of elevated blood pressure as whites; high blood pressure, in turn, is a risk factor for coronary heart disease.

Age: the mortality rate from heart attack increases with age; however, twenty-five percent of all heart attack deaths occur in individuals under the age of 65; one in six deaths resulting from strokes occur in individuals less than sixty-five years of age.

Abnormalities in organ systems: examples are renal disease and hypothyroidism.

Risk Factors That Can Be Altered Through Medical Intervention:

Serum cholesterol: cholesterol can be lowered through drugs, as well as through diet.

Hypertension: a variety of drugs can control hypertension in susceptible individuals.

Diabetes: diabetes, or the inherited tendency toward diabetes, a risk factor associated with coronary heart disease, can be controlled by drugs, diet regimens, and a combination of weight-control and exercise programs.

Risk Factors That Can Be Changed by Individual Actions:

Cigarette smoking: the mortality rate from cardiovascular disease of smokers who stopped smoking is almost as low as that of those who never smoked.

Dietary factors: a well-balanced diet low in saturated fat and cholesterol and containing calories at a level to maintain optimal body weight tends to lower serum lipids and reduce the risk of coronary heart disease.

Stress: many studies indicate that stress is a potent risk factor; the identification and modification of stressful situations may reduce the potency of this risk factor.

Lack of exercise: individuals who take regular exercise have been shown, in some studies, to have a lower risk of coronary heart disease than do those who lead sedendary lives.

---

may not be risk factors on an individual basis. The converse also holds true. Figure 7–4 illustrates the relationship of single and combined risk factors in cardiovascular disease.

Identifying individuals at high risk for the development of coronary heart disease involves assessing arbitrarily defined "abnormal" levels of risks. Thus, an individual at high risk for a number of these factors, such as cigarette smoking and hypertension, is at a compounded risk, as the risk increases with increased number of risk factors.

Such a process of risk assessment is not always the most reliable way to approach the prevention of coronary heart disease. An individual with a number of relatively high risk levels (which may not be detected by the normal screening) may in fact be at higher risk than an individual with only one significant risk factor.

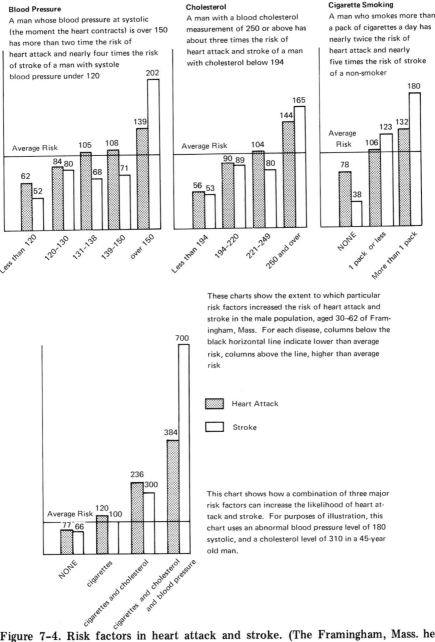

Blood Pressure

A man whose blood pressure at systolic (the moment the heart contracts) is over 150 has more than two time the risk of heart attack and nearly four times the risk of stroke of a man with systole blood pressure under 120

Cholesterol

A man with a blood cholesterol measurement of 250 or above has about three times the risk of heart attack and stroke of a man with cholesterol below 194

Cigarette Smoking

A man who smokes more than a pack of cigarettes a day has nearly twice the risk of heart attack and nearly five times the risk of stroke of a non-smoker

These charts show the extent to which particular risk factors increased the risk of heart attack and stroke in the male population, aged 30–62 of Framingham, Mass. For each disease, columns below the black horizontal line indicate lower than average risk, columns above the line, higher than average risk

▨ Heart Attack

☐ Stroke

This chart shows how a combination of three major risk factors can increase the likelihood of heart attack and stroke. For purposes of illustration, this chart uses an abnormal blood pressure level of 180 systolic, and a cholesterol level of 310 in a 45-year old man.

Figure 7-4. Risk factors in heart attack and stroke. (The Framingham, Mass. heart study, American Heart Association)

It is important that the complex of factors responsible for disease be considered. As W. G. Kannel emphasized:

it is a mistake to conceptualize the atherosclerotic diseases as the product of any single etiological agent. It is clear that in different populations, such as those in the United States, everyone has enough lipid to manufacture atheromata, but the rate of its development appears to depend upon multiple contributing factors as well as the degree of elevation of the blood lipid content.[18]

There is no general consensus about what is "normal." It is difficult to state where normal stops and abnormal begins for any of the factors predisposing an individual to coronary heart disease. Suggested "normal" limits for certain biochemical values have been formulated as an aid in identifying high-risk individuals. Normal limits are not to be confused with "safe" limits. The serum lipid levels used to establish genetic abnormalities tend to be higher than the values derived from epidemiological studies. Within the "upper" limits, the risk of developing coronary heart disease increases as the serum cholesterol levels increase. The National Heart Lung and Blood Institute suggested concentrations of serum cholesterol, as well as triglycerides and low-density lipoproteins (LDL) that, if exceeded, "clearly indicate an excess."[19] This is presented in Table 7–3. Most Americans who develop coronary heart disease have serum cholesterol levels in the range of from 220 mg/100 ml to 280 mg/100 ml.[20] Serum cholesterol levels beyond 250 mg/100 ml are associated with as high as a three- to fourfold increase in risk of developing coronary disease.[21]

The National Cooperative Pooling Project collected data from a number of studies relating serum cholesterol levels to the incidence of coronary heart disease in various populations. The studies pooled were those from the Framingham, Albany, Chicago, and Western studies; about 11,000 men were represented in the project. Results suggested that individuals whose serum cholesterol levels ranged from 225 mg/100 ml to 250 mg/100 ml were at no greater risk, statistically speaking, to develop heart attacks than those with serum cholesterol levels between 175 mg/100 ml and 200 mg/100 ml.[22] However, as levels exceeded 250 mg/100 ml there was increased risk. In the group with serum cholesterol levels from 250 mg/100 ml to 275 mg/100 ml, the incidence was 11 attacks per 1,000 males annually, whereas in the group with levels above 300 mg/100 ml, the incidence of heart attacks was approximately 16 per 1,000 males. It seems reasonable to conclude that serum cholesterol levels above 235 mg/100 ml or 240 mg/100 ml may be regarded as a risk factor.[23]

Only an estimated one third of the North American male population can maintain serum cholesterol levels of 220 mg/100 ml or less while consuming their typical, habitual diets.[24]

Table 7–3

Concentrations of Cholesterol, Triglycerides or Low-density Lipoproteins Which, if Exceeded, Clearly Indicate Hyperlipidemia

Age	C (mg per 100 ml)	LDL (mg per 100 ml)	TG
1–19	230	170	150
20–29	240	170	200
30–39	270	190	200
40–49	310	190	200
50–	336	210	200

Source: National Heart and Lung Institute. *Dietary Management of Hyperlipoproteinemia*, Publ. No. (NIH) 76–110. Bethesda, Md.: U.S. Department of Health, Education, and Welfare, 1974.

DIET-LIPID HYPOTHESIS

Despite the uncertainty about the nature, etiology, and course of the disorder, it seems relatively clear that some type of abnormality in lipid metabolism is the "one common denominator through which the multiple contributors to atherosclerosis operate."[1] The data suggesting that some type of lipid metabolic aberration is implicated are vast, consistent, and theoretically valid. Evidence from human metabolic studies, clinical investigations, epidemiological data, autopsy studies, and animal studies corroborate the validity of the premise.

In general, these lines of research have led to a working hypothesis suggesting the following:[25]

Diet (excessive consumption of dietary cholesterol, saturated fats, calories, refined sugar, and a low intake of polyunsaturated fats, fiber, and certain trace minerals).

Serum lipid abnormalities (elevated serum cholesterol, triglycerides, low-density lipoproteins, reduced high-density lipoproteins).

Lipid accumulation in coronary arteries.

Atherosclerotic coronary heart disease.

The theory suggests that

1. Atherosclerosis is present and responsible for the development of coronary heart disease.

2. Atherosclerotic plaque contains high levels of lipid material, especially cholesterol.

3. The excess cholesterol is obtained from circulating plasma lipoproteins. These lipoproteins can be distinguished on the basis of their physical characteristics and are differentiated according to their density. (See Figure 7-5).

    a. Chylomicrons are 80–95 per cent triglyceride, 2–7 per cent cholesterol, 3–6 per cent phospholipid, and 1–2 per cent protein.

    b. Very-low-density lipoproteins (VLDL) or pre-beta lipoproteins are about 50–80 per cent triglycerides, 7–16 per cent cholesterol, and 2–13 per cent protein.

    c. Low-density lipoproteins (LDL) are about 10 per cent triglycerides, 30 per cent cholesterol, and 20–25 per cent protein.

    d. High-density lipoproteins (HDL) or alpha-lipoproteins are 45–55 per cent protein, 5–8 per cent triglyceride, and 18 per cent cholesterol.

4. Premature atherosclerosis is characterized by elevated serum cholesterol. Although triglycerides are often elevated, the association of serum tryglycerides with the risk of coronary heart disease is weaker than that of serum cholesterol.

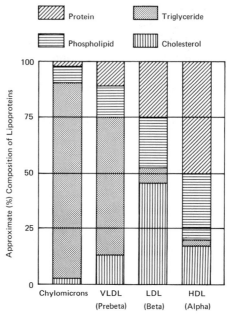

Figure 7-5. Composition of lipoproteins.

Plasma high-density lipoprotein (HDL) has been found to retard the progression of atherosclerosis. Recent research suggests that the way in which cholesterol is transported in the blood (LDL versus HDL) is a more important determinant of coronary heart disease than is total plasma cholesterol.[26,27] The HDL concentration is considered by some to be the single most potent lipid predictor of coronary heart disease.[28] Levels of HDL tend to decrease with diets very high in carbohydrate (higher than 80 per cent of calories); niacin, regular exercise, modest alcohol consumption, and estrogens have been found to increase HDL cholesterol levels. Thus, the LDLs are positive predictors of heart disease, and the HDLs are negative predictors.

Elevated serum cholesterol levels must be interpreted with caution; the total cholesterol may be high because of the elevation in LDL cholesterol, but it may also be high as a result of elevated HDL cholesterol. The assessment of risk should ideally consider LDL and HDL levels in addition to total serum cholesterol levels.

5. Habitual dietary patterns of high fat and cholesterol content are considered to be risk factors for the development of atherosclerosis. These diet patterns may act synergistically with other risk factors in the development of coronary heart disease. Table 7-4 summarizes the effect of various dietary components on serum cholesterol concentrations.[29]

Although this theory has become the generally accepted research paradigm, there is considerable controversy relating to the premises that

1. Dietary components are key determinants of serum lipid levels.

Table 7–4
Effect of Dietary Components of Serum Cholesterol Concentrations

Dietary Factor	*Effect on Lipoprotein*	*Net Effect on Serum Cholesterol*
Weight gain	Often leads to increased VLDL; other lipoproteins may decrease or be unchanged	No change or increase
Saturated fat	Leads to increased LDL; others remain unchanged	Leads to elevated serum cholesterol
Monounsaturated Fat		No Direct Effect
Polyunsaturated fat	Often leads to decrease in LDL; other fractions usually unchanged	Leads to decrease in serum cholesterol
Dietary cholesterol		Variable depending on level of cholesterol intake; persons on intake > 400 mg/day may not show increase in serum cholesterol levels with increased dietary intake; Persons on high cholesterol intake (600–700 mg/day), when they decrease intake to < 300 mg/day have a reduction in serum cholesterol

Source: O. B. Zilversmit. Questions about diet and atherosclerosis, in *Professional Perspectives*. Ithaca, N.Y.: Cornell University, April 1977.

2. Correction of abnormal serum lipid levels constitutes an appropriate preventive measure for coronary heart disease.

It is beyond the scope of the current discussion to review all the studies supporting or refuting this theory. However, a brief consideration of selected examples from epidemiological and clinical studies will illustrate some of the complexities involved.

EPIDEMIOLOGICAL DATA

Worldwide population studies have associated diets high in calories, cholesterol, saturated fat, sugar, and animal products (meat and eggs) with elevated serum lipid levels. Elevated serum lipid levels have in turn been associated with the prevalence of coronary heart disease in various population groups.

Conversely, populations with low serum lipid levels are associated with intakes of protective, nonincriminated foods, such as whole grain breads and cereals, vegetables, fruit, and fish. These populations exhibit lower coronary death rates. Data from these epidemiological studies are vast, are generally consistent, and are available from many sources. Furthermore, the correlations persist when the influence of other variables is considered. Individuals who move from a region of low cholesterol values to one of high values typically alter their diet to conform more to their new environment; subsequently, these migrants evidence higher cholesterol levels than their counterparts at home.

In the late 1800s, W. Osler described the disorder of angina pectoris and other disorders related to atherosclerosis. He suggested that physicians rarely saw a patient suffering from such disorders in the hospitals of Philadelphia, Baltimore, or Montreal but that there was a higher prevalence among businessmen and professional men who did not come to the more public "hospitals." Osler's prescription for treatment was a diet restricting rich foods. He concluded, "Angiosclerosis . . . is the Nemesis through which Nature exacts retributive justice for the transgression of her laws."[30]

Findings from more recent studies from the World Health Organization have tended to support the conclusion that atherosclerosis is most prevalent among populations whose diets contain high levels of cholesterol and saturated fats. One such study involved 1964 mortality data from 22 different developed nations. Food balance sheet information on nutrient availability was assessed in relationship to mortality rates and the prevalence of atherosclerotic disease. The study noted significant correlations between CHD mortality rates for middle-aged men and a variety of nutrients — total calories, total protein, sucrose, fat, saturated fat, and cholesterol.[10,31]

The International Cooperative Study on the Epidemiology of Cardiovascular Disease, a prospective international study, involved 18 populations in 7 different nations — Finland, Greece, Italy, Japan, the Netherlands, the United States, and Yugoslavia. Approximately 12,000 males originally aged 40 to 59 were studied over a ten-year period. The highest CHD incidence rates were noted for men from eastern Finland and the United States, whereas men in Greece and Japan demonstrated lower rates.[32]

The type and amount of typical fat in the diet, particularly saturated fat and cholesterol, differed significantly among the various population groups studied. For example, in Japan (Kyushu) total fat accounted for about 9 per cent of total calories, and polyunsaturated fat accounted for about 3 per cent. In some of the European populations, the saturated fat intake was similarly low (7–10 per cent of calories), whereas polyunsaturated fat was 3–7 per cent. However, among Finnish and North Americans, saturated fat intake was high, at 17–22 per cent of total calories, whereas total fat intake was 35–40 per cent of calories and polyunsaturated fat was 3–5 per cent. Males from eastern Finland presented the highest level of saturated fat intake, averaging 22 per cent of total calories.

Data from this study suggested that 80 per cent of the variance in mean serum cholesterol levels between various population groups could be accounted for by differences in typical dietary intake and that 70 per cent of the variance in the incidence of CHD could be explained by habitual differences in dietary saturated fat consumption.

For populations demonstrating high mean serum cholesterol levels and a high prevalence of CHD, the proportion of dietary calories from saturated fat was 15 per cent or more. In contrast, for those populations demonstrating a low prevalence of coronary heart disease, the saturated fat content of the diet averaged about 10 per cent of total calories. There were no significant associations between monounsaturated and polyunsaturated fat consumption, total calories, or blood lipid levels, and prevalence of CHD.[32]

Further analysis of the data illustrates the relationship between widespread CHD and habitual diet. In populations in which the national diet pattern was low in consumption of saturated fat and dietary cholesterol, the widespread problem of CHD was not found. For example, in Japan, despite the fact that hypertension among the population is high (20–30 per cent of adults) and smoking is widespread, the incidence of CHD was not great (in the late 1960s). The average carbohydrate intake in Japan ranged around 75 per cent of total calories, whereas total fat content of the diets was the lowest of industrial nations (10 per cent), and saturated fat intake was similarly low (3 per cent).[32]

In contrast to the Japanese, the population of Finland is burdened with the highest prevalence of atherosclerotic heart disease of those countries studied. The typical Finnish diet is 22 per cent saturated fat calories, and other risk factors, such as cigarette smoking and hypertension, parallel those of other nations in central and southern Europe.

However, not all data support these findings. The Ireland-Boston Heart Study reported by J. Brown et al. illustrates the significance of different epidemiological factors related to atherosclerotic heart disease.[33] Much of the study concerned pairs of brothers, one of whom lived in Boston, the other in Ireland. Those men who lived in Boston consumed fewer calories, but a higher proportion of the calories was contributed by simple sugars. The percentage of calories from fat and cholesterol was similar in both groups, but the Boston residents had a higher proportion of polyunsaturated fatty acids. Boston residents drank more coffee, whiskey, and gin, but less tea, beer, and stout than the Irish. The Boston residents also consumed less magnesium, weighed more, and were less physically active than their Irish counterparts. Autopsy studies on other residents from both areas indicated that more serious atherosclerotic lesions appeared at an earlier age for the Boston residents. Serum cholesterol values did not greatly differ among the two groups. These findings suggest that the amount and type of dietary fat and cholesterol may not be the determining factors of CHD among the subjects studied. The study underscores the importance of looking at a complex of variables in a total ecological way.[33]

The Framingham study, perhaps the most frequently cited diet-heart study in the United States, represents an extensive prospective population study of coronary heart disease and the associated risk factors. The study has included a biannual follow-up since its start in 1948. A total of 2,283 men and 2,844 women aged 30 to 62 years were included in the initial sample.

The dietary factors studied were total calories, protein, total fat, animal and vegetable fat, saturated and polyunsaturated fatty acids, cholesterol, iron, and simple and complex carbohydrates. The study found a positive correlation between serum cholesterol levels and the development of CHD in the diet study group, as well as in the entire population sample.

Individuals with cholesterol levels greater than 260 mg/100 ml were three times more likely to develop heart disease than were individuals whose cholesterol levels were less than 200 mg/100 ml. For males studied at autopsy, the serum cholesterol measurements made from five to nine years before death were significantly higher in those men who had the most severe atherosclerotic lesions.[34]

Elevations of plasma triglycerides associated with the pre-β-lipoprotein fractions were also significantly related to the risk of coronary heart disease when accompanied by an elevated cholesterol level. The Framingham data confirm the notion that the HDL concentration is a potent lipid predictor of coronary heart disease.[28]

However, the study has not been able to confirm the relation between the development of coronary heart disease and the dietary variables studied; neither could these dietary variables be correlated with serum cholesterol levels. The study concluded that, if there was a link between diet and serum cholesterol levels among those in the Framingham study population, the link was weak. No positive relationship was found between diet and the incidence of coronary heart disease.

A number of factors must be considered in interpreting the results from the Framingham study. Complications resulted from the way the study sample was finally selected and obtained. Originally, 3,086 men (referred to as being aged 30 to 59 years old) were asked to participate in the study — only 66 per cent responded (2,036) with the higher percentages being in the higher age levels. To increase the study participants, 312 healthy volunteers were added to the final sample. Of the participants, 2,283 men were found to be free of CHD on initial examination. This group, which formed the basis for the Framingham study results, cannot be considered to represent the American male population.

There is also a difficulty in judging results because of the wide age ranges of the sample. Although risks have been calculated for various age groups, this is a difficult task especially for cardiovascular disorders that have a marked age dependence.

A further difficulty in obtaining a clear idea of study results is that they have usually been presented in a different way for each follow-up period. Thus, it is hard to compare published study results of different time periods.

Conclusion of Epidemiological Studies

Atherosclerotic coronary heart disease is a public health problem that is encountered largely in affluent, industrialized societies. The data available suggest that mass, widespread hyperlipidemia in the population is associated with widespread atherosclerosis. The typical and habitual diet of a society seems, in turn, to be an important factor associated with mass hyperlipidemia. As H. Blackburn pointed out, "Composition of the habitual diet is the principal contributor to population levels of blood lipids, in contrast to the predominant influence of non-dietary factors on an individual's usual lipid level. Changes in population levels of blood lipids are generally predictable and safely attainable from changes in habitual diet."[17] Widespread hyperlipidemia is also thought to be a function of excessive caloric intake and of consequent obesity, which, in turn, can lead to hypertension, a significant risk factor for the development of atherosclerosis.

ANIMAL AND CLINICAL STUDIES

Data from epidemiological studies are confirmed by animal and human clinical investigations. No animal responds to dietary modification as humans do. However, both animal and human studies have established that dietary cholesterol and fat can induce hypercholesterolemia and atherosclerosis. Other factors implicated in elevation of serum cholesterol include excessive calories, sugar, and alcohol. There is also evidence that dietary modification relative to total fat, saturated fat, and cholesterol can reduce serum cholesterol values and possibly cause the regression of established atherosclerotic lesions.[32]

Pathologic-isotropic studies further confirm the role of a lipid abnormality in the development of atherosclerosis. Autopsy studies among victims who have died of heart disease indicate that the myocardial infarction was usually the result of reduced blood flow to the heart due to a blockage in the artery. Such studies have presented evidence that the atherosclerotic coronary arteries are heavily laden with cholesterol.[35]

However, not all research supports the relationship between high serum cholesterol levels and diet. J. Barboriak et al. reported that, by balancing the experimental diets of rats very carefully, they were able to nullify the effects of high dietary cholesterol. In other words, the composition of the rest of the diet appeared to offset the high dietary cholesterol content.[36]

S. Naimi et al. confirmed these results in animal studies in which high butter diets (65 per cent of total calories) were found to produce gross obesity but no significant changes in serum cholesterol levels or in cardiovascular lesions. These investigations thus suggest that obesity per se may be of little importance in causing cardiovascular disease.[37]

Many metabolic-ward studies in humans have suggested that mean serum cholesterol rises considerably and predictably with modifications in dietary lipids — that is, increased dietary cholesterol and saturated fat and decreased polyunsaturated fat.[38] But, again, many human studies have failed to demonstrate a relationship (linear) between atherosclerosis and dietary cholesterol. Beveridge,[39] Connor,[40] and Hegstad[41] and their colleagues, in a series of studies, showed an almost linear relationship between dietary cholesterol intake and elevated serum cholesterol levels, for intakes up to 400 mg daily. When cholesterol intake was greater than 400 mg daily, the relationship was quite variable. This finding has been repeated in later studies. F. Mattson suggested that each 100 mg of cholesterol consumed per 1,000 kcal will produce an average elevation of 12 mg cholesterol per 100 ml of serum.[38]

Some studies on the effects of dietary cholesterol have not been able to demonstrate a correlation with serum cholesterol levels.[42] However, individual variation is very marked in plasma cholesterol response to dietary cholesterol challenges. Further, because the typical cholesterol intake of the population in the United States is at a very high range (averaging 600 mg daily or more), this may explain the lack of relationship.

Some individuals have either extremely low or extremely high responses to dietary cholesterol. Such individuals have been termed either hypo- or hyper-responders.[43] Individuals may have an inherited defect that leads them to have high serum cholesterol levels and to develop atherosclerosis, even in the absence of high levels of dietary cholesterol.

Since the 1950s investigators have been intent on running controlled experiments with normal subjects and survivors of CHD to study the possibility of modifying diet to lower serum cholesterol and ultimately to treat or prevent atherosclerotic heart disease. These studies have investigated the effectiveness of diet in

1. Primary prevention — studying those with no previous history of heart disease.

2. Secondary prevention — studying those who suffered previous myocardial infarctions.

3. Community intervention — determining the feasibility of implementing a strategy of prevention in the general community.

PRIMARY PREVENTION

Illustrative of the type of studies aimed at primary prevention is the Anti-Coronary Club Trial (officially named the Diet and Coronary Heart Disease Study Project of the Bureau of Nutrition of the Department of Health of the City of New York), which was begun in 1957.[44] The trial attempted to demonstrate the benefit of simultaneously correcting a variety of risk factors — such as obesity, hypertension, and hypercholesterolemia — through weight reduction, sodium restriction, and a modified-fat diet and through psychological benefits of medical supervision in protecting against heart disease. The experimental group included 814 males; 463 were in the control group, and all were between the age of 40 and 59 and evidenced no coronary heart disease. The control group consumed a "prudent diet" (a maximum of four meals per week of lean beef, pork or mutton, four or five meals of poultry and veal, and five meals of fish); high-fat dairy products and saturated shortenings were eliminated and replaced by skim milk and diet margerine. The P/S ratio of the diet was 1.25 to 1.50; average daily cholesterol intake was 400 mg and that of sodium was 1600 mg.

After a five-year period, the obesity and hypertension of the experimental group were greatly corrected; serum cholesterol levels were reduced 10–13 per cent. In the control group, these factors were increased. The incidence of diagnosed coronary heart problems in the experimental group was about 50 per cent that of the control group. However, more than half these coronary disorders were fatal in the experimental group; none was fatal in the control group.

It is clear that the beneficial dietary effects were not merely the result of modified-fat diets; the benefits were most likely improved by the simultaneous correction of obesity, hypertension, serum lipid levels and psychological factors.[44]

SECONDARY PREVENTION

Various studies have been undertaken to investigate the benefits of dietary intervention as part of the treatment in the secondary prevention of heart disease. P. Leren, in a study in Oslo, Norway, studied over 400 males under the age of 28 years who had survived a myocardial infarction for an average of 20 months previous to the study. The subjects were randomly assigned to either a control or a dietary intervention group. The experimental diet was intended to reduce serum lipids through a reduction in dietary saturated fat and cholesterol and an increase in polyunsaturated fat. Those in the experimental group attained a mean reduction in serum cholesterol of 17.6 per cent; this reduction was sustained for a five-year-period. The control group also demonstrated a small decrease in serum cholesterol (3.7 per cent). During the five-year study period, there were significantly fewer incidences of new infarctions in the experimental, as compared with the control, group.[45] But the incidence of sudden death was the same in both groups.

A more recent study conducted in two Finnish mental hospitals attempted to determine whether the consumption of a diet designed to lower serum cholesterol would reduce the incidence and mortality of CHD. A cross-over design was used; individuals in two hospitals were placed on either a control or an experimental diet for a period of six years; then the diet pattern was reversed for another six years.[46]

There was an association between lower serum cholesterol levels and the experimental diet in both hospitals; the reduction was an average of 15 per cent for the hospital on the experimental as compared with the hospital on the control diet. The effect was most noticeable for men; the use of the cholesterol-lowering diet regimen was related to an average of 53 per cent CHD mortality reduction. The reduction in the women was not significant. The investigators concluded that, for males, a diet designed to lower serum cholesterol greatly reduced CHD mortality; the results for women did not permit definitive conclusions.

Because species vary in response to dietary modifications, these studies do not prove conclusively that the diet is of value in preventing coronary disease; however, the studies do support the hypothesis that dietary modification designed to reduce serum lipids can be helpful in reducing the risk of coronary heart disease.

COMMUNITY TREATMENT

Various models have been used to improve community cardiovascular disease status. One model involves identification of risks and intervention into the risk factors plus the use of mass media campaigns to improve the risk factors in high-risk families. The Stanford Three-Community Study illustrates the success of such an approach. This study compared the results from such a multistrategy intervention approach to those obtained as a result of a three-year mass media campaign alone. These results, in turn, were compared to results obtained in a sample in which only health surveys were conducted. The multistrategy approach stimulated the greatest amount of positive health behavior. The study illustrates the significant community changes in health behavior, food habits, and risk factors that result from the multistrategy program; the changes were found to be a function of the degree of exposure to the health campaign and intervention program — mass media and face-to-face interventions contributed significantly to changes in health and nutrition behavior.[47,48]

Still another model illustrating the modification of health and nutrition behavior at the community level is that conducted in North Karelia — in Finland — a community having the highest measured CHD rate in the world. A total community effort was undertaken to combat the health problems; intervention included large and small mass media campaigns, town meetings, health education, screening populations for detection of high risk, improving hypertension clinics, interpersonal interventions, and direct action on the environment to modify such life-style factors as smoking and the availability of, and consumption of, high-fat, high-cholesterol foods. For example, local creameries were motivated to increase the availability of low-fat products, and local meat retailers were persuaded to reduce the fat content of meats such as sausage. Results of the study demonstrated significant changes in health behavior; the consumption of low-fat milk tripled, serum cholesterol levels were dramatically reduced, and the rate of CHD decreased.[49]

Experience with these and other programs suggests that the "prudent" diet is successful in reducing mass hyperlipidemia in a free-living population that follows the diet. Weight gain and weight loss are important determinants of the degree to which serum lipid levels can be reduced — in persons who lose weight there is a significant and a sustained reduction in total serum cholesterol. In those persons who do not lose weight, but who do follow the prudent diet, serum cholesterol levels do not respond so significantly but usually are reduced to a degree. Experience has demonstrated that, if the framework for such programs is provided via the medical establishment and if the program is implemented in a planned, systematic way, involving the target population in every step of program operation, very real and significant modifications in health behavior and nutrition behavior can be achieved, and consequently, risk factors can be significantly reduced.[47]

OTHER DIETARY FACTORS

Recent studies on diet and heart disease consider a number of dietary components in the context of the total dietary pattern. Dietary interactions have been identified as significant;[50] trace mineral imbalances have been correlated with serum cholesterol levels and, hence, with CHD; types and amount of dietary carbohydrates have been related to coronary heart disease;[51,52] and dietary fiber has been suggested to have a protective effect.[53] Total calorie intake and energy balance has frequently been identified as a risk factor.[54]

Trace Elements

The hardness of water has been associated with coronary heart disease, in that mortality rates from coronary heart disease have been suggested to be inversely related to water hardness.[55] It has been hypothesized that soft water causes the removal of cadmium and perhaps other minerals from the water and the lead from plumbing, which may result in metal intoxication that is related to CHD.

The role of trace elements in the development of coronary heart disease is receiving increased attention. Some studies have suggested that magnesium deficiency, along with an accompanying excessive retention of calcium and sodium, is related to the development of atherosclerosis.[25,56] Other possible mineral relationships to atherosclerotic heart disease are summarized in Table 7–5. Most of the evidence for these associations has

Table 7–5

Summary of Current Concepts Relating Mineral Deficiencies to Atherosclerotic Heart Disease

Metal Deficiency	Measured Biologic Effect
Calcium	Decreased excretion of fatty acid, if fat intake is largely saturated fat. Increased serum lipid. Depletion of cardiac calcium promotes infarction. Myocardium is more excitable. Endothelium and platelets are more adhesive.
Cadmium	May be a positive factor in development of hypertension.
Chromium	Glucose tolerance is impaired.
Lithium	A possible negative lithium AHD correlation may be significant protective factors in hard water.
Magneisum	Depletion of cardiac magnesium promotes myocardial infarction Failure of protection against cardiotoxins Clotting time tends to be decreased. Endothelium and platelets are more adhesive.
Vanadium	Hepatic synthesis of cholesterol is not controlled. The oxidation of brain monoamines and their precursors is then catalyzed. Fatty acid is not desaturated.
Zinc	Atherosclerosis is promoted. Cadmium-induced hypertension is not prevented.

Source: W. A. Krehl. The nutritional epidemiology of cardiovascular disease, in N. H. Moss and J. Mayer, eds., *Food and Nutrition in Health and Disease.* New York: New York Academy of Sciences, 1977.

resulted from animal studies. Conclusive evidence has not yet been developed to suggest that the same relationships hold true in the human population.[25]

Dietary Fiber

Animal studies have demonstrated that animals who are given a fiber-free diet (synthetic diet to which saturated fat is added) develop atheroma. However, if similar animals are fed the same diet to which a level of fiber is added, no atheroma develops.[57] In a similar fashion, certain types of vegetable fiber appear to be protective to rats who are fed a diet that would otherwise induce atheroma.[58]

Fiber not only reduces the absorption of cholesterol eaten in food but it may also modify the amount of endogenous cholesterol formed in the liver and may change the chemical composition of the bile. This has been suggested to be the mechanism through which fiber is related to many diseases, such as heart disease, that are so common in industrialized populations.

Various forms of fiber have different effects on serum cholesterol. For example, pectin is usually more effective in lowering serum cholesterol levels than is the fiber in wheat bran. In general, cholesterol levels have been lowered by pectin; rolled oats; guar gum; a mixed diet of fruits, vegetables, and legumes; legumes; and beans. The serum cholesterol levels are often not lowered by wheat fiber; bagasse; cellulose; or a diet of whole maize, wheat, and vegetables.[58]

Fiber is usually more effective in lowering serum cholesterol levels of subjects who had elevated serum levels as a result of their previous high-fat or high-cholesterol diets, but it appears to be less effective when added to diets of patients suffering from other types of hyperlipoproteinemia.[58] There is also little evidence that fiber is beneficial in lowering serum triglycerides or other blood lipid levels.[58] The actions of fiber are discussed in greater detail in Chapter 8.

Carbohydrates

Some researchers, notably J. Yudkin[51] and T. Cleave, and G. Campbell,[52,59] suggest that sugar and refined carbohydrates are significantly related to the etiology of coronary heart disease. Cleave and Campbell based such a belief on the epidemiological data from various cultures. They noted that native Africans living in traditional villages did not suffer from diabetes, coronary thrombosis, varicose veins, or coronary heart disease, and suggested that ethnic factors did not enter the relationship between diet and disease because the incidence of these diseases dramatically increased when the native Africans migrated to Western regions, or adopted Westernized life-styles. The diets of these Africans differed significantly from those of Westernized populations. Campbell and Cleave noted no correlation between fat intake and disease pattern, but suggested that the absence of sugar and refined carbohydrates was a factor common to all tribal diets. However, these studies have been criticized on methodological and statistical grounds.[32,60]

Other epidemiological studies have noted positive statistical correlations between sucrose intake and heart disease mortality rates.[60,61] However, other researchers using similar types of data have failed to find a positive correlation between CHD and intake of sugar and refined carbohydrates.[62]

Another type of data relating sucrose consumption to atherosclerosis is obtained from comparing sucrose intake of CHD patients with the intakes of healthy controls. F. Grande analyzed nine reports in the literature relating sugar consumption to the incidence of CHD among patients. He found that only two of these reports demonstrated significant differences between coronary patients and controls relative to sugar intake, and in both instances the sugar intake of the coronary patients was lower than that of the controls. Although there was significant variation in sugar intake among coronary patients, it could not be concluded that sugar intake and coronary heart disease were causally related.[63] Many of the differences were associated with differences in smoking and in the consumption of sweet drinks such as cocoa and coffee. Similar results have been noted by others.[64] Studies attempting to relate intake of sugar with blood lipids have also been unsuccessful.[65] Thus, although many studies have demonstrated correlations between sucrose and heart disease, other studies have failed to demonstrate this correlation. Further, correlations merely indicate an association between the variables and do not imply cause-and-effect relationships between variables.

A number of animal research models have been used to clarify the relationship between refined carbohydrates and coronary heart disease. A considerable literature reports on the results of these investigations,[66] which have not been conclusive. Animal studies have uncovered a variety of factors that mediate the influence of sucrose on the development of atherosclerosis. The effects of sucrose vary with species, strain, sex, age, adaptive capacity, and other dietary components. Human studies have produced other conflicting results relative to the relationship between sucrose and heart disease.[67-70] Whereas some researchers have reported that sucrose exerts a significant lipid elevating effect,[67] others disagree.[68,69]

In general, the following conclusions can be made concerning the relationship between sucrose consumption and coronary heart disease:[23]

1. A moderate- to high-fat diet (high in saturated fats and cholesterol) will act synergistically with sugar to elevate serum lipids. Complex carbohydrates are less effective in influencing serum lipids.

2. In diets low in fat and cholesterol, sucrose apparently exerts less influence on serum lipids. Thus, sucrose, because of its synergistic interaction with other dietary components, such as cholesterol and triglycerides, may be regarded as a risk factor in the etiology of atherosclerosis.

3. Some individuals have a genetic predisposition to the production of a large and permanent elevation in serum lipids when consuming diets containing sugar. It is estimated that about 9 per cent of the United States population have a genetic predisposition that results in elevated

blood lipids on high carbohydrate diets.[70] In these individuals, sucrose must be regarded as an important factor in the etiology of heart disease.

CONCLUSIONS — DIET/HEART HYPOTHESIS

What can be reasonably concluded about the relationship between diet, serum lipids, and coronary heart disease? A questionnaire sent to 214 "outstanding" scientists from 22 different countries found near unanimity on the relationship between diet and coronary heart disease, between diet and plasma lipoprotein concentrations, and between plasma cholesterol and the development of coronary heart disease. There was a degree of disagreement on the role of triglycerides in coronary heart disease.[71]

The scientists were asked to list their priorities about what should be recommended to the general population to prevent CHD. The following is a list of recommendations in order of priority:

1. fewer calories,

2. less dietary fat,

3. less saturated fat,

4. less dietary cholesterol,

5. increased polyunsaturated fat,

6. less sugar,

7. less salt,

8. more fiber, and

9. more starchy, complex carbohydrate foods.

The survey revealed strong agreement on some issues but disagreement on others. Most experts were in agreement that the current state of knowledge allows some general nutrition policy statements. Results of some of the survey answers are listed in Table 7–6.

Although the diet receives primary emphasis in the prevention of atherosclerosis and certain dietary components such as saturated fatty acids and cholesterol have been implicated in the development of the disease, no single isolated factor has alone been found to be the single primary factor influencing the development of CHD. In spite of vast research and study, there is still no well-accepted empirical evidence that habitual dietary intake of saturated fat and cholesterol will cause CHD in an *individual*; similarly there is no definitive evidence to suggest that increasing the level of polyunsaturated fatty acid will prevent, alleviate, or cure CHD.

Critics have charged that past studies that attempted to relate diet to serum cholesterol levels were of poor experimental design and poor statistical analysis.[72] These critics have even suggested that the better the experimental design the less was the effect the experimental diet had on the development of CHD.

Indirect evidence, derived from epidemiological and population studies, suggests that curbing caloric intake to maintain a desirable body weight,

Table 7-6

Responses of Scientists to Questions about the Relationship Between Diet
and Heart Disease

Question	Percentage Yes	Percentage No
Is there a connection between diet and development of coronary heart disease?	99.4%	0.6%
Is there a connection between diet and plasma lipoprotein concentration?	98.9	1.2
Is there a connection between plasma cholesterol concentrations and the development of coronary heart disease?	98.9	1.2
Is there a connection between plasma triglyceride concentrations and development of coronary heart disease?	77.9	22.1
Is your knowledge of diet and coronary heart disease sufficient for recommending a moderate change in the diet of the population in our society?	91.9	8.1

Source: K. Norum. *Report to the Storting No. 32 (1975–1976) on Norwegian Nutrition and Food Policy.* Oslo: Royal Norwegian Ministry of Agriculture, 1975. (Also, *J.A.M.A.,* June 1977).

and taking measures to prevent abnormally high lipid levels, may be useful in protecting against CHD. However, factors such as individual variation, environment, life-style, past nutritional status, and the presence of other risk factors may modify the influence of diet on heart disease, making it difficult to categorically state that an individual's modification of diet will necessarily improve his or her risk of CHD.

It is, however, possible to identify those individuals prone to coronary heart disease on the basis of elevations of serum lipid and cholesterol patterns. The data from the Framingham study were used to develop a *Coronary Risk Handbook.* This tool can aid in the estimation of the risk of coronary heart disease in individuals for whom significant risk factors have been identified.[73]

CHALLENGES TO THE TRADITIONAL VIEW

Several challenges have been made recently to the traditional view that correcting specified risk factors (in particular dietary) will reduce the prevalence or severity of coronary arteriosclerosis.[3-5]

W. B. Kannel, one of the principal researchers in the Framingham study, stated, "There are few prophylactic measures of proved efficacy in coronary heart disease. This applies to primary and secondary prevention. Neither hygienic, pharmacologic, nor surgical measures have been shown conclusively to delay acute episodes or to prolong life."[3]

An editorial in *Lancet* declared:

So far, despite all the effort and money that have been spent, the evidence that eliminating risk factors will eliminate heart disease adds up to little more than zero in terms of preventing heart disease on a public scale. . . . A key test is to show that selectively reducing serum cholesterol reduces clinical atherosclerotic cardiovascular disease. The evidence in man is hopeful, but miniscule in comparison with the general aura of faith in such therapy.[6]

An even stronger challenge was made by the National Health and Lung Institute report:

Despite evidence that combinations of risk factors increase the risk of atheriosclerosis and its complications there is, as yet, no conclusive evidence that intervention with respect to normalizing these risk factors will reduce the risk of arteriosclerosis.[4]

G. V. Mann, writing of the "end of an era" of the diet-heart hypothesis, noted that years of research have not resolved the controversy. Those taking this position suggest that the era in which dietary fat is the focus of arteriosclerosis may soon end.[7]

If we attempt to promote health through nutrition, we must be aware of the state of knowledge relating diet to heart disease. The following section reviews research strategies into various aspects of coronary heart disease and opposing sides of the diet-heart controversy.

RESEARCH STRATEGIES

The current state of knowledge about the cause and prevention of coronary heart disease makes it imperative that continuing research studies be carried out. The multifactorial etiology of coronary heart disease is well established. It is also agreed that a number of risk factors have been identified but that these factors may be of different importance to various individuals and population groups. Further, the evidence establishing the importance of risk factors needs to be strengthened. Thus, additional research in the areas of epidemiological, clinical, and basic studies is essential.

The National Heart, Lung, and Blood Institute (NHLBI, USDHEW) supports much research designed to determine nutritional and behavioral influences on heart disease. Three programs of particular importance are the Multiple Risk Factor Intervention Trial (MRFIT), the Specialized Centers for Research (SCOR) in Arteriosclerosis Program, and the Lipid Research Clinics Program (LRC).[74,75]

Multiple Risk Factor Intervention Trial (MRFIT)[74]

In 1970 the Inter-Society Commission for Heart Disease Resources suggested "that a strategy of primary prevention of premature atherosclerotic diseases be adopted as long-term national policy for the United States." A year later, in response to a call by the National Heart and Lung Institute for research on the relationship between multiple risk factors and heart disease in high-risk individuals, the MRFIT was initiated.

The MRFIT involves a six-year primary prevention clinical trial with about 12,000 males aged 25 to 57. The participants have been identified as being in the upper 15 per cent of the population distribution for risk of heart disease as determined by their elevated serum cholesterol levels, elevated blood pressure, and cigarette smoking. Not included in the study were men with existing clinical evidence of the disease. The participants were divided into two groups; half the sample received their usual medical care, and half were provided with specific intervention into the risk factors. Intervention included dietary instruction designed to reduce serum cholesterol levels by about 10 per cent. The general daily diet was designed to include approximately 30–35 per cent calories from fat (less than 10 per cent from saturated fatty acids, 10–13 per cent from polyunsaturated fatty acids), about 300 mg daily of dietary cholesterol, and modification of carbohydrates as appropriate for each individual.

Drugs to reduce blood pressure and techniques to achieve cessation of smoking were also included as interventions. The basic intervention approach was a series of ten group counseling and discussion sessions, which were followed by reinforcement sessions.

Although it is too early to fully evaluate the success and results of the program, a number of lessons have been learned from this large-scale undertaking:

1. A complex project such as the MRFIT is possible; it can survive planning, revision, compromise, and controversy and be successfully implemented.

2. The trial has offered a tremendous opportunity for a cooperative, multidisciplinary venture between a broad range of professionals, policymakers, politicians, and the public.

3. Mass media response was generally favorable and encouraging.

4. The assistance provided by centers for data coordination, analysis, and evaluation was essential.

5. The process of developing materials and resources for the project was lengthy and often frustrating.

6. In general, however, the undertaking can serve as a prototype for the design and implementation of a large-scale population study on the various risks influencing the development of coronary heart disease.

Specialized Centers for Research (SCOR)[75]

The SCOR programs differ from the MRFIT and the Lipid Research Programs in that these centers do not follow a rigid, particular study design. Rather, they undertake many different studies involving both human and animal experiments. Activities conducted include those dealing with nutrition and behavioral techniques as they relate to compliance with prescribed treatment, risk factors, and motivation. Other activities include prevalence and longitudinal studies of lipid levels, blood pressure, growth and development in infants and youth, and research on the role of risk factors on hyperlipidemia.

Lipid Research Clinics Program (LRC)[75]

This program is a national research effort that was developed to obtain further understanding of the etiology, diagnosis, and management of lipid disorders, particularly those related to premature vascular disease.

The program is designed to determine the prevalence of different types of blood lipid disorders and the relationship of these disorders to diet, to increase the knowledge of the diagnosis and management of serum lipid abnormalities, and to implement an intervention study to determine the effect of lowering blood lipids in high-risk patients relative to the development, mortality, and morbidity of cardiovascular disease.

DIETARY RECOMMENDATIONS FOR PREVENTION

There is no question that the preventive approach is appropriate, but scientific controversy exists as to certain issues, including: (1) the adequacy and validity of scientific evidence about identified risk factors, (2) the validity of applying questionable data to recommendations aimed at patients or the public as a whole, and (3) the possible hazards of some of the proposed recommendations.

Opinions about these issues have polarized in two general directions. One school of thought espouses the role of advocating any possible modes and activities that might enhance prevention. Advocates demand immediate action and suggest that the appropriate strategy in dealing with public health matters of such importance is to act upon available information, while admitting the possibility that future knowledge will be forthcoming. This approach acknowledges the limitations of existing knowledge, but it suggests that the consequences of the disease are so damaging, and the possible adverse consequences of preventive measures are either minimal or nonexistent, that the prudent course of action is to act on available evidence.

The other school suggests that immediate action on the basis of inconclusive information, and in the face of possible risk, is not called for. Advocates of this position call for further research, fearing that promises or suggestions to the effect that intervention into uncertain risk factors that may improve health are unwise. If a gullible public is convinced to change their diets on the belief that better health will result, and if such modifications do not reap tangible and speedy rewards, the public will be lost to future preventive recommendations.

Groups such as the American Heart Association, the American Health Foundation, and the Inter-Society Commission for Heart Disease Resources recommend that the entire population make moderate changes in their diets. The American Heart Association recommendations are summarized as follows:[76]

1. Caloric intake adjusted to achieve and maintain ideal body weight.

2. A reduction in total fat calories achieved by a substantial reduction in dietary saturated fats — the recommended reduction is from the current average of 40–45 per cent of total calories from fat to no more

than 35 per cent. Of this, 10 per cent of total calories are to be poly-unsaturated and less than 10 per cent are to be saturated fatty acids. It is preferable to distribute fat calories throughout the day; a heavy intake of fat calories at one time is ill-advised.

3. Substantial reduction in dietary cholesterol — the recommendation is an average daily intake of cholesterol approximating 300 mg.

4. Dietary carbohydrates — the emphasis should be on foods high in naturally occurring, complex carbohydrates, such as vegetables, breads, and cereals. Refined sugar foods, such as desserts, candy, soft drinks, and sweets should be limited. The previous recommendation of limit-ing total fat intake necessitates a slight increase in the calories from dietary carbohydrates. However, this is not expected to greatly affect serum lipid levels of most people, as the suggested increase is in com-plex carbohydrates.

5. Salt intake — the association between atherosclerosis and hypertension is recognized, whereas the relationship between dietary high salt intake and elevated blood pressure is not so well established.

6. Other dietary factors of interest — trace minerals, hardness of water, vitamin intake, and fiber content of the diet. Available evidence does not permit the formulation of specific recommendations relative to these factors.

This model for promoting the general health of the public through di-etary modifications assumes that the practical application of carefully developed recommendations may not necessitate more sophisticated knowledge of various disease processes. The model allows for the possibil-ity of increased scientific knowledge and acknowledges the importance and desire to define more precisely those factors related to disease. But the practical approach suggests that these future data will not invalidate the conclusions that: (1) an habitual, public dietary pattern high in satu-rated fat and cholesterol is a prerequisite for widespread CHD, and (2) a shift to diets lower in saturated fat and cholesterol are important parts of public health prevention of CHD.[76,77]

The Council on Foods and Nutrition of the American Medical Associa-tion, the American Academy of Pediatrics, and the Food and Nutrition Board (NRC, NAS) take the more traditional approach,[24,78] urging that high-risk individuals be identified early and that these individuals then modify their diets in accord with the current knowledge relative to secondary prevention or tertiary prevention. The general public should not be subjected to dietary alterations until conclusive answers are avail-able that indicate the specific changes that are to be made.[24]

The Food and Nutrition Board of the National Academy of Sciences, National Research Council, and the Council on Foods and Nutrition of the American Medical Association issued a joint statement on diet and coronary heart disease in 1972. They recommended that:[24]

1. Measurement of plasma lipid profile, particularly plasma cholesterol, become a routine part of all health maintenance physical examinations.

2. Persons in "risk categories" on the basis of plasma lipid levels be made aware and be given suitable dietary counseling.

3. Care be taken to ensure that dietary advice allows for intake of essential nutrients.

4. Modified and ordinary foods useful for the purpose be available on the market, reasonably priced, and easily identified by appropriate labeling.

5. High priority be given to research to determine reliably the effect of dietary modifications on CHD.

On the face of it, this stance may appear to be the wise course of action. However, to follow this approach, it is necessary to have techniques and capabilities to identify individuals who are at risk. The FNB and the AMA concede that "the average level of plasma lipids in most American men and women is undesirably elevated."[24] Teenagers and adults are often disinclined to visit a health care facility unless they have a particular problem that deserves medical attention, thus complicating possible mechanisms by which early detection might be implemented. Even if high-risk individuals could be identified early, it is questionable whether they could be motivated to consume a diet that is different from that served to other family members.

POSSIBLE HAZARDS OF THE PRUDENT DIET

The recommendations of the prudent diet — reducing consumption of high-fat foods, but retaining meat protein in the form of lean meats and retaining milk protein in the form of skim milk products — do not seem to imply a danger if a balance of calories is achieved. There is, however, a potential hazard for those who sustain a prolonged weight loss. For those attempting to reduce, the consumption of additional fruits and vegetables and whole grain products — all of which are high in vitamins and minerals — instead of an excess of high-fat and high-sugar foods is thought to be advantageous to general health.

One frequently cited "danger" is that which results from an excess of polyunsaturated fats. Some investigators have noted a relationship between diets that are high in polyunsaturated fatty acids with the formation of gallstones[79] and certain kinds of cancer.[80-82] No conclusive evidence has been obtained of such danger from experiments of a relatively large population size and over a long time period. Epidemiological data indicate that cultures in the Mediterranean Basin, Japan, and other areas of apparently healthy individuals who typically consume a diet similar to the prudent diet do not suffer from health hazards.

The United States is not the only nation engaged in recommending dietary modification to the general public. Table 7-7 summarizes the recommendations of various organizations that are involved in suggesting changes in national diet as a preventive approach to disease. The striking similarity in recommendations is clear. Most of these recommendations include a call for a return to the dietary habits that are characteristic of

Table 7-7
Recommendations of 16 Expert Committees on Dietary Fat and Coronary Heart Disease

Country and Organization of Origin	Source Reference	Recommendations for (GP) General Populations of (HR) High-risk Groups	Recommended Fat as Percentage of Total Calories	Recommended Increased PUFA	Recommended PUFA–SAFA Ratio	Recommended Daily Dietary Cholesterol (mg)	Recommended Reduction of Sugar	Recommended Labeling of Fat Content of Foods
Scandinavian countries official report, 1968	(29)	GP	25 to 35	Yes			Yes	Yes.
United States, 1970, Intersociety report	(23)	GP HR	Less than 35	Yes	1.0	Less than 300		Yes.
New Zealand, 1971, Heart Foundation	(46)	GP HR	35 35	Yes	1.0	300 to 600 do	No	Yes.
United States, 1972, American Health Foundation	(4)	GP	35	Yes	1.0	300	Yes	Yes.
United States, 1972, American Medical Association and National Academy of Sciences	(5)	HR	Substantial decrease in saturated fat.	Yes		Reduce		Yes.
International Society of Cardiology, 1973	(24)	HR	Less than 30	Yes	Less than 1.0	Less than 300		Yes.
United States, 1973, American Heart Association	(6)	GP	35	Yes	1.0	300	Yes	Yes.
The Netherlands, 1973, Nutritional Council	(42)	GP	35	Yes	1.0	250 to 300	Yes	Yes.
United States, 1973, White House Conference	(64)	GP	35	Yes		Less than 300		Yes.
Australia, 1974, National Heart Foundation	(45)	GP HR	30 to 35 do	Yes Yes	1.5 1.5	300 300	Yes	
United Kingdom, 1974, Dept. of Health and Social Security	(2)	GP	Reduce saturated fat	No			Yes	
Germany, 1975, Federal Republic report	(56)	GP	do	Yes	0	300		
Australia, 1975, Academy of Science	(8)	GP	35	Yes	1.0	Less than 350	Yes	Yes.
United Kingdom, 1976, Royal College of Physicians and British Cardiac Society	(51)	GP	Toward 35	Yes		Reduce	Yes	Yes.
Norway, 1976, Ministry of Agriculture	(41)	GP	35	Yes			Yes	Yes.
United States, 1977, Senate Committee on Nutrition	(61)	GP	30	Yes	1.0	300	Yes	Yes.

earlier times in history: increased complex carbohydrates, reduced intake of high-fat foods and sugar, and increased consumption of foods higher in polyunsaturated fatty acids. Some of the reports also suggest a reduction in salt consumption.

ALTERNATIVE STRATEGIES TO INDIVIDUALLY MOTIVATED DIETARY CHANGES

These recommended dietary changes present an almost impossible task: motivating an individual to give up pleasures of the present for an uncertain and possible nonexistent reward in the distant future, and in an environment that offers almost continuous enticements and temptations. It is easier, perhaps, to work toward the goal of dietary modification by adjusting the availability of different foods, while at the same time attempting to promote an increased understanding, awareness, and appreciation of the positive benefits to be gained from altering eating habits.

It is possible to significantly alter the amount and composition of fat in animal products.[86] Milk fat, for example, can be modified during processing. It is also possible through feeding modification to modify the fatty acid content of animal fat. T. Scott et al. reported that the polyunsaturated fatty acid content of the fat in goat milk could be increased from 2 per cent to 30–35 per cent.[83] There have also been significant increases in the polyunsaturated fatty acid composition of cow's milk[84] as well as of the content of body fat of ruminants and nonruminants, such as swine and poultry.[85]

The food industry has become very interested in the problem of modifying dietary fat, and in recent years that industry has placed numerous new products on the market. Much consideration has been devoted to the production of sunflowers and other oil plants that yield fat of high quality and are rich in linoleic acid vegetable oils. The status of other activities directed at modifying diets by adjusting the availability of various foods includes the following:[86]

Meat product changes	Meat product fat limits set by USDA; soy protein products availability and use; beef grading changes of "Good" to "Choice"; beef freeze demonstration of a beef-free society; grain shortage and increased range feeding; "The Poly Cow" development in beef culture with coated grains; beef breeding for leanness including the "Beefalo"; pork breeding for leanness, a long success story.
Dairy product changes	Increased low-fat dairy consumption; increased low-fat product availability; improved low-fat product acceptability; no change in breeding or grading for low-fat milk; FTC egg trial discouraged misleading ads.

Cooking fats

Vegetable oil boom; soft margarine boom; soft shortening availability.

Food labeling

Legislation, voluntary labeling of fat.

Food advertising

Increased FDA-FTC responsiveness to nutrition-health concerns; hearings on health claims.

Government food programs

Little progress in reducing fat in school lunches or institutional diets.

PEDIATRIC CONSIDERATIONS

Although some authorities have reached tentative agreement about preventive measures for adults, they have not reached agreement about appropriate preventive measures for infants and children. The controversy over recommendations for infants and children centers around such considerations as

— Measures appropriate for adults may not be suitable for infants or children since the threat of atherosclerosis will usually be felt several years later.

— It may be possible that preventive measures instituted during the early adult years are adequate to protect against atherosclerosis.

— Infants and children may suffer certain risks, such as impaired growth or development, from dietary modifications that are suitable for adults.

The development of advanced atherosclerotic lesions is thought to occur gradually and over periods of many years. It has long been recognized that fatty streaks, or abnormal lipid accumulation in the intima of the coronary arteries, occur in children and even in infants. Such deposits appear to represent early stages in the long process of the development of atherosclerosis. Current thinking supports the hypothesis that these fatty streaks progress in later years to accumulate increased lipid and to cause changes in coronary tissues. These changes eventually lead to advanced atherosclerotic lesions.

Aortic fatty streaks have been found within months of birth. By the age of three years, most children present some evidence of these streaks, and individuals in certain countries show stress in from 5 per cent to almost 100 per cent of aortic intimal surface by the age of ten to twenty years.[87] In the U.S. population, the prevalence of atherosclerosis has been reported to be at least 45 per cent among American men under the age of thirty who were killed during wartime.[88] Of this percentage, 5 per cent were found upon autopsy to evidence severe coronary atherosclerosis.

Research has not yet identified consistent correlations between these fatty streaks in children and other factors, such as environment, dietary patterns, and geography, that are commonly associated with advanced lesions in adulthood.[87] However, lipid abnormalities are considered to be a possible risk factor. Screening programs for the risk of cardiovascular disease have suggested that a significant number of children have elevated serum cholesterol levels.[89] There is no general consensus as to the desired serum cholesterol level in children, although I. Wright has suggested that the desired level should not be greater than 160 mg/100 ml.[90]

Several studies indicate a disturbing number of children with elevated levels of serum cholesterol that may predict an early onset of coronary heart disease. Children with persisting elevated serum cholesterol levels more frequently come from families with a high risk of coronary heart disease development. Thus, it may be advisable to introduce dietary modification for these children.[91]

INFANT DIETS

Diets of infants in the United States can be described in only general patterns because of the vast differences among socioeconomic, cultural, racial, ethnic, and religious groups. However, a fairly comprehensive survey of infant dietary patterns and nutrient intakes by G. Purvis indicated that during the first 3 months of life, the infant typically consumes either breast milk or infant formula. Both types of foods are greatly reduced by the age of 6 months and are usually discontinued by the age of 12 months.[92]

By 6 months of age, close to 50 per cent of infants in the United States consume whole, 2 per cent skim cow's milk, or skim cow's milk. Most infants drink one of these milks by the age of 1 year. Commercial baby foods and cereals are largely used between the age of 4 to 9 months; by the age of 1 year the principal calorie intake of the infant comes from table food. Dietary cholesterol and fat intakes are greatly related to the type of milk and other foods that are provided to the infant. Relative to human or cow's milk, most infant formula contains approximately 15–20 per cent of the amount of cholesterol and five to fifteen times the amount of polyunsaturated fatty acids; total fat contents are comparable. Infant formula typically supplies a high proportion of fatty acids in the form of linoleic acid, which constitutes 15–60 per cent of total fatty acids in commercial formula. The P/S ratio of infant formula is usually higher than that of human or cow's milk.

In view of the previously mentioned study indicating that close to 80 per cent of infants in the United States receive infant formula during the first 3 months and about 40 per cent continue to receive formula until the age of 6 months, a high proportion of infants in this country are receiving diets that are relatively low in cholesterol and fatty acids but high in polyunsaturated fatty acids.

The long-term consequences of these trends are not known. Plasma cholesterol levels in normal infants who are fed either breast or cow's milk at the age of 3 to 6 months range from 150 mg/100 ml to 190 mg/ml; in contrast, infants who are fed commercial infant formula have plasma cholesterol levels ranging from 120 mg/100 ml to 150 mg/100 ml.

Surveys have indicated that normal children who are fed low (less than 300 mg) cholesterol diets between 6 and 12 months tend to have plasma cholesterol levels 10–15 mg/100 ml lower than those who are fed cholesterol levels closer to 600 mg/day.[93] The advantages and disadvantages of maintaining infants on diets restricted in cholesterol during their first year are controversial and widely debated. One hypothesis based upon animal studies, suggests that physiological systems for the degradation of cholesterol need a type of "priming" with dietary cholesterol in early life so that the enzymes and metabolic pathways involved can develop to function normally in later life.

Other studies, however, have found no evidence to support this hypothesis as the case in human infants, and some have reported that children who are fed diets that are very low in cholesterol in early months of life tended to have low cholesterol levels by the age of 8 or 9 years. Many more longitudinal studies are needed to document the validity of both positions.

Much of the concern about the safety of infants' and children's diets that are low in cholesterol and in saturated fatty acids focuses on certain considerations:

1. Cholesterol seems to be an essential dietary component in the early years; it appears that the body needs more than that supplied from endogenous sources.

2. It is possible that a drastic reduction in dietary cholesterol in the diets of infants and children may cause these diets to be limited in essential nutrients.

3. We may not yet know all essential elements for optimal growth and development; a drastic modification in diet may result in harmful consequences that are not now known.

What are the implications for prevention? At present it does not appear possible to prevent fatty streaks in children. The fatty streak seems to be universal in children from all geographical, socioeconomic, and cultural and genetic origins; further, as long as it remains a fatty streak, it may be harmless. Thus, the optimal point for implementing preventive methods appears to be the prevention of fibrous plaque formation — successful intervention may be practical during the late adolescent years, or even sooner.[87]

Many experts agree that, for infants in families without familial hyperlipoproteinemia, the restriction of dietary cholesterol and saturated fatty acids is not necessary. Because human milk is relatively high in cholesterol, to suggest that dietary cholesterol in infants should be limited would be paramount to recommending against the use of breast milk.

There is a lack of agreement about recommendations for children. The Subcommittee on Atherosclerosis, Council of Rheumatic Fever and Congenital Heart Disease of the American Heart Association and the American Academy of Pediatrics recommend against the widespread modification of the diets of American children.[78,94] Because of the lack of understanding about how atherosclerosis develops, the specific mechanisms of its prevention, as well as the fact that the restriction of dietary intake during childhood has an uncertain effect on the future risk of developing coronary heart disease, the subcommittee suggests that dietary restriction is not warranted at this time.

Others, however, believe that changes in infant and childhood eating patterns are warranted. For example, S. Blumenthal has suggested that:

> Atherosclerosis appears to begin in childhood. . . . There is little evidence that advanced lesions regress. Until such evidence is available, primary prevention will be essential, especially for those whose initial symptom of the disease is a fatal event. If it is true that advanced lesions are not apt to regress, prevention should be instituted early in life.[95]

Until more evidence is in, a middle-of-the road approach may be most acceptable and probably most likely to be followed:

> Until more data on the efficacy of preventive measures become available, the practicing physician must decide for himself. . . . He must weigh the hazards against the potential benefits. . . . If he elects to proceed on the incomplete evidence available, he can take comfort in the fact that the measures advocated are good health practices and have other benefits.[96]

The pediatrician can play an active role in preventing coronary heart disorders by identifying infants and children (an estimated 7 per cent of the children in the United States) with genetic lipoprotein disorders and then implementing treatment for this high-risk group.[97] Health professionals should take careful family medical histories to determine possible familial hypertension, hyperlipidemia, angina pectoris, myocardial infarction, stroke, diabetes, and obesity. When such disorders are noted, the child as well as the family should be given advice about prevention, and, where appropriate, they should be tested for elevated serum cholesterol and triglyceride levels.

CONCLUSIONS

It is often necessary to make a decision on the basis of knowledge sufficient for action but insufficient to satisfy the intellect.

— I. Kant

The problems inherent in attempting to make dietary recommendations for the public are, of necessity, complex — there are no easy answers. Indeed, quick and easy answers may be, in the long run, counterproductive.

It can be stated unequivocally that we do not have enough knowledge to provide conclusive answers to these complex problems. We cannot write the final chapter to the complete volume on the diet-heart relationship. But we *do* have much evidence and a degree of scientific consensus on many of these issues. The practical approach, as a matter of prudence, is to act in the direction indicated by current knowledge.

People, behavior, food habits, and health status are dynamic and constantly changing. Policymakers are constantly making policies and decisions, with or without the benefits of scientifically informed public recommendations. There is a very real responsibility for those in a position to shape public policy to be "up front" about the current state of science, nutrition, and health and to acknowledge the gaps and limitations of present knowledge.

GLOSSARY OF TERMS USED IN CARDIOVASCULAR DISEASE

aneurysm   A sac or ballooning of the wall of an artery or vein resulting from weakness of the wall.

angina pectoris   A sudden severe pain in the chest and often in the left arm and shoulder. When the arteries supplying the heart muscle become narrowed, there is insufficient blood supply and pain results. It tends to appear during stress of any kind.

angiography   Injection of opaque substance into the circulation and x-ray films are taken of the heart and great blood vessels.

anticoagulant   A substance that inhibits blood clotting, such as heparin and dicumarol.

arrhythmia   An irregular rhythm of the heart beat.

arteriosclerosis   A thickening, hardening, and loss of elasticity of arteries.

atherogenesis   The formation of atheromatous lesions in the walls of the artery.

atheroma   A deposit of lipid and lipidlike substances in the intima of the artery.

atherosclerosis   A deposit of lipid and lipidlike substances in the wall of the intima in the large and small arteries (atheromata), which decrease the diameter of the lumen of the arteries. This is a form of arteriosclerosis.

blood pressure   The pressure of the blood on the walls of the arteries. Systolic pressure is the pressure when the heart muscle is contracted, while diastolic pressure is the pressure during the resting phase. Blood pressure is expressed as the systolic and then diastolic pressure, for example 115/80.

cerebrovascular accident   A decreased blood supply to the brain caused by a thrombosis, hemorrhage, embolism, or pressure on a blood vessel. It is commonly called a stroke.

congestive heart failure   When the heart is unable to maintain an adequate blood flow to the tissues, blood backs up in the veins leading to the heart; as a result, fluid accumulates in various parts of the body.

coronary arteries   Two arteries (left and right) that start at the aorta and branch down and carry blood into the heart.

coronary care unit (CCU)   This unit in the hospital originally was designed to provide effective means of resuscitation for cardiac arrest patients. The major efforts are now directed toward prevention of complications by continuous surveillance and immediate therapy.

coronary occlusion   Generally, a clot in one of the coronary arteries. Due to the lack of blood, this part of the heart dies. This is also called a heart attack.

coronary thrombosis   A clot in one of the coronary arteries. It is also called coronary occlusion.

diuretic   A substance that increases the secretion of urine.

electrocardiogram (ECG or EKG)   Graphic tracing of the electric current resulting from the contraction of the heart muscle.

embolism   The blocking of an artery or vein by a substance that was carried to that place.

embolus   A foreign substance present in the blood, such as air, a clot, fat, and cells, that circulates and finally blocks a small vessel.

essential hypertension   High blood pressure for which the cause is unknown.

fatty streak   A fatty lesion in the intima of a blood vessel.

heart attack   See Coronary occlusion.

hypercholesterolemia   Elevated blood cholesterol levels.

Source: V. Thiele: *Clinical Nutrition.* St. Louis: C. V. Mosby Co. 1976.

hyperlipemia A general term that refers to an excess of fat in the blood.

hyperlipidemia A nonspecific term that refers to the increase of one or more blood lipid components.

hyperlipoproteinemia An elevation of blood lipoproteins.

hypertension An elevation of blood pressure. It is often called high blood pressure.

hypokalemia Low blood levels of potassium.

hyponatremia Low blood levels of sodium.

infarct Death of tissue because of an insufficient supply of blood.

intima The innermost layer of a blood vessel.

ischemia A local temporary deficiency of blood that is caused by an obstruction.

morbidity The prevalence of a disease. It is usually expressed as the number of cases of a given disease in a given population.

mortality The rate of which is expressed as the number of deaths from a given disease in a given population.

myocardial infarction The death (necrosis) of part of the myocardium because of a decrease in blood supply to that area.

myocardial insufficiency Inability of the heart to maintain normal blood flow.

myocardium The middle layer of the three layers of the heart.

plaque An elevated lesion on the intima. The base of fat is covered with a fibrous connective tissue cap.

primary hypertension Essential hypertension.

risk factor A characteristic that appears with a greater incidence in a given disease.

sclerosis Hardening caused by the growth of fibrous tissue.

secondary hypertention High blood pressure that is the result of a given disease.

stroke See Cerebrovascular accident.

thrombosis The formation of a clot.

thrombus The formation of a plug or clot in a blood vessel or the heart resulting from coagulation of the blood. It remains at the site of formation.

xanthoma A yellowish or orange growth on the skin occurring as a flat or slightly raised patch because of deposits of lipid.

REFERENCES

1. Kannel, W. B. The disease of living. *Nutr. Today* 6 (1971): 2.
2. Levy, R. Press briefing on arteriosclerosis program goal. Washington, D.C.: U.S. Department of Health, Education and Welfare, July 13, 1977.
3. Kannel, W. B. Prevention of coronary heart disease by control of risk factors. *J.A.M.A.* 227 (1974): 338.
4. National Heart and Lung Institute Task Force on Arteriosclerosis. *Arteriosclerosis: A Report by the National Heart and Lung Institute Task Force.* Vol. II. Washington, D.C.: Government Printing Office, June 1971.
5. Corday, E., and S. R. Corday. Prevention of heart disease by control of risk factors: The time has come to face facts. *Am. J. Cardiol.* 35 (February 1975): 330.
6. Editorial. Can I avoid a heart attack? *Lancet* 1 (1974): 605.
7. Mann, G. V. Diet-heart: End of an era. *N. Eng. J. Med.* 297 (1977): 644-649.
8. American Heart Association. *Heart Facts.* Dallas, Texas: American Heart Association, 1978.
9. Inter-Society Commission for Heart Disease Resources, Atherosclerosis Study Group and Epidemiology Study Group. Primary prevention of atherosclerotic disease. *Circulation* 42 (1970): A55.
10. Stamler, J., D. M. Berkson, and A. Lindberg. Risk factors: Their role in the etiology and pathogenesis of the atherosclerotic diseases, in The American Association of Pathologists and Bacteriologists, *The Pathogenesis of Atherosclerosis*, Bethesda, Maryland, 1972.
11. Stamler, J. In U.S. Senate Select Committee on Nutrition and Human Needs, *Diet Related to Killer Diseases, Part 2.* Washington, D.C.: Government Printing Office, February 1-2, 1977.

12. Rice, O. Deaths from both heart disease and stroke. *The Nation's Health*, December 1977, p. 12.
13. Brody, J. E. Heart disease goes out of style. *The New York Times*, December 11, 1977.
14. Walker, W. J. Changing United States life-style and declining vascular mortality: Cause or coincidence? *N. Eng. J. Med.* 297 (1977): 163–165.
15. Strasser, T. Atherosclerosis and coronary heart disease: The contribution of epidemiology. *WHO Chron.* 26 (1972): 7.
16. Kritchevsky, D. Dietary interactions, in American Dairy Science Association, American Society of Animal Science, *Diet, Blood Lipids, and Cardiovascular Disease*, Champaign, Illinois, 1972.
17. Blackburn, H. Prevention of heart disease. II. *Am. J. Cardiol.* 37 (1976): 450.
18. Kannel, W. B. Lipid profile and the potential coronary victim. *Am. J. Clin. Nutr.* 24 (1971): 1074.
19. U.S. Department of Health, Education, and Welfare. *Dietary Management of Hyperlipoproteinemia*, Publ. No. (NIH) 76-110. Bethesda, Md.: National Heart and Lung Institute, 1974.
20. Connor, W. D., and S. L. Connor. The key role of nutritional factors in the prevention of coronary heart disease. *Prev. Med.* 1 (1972): 49.
21. Stamler, J. *Lectures on Preventive Cardiology*. New York: Grune and Stratton, 1967, pp. 109, 1023.
22. Blackburn, H. Progress in the epidemiology and prevention of coronary heart disease, in P. N. Yu and J. F. Goodwin, eds., *Progress in Cardiology*. Philadelphia: Lea and Febiger, 1974.
23. Reiser, R. Normal vs. pathological variations in serum cholesterol levels, in L. Hofmann, ed., *The Great American Nutritional Hassle*. Palo Alto, Calif.: Mayfield Publishing Co., 1978, p. 269.
24. National Academy of Sciences, Food and Nutrition Board, et al. Diet and coronary heart disease. *J. Am. Diet. Assoc.* 61 (1972): 379.
25. Krehl, W. A. The nutritional epidemiology of cardiovascular disease, in N. H. Moss and J. Mayer, eds., *Food and Nutrition in Health and Disease*. New York: New York Academy of Sciences, 1977, p. 335.
26. Gotto, A. Is atherosclerosis reversible? *J. Am. Diet. Assoc.* 74 (1979): 551.
27. Gordon, T., W. Castelli, M. Hjortland, et al. High-density lipoprotein as a protective factor against coronary heart disease: The Framingham Study. *Am. J. Med.* 62 (1977): 707.
28. Castelli, W. P., J. T. Doyle, T. Gordon, et al. HDL cholesterol and other lipids in coronary heart disease: The cooperative lipoprotein phenotyping study. *Circulation* 55 (1977): 767.
29. Zilversmit, O. B. Questions about diet and atherosclerosis. *Professional Perspectives*. Ithaca, N.Y.: Cornell University, April 1977.
30. Osler, W. Lectures on angina pectoris and allied states. I. Diagnosis, prognosis, and treatment of angina pectoris. *N.Y. Med. J.* 64 (1896): 800.
31. Stamler, J., R. Stamler, and R. Shekelle. Regional differences in prevalence, incidence, and mortality from atherosclerotic coronary heart disease, in J. H. de Haas, H. Hemker, and H. Snellen, eds., *Ischaemic Heart Disease*. Leiden, The Netherlands: Leiden University Press, 1970, p. 84.
32. Keys, A. Coronary heart disease in seven countries. *Circulation* 41 (1970): suppl. 1, 1–211.
33. Brown, J., G. J. Bourke, G. F. Gearty, A. Finnegan, et al. Nutritional and epidemiologic factors related to heart disease. *World Rev. Nutr. Diet* 12 (1970): 1–42.
34. Feinleib, M., W. B. Kannel, C. G. Tedeschi, T. K. Landau, and R. J. Garri-

son. The relation of ante mortem characteristics to cardiovascular findings at necropsy: The Framingham Study. Council on Epidemiology Conference on Cardiovascular Disease Epidemiology. San Diego, Calif.: American Heart Association et al., March 1-2, 1971.

35. Moore, M. C., M. A. Guzman, P. E. Schilling, and J. P. Strong. Dietary atherosclerosis study on deceased persons: Further data on the relation of select nutrients to raised coronary lesions. *J. Am. Diet. Assoc.* 70 (1977): 602.

36. Barboriak, J. J., W. A. Krehl, G. H. Cowgill, and A. D. Wheldon. Influence of high-fat diets on growth and development of obesity in the albino rat. *J. Nutr.* 64 (1958): 241–249.

37. Naimi, S., G. F. Wilgram, M. M. Nothman, and S. Proger. Cardiovascular lesions, blood lipids, coagulation, and fibrinolysis in butter-induced obesity in the rat. *J. Nutr.* 86 (1965): 325–332.

38. Mattson, F. H., B. A. Erickson, and A. M. Kligman. Effect of dietary cholesterol on serum cholesterol in man. *Am. J. Clin. Nutr.* 25 (1972): 589.

39. Beveridge, J. M. R., W. F. Connell, H. L. Haust, and G. A. Mayer. Dietary cholesterol and plasma cholesterol levels in man. *Canad. J. Biochem. Physiol.* 37 (1959): 575–582.

40. Connor, W. E., R. E. Hodges, and R. E. Bleiler. The serum lipids in men receiving high-cholesterol and cholesterol-free diets. *J. Clin. Invest.* 40 (1961): 894–901.

41. Hegsted, D. M., R. McGandy, M. Meyers, and F. J. Stare. Quantitative effects of dietary fat on serum cholesterol in man. *Am. J. Clin. Nutr.* 17 (1965): 281.

42. Alfin-Slater, R. B. *Nutrition — Styled to Protect against Heart Disease: The Moderately Styled Approach.* Los Angeles, American Dietetic Association Annual Meeting, October 1977.

43. Lofland, H. B., T. B. Clarkson, R. W. St. Clair, and N. D. M. Lehner. Studies on the regulation of plasma cholesterol levels in squirrel monkeys of two genotypes. *J. Lipid Res.* 13 (1972): 39–47.

44. Christakis, G., S. H. Rinzler, M. Archer, G. Winslow, S. Jempel, J. Stephenson, G. Friedman, H. Fein, A. Kraus, and C. James. The Anti-Coronary Club: A dietary approach to the prevention of coronary heart disease — A seven-year report. *Am. J. Publ. Health* 56 (1966): 299.

45. Leren, P. The Oslo Diet Heart Study, eleven-year report. *Circulation* 42 (1970): 935.

46. Turpeinen, O. Effect of cholesterol-lowering diet on mortality from coronary heart disease and other causes. *Circulation II* 56 (1977): 111–112.

47. Blackburn, H. Community implementation of CHD prevention programs, in Peter Schnohr, ed., *Proceedings of the International Symposium on the Strategy of Postponement of Ischemic Heart Disease.* Copenhagen, Denmark, August 13-14, 1976.

48. Farquhar, J., W. P. Wood, H. Breitrose, et al. Community education for cardiovascular health. *Lancet* 1 (1977): 1192–1195.

49. Puska, P., J. Tuomilehot, J. Salonen, and H. Mustaniemi. Community control of acute myocardial infarction in North Karelia. Paper presented at the International Cardiovascular Congress I. Scottsdale, Ariz., March 28–30, 1977.

50. Kritchevsky, D. Dietary interactions, in American Dairy Science Association, American Society of Animal Science, *Diet, Blood Lipids, and Cardiovascular Disease*, Champaign, Illinois, 1972.

51. Yudkin, J. Sucrose and cardiovascular disease. *Proc. Nutr. Soc.* 31 (1972): 331.

52. Cleave, T. L. *The Saccharine Disease.* Bristol, England: John Wright and Sons, 1974.
53. Trowell, H. Ischemic heart disease and dietary fiber. *Am. J. Clin. Nutr.* 25 (1972): 926.
54. American Heart Association. *Diet and Coronary Heart Disease.* Dallas, Texas, 1973.
55. Anderson, T. W., L. C. Neri, G. B. Schreiber, F. D. Talbot, and A. Zdrojewski. Ischemic heart disease, water hardness, and myocardial magnesium. *Canad. Med. Assoc. J.* 113 (1975): 199.
56. Masironi, R., ed. Trace elements in relation to cardiovascular disease. *WHO Offset Publ.* (Geneva) 5 (1974): 1–42.
57. Kritchevsky, D., and S. A. Tepper. Experimental atherosclerosis in rabbits fed cholesterol-free diets: Influence of chow components. *J. Atheroscler. Res.* 8 (1968): 357.
58. Kelsay, J. L. A review of research on effects of fiber intake on man. *Am. J. Clin. Nutr.* 31 (1978): 142.
59. Cleave, T. L., and G. D. Campbell. *Diabetes, Coronary Thrombosis, and the Saccharine Disease,* 2d ed. Bristol, England: John Wright and Sons, 1969.
60. Keys, A. Sucrose in the diet and coronary heart disease. *Atherosclerosis* 14 (1971): 193–202.
61. Albrink, M. J. In I. Macdonald, ed., *Effect of Carbohydrates on Lipid Metabolism.* New York/Basel: S. Karger, 1973.
62. Wretlind, A. World sugar production and usage in Europe, in H. L. Sipple and K. W. McNutt, eds., *Sugars in Nutrition.* New York: Academic Press, 1974, p. 91.
63. Grande, F. Sugars in cardiovascular disease, in H. L. Sipple and K. W. McNutt, eds., *Sugars in Nutrition.* New York: Academic Press, 1974, pp. 401–437.
64. Bennett, A. E., R. W. Howell, and R. Doll. Sugar consumption and cigarette smoking. *Lancet* 1 (1970): 1011–1014.
65. Nelson, R. A. In National Academy of Sciences, Academy Forum, *Sweeteners: Issues and Uncertainties.* Washington, D.C., 1975, p. 110.
66. Reiser, S. Metabolic effects of dietary carbohydrates — A review, in A. Jeanes and J. Hodge, eds., *Physiological Effects of Food Carbohydrates.* Washington, D.C.: American Chemical Society Symposium Series 15, 1975.
67. Walker, A. R. P. Sugar intake and coronary heart disease. *Atherosclerosis* 14 (1971): 137.
68. Mann, J. I., and A. S. Trusswell. Effects of isocaloric exchange of dietary sucrose and starch on fasting serum lipids, postprandial insulin secretion, and alimentary lipaemia in human subjects. *Brit. J. Nutr.* 27 (1972): 395–405.
69. Dunnigan, M. G., T. Fyfe, M. T. McKiddie, and S. M. Crosbie. The effects of isocaloric exchange of dietary starch and sucrose on glucose tolerance, plasma insulin, and serum lipids in man. *Clin. Sci.* 38 (1970): 1.
70. Wood, P. D., M. P. Stern, A. Silver, C. M. Reaven, and J. van der Groeben. Prevalence of plasma lipoprotein abnormalities in a free-living population in the Central Valley, California. *Circulation* 45 (1972): 114–126.
71. Norum, K. *Report to the Storting No. 32 (1975–1976) on Norwegian Nutrition and Food Policy.* Oslo: Royal Norwegian Ministry of Agriculture, 1975. (Also, *J.A.M.A.,* June 1977).
72. Cornfield, J., and S. Mitchell. Selected risk factors in coronary disease: Possible intervention effects. *Arch. Environ. Health* 19 (1969): 382–394.

73. Gordon, T., and W. B. Kannel. In American Heart Association, *Coronary Risk Handbook. Estimating Risk of Coronary Heart Disease in Daily Practice: Framingham Study, 16-Year Follow-up.* Dallas, Texas, 1973, pp. 1–35.

74. The multiple-risk factor intervention trial (MRFIT): A national study of primary prevention of coronary heart disease. *J.A.M.A.* 235 (1976): 825.

75. U.S. Department of Health, Education, and Welfare. *Proceedings of the Nutrition-Behavioral Research Conference,* Publ. No. (NIH) 76-978. Bethesda, Md.: National Heart and Lung Institute, April 29–30, 1975.

76. American Heart Association, Commission on Nutrition. Diet and coronary heart disease. *Nutr. Today* 9 (May–June 1974): 26.

77. American Health Foundation. Position statement on diet and coronary heart disease. *Prev. Med.* 1 (1972): 255.

78. American Academy of Pediatrics, Commission on Nutrition. Childhood diet and coronary heart disease. *Pediatrics* 49 (1972): 305.

79. Sturdevant, R. L., M. L. Pearce, and S. Dayton. Increased prevalence of cholelithiasis in men ingesting a serum-cholesterol-lowering diet. *N. Eng. J. Med.* 288 (1973): 24.

80. Pearce, M. L., and S. Dayton. Incidence of cancer in men on a diet high in polyunsaturated fat. *Lancet* 1 (1971): 464–467.

81. Rose, G., H. Blackburn, A. Keys, H. L. Taylor, W. B. Kannel, O. Paul, D. D. Reid, and J. Stamler. Colon cancer and blood cholesterol. *Lancet* 1 (1974): 181.

82. Rose, G. A., W. B. Thomson, and R. T. Williams. Corn oil in treatment of ischaemic heart disease. *Brit. Med. J.* 5449 (1965): 1531–1533.

83. Scott, T. W., L. J. Cook, K. A. Ferguson, I. W. McDonald, R. A. Buchanan, and G. L. Hills. Production of polyunsaturated milk fat in domestic ruminants. *Aust. J. Sci.* 32 (1970): 291–293.

84. Plowman, R. C., J. Bitman, C. H. Gordon, and L. P. Dryden, et al. Milk fat with increased polyunsaturated fatty acids. *J. Dairy Sci.* 55 (1972): 204–207.

85. Scott, T. W., and L. J. Cook. Production of ruminant meats containing high proportions of polyunsaturated fats. *Food Technology in Australia,* July 1972, p. 328.

86. Blackburn, H. In U.S. Senate Select Committee on Nutrition and Human Needs, *Diet Related to Killer Diseases, Part 4.* Washington, D.C.: Government Printing Office, July 26, 1977, pp. 101–129.

87. McGill, H. G. Arterial fatty streaks in childhood and atherosclerosis, in *Atherosclerosis No. 9.* Columbus, Ohio: Ross Laboratories, March 1974, pp. 2–6.

88. McNamara, J., M. A. Molot, J. F. Stremple, and R. T. Curring. Coronary artery disease in combat casualties in Vietnam. *J.A.M.A.* 216 (1971): 1185.

89. Friedman, G., and S. J. Goldberg. Normal serum cholesterol values: Percentile ranking in a middle-class pediatric population. *J.A.M.A.* 225 (1973): 610.

90. Wright, I. S. Correct levels of serum cholesterol: Average vs. normal vs. optimal, *J.A.M.A.* 236 (1976): 261–262.

91. Cardiac risk factors are also important in children. *J.A.M.A.* 237 (1977): 1543.

92. Purvis, G. A. What nutrients do our infants really get? *Nutr. Today* 8 (1973): 28.

93. Winick, M., ed. *Year One: Nutrition, Growth, Health.* New York: Medcom Inc., 1975.
94. Mitchel, S., S. G. Blount, Jr., S. Blumenthal, M. J. Jesse, and W. H. Weidman. The pediatrician and atherosclerosis. *Pediatrics* 49 (1972): 165.
95. Blumenthal, S. Prevention of atherosclerosis. *Am. J. Cardiol.* 31 (1973): 591.
96. Kannel, W. B. Prevention of coronary heart disease by control of risk factors (questions and answers). *J.A.M.A.* 227 (1974): 338.
97. McBean, D., and E. W. Speckman. An interpretive review: Diet in early life and the prevention of atherosclerosis. *Pediatr. Res.* 8 (1974): 837.

8

Diet, nutrition, and cancer

Reader Objectives

After completing this chapter, the reader should be able to
1. Describe the public health significance of cancer in the United States.
2. State the possible influence of diet on the development of cancer.
3. State the fiber hypothesis as it relates to the development of cancer.
4. Define *dietary fiber, crude fiber,* and *fiber.*
5. State the research conclusions on the relationship between
   — dietary fiber and the development of cancer.
   — fat intake and cancer.
   — calorie intake, body weight, and cancer.
   — protein intake and cancer.
   — other nutrient imbalances and cancer.
6. List the objectives of the Diet, Nutrition, and Cancer Program.
7. List the general dietary recommendations for preventing cancer.

PUBLIC HEALTH SIGNIFICANCE

Cancer, the second leading cause of death in the United States, is responsible for 10–21 per cent of total deaths. An estimated 19–20 per cent of these deaths are attributed to colonic cancer, which is responsible for 2–4 per cent of all deaths in the United States. Mortality rates for other developed industrialized nations are similarly high, but there are differences among socially and economically advanced nations. For example, Finland has a low mortality rate from cancer; mortality rates from cancer are falling in countries such as Scotland but are increasing in other nations, such as Denmark.[1] Cancer statistics for the United States by site and sex are presented in Figure 8–1.

The World Health Organization estimates that up to 85 per cent of all cancer is the direct result of exposure to environmental factors of one kind or another. In most cases, these factors are self-inflicted by habits such as overeating, smoking, overdrinking, excessive exposure to sunlight, and dangerous chemicals in the environment. These environmental factors provide targets at which to aim cancer prevention programs.

Environmental factors are responsible for certain kinds of cancer, but they are also responsible for influencing factors that enhance tumor formation of apparently organic origin (e.g., hormones, metabolic, or dietary imbalances). More than three fourths of human cancers are thus environmentally influenced, including tumors of the skin, mouth, respiratory, gastrointestinal and urinary tracts, breast, thyroid, uterus, and hematopoietic and lymphpoietic systems. In view of these considerations, it appears that much human cancer is preventable.[1]

Cancer Deaths by Site and Sex, 1977

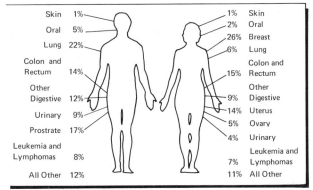

Cancer Incidence by Site and Sex
Excluding non-melanoma skin cancer and carcinoma in situ of uterine cervix.

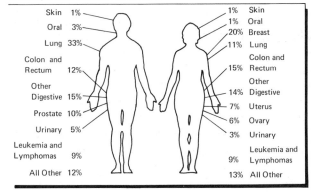

Figure 8-1. Cancer deaths and cancer incidence, by site and sex, 1977. (American Cancer Society, *A Cancer Journal for Clinicians*, 27 (January-February, 1977):27.

DIET AND CANCER OVERVIEW

A vast literature of epidemiological as well as laboratory data suggest strong correlations between higher cancer prevalence for specific organs and nutrient imbalances.[2] It has been estimated that the proportion of total cancers in the United States related specifically to diet or nutrition is 60 per cent for females and 40 per cent for males.[3] Table 8-1 and Figure 8-2 illustrate this estimation for various types of cancer.

This does not imply that cancer is caused by diet. The prevalence of cancer depends on a variety of factors — those related to the environment and those related to individual personal and genetic variables. Acting in concert, these various factors can lead to alterations in cellular metabolic processes and increased susceptibility to the development of tumors.

Nutrition can influence the development of cancer in a variety of ways. There are specific food carcinogens, either naturally occurring or added artificially. Examples of currently known carcinogens are mycotoxins; cycasin (a plant product) implicated in cancer of the liver; nitrates, nitrites, nitrosamides implicated in cancer of the stomach; nitrosamines implicated in other forms of cancer; and synthetic food additives and residues. With the exception of certain substances, such as aflatoxin, these

Table 8–1
Diet and Cancer Incidence (estimates)

	Incidence Related to Diet	
Site	*Male*	*Female*
Stomach	12,600	6,230
Colon and rectum	40,080	48,960
Liver	5,220	5,100
Kidney	5,520	4,560
Breast	—	79,200
Prostate	50,400	—
All sites	138,695	201,836
% of total incidence	40	60

Source: NCI, unpublished data, 1976.

food carcinogens are thought to play a relatively small role in total human cancer, but their exact effect on the etiology of cancer is currently largely unknown.[4]

Diet composition and nutrition may also affect the development of cancer by altering patterns of enzyme activity and other metabolic factors that influence the number of naturally occurring or induced tumors. It is the latter relationship between diet and cancer that is reviewed here.

Many hypotheses relate diet to various types of cancer. The typical dietary profile of populations living in communities with a low prevalence of cancer includes diets that contain less fat, protein, cholesterol, and sugar but more bulk-containing and bulk-forming foods than in cancer-prone communities. However, within the populations of "civilized" affluent and industrialized nations, there seem to be minimal dietary differences among individuals who have cancer and their healthy controls.[5] Cancer has also been related to certain vitamin and mineral imbalances. (See p. 296.)

EPIDEMIOLOGICAL STUDIES

At present, most of the data supporting the diet-cancer hypothesis are the result of epidemiological studies. Although an exhaustive review of such

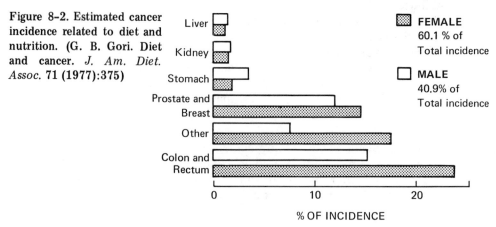

Figure 8-2. Estimated cancer incidence related to diet and nutrition. (G. B. Gori. Diet and cancer. *J. Am. Diet. Assoc.* 71 (1977):375)

FEMALE
60.1 % of
Total incidence

MALE
40.9% of
Total incidence

% OF INCIDENCE

research is beyond the scope of the chapter, a brief review of some of the reports is useful.

As early as the first written medical records, physicians and lay people alike suggested a link between diet and cancer.[6] This relationship has been a stimulus to vast scientific research as well as to the activities of food faddists who are intent upon influencing uncritical and unsuspecting victims. Of recent interest to clinicians has been the development of gastrointestinal lesions and colonic cancer.

Esophagus

E. Wynder and I. Bross investigated the possible dietary and environmental influences on cancer of the esophagus in New York City victims and reported that the incidence was associated with heavy smoking and alcoholic beverage intake and was inversely related to consumption of milk, eggs, and green and leafy vegetables. Other studies have also established associations between esophageal cancer and alcohol consumption.[7]

Stomach

Cancer of the stomach is four or more times as prevalent in Japan, Chile, Austria, Finland, and Iceland as in the United States.[8] Moreover, gastric cancer appears to be more prevalent among low-income groups. Suggestions about possible dietary factors are controversial. It has been postulated, for example, that gastric cancer is a function of use of laxatives, mineral oil, alcohol consumption, smoked food, low vitamin C intake, or other dietary contaminants.

Cancer of the stomach has also been negatively correlated with raw vegetable and milk intake. As an illustration, the consumption of milk and milk products in Japan increased more than 20 times from 1949 to 1971, whereas the incidence of gastric cancer decreased and continues to decrease.[9]

T. Hirayama reported that cancer patients tended to consume less milk and more highly salted foods than did healthy controls.[9] It has also been noted that Japanese-type pickled vegetables and dried salt fish products may be related to the high prevalence of stomach cancer in Japan.[10]

Diets that contain high starch and low fat levels, such as those consumed by economically poor Japanese or Colombians, may also be related to the incidence of stomach cancer and may be negatively related to colonic cancer.[11]

Colon and Breast

There are also striking differences in the prevalence of colon cancer among various populations. Cancer of the colon is usually prevalent among population groups where gastric cancer is rare and, conversely, is rare where gastric cancer is common. Thus, in the United States and in England, cancer of the colon is responsible for more deaths than any other type of cancer with the exception of lung cancer.

Global differences in fat consumption have been related to colonic cancer. For example, in nations such as New Zealand, the United States, England, Wales, Belgium, and Denmark, where high fat consumption is

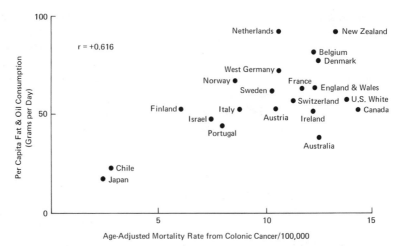

Figure 8–3. Bowel cancer mortality and dietary fat and oil consumption. (E. L. Wynder. The epidemiology of large bowel cancer. *Cancer Res.* 35 (1975):3388–3394)

typical, mortality rates for colonic cancer are significant. In contrast, in countries such as Japan and Chile, where fat intake tends to be low, colonic cancer is less prevalent.[12] Figure 8–3 illustrates the relationship between bowel cancer mortality, dietary fat, and oil consumption for selected countries. Similar relationships between fat consumption and female breast cancer have been reported.[13]

Mortality rates from cancer of the colon have also been highly correlated with meat consumption; however, the specific nutrient component in meat responsible for such a correlation is disputed. In countries such as the United States and Canada, where high meat consumption is typical, mortality from cancer of the colon is high in contrast to countries such as Japan and Chile, where consumption of meat, as well as mortality rates from cancer of the colon, are lower. Similarly, populations of Seventh-Day Adventists, who consume little meat demonstrate lower rates of mortality from colonic cancer than their non-Seventh-Day Adventist American counterparts.

R. L. Phillips reported the findings of a case-control investigation of colon and breast cancer among the SDA population. The relative risks for colon cancer were 2.8 for previous meat use. For current food use, the significant relative risks reported were:[14]

Beef, 2.3

Lamb, 2.7

Combination of highly saturated fat foods, 2.1

The author suggested that the lactoovovegetarian* diet may provide protection against colon cancer.

B. Drasar and D. Irving correlated the colonic cancer rates in 37 nations with a variety of variables indexing life-style of the population and the

*A lactoovovegetarian is a vegetarian who eats no animal flesh but does eat animal products such as milk, cheese, and eggs.

degree of economic development. Among the variables studied were per capita income, cars, radios, television sets, and dietary factors of average fat, animal protein, sugar, and high-fiber carbohydrate consumption. The most significant correlations noted were between colonic cancer and dietary factors; the correlation was significant for total fat intake and for animal protein; sugar and fiber variables were not significantly related to colonic cancer.[15]

In the same vein, G. A. Leveille who reviewed the relationship between diet and colonic cancer in Connecticut males, noted high positive correlations with intake of beef, other meat, poultry, and fish and negative correlations between cancer and intake of cereals and potatoes.[16]

Low intakes of dietary fiber have also been implicated in the etiology of colonic cancer on similar epidemiological grounds. For example, cancer of the colon in India has been reported to be less prevalent in northern Indians than in southern Indians; the prevalence differences have been explained by the fact that the northern Indians enjoy diets high in "roughage, cellulose and vegetable fibers," whereas the diets of the southern Indians are deficient in such fibers. When the researchers examined the feces they found abundant vegetable fibers in the stools of the northern Indians, and virtually no such fibers in the stools of the southern Indians.[17]

Lower fiber intake and higher beef consumption among cancer patients has also been noted. However, others have noted no dietary differences, with the exception of less fat consumption by patients with diverticulitis, as compared with patients with cancer and normal controls.[18]

Studies of the relationship between dietary factors and cancer prevalence among immigrant populations provide additional helpful information. The prevalence and the mortality rates for cancer among the migrants typically parallel the experiences of the host country rather than those of the native homeland. One of the classic illustrations of this concerns Japanese immigrants to the United States. Mortality rates in Japanese immigrants from cancer of the stomach, breast, and colon tended to shift toward those patterns of the United States in as early as the first generation. After the second generation, the rates were identical with those of the United States. Explanations for these patterns have centered around the vast dietary changes in calories and fat consumption as the immigrants adopt the American diet.[19]

Similar trends have been reported by investigators studying other migrant populations. Breast cancer in females and cancer of the large intestine in both sexes is far greater in the United States than in Poland. However, when the Polish immigrated to the United States, after a short period of time, the prevalence rates of cancer in the Polish immigrants were identical to those of native Americans. Similarly, there was a wide difference between the immigrants' prevalence rates and those of their counterparts in Poland.[20]

Despite the fact that epidemiological data do not prove a cause-and-effect relationship between dietary factors and cancer, they clearly raise significant questions and suggest that the average American diet, high in fat, refined carbohydrate, and calories but low in complex carbohydrates and fiber, may be related to the development of certain types of cancer.

The following sections consider other evidence pertaining to diet and cancer.

THE FIBER HYPOTHESIS

In 1920 J. H. Kellogg published a book entitled *The Itinerary of a Breakfast.* He began the preface by stating,

> Modern medical research has clearly incriminated the colon as the source of more disease and physical suffering than any other organ of the body. The artificial conditions of civilized life, sedentary habits, concentrated foodstuffs, false modesty, ignorance, and neglect of bodily need have produced a crippled state of the colon as an almost universal condition among civilized men and women.[21]

As a suggested remedy for the problem, Dr. Kellogg, then the medical director of the Battle Creek Sanatarium, suggested his "antitoxic diet," which consisted of fruits, cereals, and fresh vegetables. Especially favored were potatoes, dates, carrots, wheat bran, and old-fashioned Scotch oats and nuts.

Almost 60 years after his little volume appeared, there is an upsurge of interest in the helpful role of fiber in the human diet. Diets low in fiber have been related not only to certain types of cancer but also to ischemic heart disease, diabetes, diverticular disease, gastrointestinal disorders, and other diseases.

Definitions of Fiber

There is no general consensus about the definition and terminology for fiber.[22,23] In fact, there is considerable controversy and disagreement, as well as objection to the term *fiber*, a term that has been used to describe plant cell walls for over 200 years. Many have suggested that the term be retired.

Crude fiber (CF) has been defined as "the residue of plant food left after sequential extraction with solvent, dilute acid, and dilute alkali." This is the term usually used in reporting food fiber content in food composition tables.[22]

Dietary fiber (DF) has been defined "in terms of physiology as the remnants of plant cells resistant to hydrolysis by the alimentary enzymes of man."[24] More recently, dietary fiber has been redefined to include "undigested storage polysaccharides, present within the contents of the cell, as well as undigested polysaccharides and lignin present in the cell wall."[22]

D. M. Hegsted has suggested that the correct definition for the present should be stated in functional terms, that is, "Dietary fiber is the material in foods which decreases the transit time, increases the fecal volume, fecal water content, etc."[25] The controversy is evident. Until there is a generally accepted definition of dietary fiber, there is no clear direction as to what should be studied.

Determination of Fiber Content in Foods

There is also a lack of consensus about how to determine quantitatively the fiber in human foods. Early approaches were based on methods developed in the 1800s, in which the residue remaining after extraction with solvent, dilute acid, and alkali represented the indigestible material.

Cellulose, hemicellulose, lignin, and pectin are the major forms of fiber in which nutritionists and health researchers are interested.[26] There are various methods for determining these different types of fiber in foods, many of which are grossly inaccurate and not highly satisfactory. For example, the common method involves crude fiber determination by which 80 per cent of the hemicellulose, 50–90 per cent of the lignin, and 50 per cent of the cellulose is destroyed.[23] Thus, values for crude fiber exclude significant amounts of dietary fiber.

Estimating the fiber content in foods by determining the "difference" of roughage involves an estimation of roughage from the fat-free alcohol-insoluble residue remaining after subtraction of available carbohydrate and protein.[27] A number of other researchers have developed methods for determining various forms of fiber in foods.[28-30] The resulting values for various forms of fiber may differ dramatically, depending upon the method for determination. This is illustrated in Table 8-2. As can be seen, only 20–50 per cent of the total dietary fiber is crude fiber. Most of the crude fiber determined by various methods seems to come from fruits and vegetables rather than from cereals and legumes.[26]

Consumption of Fiber

Consumption of dietary fiber varies widely on a worldwide basis. As illustrated in Figure 8-4, peoples in the developing nations consume approximately 75 per cent of their daily energy intake as starchy foods that are either unrefined or minimally refined fiber-rich foods. They contain about 1.0–1.5 gm crude fiber per megajoule (240 kcal). In these developing nations, the mean adult fiber intake from starchy foods is 10–15 gm crude fiber daily.[22]

In contrast, populations in the Western "civilized" nations consume about 30 per cent of their daily dietary energy in the form of starchy foods. These starchy foods tend to be more refined and contain minimal

Figure 8-4. World consumption of dietary fiber in countries with various gross domestic product totals. UV: unsaturated vegetable fats; SV: saturated vegetable fats; UA: unsaturated animal fats; VP: vegetable protein; AP: animal protein. (Trowell, *Nutr. Rev.*, 35:6, 1977)

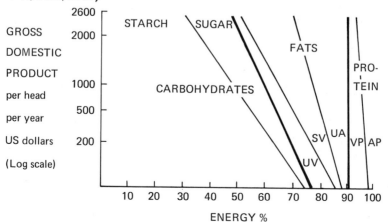

Table 8-2
Fiber Content of Food (g/100g)

Food	Southgate Method (23)				Van Soest Method (24)		Indigestible Residue
	Crude Fiber	Cellulose	Hemicellulose	Lignin	ADF[a]	Lignin	
Apple	1.0	0.47	0.66	0.18	0.99	0.18	
	0.66						1.15[b]
							1.7–2.4[c]
		0.67	0.52	0.40			
Banana	0.5						3.4[c]
		1.00	6.10	0.20			
Beans, brown	1.5						12.1[b]
cooked	2.2						5.1[c]
Cabbage	0.8						
		1.04	0.92	0.24	1.19	0.14	
	1.46						1.64[b]
							2.2–3.4[c]
		0.81	0.29	0.08			
Carrots	1.0						
	1.01						1.64[b]
							2.9–3.1[c]
Celery	1.0						
		0.91	0.65	0.16	0.91	0.16	
							1.8[c]
Rolled oats	1.2						
dry	1.5						6.9[b]
Peas	2.0						
	0.57						3.29[b]
							5.2[c]
		3.06	1.42	0.33			
Turnips	0.9						
		0.66	0.41	0.11	0.72	0.14	
	0.98						1.3[b]
							2.2–2.8[c]
Wheat bran	9.1						
		9.3	21.7	4.3	12.2	2.8	
	9.1						48.8[b]

[a] Acid Detergent Fiber.
[b] Enzymatic determination. Values have been calculated for wet weight, using figures for indigestible residue and % dry matter.
[c] Roughage "by difference", after subtraction of fat available carbohydrate and protein.
Source: (Kelsay, 1978, Am. J. Clin. Nutr.)

fiber. In these affluent nations, the average adult intake of starchy fiber is about 1.0–1.5 gm of crude fiber daily. Populations in both developing and developed nations consume differing amounts of fruit and vegetables and receive from 2–10 gm of crude fiber daily from them.

Let us look at this situation in a slightly different way. As can be seen from Figure 8-5, populations in developing nations receive more than 80 per cent of their dietary energy from fiber-containing foods; this compares with only 32 per cent of energy from fiber-containing foods for

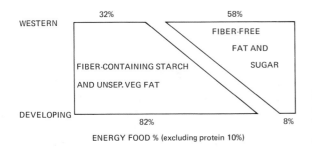

WESTERN

32%   58%

FIBER-FREE

FAT AND

FIBER-CONTAINING STARCH   SUGAR

AND UNSEP. VEG FAT

DEVELOPING

82%   8%

ENERGY FOOD % (excluding protein 10%)

Figure 8-5. Dietary fiber as percent of energy foods in developing and Western nations. (Trowell, *Nutr Rev.* 35:6, 1977)

inhabitants of developed nations. At the same time, in developing nations, approximately 8 per cent of fiber-free energy foods are consumed, whereas the comparable figure for developed nations is 58 per cent, chiefly in the form of oils and sugars.[22]

J. Scala reported a 20 per cent decline in the consumption of fiber from fruits and vegetables and a 50 per cent decline from cereals and grains in the U.S. population over the past century. It is difficult to suggest average levels of fiber intake in the population because of the difficulties in defining fiber and in determining the fiber content of various foods.[31] M. Hardinge et al. reported that nonvegetarians consumed approximately 8–12 gm crude fiber daily, or 16–60 gm of total fiber.[32] There is considerable question as to how typical these intakes are. Many individuals may consume minimal amounts of whole grain cereals, legumes, fruits, and vegetables, and, hence, their diets may be dramatically lower in fiber.

Actions of Fiber

Diets that are high in fiber content are associated with more rapid intestinal transit times and often with greater stool weights. In contrast, communities consuming low-residue diets, typified by modern foods of Western Europe and North America, have a slower intestinal transit time and stools that are firm, small, and lower in weight.[33–37]

The lack of dietary fiber has been related to two broad disease conditions according to the physiological functions of fiber.[38] These two functions are postulated to include:

1. *Fiber as a chelater* — the ability of various types of fiber to bind bile salts and sterols such as cholesterol is postulated to be responsible for the ability of fiber to reduce serum cholesterol. For instance, the increased binding and hence elimination of bile acids provides a mechanism by which hepatic cholesterol can be removed and serum cholesterol reduced. By binding bile acids, fiber may also reduce their bacterial conversion to secondary bile acids that are potential carcinogens. Fiber may also bind ingested toxins and promote their excretion in the feces. The adsorption-related diseases, which include stroke, thrombosis, and heart disease, are so named because they appear to be caused, in part, by the lack of fiber able to adsorb materials that reduce serum cholesterol.

2. *Water binding* — the water-binding capacity of fiber results in increased stool weight and decreased stool transit time — simply stated, it results in more frequent and softer stool elimination. Thus, it is postulated that intracolonic pressure is reduced and the predisposition to diver-

ticular disease and related disorders is minimized. Diseases related to water binding include diverticulitis, colonic cancer, and hemorrhoids. These diseases are influenced by the physical properties of the intestines.

The fiber-related functions in reducing cancer incidence among populations consuming high-fiber diets are suggested to result from increased stool velocity and volume. Cancer-causing agents can be more readily adsorbed to the fiber and hence can be eliminated more quickly. It has been suggested that dietary fiber results in an altered type of microflora in the gut that tends to be more aerobic and, hence, less likely to produce carcinogenic bile acid metabolites. Also being investigated are the satiety value of fiber and the time required for chewing the fiber that may thus help to reduce overall food intake.

Although a considerable body of experimental animal evidence suggests that fiber has a beneficial effect on cholesterol and bile acid metabolism, evidence from human studies is limited and sometimes conflicting. Critics note that a higher actual concentration of carcinogens in the stool with a refined diet has not been satisfactorily proven. A more rapid stool passage rate does not necessarily mean that at a given point the colon wall receives less exposure to carcinogens; the end result of frequent short exposures to carcinogens may be as great as that from fewer, longer exposures.

Recent studies have shown that the intestinal flora of individuals seems to be very stable and that no greatly significant changes are found to result from changes in the fiber content of the diet.[39]

Other studies have investigated the response of serum lipids to dietary bran, a form of fiber easily added to the diet.[40–41] None of the researchers found changes in serum lipid levels in response to the added bran. However, other experiments found that the addition of pectin or guar gum to the diet could lower serum cholesterol levels.[42]

Studies on the effect of fiber in increasing stool transit time are not definitive. Although some studies have demonstrated a positive relationship between transit time and fiber, other studies have demonstrated no effect, or even decreased transit time.[26] The variation in results may be due to different intakes of fiber, different health statuses of the subjects, different ages, different sexes, or other variables. Another possible explanation may lie in the fact that the studies did not allow sufficient time on the fiber-supplemented diet to produce measurable changes. Factors such as psychological disposition and emotions may also affect transit time.

J. L. Kelsay reviewed more than 50 studies in which varying amounts of fiber from different food sources were studied in human subjects. Some of the studies suffered from poor design and from lack of control over other variables. The results of different studies were difficult to generalize or to compare because of varying definitions of fiber and different methods of fiber determination. In view of these considerations, Kelsay suggested some tentative conclusions about the current state of knowledge concerning fiber in the diet of humans:[26]

1. The inclusion of fiber in the diet results in increased bulk of stools.

2. Stool transit times are not always influenced by dietary fiber.

3. Fecal bile acids are often increased as a result of increased dietary fiber.

4. More carefully controlled, well-designed studies are needed to provide objective information about the relationship between dietary fiber, diverticular disease, irritable bowel syndrome, blood glucose levels, and calcium and iron levels.

5. Serum cholesterol levels are often lowered by the addition of pectin to the diet, but are not highly sensitive to the addition of other fiber-containing foods.

6. Serum triglyceride levels appear to be minimally sensitive to dietary fiber.

7. Consumption of dietary fiber appears to be inversely related to consumption of dietary energy, fat, nitrogen, and mineral absorption. If diets contain protective levels of minerals and other nutrients, there may be no problem, but care must be taken in populations in which such nutrients are low.

Other Fiber-related Diseases

D. P. Burkitt suggested that over 33 "Western" diseases are common in "civilized" nations but are rare in developing countries. He theorized that diets low in fiber as well as in starch but high in calories, sucrose, fat, and animal protein are the "common cause of these characteristically Western diseases." Burkitt noted that these diseases are related to one another in different ways, including their order of emergence. This order, with increasing age in Western nations, is similar to that of their emergence with time after the impact of Western culture in developing nations. These diseases include:

Colonic

Constipation, appendicitis, diverticular disease, hemorrhoids, irritable colon, ulcerative colitis, cancer of colon and rectum, polyps. Also hiatus hernia.

Metabolic and Cardiovascular

Obesity, diabetes, ischemic heart disease, peripheral arterial disease of legs, angina, varicose veins, deep vein thrombosis, pulmonary embolism, gallstones, kidney stones, gout.

Endocrine, Auto-Immune, and Other Diseases

Thyrotoxicosis, myxedema, Hashimoto's thyroiditis, Addison's adrenal hypocorticalism, hypoglycemia, rheumatoid arthritis, multiple sclerosis, senile osteoporosis, osteitis deformans (Paget's), pernicious anemia, subacute combined degeneration. Also breast cancer in women.

Essential Hypertension and Strokes

Previously rare in a few areas such as east Africa, when salt intake was less than 3 grams per day and the diet was high fiber, very high starch.[36,37]

Conclusions about the Diet-Fiber Hypothesis

Evidence linking diet with these diseases is primarily based on epidemiological studies. There is clinical and pharmacological evidence that supports the importance of dietary fiber in diverticular disease. Researchers have found that supplementation of low-fiber diets with fiber in the form of whole-meal bread, bran, and the like often offers relief.[44]

A. Brodribb and D. Humphreys report that patients with diverticular disease tend to consume less fiber than do healthy controls.[45] Gastroenterologists frequently recommend high-fiber diets in the treatment of diverticulitis.

However, there is a lack of definitive scientific evidence relating dietary fiber to the etiology of most of these diseases. A. I. Mendeloff, for example, suggests that there is no evidence that such diseases are related to fiber as a causative factor.[46]

In discussing the validity of the fiber hypothesis, L. Galton narrates the following:

> An old tale — true — has it that Charles Darwin observed that only bumblebees with their long tongues could pollinate red clover effectively and that the prime enemies of bumblebees are field mice that devour both larvae and honeycombs. The better crops of clover near villages, Darwin remarked, had much to do with the control of mice by the village cats.
> But another scientist went further, suggesting that since red clover was the staple diet of British cattle and bully beef the staple of the British sailor, a relationship might be shown between British naval victories and keeping cats.[47]

His point is that associations are often made between very indirect events and that such hypothesized relationships may in reality be fallacious. The fiber hypothesis is based on relationships in time, region, and environmental conditions. But there are conflicting data, such as the observation that people with chronic constipation do not have a higher incidence of colon cancer than those without.[46] The hypothesis is not a fact, proved beyond doubt. But what the proponents of the hypothesis suggest is that a fiber-depleted diet may be one factor common to the etiology of cancer and other "civilized diseases." As such, the hypothesis deserves further attention and careful research.

FAT INTAKE AND CANCER

Dietary fat, both saturated and unsaturated, is the agent that is principally blamed for the high incidence of colorectal cancer.[48] The International Union Against Cancer Report on Colorectal Cancer, on the basis of correlational analysis, suggested that "meat and fat are of major importance . . . deficiency of dietary fiber has not been validated as a contributing factor" in the etiology of colonic cancer.[49]

As noted previously, many epidemiological studies have reported that the principal variations in prevalence of cancer of the colon, breast, and prostate are statistically correlated with variations in the dietary intakes of fat and fat-related variables. Animal studies appear to support the hypothesized relationship between cancer and high-fat diets. Both saturated and unsaturated fats have been shown to enhance tumor growth and to increase tumor incidence in rats.[50]

A number of studies have demonstrated that increasing the fat content of a diet to 20–27 per cent of total calories will result in increased incidence of cancer of the skin, breast, and liver. In addition, these cancers appear earlier in the animals that are fed such high-fat diets than in control groups of animals. High-fat diets have also been associated with increased incidence of colonic tumors in animals.[51,52]

The type of fat, as well as the amount, appears to influence tumor formation. A number of animal studies indicate that polyunsaturated fatty acids enhance the development of cancerous tumors more than do saturated fatty acids. Human studies indicate that individuals on cholesterol-lowering diets (i.e., diets high in polyunsaturated fatty acids) increase cancer incidence as compared with those on diets that are higher in saturated fat. But these data are, for the most part, an analysis of previous clinical trials.[53] Other studies have found no increased incidence of cancer with diets that were high in polyunsaturated fatty acids.[54]

Mechanisms to explain the role of dietary fat in tumor growth and development are not well developed. One theory suggests that fat enhances the formation of bile salts, thereby increasing carcinogenic substances and risk. Another suggestion is that fat promotes tumor formation by altering the rate of carcinogen transfer, or through an effect on forming tumor cells.[53] It has also been hypothesized that dietary fat provides breast cancer procarcinogens that may be contained in breast fluid and that influence hormones to serve as permissive agents in the transformation of cells into cancerous cells in the breast ducts.[4,53]

Another hypothesis is that polyunsaturated fatty acids have an inhibitory effect on the response of lymphocytes to antigens. This might result in suppressed immune system reaction to cancer and, thus, enhance the development of cancer.[55]

Cholesterol has also been implicated in the etiology of malignant tumor development. However, studies attempting to relate high cholesterol levels to the development of cancer report conflicting and inconsistent results.[53]

CALORIC INTAKE, BODY WEIGHT, AND CANCER

Chronic calorie restriction has been found to inhibit many types of tumor formations; the time of tumor appearance and the prevalence of tumors is reduced. Early studies on rats suggested that underfeeding, that is, restricting all dietary components, inhibited the development of spontaneous tumors, the degree of inhibition being influenced by the type of tumor, the level of dietary restrictions, and the presence or absence of other carcinogenic factors.[56] There are exceptions; for example, the induction of hepatic tumors may be enhanced by calorie restriction.[53]

More recent studies confirm these findings. For example, M. Ross and G. Bras, in a long-term study involving various diets differing in protein, carbohydrate, and total calories, reported that the final risk of tumor development was directly related to the level of calories. Further, the heavier-weight rats were more prone to tumor development than were the lighter-weight rats. Some specific tumors were found to be related to protein intake; for example, malignant lymphomas were greater among rats that were fed high-protein diets, whereas fibromas were more frequent in rats on low-protein intakes. Diets that were low in protein, carbohydrate, and total calories resulted in the lowest incidence of tumors, the greatest delay in the time of their appearance, the absence of malignant epithelial tumors, and the greatest life expectancy of the rats.[57]

A similar study reported that, under restricted conditions, the incidence of tumors was directly associated with the calorie level of the diet. Both restricted calorie and protein intakes resulted in reduced incidence of tumors, whereas the body weight of the rat, early in life, was related to the development of tumors in later life.[58]

In relating body weight to cancer, A. Tannenbaum summarized statistics derived from life insurance records. The statistics showed a positive correlation between the incidence of increasing cancer deaths with increasing weights. In a few studies an attempt was made to correlate cancer according to site.[56] Cancer of the intestinal tract, liver, gallbladder, and genitourinary tract were positively associated with weight to a greater degree than those in other sites. Body mass has also been related to cancer of the endometrium, breast, gallbladder, uterus, and colon.

One possible mechanism developed to explain the relationship between calorie intake and tumor formation suggests that mitotic cell activity is inhibited by restricted calories; the result may be reduced tissue growth. Restricted calorie intake may result in diminished hormonal activity, altered tissue response to hormones, diminished hormone production or altered hormonal interactions, all of which may play a role in altered cell growth and the development and risk of cancer.

PROTEIN

Animal research suggests that the protein/caloric ratio of the diet influences the risk of incurring a variety of spontaneous tumors. Caloric restriction and marginal protein deficiency resulted in an increased prevalence of tumors of the adrenal glands and the lymphoid organs but a decrease of tumors in the endocrine glands and endocrine-dependent organs (pituitary, thyroid, parathyroid, adrenal, pineal body, gonads, and pancreas). The degree of inhibition or enhancement depended on the severity of protein restriction.[57,58] Other studies found no relationship between protein intake and tumors of the skin, mammary tumors, and sarcoma.[56]

Some amino acid deficiencies may suppress tumor formation. For example, low intakes of the sulfur amino acid, cystine, inhibited the induction of leukemia in mice.[53]

B. Worthington noted that a sufficiently severe protein deficiency will inhibit the formation of circulating antibodies. This phenomenon has been observed in laboratory animals and in a large number of children suffering from protein/calorie malnutrition. Dietary regimens with inadequate protein have proved to be most detrimental to the immune response of the host.[59]

The part that immunity plays in cancer development is controversial at present. Cell-mediated immunity may be a defense against cancer. On the other hand, the formation of antibodies may protect the tumor from the body's immune activities and, hence, support tumor development.[59]

Dietary protein has also been theorized to be related to the development of cancer because of the increased production of ammonia.[60] Ammonia can destroy cells, alter nucleic acid synthesis, alter growth of transplantable tumors, discriminate against noncancerous cells more than cancerous cells in a culture, and increase viral infections. These actions are all related to the cancer process. Ammonia is released by cell metabolism and by digestive and microbial processes whenever protein is consumed. Because ammonia destroys cells, more cells must be formed to repair tissues. Thus, there are more cells at risk to undergo cancerous change. It has been shown that tumors produced in animals can be reduced by feeding amino acids that reduce tissue ammonia concentrations. The amount of ammonia released in metabolism and by intestinal microorganisms is increased when total protein intake is increased. The greater amount of protein taken in, the greater amount of ammonia in the bowel. Although ammonia has not been shown to convert normal cells to malignant cells, it has the ability to increase viral infections, and viruses have been shown to produce cancer in animals. Ammonia has also been shown to change the ribonucleic acid (RNA) of the cell. Figure 8-6 illustrates a hypothesized relationship between cancer and protein intake.[60]

Figure 8-6. Hypothesized relationship between dietary protein and cancer. (From W. J. Visick. Evidence supporting the hypothesis that ammonia increases cancer incipience. Unpublished paper. Ithaca, N.Y.: Cornell University, 1975)

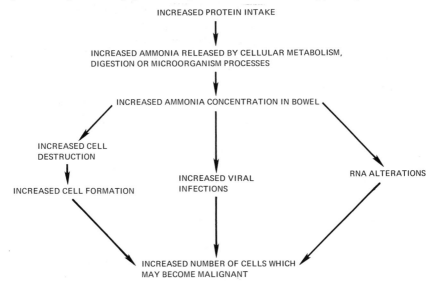

INCREASED PROTEIN INTAKE

INCREASED AMMONIA RELEASED BY CELLULAR METABOLISM, DIGESTION OR MICROORGANISM PROCESSES

INCREASED AMMONIA CONCENTRATION IN BOWEL

INCREASED CELL DESTRUCTION

INCREASED CELL FORMATION

INCREASED VIRAL INFECTIONS

RNA ALTERATIONS

INCREASED NUMBER OF CELLS WHICH MAY BECOME MALIGNANT

OTHER NUTRIENT IMBALANCES

Deficiencies of certain essential nutrients have also been implicated in the development of cancer. Iron deficiency has been related to cancer of the upper alimentary tract, which has been shown to be reduced by the addition of iron and vitamin supplements.[61] Similarly, alcoholism and a deficiency of riboflavin have been related to cancer of the upper gastrointestinal tract, vitamin A deficiency has been related to cancer of the cervix and stomach, and pyridoxine deficiency has been related to hepatic cancer.[4]

Whereas a deficiency of vitamin A has been associated with the development of tumors of the salivary gland, gastric mucosa, and colon in rats, high vitamin A intake has reportedly had a cancer-enhancing effect in some instances. Data on the relationship between vitamin A intake and tumor formation, however, are controversial, and the enhancing and inhibiting effects of high vitamin A levels have both been reported relative to tumors of the respiratory tract.[53,62]

Vitamin A administration has reportedly moderated the carcinogenic effects of certain polycyclic hydrocarbons. Retinoids, which are vitamin A analogs, seem to have an inhibitory effect on tumor development, but this finding is disputed by others.[51,52] It has been demonstrated, however, that the administration of vitamin A does inhibit stomach tumor growth in hamsters.[63]

Deficiencies of folic acid, vitamin B_{12}, and choline have been associated with tumor-enhancing effects in the liver, colon, and esophagus.[51,52] Vitamin B_{12} excess has also been found to enhance cancer development in rats that were fed diets deficient in methionine.[64]

The effect of vitamin C on cancer is controversial. E. Cameron and L. Pauling have suggested that high ascorbic acid intakes might offer protection against cancer, but this hypothesis remains to be substantiated.[65]

Excess amounts of certain minerals (arsenic, beryllium, chromium, radium, lead, nickel, and cadmium) have been implicated as cancer-causing.[56] These elements, however, are not usual dietary components. Evidence relating sodium, potassium, calcium, magnesium, and selenium to tumor development is also controversial. Iodine deficiency has been related to increased thyroid cancer, and magnesium deficiency has been related to thymoma.[53]

The mechanisms by which these dietary components influence the development and growth of tumors are still uncertain. W. S. Bullough has suggested that the inhibition of tumors by a dietary deficiency is related to a decrease in normal tissue mitotic activity.[66] When a deficiency results in tumor development, the converse may happen, with an increase in tissue mitosis resulting in the growth of cancerous cells.

SUGGESTED RESEARCH

The relationship between diet and cancer is by no means clear. The following directions for future research are indicated by the current state of knowledge:

1. An identification of the confusing epidemiological situation, which indicates, for example, a high prevalence of colonic cancer mortality rates in Scotland and a low prevalence in Finland. What are the factors that contribute to this differential?

2. A study of population groups evidencing a low prevalence of cancer, but living within pockets of high prevalence; for example, the Seventh-Day Adventists or the Mormons. What specific factors act to protect these groups from cancers that are so prevalent among their geographically close neighbors?

3. Investigations into possible hazardous effects that may result from a diet of high bulk-forming agents. For example, is mineral absorption impaired by a high-fiber diet? If so, what minerals are affected?

4. Elucidation of a plausible model explaining the relationship of diet and bowel habits (transit time, concentrations of fecal bile acids, stool size, and others) and the development of the so-called civilized diseases. This would require an investigation into the roles of diet, genetic predisposition, and modifying environmental factors in individuals who are prone or not prone to such disorders.

The challenge has been well stated by G. B. Gori:

> The task, then, is to define the mechanisms involved in dietary enhancement of disease and to develop a nutritional approach for health maintenance. If dietary imbalances are important in the multifactorial events of cancer development, we must determine the desirable dietary proportions of various nutrients. The definition of desirable dietary intake should not be aimed at generalized statistical levels, but must be formulated to be applicable to varying individual requirements, considering somatic, behavioral and environmental factors.[3]

It is important that diagnostic techniques and assessment methods of individual nutritional status be refined and sophisticated. In addition, other cancer-related factors that may be mediated by nutrition, such as toxins, hormones, and immune capacity, must be investigated, and their relationship to the human diet must be clarified.

DIET, NUTRITION, AND CANCER PROGRAM

The Diet, Nutrition, and Cancer Program of the National Cancer Institute was established to coordinate the efforts of cancer specialists to research priorities of nutrition and cancer. The primary objectives of this program include research into the prevention of nutrition-dependent cancer and the utilization of optimal nutritional support in the treatment of cancer. The expertise of specialists from universities, industry, private and government organizations, as well as federal agencies, such as the National Heart, Lung, and Blood Institute, the Food and Drug Administration, the U.S. Department of Agriculture, and the National Institutes of Health, are coordinated by the program. The recommendations for policy changes and education to prevent and treat cancer will come from the research sponsored by the program.

The research activities of the program are sponsored through contracts and grants directed toward achieving specific goals. These goals include the following:[3]

1. To assess the role of nutrition in the etiology and prevention of cancer — this knowledge will aid in formulating public health strategies aimed at disease prevention.

2. To define nutritional and dietary requirements as they are specifically related to individual and environmental factors. This will enable the prediction of individual diet consumption and the estimation of the role dietary imbalances play in cancer; it will also facilitate the formulation of food production and processing methods.

3. To define the nutrient value of foods. This information will aid in matching diet recommendations to individual dietary needs and will assist food processors and producers in identifying alternate food sources.

4. To develop methods to assess individual nutritional status. This knowledge and skill will aid in determining the nutritional needs of individual population groups, in recommending nutrition intervention methods, and in formulating national and international nutrition policy.

5. To study the use of diet and nutrition in cancer and other disease treatment and therapy. This knowledge will provide insight into the use of nutrition in cancer therapy. This line of research will investigate the possibility of changing taste perception in the cancer victim, in modifying food taste, in designing behavioral strategies in improving the nutritional status of the cancer patient, and in developing improved methods of artificial alimentation.

6. To develop educational programs aimed at the health professionals and the general public. The focus of these efforts will be on promoting sound and prudent dietary habits.

CONCLUSIONS — PREVENTIVE DIETARY RECOMMENDATIONS

Although the current state of knowledge does not allow conclusive specific dietary recommendations, evidence is sufficient to recommend general dietary prudence to the public. Further, recommendations cannot be applied to specific individuals because of the uncertainty of individual dietary requirements, environmental, and other factors that influence individual nutritional status.

But from the point of public benefit, current knowledge suggests that cancer prevention would be advanced if the American public made certain dietary changes including the consumption of fewer calories, especially calories from high-fat foods and empty calories. Further, disease prevention also suggests that food additives and contaminants should be limited.

The ideal approach to disease prevention involves a "partial return to the pattern of diet and manner of life of our ancestors and of developing populations."[67] This approach would involve an increased dietary intake of unrefined foods, with a concomitant reduction in refined carbohydrate products, calories, and animal products. An increase in physical activity, a reduction in social stress, and a slower-paced life-style are suggested to have both desirable nutritional and health consequences.

There is no general consensus about the optimum consumption of fiber. It is probably preferable to consume the fiber in the form found in a variety of fresh fruits and vegetables. M. Painter et al. have recommended a supplement of 2 teaspoons of bran taken three times daily, an added 16 gm of bran a day.[68] Others have suggested that, for satisfactory laxation, fiber in the range of 90–100 mg/kg of body weight daily is preferable.[69,70] For a 70-kg individual, this would amount to an intake of 6.3–7.0 gm of crude fiber, or 13–35 gm of total fiber daily.[26] Still another recommendation is an intake of an additional 1 oz of bran daily (about 40 mg of crude fiber) per kilogram of body weight.[71]

A number of nutrition researchers advocate the "prudent diet" not only for the prevention of coronary heart disease but also for certain types of cancer and other so-called "civilized diseases."[72]

Not all agree that this is a realistic or even a possible approach. It is very difficult to convince people to reduce their consumption of fat, protein food, animal foods, or any given and highly desired food to avoid cancer. Coronary heart disease is responsible for ten times the number of deaths as cancer, and numerous expert groups suggest a reduction in dietary fat as a possible preventive measure. Many studies aimed at the prevention of coronary heart disease that involved a reduction in fat intake revealed promising results. But we are unable to get people to significantly reduce their fat intake. The North American public still prefers a diet high in animal foods and hence high in saturated and total fat. A significant dietary change to reduce the risk of cancer is probably also unlikely.

D. P. Burkitt summarized the rationale behind suggesting that a preventive approach to dietary counseling be taken:

> The most reasonable approach would be to see what important cause is most easily removable. . . . If an invading army has to cross a multi-span bridge, only one span need be blown up to impede progress. If the spans vary in strength, the weakest is naturally chosen for destruction. The same approach should be adopted with regard to disease prevention. . . . Genetic factors, which probably always play a role, are currently unassailable. A reduction in dietary fat which, on the whole has been unsuccessfully recommended for reducing heart disease, is hard to achieve. We cannot be expected to change our manner of life radically, or even our eating habits. But it is the easiest thing in the world to increase our fiber intake to destroy the bridge span representing fiber deficiency.[36]

This is illustrated in Figure 8-7.

Perhaps the wisest recommendation is first to focus educational efforts on dietary modifications that are likely to be accepted and adopted, such as increasing dietary fiber. It is relatively easy to increase dietary fiber, and this change does not need to involve drastic changes in dietary habits. Positive health results from this will provide the impetus for the acceptance of more difficult dietary changes, such as reducing fat intake or reducing cholesterol consumption and calories.

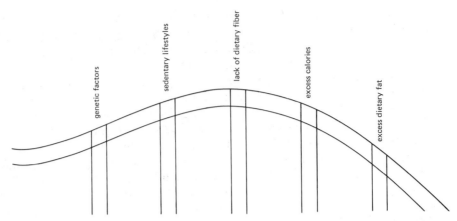

Figure 8-7. Multispan "life bridge" represents the spans that need to be modified to promote health. (adapted from D. P. Burkitt. Economic development not all bonus. *Nutr. Today* 11:6, 1976

REFERENCES

1. Special subject: Cancer of the oesophagus, stomach, intestine, and rectum: International mortality patterns and trends. *World Health Stat. Rep.* 28 (1975): 473.
2. Tannenbaum, A. Nutrition and cancer, in F. Homburger, ed., *Physiopathology of Cancer*, 2d ed. New York: Hoeber-Harper, 1959, pp. 517–562.
3. Gori, G. B. Diet and cancer. *J. Am. Diet. Assoc.* 71 (1977): 375.
4. Wynder, E. L. The dietary environment and cancer. *J. Am. Diet. Assoc.* 71 (1977): 385.
5. Hegsted, D. M. Summary of the conference on nutrition in the causation of cancer. *Cancer Res.* 35 (1975): 3541.
6. Hoffman, F. L. *Cancer and Diet*. Baltimore, Md.: Williams and Wilkins, 1937.
7. Wynder, E. L., and I. J. Bross. A study of etiological factors in cancer of the esophagus. *Cancer* 14 (1961): 389–413.
8. Correa, P., and W. Haenszel. Comparative international incidence and prevention, in S. G. Stewart, ed., *Cancer Epidemiology and Prevention*. Springfield, Ill.: Charles C Thomas, 1975.
9. Hirayama, T. Epidemiology of cancer of the stomach with special reference to its recent decrease in Japan. *Cancer Res.* 35 (1975): 3460.
10. Haenszel, W., M. Kurihara, M. Segi, and R. K. C. Lee. Stomach cancer among Japanese in Hawaii. *J. Nat'l Cancer Inst.* 49 (1972): 969–988.
11. Haenszel, W., and P. Correa. Developments in the epidemiology of stomach cancer over the past decade. *Cancer Res.* 35 (1975): 3452.
12. Wynder, E. L. The epidemiology of large bowel cancer. *Cancer Res.* 35 (1975): 3388–3394.
13. Carroll, K. K., and H. T. Khot. Dietary fat in relation to tumorigenesis, in *Progress in Biochemical Pharmacology*. Vol. 10. *Lipids and Tumors*. White Plains, N.Y.: S. Karger, 1979.
14. Phillips, R. L. Role of life-style and dietary habits in risk of cancer among Seventh-Day Adventists. *Cancer Res.* 35 (1975): 3513.

15. Drasar, B. S., and D. Irving. Environmental factors and cancer of the colon and breast. *Brit. J. Cancer* 27 (1973): 167.
16. Leveille, G. A. Issues in human nutrition and their probable impact on foods of animal origin. *J. Animal Sci.* 41 (1975): 723.
17. Malhotra, S. L. Geographical distribution of gastrointestinal cancers in India with special reference to causation. *Gut* 8 (1967): 361.
18. Floch, M. H. Discussion, in R. W. Reilly and J. B. Kirsner, eds., *Fiber Deficiency and Colonic Disorders.* New York: Plenum Press, 1975, pp. 23, 156.
19. Howell, M. A. Diet as an etiological factor in the development of cancers of the colon and rectum. *J. Chronic Dis.* 28 (1975): 67.
20. Staszewski, J., and W. Haenszel. Cancer mortality among the Polish-born in the United States. *J. Nat'l Cancer Inst.* 35 (1965): 291.
21. Kellogg, J. H. *The Itinerary of a Breakfast.* New York; Funk and Wagnalls, 1920.
22. Trowell, H. Food and dietary fibre. *Nutr. Rev.* 35 (1977): 6.
23. Van Soest, P. J., and R. W. McQueen. The chemistry and estimation of fibre. *Proc. Nutr. Soc.* 32 (1973): 123. See also Van Soest, P. J., Dietary fibres: Their definition and nutritional properties. *Am. J. Clin. Nutr.* 31 (1978): 512.
24. Trowell, H. Definitions of fibre. *Lancet* 1 (1974): 503.
25. Hegsted, D. M. Food and fibre: Evidence from experimental animals. *Nutr. Rev.* 35 (1977): 45.
26. Kelsay, J. L. A review of research on effects of fiber intake on man. *Am. J. Clin. Nutr.* 31 (1978): 142.
27. McCance, R. A., E. M. Widdowson, and L. R. Shackleton. *The Nutritive Value of Fruits, Vegetables, and Nuts.* London: Medical Research Council Special Rept. No. 213, 1936.
28. Southgate, D. A. T. Dietary fiber: Analysis and food sources. *Am. J. Clin. Nutr.* 31 (1978): 5107.
29. Goering, H. K., and P. J. Van Soest. Forage fiber analyses. *Agriculture Handbook No. 379.* Washington, D.C.: Government Printing Office, 1970.
30. Hellendoorn, E. W., M. G. Noordhoff, and J. Slagman. Enzymatic determination of the indigestible residue (dietary fibre) content of human food. *J. Sci. Food Agri.* 26 (1975): 1461.
31. Scala, J. Fiber: The forgotten nutrient. *Food Technol.* 28 (1974): 34.
32. Hardinge, M. G., A. C. Chambers, H. Crooks, and F. J. Stare. Nutritional studies of vegetarians. III. Dietary levels of fiber. *Am. J. Clin. Nutr.* 6 (1958): 523.
33. Burkitt, D. P. Epidemiology of cancer of the colon and rectum. *Cancer* 28 (1971): 3.
34. Burkitt, D. P. Epidemiology of large bowel disease: The role of fibre. *Proc. Nutr. Soc.* 32 (1973): 145.
35. Burkitt, D. P. Some neglected leads to cancer causation. *J. Nat'l Cancer Inst.* 47 (1971): 913.
36. Burkitt, D. P. Economic development not all bonus. *Nutr. Today* 11 (1976): 6.
37. Burkitt, D. P., and H. Trowell. *Refined Carbohydrate Foods and Disease.* London: Academic Press, 1975.
38. Scala, J. Fiber and food technology, in *The Role of Fiber in the Diet.* Tenth Annual Symposium, Western New York Section of the Institute of Food Technologists. Ithaca, N.Y.: Cornell University, March 1976, pp. 3-4.
39. Finegold, S. M., and V. L. Suther. Fecal flows in different populations, with special reference to diet. *Am. J. Clin. Nutr.* 31 (1978): 5116.

40. Kritchevsky, D. Fiber, lipids, and atherosclerosis. *Am. J. Clin. Nutr.* 31 (1978): 565.
41. Durrington, P. A., A. C. Wicks, and K. W. Heaton. Effect of bran on blood lipids. *Lancet* 2 (1975): 133.
42. Jenkins, D. J., C. Newton, A. R. Leeds, and J. H. Cummings. Effect of pectin, guar gum, and wheat fibre on serum cholesterol. *Lancet* 1 (1975): 1116.
43. Burkitt, D. P. Colonic-rectal cancer: Fiber and other dietary factors. *Am. J. Clin. Nutr.* 31 (1978): 558.
44. Painter, N. S. *Diverticular Disease of the Colon: A Deficiency Disease of Western Civilization.* London: Heinemann Medical Books, 1975.
45. Brodribb, A. J. M., and D. M. Humphreys. Diverticular disease: Three studies. *Brit. Med. J.* 1 (1976): 424.
46. Mendeloff, A. L. Dietary fiber, in The Nutrition Foundation, *Present Knowledge in Nutrition.* Washington, D.C., 1976.
47. Galton, L. Fiber in your food: Assessment and guidelines, in L. Hofmann, ed., *The Great American Nutrition Hassle.* Palo Alto, Calif.: Mayfield Publishing Co., 1978, pp. 274–280.
48. Medical News. Fat and forty is no joke for colorectal cancer victims. *J.A.M.A.* 238 (1977): 843.
49. *Colorectal Cancer,* Geneva: IUCC Technical Report Series, Vol. 19, No. 2, 1975.
50. Carroll, K. K., and H. T. Kohr. Effects of dietary fat and dose level of 7, 12-dimethylbenz (α) anthracene on mammary tumor incidence in rats. *Cancer Res.* 30 (1970): 2260.
51. Rogers, A. E., and P. M. Newberne. Dietary effects in chemical carcinogenesis in animal models for colon and liver tumors, in *Nutrition in the Causation of Cancer.* Key Biscayne, Fla., May 1975.
52. Rogers, A. E., and P. M. Newberne. Dietary effects in chemical carcinogenesis in animal models for colon and liver tumors. *Cancer Res.* 35 (1975): 3427.
53. Alcantara, E. M., and E. W. Speckmann. Diet, nutrition, and cancer. *Am. J. Clin. Nutr.* 29 (1976): 1035.
54. Ederer, F., P. Leren, O. Turpeinen, and I. D. Frantz. Cancer among men on cholesterol-lowering diets. *Lancet* 2 (1971): 203.
55. Mertin, J. Polyunsaturated fatty acids and cancer. *Brit. Med. J.* 4 (1973): 357.
56. Tannenbaum, A. Nutrition and cancer, in F. Homberger, ed., *Physiopathology of Cancer,* 2d ed. New York: Hoeber-Harper, 1959, pp. 517–562.
57. Ross, M. H., and G. Bras. Tumor incidence patterns and nutrition in the rat. *J. Nutr.* 87 (1965): 245–260.
58. Ross, M. H., G. Bras, and M. W. Ragbeer. Influence of protein and caloric intake upon spontaneous tumor incidence of the anterior pituitary gland of the rat. *J. Nutr.* 100 (1970): 177–189.
59. Worthington, B. Effect of nutritional status on immune phenomena. *J. Am. Diet. Assoc.* 65 (1974): 123.
60. Visick, W. J. Evidence supporting the hypothesis that ammonia increases cancer incidence. Unpublished paper. Ithaca, N.Y.: Cornell University, 1975.
61. Larsson, L. B., A. Sandström, and P. Westling. Relationship of Plummer Vinson disease to cancer of the upper alimentary tract in Sweden. *Cancer Res.* 35 (1975): 3308.

62. Smith, D. M., A. E. Rogers, B. J. Herndon, and O. M. Newberne. Vitamin A (retinyl acetate) and benzo (α) pyrene-induced respiratory tract carcinogenesis in hamsters fed a commercial diet. *Cancer Res.* 35 (1975): 11.

63. Chu, E. W., and R. A. Malmgren. An inhibitory effect of vitamin A on the induction of tumors of forestomach and cervix in the Syrian hamster by carcinogenic polycyclic hydrocarbons. *Cancer Res.* 25 (1965): 884.

64. Poirer, L. A., and R. K. Boutwell. Current problems in nutrition and cancer. *Fed. Proc.* 35 (1976): 1307.

65. Cameron, E., and L. Pauling. Ascorbic acid and the glycosaminoglycans: An orthomolecular approach to cancer and other diseases. *Oncology* 27 (1973): 181.

66. Bullough, W. S. Mitotic activity and carcinogenesis. *Brit. J. Cancer* 4 (1950): 329–336.

67. Walker, A. R. P. Colon cancer and diet, with special reference to intakes of fat and fiber. *Am. J. Clin. Nutr.* 29 (1976): 1417.

68. Painter, N. S., A. Z. Almeida, and K. W. Colebourne. Unprocessed bran in treatment of diverticular disease of the colon. *Brit. Med. J.* 2 (1972): 137.

69. Cowgill, G. R., and W. E. Anderson. Laxative effects of wheat bran and "washed bran" in healthy men: A comparative study. *J.A.M.A.* 98 (1932): 1866.

70. Cowgill, G. R., and A. J. Sullivan. Further studies on the use of wheat bran as a laxative: Observations on patients. *J.A.M.A.* 100 (1933): 795.

71. Hoppert, C. A., and A. J. Clark. Digestibility and effect on laxation of crude fiber and cellulose in certain common foods. *J.A.M.A.* 21 (1945): 157.

72. Reddy, B. S., and E. L. Wynder. Large bowel carcinogenesis: Fecal constituents of populations with diverse incidence rates of colon cancer. *J. Nat'l Cancer Inst.* 50 (1973): 1437.

9
Obesity

Reader Objectives

After completing this chapter, the reader should be able to
1. Distinguish between obesity and overweight; describe ways to detect each.
2. List six hazards associated with obesity.
3. Outline three theories regarding the etiology of obesity.
4. Describe a general approach to the prevention of obesity.
5. List six techniques used to treat obesity; describe the advantages and disadvantages of each.
6. Outline techniques of behavior modification in the treatment of obesity.

Instead of the gong for dinner, let us hear a whistle from the Spartan fife.
— Ralph Waldo Emerson

OBESITY — DEFINITIONS AND ASSESSMENT

Obesity is generally regarded as one of the most common and serious nutritional problems confronting North Americans. Obesity has been defined as an excessive accumulation of adipose (fat) tissue in the body. It differs from "overweight," defined as "overheavy," which indicates a weight greater than that assumed to be desirable, without reference to body composition, and may or may not involve an excessive amount of body fat. Because the body is made up of different types of tissues, such as muscle, fat, organs, fluid, and bones, and because each contributes weight to the total body, an athlete, for example, may be overweight but not obese. An individual who is obese is usually overweight, but not all overweight individuals are obese. (See Figure 9–1.)

The notion of what the "ideal weight" is has greatly changed in recent years. Even today there is no universal agreement as to what is a "normal" or an "ideal" weight. Methods for estimating overweight usually involve the use of height and weight tables for adults. Early height-weight tables were based on the heights and weights of male and female life insurance policyholders aged 15 to 59 years old. These tables reflect average weight for height, as well as the ages of those individuals measured. Thus, as averages, they reflect the usual increase in weight with increasing age and should not be used as a standard for desirable weights.

More recently, revised height-weight tables give desirable weight ranges for males and females aged 25 and over, according to body frame (small, medium, or large). However, it is often difficult to determine whether an individual's frame is small, medium, or large. Appendix 1, Table I–J presents height-weight standards for adults.

Growth charts are often used to assess weights of infants and children. (See Appendix I, Table I–K) Growth charts are based on measurements

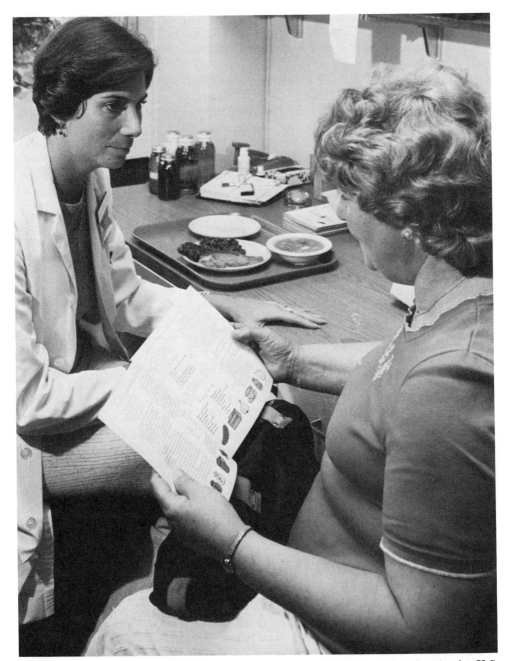

Figure 9-1. Obesity is one of the most prevalent nutrition-related disorders in the U.S. Between 25 and 45 per cent of Americans have been classified as obese. (American Dietetic Association/Doyle Pharmaceutical Company)

of large numbers of healthy infants and children; percentiles show the percentage of the surveyed population that falls below them in terms of height and weight.

The use of height-weight tables or growth charts does not necessarily identify obesity. A simple way to estimate obesity is a mere inspection of the nude body in front of a mirror. The "pinch test," in which a fold of skin and its underlying fat are lifted from the side of the lower chest or the back of the arm and pinched, can also help to estimate (in a very rough way) obesity. If the fold is more than an inch thick, the individual is probably obese.

A more sophisticated variation of the pinch test involves measuring skinfold thickness with a device called a caliper, which allows for the measurement of skinfold thickness. The most frequently measured sites are at the triceps muscle (back of the upper arm, midway between the shoulder bone and the elbow) and the subscapular region (just below the shoulder blade). See Figure 9-2. Standards or norms are available to suggest which minimum skinfold thickness measurements indicate obesity. (See Appendix I, Table L.)

The only direct way to measure total body fat is to measure the fat content of the cadaver. About fourteen per cent of the male body is fat, while a slightly higher percentage, about 22 per cent of the female body is fat. Thus, values greater than 25 per cent of body weight for males and thirty per cent for females are considered to indicate obesity.[1]

Other methods are used to identify the nonfat components of the body and then to estimate body fat content. These methods include sophisticated techniques, such as measuring body density, total body water, or whole body potassium. These methods are more precise than skinfold measurements, but are rarely available in a clinical setting. Thus, skinfold thickness or the overweight percentages relative to standards are the methods commonly used to assess overweight and obesity.

Figure 9-3 presents statistics on the prevalence of obesity in the United States. Depending upon the criteria for determining obesity, the percentage of the United States, adult population considered to be obese ranges from 25 to 45 per cent.[2]

Obesity includes such a diverse set of conditions that it is more correct to refer to the "obesities" rather than to obesity per se. For example, obesity may be differentiated according to the age of onset. Juvenile onset obesity, which usually develops before the child is ten years old, is generally very severe, is extremely difficult to treat, and has a poor response to therapy. It occurs twice as frequently in girls as in boys. On the other hand, adult onset obesity develops with increased age and is characterized by a constant level of food intake and a slowly declining energy expenditure in both activity and metabolism.

Distinctions can also be made according to the mechanism behind the development of obesity. Regulatory obesity usually refers to a psycho-

Figure 9-2. Skinfold calipers. (Reproduced with permission of *Nutrition Today* magazine, 703 Giddings Avenue, Annapolis, Maryland 21404 © March/April 1975)

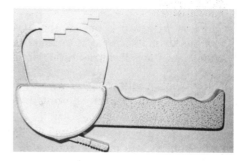

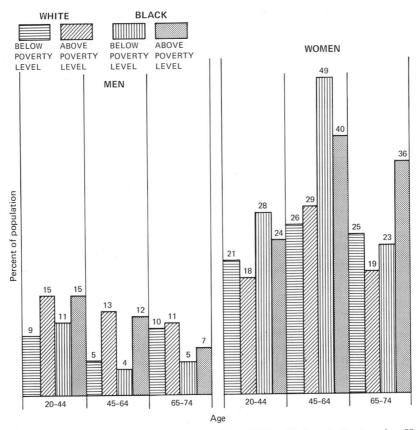

Figure 9-3. Adults classified as obese, 1971-1974. (National Center for Health Statistics)

logical or physiological defect in the regulation of food intake, relative to energy expenditure. There is no metabolic defect involved. Metabolic obesity refers to an underlying metabolic defect that may be enzymatic, hormonal, or neurologic. Constitutional obesity is caused by an increased number of fat cells (hyperplasia) in contrast to an increased size of fat cells (hypertrophy).

CHILDHOOD OBESITY

Childhood obesity is a special health concern in the United States. Children now are larger and taller than they were 20–30 years ago and also have a lower age of puberty. It is hard to precisely quantify the extent of childhood obesity. In Western Europe it is thought that 2–6 per cent of school children are obese. The figures are higher in the United States where 15 per cent prevalence rates of obesity have been reported in 6- to 16-year-old children. These statistics are higher only in Dortmund, Germany, where 23 per cent of the boys and 27 per cent of the girls were considered obese as measured by subcutaneous fat.[3]

The Ten-State Nutrition Survey, applying an arbitrary triceps skinfold measure to diagnose obesity, identified considerable prevalences of obesity among children and adolescents. For example, among children aged 12 and 13 years, 17 per cent of white males, 9 per cent of black males, 12 per cent of white females, and 11 per cent of black females were obese. Children in older age groups evidenced even higher percentages of obesity.[4]

EFFECT OF CHILDHOOD WEIGHT ON ADULT WEIGHT

The two factors that are most significant in predicting adult obesity appear to be childhood obesity and parental weights.[5] A number of studies confirm that overweight infants tend to become overweight children, adolescents, and adults.[6-8]

S. J. Fomon has suggested that "there can be little question that the obese child has a high likelihood of becoming an obese adult."[5] For example, S. Abraham et al. noted that 86 per cent of the overweight males and 80 per cent of the overweight females became overweight adults. In contrast, only 42 per cent of the average-weight males and 18 per cent of the average-weight females were overweight as adults.[8] A. Stunkard and V. Burt have suggested that the odds against an overweight adolescent being of normal or average adult weight were 28 to 1.[9] I. Rimm and A. Rimm estimated that about 24 times more obese women than normal weight women were obese as children.[7] Fisch et al. studied 300 babies at birth, at 4, and at 7 years to determine the relationship among weights at different ages. They found that the obese babies and 3-year-olds had a significantly higher than average birth weight. Mothers of the obese children tended to be obese before pregnancy and gained more weight during the pregnancy than did mothers of the slender children. Beyond these relationships, however, parental characteristics seemed to bear little association to the child's weight in later life.[10]

The results of other studies, however, disagree with these findings.[11,12] E. Poskitt, in a study of 203 children, found that the majority of the overweight infants did not become overweight children, but, rather, reached the average weight for their age and size and then maintained that weight.[11] S. J. Fomon reviewed a variety of studies indicating a relationship between infant weight patterns and childhood obesity. Several studies present difficulties in interpretation or design.[5] T. Mellbin and J. Vuille suggested, on the basis of limited studies of satisfactory design, that "only 10–20 per cent of the variation in weight for height (at age 7 years) can be explained by factors whose effect was detectable in infancy."[13]

HAZARDS ASSOCIATED WITH OBESITY

Many hazards are associated with obesity. The additional weight may add mechanical stress to the body frame and to the circulatory system, and, hence, strain the physiological system and ultimately place the individual at a higher risk of poor health. In addition, the excess food intake may increase the risk of consumption of either noxious or harmful substances, such as an excess of fat or cholesterol. Further, the obese or overweight individual is often inactive, and this in turn may aggravate existing health problems, such as heart disease.

Obesity is associated with an increased risk of cardiovascular-renal disease, osteoarthritis, hypertension, atherosclerosis, hernia, gallbladder disease, liver disorders, diabetes, appendicitis, and biliary calculi. It may also cause postural derangement or, in severe instances, may be the cause of pulmonary insufficiency. Obesity increases the hazards of surgery. Medio-actuarial statistics indicate that the life span of the obese individual is reduced; the principal causes of death among the obese are cardiovascular-renal disorders, diabetes, and liver or gallbladder disease.[14] The effects of obesity on existing diseases are also significant. Figure 9-4 illustrates the effects of obesity on susceptibility to selected diseases.

Gain in body weight is often accompanied by changes in serum lipids, blood pressure, uric acid, and carbohydrate tolerance. Conversely, reduction of the obesity is often accompanied by lowered blood pressure, improved glucose tolerance, and a decrease in the concentration of serum lipids. Data from the Framingham study suggest that each 10 per cent in weight reduction in males aged 33 to 35 years old would result in a 20 per cent reduction in the incidence of coronary heart disease. On the other hand, each 10 per cent increase in weight would result in a 30 per cent increase in the incidence of coronary heart disease. B. Winikoff suggested that, if a 20 per cent reduction in the prevalence of obesity occurred in the United States population, and if this resulted in a 20 per cent decrease in overall mortality, about 170,000 lives would be saved per year.[15]

Obesity among children and adolescents is often associated with particularly devastating effects. Some of the most commonly reported include

Figure 9-4. Effects of obesity on susceptibility to various diseases. Shaded bars represent increased susceptibility in overweight individuals. (From H. H. Marks. Influence of obesity on morbidity and mortality. *Bull. N.Y. Acad. Med.* **36** (1960):296–312)

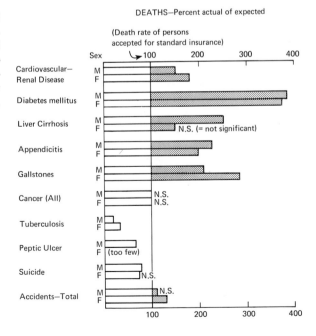

the increased risk of such physical and psychological problems as depressed growth hormone release, increased insulin release, intolerance to carbohydrates, and elevated blood pressure. Increased coronary risk factors, such as elevated blood lipid levels, have also been reported, suggesting that obesity per se may contribute an independent risk factor for CHD among children and adolescents. Females who were obese during their adolescent years are also more likely than those of normal weight to develop cancer of the uterus.[16]

The psychological and emotional burden suffered by the obese is frequently a heavy one. The young are especially subject to peer criticism, lack of acceptance, and other social/psychological problems that result in long-lasting social adjustment problems. Disturbed body images, poor self-concepts, and personality disturbances often result from social and psychological difficulties that are experienced by the obese.[16]

ETIOLOGY

The origins of obesity can be traced to a variety of factors including early overfeeding, reduced physical activity, and psychological and social factors. In the United States, social forces may be the most significant contributors to obesity. Obesity may also result from genetic, hypothalamic, central nervous system, or endocrine disorders.

A number of theories have been proposed to explain the etiology of obesity[17-20]. The reader is referred to J. Mayer[19] for a more detailed discussion of some of the theories on the etiology of obesity. This section focuses on theories of obesity as they particularly relate to the diet and the prevention of obesity.

The traditional theory of obesity suggests that if caloric input is greater than caloric output, body weight is gained. The basic cause of obesity results from a positive energy balance — consumption or metabolism of more calories than are used in body activities.

Most people agree that the etiology of obesity involves both genetic and environmental factors.[18-20] Some of the most important environmental components involve the way food is presented as being desirable, magic, status giving, fun, good tasting, and the like. As J. Stamler noted: "We have a culture that is calorie rich, and a culture that [includes] T.V. and automobile, so we have lifestyles that combine caloric excess relatively with sedentary living, leading to the frequency of obesity in childhood in our society today".[18] This is especially the case where other factors such as genetics, culture, or responses to stress predispose an individual to being overweight.[19]

Some investigators suggest that a particular type of diet plays a key role in the etiology of obesity. J. Gates et al., for instance, noted that those classified as obese tended to select more servings of food and more foods of the high-energy, low-nutrient type than did individuals of average weight.[21] However, other data on the relationship between body fat, diet, and physical activity reveal little correlation between caloric intake and the degree of body fatness. In addition, no correlation was found between degree of body fatness and eating frequency or consumption of half of total daily calories at one meal.[19]

In contrast to the traditional caloric theory, the QQF theory suggests that obesity is a function of the quality (Q) and the quantity (Q) of the diet as well as the frequency (F) of eating. Akin to this notion is the idea that the size and number or frequency of meals affects lipid metabolism. Small meals are thought to be associated with greater weight loss and reduced cholesterol levels in obese patients. Equicaloric intake in one or two large meals is associated with elevated cholesterol levels, impaired glucose tolerance, increased lipogenesis, and a greater tendency to obesity.[22] This QQF hypothesis is, at present, nothing more than that — a hypothesis. Some studies have confirmed the data, whereas others have produced data that dispute the theory.

Based on data from the Ten-State Survey, S. Garn and D. Clark[20] suggested that some fatness trends were a part of normal development. However, other trends to fatness occur in particular socioeconomic groups. In many cases, obesity occurs along family lines. Although this may support the notion that obesity is of genetic origins, family-line fatness similarities may also be a reflection of culture, attitudes, and practices of eating, as well as of exercise. These practices and attitudes are learned within the home and are reinforced there.

Knowledge of parent weight trends are considered to be more useful in predicting that a child will later become overweight than are the child's infant and childhood growth patterns.[5] R. Huenemann studied 488 infants 6 months of age to determine the environmental factors associated with obesity. Factors that were noted to be associated with obesity included more rapid weight gain after birth, lower birth weight, primary birth order, questionably high-caloric intake, obesity of the mother, little nutrition knowledge of the mother, and an unconventional life-style.[23] Other factors related to overweight in infants include overly zealous feeding, early introduction of high-energy foods, and permissive parental and pediatrician attitudes to excess infant weight gain.[24,25]

M. Borjeson studied 40 monozygotic and 61 dizygotic twins of preschool age and reported that genetic disposition was of greater importance than either environment or early nutrition for the onset of obesity before puberty. Preschool environment and nutrition acted mainly in modifying existing obesity in school-aged children.[26] A similar study by S. Garn et al. also indicated similar fatness progressions between both biological and adoptive children and their parents. It appears that levels of fatness are to a significant extent familial.[27]

Only a few conclusions can be stated with assurance, relative to childhood obesity. Behavioral and social factors predominate in the etiology of childhood obesity, but biological and genetic factors also play a role.[28] The mechanism behind infant or childhood weight gain and adult obesity are not completely clear. Obesity is related to an increase in fat cell (adipocyte) size (hypertrophy) and fat cell number (hyperplasia). It appears likely that the earlier the obesity, the greater the increase in fat cell number (hyperplasia). However, it is not yet known whether hyperplasia, once it occurs, can be reversed.[29,30]

Many researchers have defined what they call "critical periods" in which an individual is especially vulnerable to weight gain because of the increased number of adipose cells. J. Hirsch identified three such periods in which nutritional factors are especially important to later weight: during the last trimester of pregnancy, the first 3 years of life, and the adolescent period.[31] Others have described different periods. J. L. Knittle terms the period through age 5 as critical;[6] Heald and Hollander suggest that "peak periods" for the development of obesity are infancy up to age 6 and adolescence.[32]

There is much controversy over whether overfeeding of the infant and young child will lead to hyperplasia. Several investigators have concluded that it does[30] whereas others suggest that this conclusion is not yet proven.[5]

Unique information of an epidemiological nature has come from studies of 19-year-old males in Holland whose mothers had suffered severe food shortages during World War II. The severe food shortage over a period of 6 months was followed by 2 years of food rationing. The weights and heights of the male babies born in cities that were subjected to the famine were determined and related to the intrauterine stage of development during the acute food shortage.

The study found that, for those males whose mothers suffered the severe shortage in midpregnancy, there was a significantly higher than expected prevalence of obesity at age 19. Where the shortage occurred at the end of pregnancy, fewer than the predicted number of males were obese at age 19. It seems possible that undernutrition during the middle of pregnancy may have altered the development of food intake control mechanisms and that undernutrition during late pregnancy may have reduced the replication of fat cells.[33]

A recent review and recalculation of published reports on the effects of early infant feeding patterns on later body size revealed "no real difference in later weight related to type of milk fed or to early or late introduction of semisolid foods." In other words, it cannot yet be stated that "fat infants become fat children."[33]

However, infant feeding patterns obviously influence infant weight status. An important factor determining food intake of the young child is the child's physiological need to satisfy hunger. The breast-fed baby thus consumes the amount of milk needed to make him or her feel full and comfortable. In contrast, the bottle-fed baby may respond to physiological cues but may also be influenced by the mother who may encourage milk consumption beyond that needed to satisfy hunger.

It is known that bottle-fed infants gain weight at a faster rate during the early days of life than do breast-fed infants. Gains in body length also tend to be greater in the early days for the bottle-fed infant. Such increased gains appear to be a function of increased caloric intake, and a statistically significant relationship between calorie consumption and growth rates can be demonstrated.

Adding to the difficulty of establishing a child's feeding pattern is the early introduction of solid foods to the infant's diet. Pediatric texts advising on the age to introduce solid foods have changed from suggesting the age of 1 year in the early 1900s to the age of 2 months in the 1970s. Changes in professional advice on solid foods seems to parallel the development of commercial infant foods.[3]

The child is often encouraged to clean his or her plate and to perhaps eat more than he or she would be naturally inclined to. The child may receive rewards for eating all the food served, and, in the process, his or her innate physiological signals governing satiety may become suppressed as he or she forms habits of overeating.

Not all infants who receive artificial formula or early introduction to solid foods become overweight, but early infant feeding patterns set the stage for later adult nutrition behavior and nutritional status.

During the later childhood and adolescent years, psychosocial factors become important influences of dietary habits. Food has many nonnutritive meanings; its use as a reward or punishment; as a substitute for love, security, and belongingness; or as a comfort in time of frustration or anxiety can lead to overeating and to an emotional rather than a physiological dependence on food, which is often an important factor in the etiology of obesity.

PREVENTION OF OBESITY

Although the prevention of childhood obesity is very difficult, it is probably our "only hope." Before obesity in the child can be prevented, we must be able to influence current eating habits of many obese parents and adults who care for and feed the children.

Parents have a tremendous influence on childrens' eating habits — not only on what food is available but also on what food is acceptable, tastes good, and is preferred and what constitutes acceptable eating habits. Children imitate what they see their parents doing and may pattern their own eating habits after those of their parents.

Successful programs using these ideas in the prevention and treatment of childhood obesity have been reported by B. Friedman[34] and H. Smiciklas-Wright and A. D'Augelli.[35]

S. J. Fomon has suggested various strategies for the prevention of obesity:[5]

1. Parents should be educated about the dangers and problems of overfeeding and wrongly using food in infant and childhood feeding; parents should be educated about the influence of childhood eating habits on later nutritional status.

2. Mothers should be encouraged to breast-feed; introduction of solid foods should be delayed, at least until the age of 3 months.

3. Physical exercise should be promoted.

4. Facilities for regular, year-round physical activity should be developed.

5. More smaller meals rather than fewer larger meals may be more effective in preventing obesity, as long as the energy value of the two patterns are similar.

6. In families of one or both obese parents, children and parents should be identified and given special help and counseling.

Obesity is preventable in most cases. The best treatment seems to be prophylaxis, which requires a heavy involvement of behavioral and social factors as well as the widespread dissemination of sound diet and nutrition information. The development of techniques to identify periods of rapid adipose cell multiplication and abnormal development of fat deposits must parallel the initiation of therapeutic techniques to modify the development of obesity before it reaches the stage of being resistant to treatment.[28]

TREATMENT OF OBESITY

It is generally agreed that obesity is becoming a serious public health problem in the United States. What cannot be agreed upon is the proper course of action to either treat or prevent the problem.

In a nation of 200 million persons of widely differing social, economic, ethnic, cultural, religious, and educational backgrounds with varying tastes, preferences, and life-styles — all factors affecting eating habits — what approach should be taken?

Significant weight losses in short periods of time are possible with rather drastic measures: drugs, fasting, fad diets. But the results are usually short-lived, and the long-term maintenance of weight loss is poor.

Experts are generally in agreement that fad diets are not the answer. Every month the public press abounds with new fad diets, "diets that work," diets that are "right for you." If these diets worked, there would be little need for, or incentive to devise, new ones.

As previously mentioned, the underlying physiological process of obesity and the psychological factors accompanying it are not well understood. Such an understanding is basic to strategies of prevention and treatment. Complicating the problem is the fact that all obesity is not the same. The large number of different types of obesity suggests that multiple causes may require multiple preventive measures.

Treatment for obesity can take a variety of forms. This section briefly discusses the following: dietary management, exercise, nonprescription weight reduction programs, fasting or semistarvation, drug therapy, and surgery. Behavior modification and weight reduction are discussed in greater detail.

Dietary Management

The treatment of obesity by diet has thus far not been impressively successful. Some clinicians believe that in future years diet therapy may be of minor importance whereas behavior modification will become increasingly important in treating obesity.[1]

The ideal weight reduction diet is based on the individual's food preferences, is well balanced, but achieves negative caloric balance, that is, calorie intake is less than the calories expended. The diet should also provide satiety, because hunger sensations will result in nonadherence to the diet. The diet should be such that it can be followed for life. In other words, it is important that the individual learn new eating habits so that any weight loss can be maintained. A suggested balanced diet for weight reduction would contain about 14 per cent protein, 30 per cent fat, and 56 per cent carbohydrate.[1]

A number of formula diets have been developed to aid in weight reduction. Although these diets provide a specific number of calories and reduce the decisions that the individual must make about food calories, there are many disadvantages. There is no bulk in the diets so that gastrointestinal symptoms may develop. But the principal drawback is that these diets do not help the individual to learn new food habits. For example, because it is very boring over any period of time, adherence to a diet of liquid formula is usually short-lived and frequently the individual immediately reverts to old food patterns and quickly regains any weight loss.

Evidence regarding the frequency of meals is conflicting. G. A. Bray has cited studies in which meal frequency was negatively associated with obesity, whereas other studies have reported no association between weight loss and frequency of meals.[36]

Exercise

Lack of exercise may aid the development of overweight in two distinct ways: (1) if exercise is limited, large amounts of calories will not be burned up, and the excess energy will be stored as fat; (2) recent data suggest that normal appetite control mechanisms do not operate properly at very low levels of physical activities.[37] Although some risk may be associated with exercise programs for some individuals, in general, exercise, in combination with diet control, will contribute to weight reduction. Exercise is also important because it aids nitrogen balance and good muscle tone.

Nonprescription Weight Reduction Programs[38]

A number of nonprescription programs have become available to help the obese in recent years. Four means by which the obese can participate in these treatments are:

1. self-help, nonprofessional groups,
2. professionally authored books,
3. popular media diets and popular media, and
4. advertisements.

1. Nonprofessional Groups

An excess of 1 million people weekly take part in nonprofessional group efforts to lose weight. Examples include Weight Watchers, TOPS (Take Off Pounds Sensibly), Diet Workshop, and Overeaters Anonymous.

These groups usually involve frequent meetings that may be free or may cost up to $600. The meetings are usually led by an individual who has been successful in losing weight on the program. Meal plans are distributed to members, and all are encouraged to discuss their weight problems, their feelings, and how they cope with losing weight. There are clearly many benefits to such programs. R. B. Stuart summarized some of them: (1) they help the individual to focus on a specific task, (2) they encourage the overweight person to have faith, which in turn builds motivation, (3) they are informal enough to meet members' social needs, (4) the peer group leaders serve as appropriate role models, (5) they can be easily entered into and then left, so that treatment can be taken when desired, (6) they "normalize" appropriate behaviors so that members can call upon their own abilities to solve their problems, (7) because the programs are of a self-help nature, individuals can attribute program success to personal growth, (8) their reliance on principles of promotion allow them to be presented in an appealing way, and (9) the cost is modest and the need to rely on third-party payments is minimized so that individual responsibility in the process is not undermined.[39]

Despite these advantages, there is a high degree of attrition in self-help programs — the attrition rates may be as high as 95 per cent a year. Thus, reports of weight losses from various groups are not always valid as the results are inflated as a result of high attrition. Available studies suggest that self-help groups can be effective in stimulating weight loss, but more study is needed before a clear picture of their effectiveness is available.

2. Professionally Authored Books

There are well over 1,000 diet books available to the public. Most are authored by individuals with some type of professional degree, thus giving credibility to the material. Many of these feature "one-emphasis diets" based on the notion that eating the primary food featured in the diet will result in weight loss.[40] The low-carbohydrate diet, for example, is featured in the *Calories Don't Count Diet*,[41] the Air Force Diet, the *Doctor's Quick-Weight-Loss Diet*,[42] and the *Dr. Atkins' Diet Revolution*.[43] These diets have been criticized because they advocate eating foods having a high level of fat and may result in ketosis.[38] At the opposite end of the diet spectrum are the low-protein, high-carbohydrate diets such as the one described in the *Doctors' Quick-Inches-Off Diet*.[44]

There is little in most of these books that would justify the use of the diets they advocate with the notable exceptions of some behavioral books that are well founded on reliable programs. Studies of the value of self-help diet manuals and books have failed to find evidence that these diets are effective aids to taking off, and keeping off, excess weight.

The ideal weight-reduction plan should be tailored to the individual according to the person's age, sex, weight, physical activity, and health status, something that is not done in these diet books. In addition, many medical and psychological hazards are associated with these diets.

3. Popular Media Diets

It is almost impossible to pick up a newspaper or a women's magazine without reading about weight reduction. In August 1978, a survey conducted on four women's magazines (*Cosmopolitan, Glamour, Mademoiselle,* and *Redbook*) found that each of these magazines contained an average of three articles on weight reduction, low-calorie meal planning, and nutrition. Some of these publication contained serializations of books dealing with weight loss. The tremendous proliferation of articles of this type in the popular press suggests that available diets have met with little or no success.[38]

4. Advertisements in the Popular Media

Advertisements for weight loss regalia may be the most damaging form of diet schemes. The previously mentioned survey of women's magazines found an average of four advertisements in each issue for diet devices, pills, schemes, meal plans, and the like. An example of these devices is Slim Skins, a sweat suit designed to be attached to a vacuum cleaner and promoted as follows:

> All new — the most phenomenal slenderizer ever conceived. Guaranteed to reduce your waist, abdomen, hips and thighs a total of 9 to 15 inches in just 3 days or your money refunded! . . . Using this newly discovered method of slenderizing the Slim Skins combine with your own vacuum cleaner to create a super new inch reducer that is infinitely more effective than any reducing method known![45]

The effectiveness (or rather lack of effectiveness) of these diet devices should be obvious, but the public continues to buy and try them.

In evaluating these nonprescription programs, K. D. Brownell notes that more is lost than just the time and money invested. These programs may be hazardous in two general ways: (1) a diet plan may be, in and of itself, dangerous, and (2) a plan may be dangerous because of its ineffectiveness.[38]

The innate overt dangers of these plans include medical hazards. The Atkins' diet, for example, or the low-calorie, high-protein diet can be dangerous and even lethal. In a recent report, the Food and Drug Administration noted that 58 deaths associated with the low-calorie protein diet were being investigated. In addition, most weight loss achieved by this diet is quickly regained.[46]

Psychological hazards are also associated with these programs. Emotional problems that occur with great frequency in patients using these diet methods include nervousness, weakness, instability, depression, anxiety, anger, frustration, and difficulty coping with work and home problems. Because the lost weight is usually regained, this adds yet another failure and compounds the emotional problems.

It is clear that, although these various nonprescription weight reduction plans may have some potential for helping people lose weight, very few of the plans have been found to be both safe and effective. The medical and psychological hazards involved in these diets may place those who participate in such programs at considerable risk. Thus, professional scrutiny is needed for these various types of programs that may be best conducted by routine monitoring of diet plans by an independent agency such as the Consumers Union or another similar and credible organization. If this were done, the public would have some way of knowing which diet plans were reliable. One example of this type of scrutiny is available in a book written by T. Berland and published by Consumers Union: *Rating the Diets: New Ways to Lose Weight*, which provides consumers information about the advantages and disadvantages of many diet plans.[47] If this type of endeavor were expanded, it could be very helpful in educating the consumer about practical and successful methods for losing weight.[38]

Fasting or Semistarvation

Fasting or starvation is sometimes used as a temporary treatment of very obese individuals who have not been successful in losing weight with other treatments. In complete fasting, only water and vitamin and mineral supplements are allowed. This treatment should be undertaken only under close medical supervision, and the patient's metabolic reactions to the treatment should be carefully monitored. Weight loss averaging about a pound per day has been achieved over a two-month period of fasting.[1]

Semistarvation diets, which allow 300 to 600 kcal daily, are an alteration of the total fasting regime. Refeeding after either total or partial fasting must be conducted carefully. Clear liquids are sometimes given for a day or two, followed by a very-low-calorie diet, given in small feedings.

There are some advantages to total fasting: the individual's rapid weight loss instills the sense of success and motivates the person to continue to try to lose weight. A sense of emotional well-being sometimes accompanies this successful weight loss. However, certain hazards include postural hypotension, impaired liver function, gout and urate stones, and cardiac complications such as atrial fibrillation.[1] Of great importance and concern is the loss of lean body mass, electrolyte disorders, and ketosis.

A modification of the starvation treatment that has recently become popular with children is the special camp at which the child or adolescent resides for a period of time. Various procedures designed to promote weight loss, such as carefully controlled diets and exercise programs, are used in conjunction with nutritional counseling. Although there are now many of these camps, there have been few controlled evaluations of them. Some studies have reported favorable results as long as the patient remains in the carefully controlled environment of the camp.[16]

For the most part, the significance and long-term success of these fasting or semistarvation approaches remain to be demonstrated. In general, these approaches do not teach the individual new eating habits under normal life situations.[16]

Drug Therapy

Various drugs used to promote weight loss include anorexic agents, drugs to prevent gastrointestinal absorption, bulk-producing agents, and hormones. The reader is referred to G. A. Bray for a comprehensive review of these substances.[36]

Anorexic agents (used to promote loss of appetite) act on the satiety center of the brain and are designed to lessen the person's impulse to eat. Because individuals vary widely in their response to these drugs, the effectiveness of the drugs can be maximized after the hunger-satiety pattern on a reducing diet is established so that the drugs may be taken throughout the day when hunger sensations are the greatest. Side effects observed with the use of anorexic agents include addiction, insomnia, hypertension, cardiac arrhythmias, dry mouth, constipation, impotence, blood disorders, and allergic reactions.[1]

It is difficult to evaluate the effectiveness of these drugs in stimulating weight loss because the rates at which individuals stop using these drugs tend to be high and the short-term efficacy of the drugs is minimal. Available evidence from controlled studies indicates a trend to regain lost weight. No one anorexic agent has been found to be consistently more successful than any other. Although these agents sometimes promote greater weight loss than would occurr without them, their total effect is usually a modest one.[40]

Other substances, such as cellulose and methyl derivatives, are sometimes used as bulk producers. Because they are not digestible and they swell in the stomach, these substances not only produce bulk but may also reduce the caloric content of the food eaten, absorb water, and thus produce a feeling of satiety.

Weight loss sometimes accompanies the use of these agents as a result of reduction in hunger sensations. The usefulness of methylcellulose has been brought into doubt because of the finding that it swells slowly in the stomach and thus acts more as a laxative than as an appetite suppressant. There are potential hazards, such as psychological dependence and abuse, that suggest that these bulk-producing agents should only be used as a short-term, interim treatment (four to six weeks) for those who have trouble adhering to a low-calorie regime.[40]

Hormones, such as human growth, thyroid, and human chorionic gonadotrophin, have also been used to treat weight problems.[1] Controlled studies of chorionic gonadotropin are not conclusive; studies of human growth hormone suggest that this may be suitable only for those individuals who are deficient in it. Thyroid therapy, although it produces minimal weight loss, may adversely affect cardiovascular health and skeletal growth.[16]

Surgery

Surgery is sometimes used in refractory cases of massive, morbid obesity when other treatments fail. Two types of surgery used are intestinal bypass and gastric bypass. Intestinal bypass has been used much longer and more widely than gastric bypass, but it also carries a greater risk of long-term complications. Medical complications include diarrhea, indigestion, liver damage, cardiac failure, pancreatic disorders, hemorrhage, and death from the surgery itself. Metabolic side effects may also result from malabsorption and loss of nutrients. However, many of these effects are also experienced with gastric surgery; neither method is without hazard.[48] The amount of weight loss depends upon initial weight and may be as great as 85 pounds the first year.

Because of this great loss of weight, the surgery often results in an improved psychosocial function (such as new self-respect and improved employment opportunities) and decreased risk factors for heart disease (such as lower serum cholesterol, blood pressure, and hyperglycemia).

Currently, surgery for obesity is investigational. Much study and evaluation is needed on its long-term effects, as well as on the medical, nutritional, economic, and psychological risks and benefits of this procedure.[40]

Behavior Modification

Recent advances in the fields of scoiology, social psychology, and experimental psychology are providing new basic science applications for a better understanding of obesity. Every social factor studied thus far by sociological techniques has been related to the prevalence and etiology of obesity. Illustrative of the social factors associated with obesity include parental socioeconomic status and ethnic background.[49,50]

Social psychological techniques have yielded data that suggest similarities between the nutrition behavior of obese humans and of experimentally obese animals. There appear to be a number of "external" environmental controls that influence eating, which are often of greater importance than "internal" factors in influencing obesity.

Many researchers have conducted experiments to illustrate this point. In one experiment, subjects who came to the laboratory at 5:00 P.M. were told that they were to take part in an experiment that was unrelated to eating behavior. Each person was left alone for 30 minutes in a room with only electronic equipment and a clock. There were two experimental conditions. The experimentor returned in 30 minutes but the clock read, for one group, 5:20 (the clock ran at half the normal rate) and for the other group it read 6:05 (the clock ran at twice the normal rate).

The latter time was the normal dinner hour for the subjects. The subjects were given a box of crackers to nibble on while they were filling out a questionnaire.

The obese people ate about twice as many crackers when they thought it was 6:05 compared with when they thought it was 5:20. The subjects who were of normal weight did just the opposite; they did not want to spoil their dinner by eating the crackers. This study demonstrated that time, an external cue, was much more important to the obese than to the normal-weight subjects.[51]

In another study, obese people who were given only a bland liquid diet dispensed freely by a machine for weeks or months dramatically reduced their normal calorie intake and lost weight. In contrast to this, normal-weight individuals maintained their weight and ate much more freely than did the obese. The study showed that when food is dull, or when there is no social interaction associated with eating, the obese person often reduces his or her food intake. In other words, the obese person does not know when he or she is "hungry" but is very responsive to visual, taste, or food-related environmental cues.[51]

Thus, the obese person needs to develop a method to alter responses to external cues. This is the principle behind the use of behavior modification techniques used to control food intake. Behavioral therapy stresses the importance of stimulus control or modifying environmental cues that affect overeating and of self-control or modifying personal responses to environmental eating cues.

Techniques

Behavioral therapy techniques have been heralded by many as a landmark in the treatment of obesity.[50] The basic premise underlying these techniques is that eating behavior is learned as a result of various social and environmental stimuli. As such, the poor eating practices can be unlearned. Related to this is the control of certain factors in an individual's immediate environment that relate to eating behavior: physical and social cues (such as food advertising, social gatherings, and family meals), feelings and attitudes about food (such as relating food to feelings of security, frustrations, relieving of depressions), and other actions, such as going to the movies and viewing television. By changing those variables related to eating in the immediate environment, behavior modification seeks to influence food consumption.

Behavior modification, a relatively new technique, is based on basic animal learning research.[52,53] The approach focuses on relating measurable activities to preceding and subsequent environmental stimuli.[54]

Of particular interest in the behavioral approach to modifying human behavior are *contingency management* and *stimulus control*.[54] Contingency management relies on the notion that the results of behavior determine future behavior patterns. Behavioral consequences, or reinforcing stimuli as they are termed, make future behavior more likely to resemble previous reinforced behavior. For example, a reward offered for a particular behavior reinforces that behavior pattern, making it more likely to be repeated.

The concept of stimulus control analyzes the ways in which given stimuli affect future behavior. A stimulus can affect behavior if it is associated with a reinforcer. The use of the stimulus-control analysis involves a record of current activity, mood, location, and environmental factors associated with current behavior. For example, a record made of food patterns, including where the food was eaten, the circumstances surrounding the eating, the individual's mood, and the social context, is used as a tool for modifying undesirable eating behavior.

Behavior modification techniques used to treat obesity include: (1) analyzing the stimulus-control mechanism, including the use of a written record of eating behavior and associated environmental factors; (2) eliminating certain cues associated with eating; (3) changing the antecedents of eating behavior or the consequences of eating, (4) suppressing certain cues associated with undesirable eating, (5) strengthening or accelerating desirable results, and (6) weakening or decelerating undesirable consequences or responses.[50,55] Examples of these procedures are listed in Table 9–1. Table 9–2 summarizes the techniques of behavior modification and some of the advantages of these techniques are presented in Table 9–3.

Few well-designed studies have evaluated the use of behavior modification techniques in producing long-term weight changes. Those studies that have been done, however, suggest that the treatment is promising, at least in achieving short-term weight loss.

Many studies have reported the effectiveness of such techniques. In one study, in which nutritionists were used as therapists, therapist training on the use of behavioral techniques was conducted through self-study. A

Table 9-1

Examples of Procedures Used in the Use of Behavior Modification to Treat Obesity

Modifications	Procedures
Eliminating of undesirable cues	Restrict eating to one room. Do nothing else while eating Make available only appropriate foods; shop from a list; do not shop when hungry Clear plates directly into the garbage; do not nibble leftovers
Suppressing undesirable cues	Make meals a social occasion Serve small amounts of food Eat slowly Save part of the meal for later
Strengthening desirable cues	Keep detailed food and weight record Allow extra money for appropriate low-calorie foods Prepare foods attractively Post a picture of desired look or clothes List activities that will be possible with weight loss
Reducing the strength of un-desirable responses	Swallow food already in mouth before eating more Drink sparingly with meals
Increasing the strength of de-sirable responses	Count to 5 after every bite Chew food slowly and thoroughly; savor every bite Concentrate on the food eaten
Decelerating consequences	Display caloric values of foods eaten Keep a chart of weight changes Have overeater analyze failures and plan alternative techniques that might have succeeded
Accelerating consequences	Display calorie value of food eaten Chart weight changes Develop mechanism for social feedback with success from family, friends, peers, other weight watchers, or professionals Devise reinforcement schedule for successes

Source: R. B. Stuart. Behavioral Control of Overeating. *Behav. Res. and Ther.* 9 (1971): 182.

total of 57 women who were at least 10 per cent overweight were directed to a multiple technique behavioral program, a food exchange treatment, or a delay treatment control group. The study period lasted 10 weeks.[56] The weight losses assessed at the end of the study period were 3.0 kg, 2.2 kg, and 1.0 kg, respectively. When the treatment was later provided to the control group, the average weight loss was 2.7 kg. One year later the subjects who had received the behavior treatment maintained 70 per cent of the weight loss achieved during the treatment; the other groups maintained less than half their weight loss.[56]

A second study compared the multiple treatment technique used in the first study to a program built around the concept of stimulus control. Both treatments included nutrition information. The stimulus-control treatment was found to be more effective in initial weight loss as well as

Table 9-2

Techniques of Behavior Modification in the Treatment of Obesity

---

1. Initial Assessment — Functional Analysis of Eating Patterns to Describe:

   Food habits and their patterns of occurrence: types, quantity, caloric value of food, when, where, with whom; social responses to eating.

   Antecedent conditions that signal eating: degree of hunger perceived, both before and after eating; emotional responses such as depression and boredom; situations that stimulate eating.

   Focus on observable behavior and discrete, specific behavior change.

2. Alter Eating Behavior:

   Shape new habits by providing for small, incremental changes in behavior with each step more closely approximating the final goal.

   Alter antecedent stimulus controls. Through repeated association with food, certain places and times stimulate eating; in other words, the place or time signals that eating will have rewarding or reinforcing consequences. These cues must thus be altered.

3. Program Incompatible Behaviors:

   For example, if emotional states such as boredom or depression serve as antecedents to stimulate eating, alter the behavior pattern by replacing the eating behavior with actions incompatible with eating, such as taking a walk, singing, or taking a shower.

4. Reinforce Acceptable Eating Behavior:

   Food is a potent and immediate positive reinforcer; thus, other replacement reinforcers should be substituted for food. For example, a contingency contract, a self-presentation of a certain amount of time in a valued activity, contingent on practicing the desired behavior may serve as such a substitute reinforcer. Reinforcers should be immediate; token systems may be possible.

---

in the maintenance of the achieved weight loss. Additional studies on the effects of behavior modification on weight control can be found in references 57–61.

After reviewing many of these studies, T. Coates and C. Thorensen summarized the current state of thinking about the use of behavior modification in treating obesity:

> Some beneficial results are achieved with some subjects, but maintenance of changes or continued losses may still be the rare exception rather than the rule.
>
> This approach, however, does offer two advantages not typically employed by other treatments: treatment programs are defined explicitly; and the treatment results are documented carefully on an individual basis.[16]

Table 9-3

Advantages of Behavior Modification

Patient is actively involved in his or her own treatment; the patient assumes responsibility for the modification of his or her own eating habits.

Patient is taught to become aware of discrete problem behaviors — he or she learns to implement small changes in these behaviors.

Patient learns to analyze environmental cues related to eating and to modify these as appropriate to attain his or her goal.

Patient seeks to ultimately develop sound eating habits, consistent with his or her weight goals; it is hoped that these new habits will be long lasting.

SUMMARY AND CONCLUSIONS

There is a lack of unanimity regarding the current state of knowledge about the etiology, classification, and definition of obesity. Obesity is much more than a clinical/medical problem. It is related to behavioral, psychological, cultural, social, and life-style factors. In addition, it is not yet possible to distinguish whether social/environmental factors are primary or secondary factors in the development of obesity. It is clear that there is a need for continuing research into all factors related to the etiology of obesity before strategies of prevention can be successful.

Traditional dietary counseling has been relatively ineffective in producing sustained weight reduction; although it may work in the short run, it is rarely successful in weight maintenance for long periods of time. Thus, it is suggested that dietary counseling by itself may be an inefficient use of both client and professional time.[16]

Long-term success in maintenance of weight loss is limited. The subject of the treatment of overweight and obesity has been described as "generally gloomy." By continuing to prescribe treatment methods that have been proven only marginally effective at best, we may be "fostering a deepening despair and discouragement among our patients."[16] It is important and essential that the use of ineffective techniques of weight control be discontinued.

The most effective weight reduction programs are those exhibiting high levels of structure, organization, and supervision. For programs to have long-lasting success, they themselves must be long term. It is unrealistic to expect that a six-week program of group meetings or discussions will produce significant weight loss as well as stimulate eating patterns that support a maintenance of the loss.

In general, the most successful weight reduction approach involves three components: sound dietary control, exercise, and behavior modification aimed at achieving the first two.[37] For effective and lasting correction of abnormal body weight, the therapeutic program should incorporate strategies coordinated with psychotherapy as well as with the resolution of family problems and conflicts.[60,62] The involvement of family or of "important others" is also important, as obesity frequently follows family patterns. Although these relationships may be the result of genetic influences, they are also influenced by cultural family practices and behavioral patterns.

Behavior modification techniques offer promising hope for the treatment of obesity. Particularly important components to be included in obesity prevention and treatment programs are:[49]

1. A self-evaluative, self-monitoring, self-reinforcing program emphasizing actual eating habits and environmental cues affecting these habits.

2. Provision of sound nutrition education aimed at achieving long-term weight control through a balanced and adequate diet.

3. Use of stimulus control to regulate food consumption.

4. The participation of family or friends who could provide positive reinforcement to encourage modification of eating habits.

Strategies that are successful usually require the individual to modify an eating pattern in such a way that he or she can live with the altered habits for a lifetime. Social, behavioral, cognitive, motivational, affective, and psychological variables must be considered and planned for, as they influence nutrition and dietary behavior.

One program designed to be a step-by-step approach to weight reduction is described by R. B. Stuart and B. Davis.[63] However, as these authors admonish, this should not be considered the cure for overweight; the best approach must lie in prevention. A multidisciplinary approach, including education and behavioral science techniques as well as sound nutrition principles, should be directed to prevent as well as to control the complex problem of "the obesities."

REFERENCES

1. Thiel, V. *Clinical Nutrition.* St. Louis, Mo. C. V. Mosby, 1976.
2. U.S. Public Health Service, Division of Chronic Diseases. *Obesity and Health: A Sourcebook of Current Information for Professional Health Personnel,* Rept. No. 1485. Washington, D.C.: Government Printing Office, 1966.
3. Jelliffe, D. G., and E. F. P. Jelliffe. Fat babies: Perils, prevalence, and prevention. *J. Trop. Pediatr. Child Health* 21 (1975): 123 (mono. 41).
4. U.S. Department of Health, Education, and Welfare. *Ten-State Nutrition Survey,* Publ. No. (HSM) 72-8134. Washington, D.C.: Government Printing Office, 1972.
5. Fomon, S. J. *Nutritional Disorders of Children: Prevention, Screening, and Follow-up,* Publ. No. (HSA) 77-5104. Washington, D.C.: U.S. Department of Health, Education, and Welfare, 1977).
6. Knittle, J. L. Obesity in childhood: A problem in adipose tissue cellular development. *J. Pediatr.* 81 (1972): 1048.
7. Rimm, I. J., and A. A. Rimm. Association between juvenile onset obesity and severe adult obesity in 73,532 women. *Am. J. Publ. Health* 6 (1976): 479.
8. Abraham, S., G. Collins, and M. Nordsieck. Relationship of childhood weight status to morbidity in adults. *Publ. Health Rep.* 86 (1971): 273.
9. Stunkard, A. J., and V. Burt. Obesity and the body image. II. Age at onset of disturbances in the body. *Am. J. Psychiatry* 123 (1967): 1443.
10. Fisch, R. O., M. K. Bilek, and R. Ulstrom. Obesity and leanness at birth and their relationship to body habitus in later childhood. *Pediatrics* 56 (1975): 521.
11. Poskitt, E. Overfeeding and overweight in infancy and their relation to body size in early childhood. *Nutr. and Metab.* 21 (1977): 54–55.
12. Will a fat baby become a fat child? *Nutr. Rev.* 35 (June 1977): 138.
13. Mellbin, T., and J. C. Vuille. Physical development at 7 years of age in relation to velocity of weight gain in infancy with special reference to incidence of overweight. *Brit. J. Prev. Soc. Med.* 27 (1973): 225.
14. Cooper, T. In U.S. Senate Select Committee on Nutrition and Human Needs, *Diet Related to Killer Diseases.* Washington, D.C.: Government Printing Office, July 1976.
15. Winikoff, B. In U.S. Senate Select Committee on Nutrition and Human Needs, *Diet Related to Killer Diseases.* Washington, D.C.: Government Printing Office, July 1976.

16. Coates, T. J., and C. E. Thoresen. Treating obesity in children and adolescents: A review. *Am. J. Publ. Health* 68 (1978): 143.
17. Van Itallie, T. B., and R. G. Campbell. Multidisciplinary approach to the problem of obesity. *J. Am. Diet. Assoc.* 61 (1972): 385.
18. Stamler, J. Quoted in U.S. Senate Select Committee on Nutrition and Human Needs, *Edible T.V.: Your Child and Food Commercials.* Washington, D.C.: Government Printing Office, September 1977.
19. Mayer, J. Obesity, in R. S. Goodhard and M. E. Shils, eds., *Nutrition in Health and Disease.* Philadelphia: Lea and Febiger, 1973.
20. Garn, S. M., and D. C. Clark: Nutrition, growth, development, and maturation: Findings from the *Ten-State Nutrition Survey, 1968–1970. Pediatrics* 56 (1975): 306.
21. Gates, J. C., R. L. Huenemann, and R. J. Brand. Food choices of obese and nonobese persons. *J. Am. Diet. Assoc.* 67 (1975): 339.
22. Danowski, T. S., S. Nolan, and T. Stephan. Obesity, in *World Review of Nutrition and Dietetics.* Vol. 22. Karger Gazette (31), 1975.
23. Huenemann, R. L. Environmental factors associated with preschool obesity. *J. Am. Diet. Assoc.* 64 (1974): 489.
24. Dwyer, J. T., and J. Mayer. Overfeeding and obesity in infants and children. *Bibl. Nutr. Diet.* 18 (1973): 123.
25. Weil, W. B. Infantile obesity, in M. Winick, ed., *Childhood Obesity.* New York: John Wiley, 1975.
26. Borjeson, M. The etiology of obesity in children: A study of 101 twin pairs. *Acta Paediatr. Scand.* 65 (1976): 279.
27. Garn, S. M., P. E. Cole, and S. M. Bailey. Effect of parental levels on the fatness of biological and adoptive children. *Ecol. of Food and Nutr.* 7 (1977): 91.
28. Weill, W. B., Jr. Current controversies in childhood obesity. *J. Pediatr.* 91 (1977): 175.
29. Hirsch, J., and J. L. Knittle. Cellularity of obese and nonobese human adipose tissue. *Fed. Proc.* 29 (1970): 1516.
30. Brook, C. G. D., J. K. Lloyd, and O. H. Wolf. Relation between age of onset of obesity and size and number of adipose cells. *Brit. Med. J.* 2 (1972): 25.
31. Hirsch, J. Cell number and size as a determinant of subsequent obesity, in M. Winick, ed., *Childhood Obesity.* New York: John Wiley, 1975.
32. Heald, F. P., and R. J. Hollander. The relationship between obesity in adolescence and early growth. *J. Pediatr.* 67 (1965): 35.
33. National Research Council. *Summary of a Workshop: Fetal and Infant Nutrition and Susceptibility to Obesity.* Washington, D.C.: Government Printing Office, February 28 and March 1, 1977.
34. Friedman, B. M. Atherosclerosis and the pediatrician, in M. Winick, ed., *Childhood Obesity.* New York: John Wiley, 1975.
35. Smicklas-Wright, H., and A. R. D'Augelli. Primary prevention for overweight: The preschool eating patterns (PEP) program. *J. Am. Diet. Assoc.* 72 (1978): 626.
36. Bray, G. A. *The Obese Patient.* Vol. 9. *Series of Major Problems in Internal Medicine.* Philadelphia: W. B. Saunders, 1976.
37. National Institutes of Health. *Facts about Obesity.* Washington, D.C.: Government Printing Office, 1976.
38. Brownell, K. D. The pyschological and medical sequelae of nonprescription weight reduction programs. Paper presented at the Annual Meeting of the American Psychological Association, Toronto, August 1978.
39. Stuart, R. B. Self-help for self-management, in R. B. Stuart, ed., *Behavior Self-management.* New York: Brunner/Mazel, 1977.

40. What's new in weight control? *Dairy Council Digest* 49 (March–April 1978).

41. Taller, H. *Calories Don't Count.* New York: Simon & Schuster, 1961.

42. Stillman, I. M., and S. S. Baker. *The Doctor's Quick-Weight-Loss Diet.* Englewood Cliffs, N.J.: Prentice-Hall, 1967.

43. Atkins, R. C. *Dr. Atkins' Diet Revolution.* New York: David McKay, 1972.

44. Stillman, I. M., and S. S. Baker. *The Doctor's Quick-Inches-Off Diet.* Englewood Cliffs, N.Y.: Prentice-Hall, 1969.

45. *Women's Day*, April, 1978.

46. Food and Drug Administration. Liquid protein and sudden cardiac deaths — An update. *FDA Drug Bull.* (May–July 1978).

47. Berland, T. *Rating the Diets. New Ways to Lose Weight.* New York: Consumers Union, 1977.

48. Cegielski, M. M., and J. A. Saporta. Surgical treatment of massive obesity: Current status of the art. *Obesity and Bariatr. Med.* 7 (1978): 156.

49. Stunkard, A. J., and M. J. Mahoney. Behavioral treatment of the eating disorders, in H. Leitenberg, ed., *Handbook of Behavior Modification.* New York: Appleton-Century-Crofts, 1976.

50. Stunkard, A. J. From explanation to action in psychosomatic medicine: The case of obesity. *Psychosomatic Med.* 37 (1975): 195.

51. Cues affecting eating behavior and obesity. *Nutr. Rev.* 27 (1969): 11.

52. Pavlov, I. P. *Conditioned Reflexes.* New York: Dover Publications, 1927.

53. Skinner, B. F. *Science and Human Behavior.* New York: Macmillan, 1953.

54. Bass, F. Behavior modification: A review of basic concepts and recent research, in Fogarty International Center et al., *Preventive Medicine, U.S.A.: Health Promotion and Consumer Health Education.* New York: Prodist, 1976, p. 128.

55. Stuart, R. B. Behavioral control of overeating. *Behav. Res. and Ther.* 5 (1967): 357.

56. Paulsen, B. K., R. N. Lutz, W. T. McReynolds, and M. B. Kohrs. Behavior therapy for weight control: Long-term results of two programs with nutritionists as therapists. *Am. J. Clin. Nutr.* 29 (1976): 880.

57. Rivinus, T. M., T. Drummond, and L. Combrinck-Graham. A group-behavior treatment program for overweight children: The results of a pilot study. Unpublished manuscript. Philadelphia: University of Pennsylvania, 1973.

58. Aragona, J., J. Cassady, and R. S. Drabman. Treating overweight children through parental training and contingency contracting. *J. Appl. Behav. Anal.* 8 (1975): 269.

59. Wheller, M. E., and K. W. Hess. Treatment of juvenile obesity in adolescents using behavioral self-control. *Clin. Pediatr.* 15 (1976): 920.

60. Stunkard, A. J., L. W. Craighead, and R. O'Brien. New treatments for obesity. Paper presented at Annual Meeting of American Psychiatric Association, Atlanta, Ga., May 11, 1978.

61. Bruch, H. Treatment of eating disorders. *Mayo Clinic Proc.* 51 (1976): 206.

63. Stuart, R. B., and B. Davis. *Slim Chance in a Fat World.* Champaign, Ill., Research Press, 1972.

Diet, nutrition, and dental caries

Reader Objectives

After completing this chapter, the reader should be able to
1. State the public health significance of dental caries.
2. Describe the etiology of dental caries using the epidemiological triad as a reference point.
3. Outline the effects of dietary carbohydrates on the development of dental caries.
4. Describe the other dietary influences on dental caries.
5. State the current uses of fluoride in preventing dental caries.

You may have heard the expression "a sweet tooth is a decaying tooth." Scientific studies support this claim. Since sugar was found to cause tooth decay, a notable experiment has been performed. Dr. Clive McCay, doing Naval Research, discovered that human teeth soften when they are submerged for a few days in cola drinks, due to the phosphoric acid content. . . . I am appalled at seeing children queue up daily at confectionery stores during lunchtime and after school hours to spend their allowance for candy and soft drinks. In one town where unlimited purchase of candy by school children is common, a dentist reports that it is not unusual for individual children to have thirty new cavities every year.

—L. Clark

This quote, taken from a popular nutrition book, already beyond its thirteenth printing since its original publication in 1974, illustrates some of the common, but misinformed, beliefs about tooth decay and nutrition.[1] It is clear that the process of teeth softening in acidic solutions differs from the damage that occurs after a person has consumed a sugar-containing beverage that affects the enamel of the tooth. And it is believed that phosphorous may actually inhibit caries formation. The scientific evidence relating sugar to tooth decay is, at best, controversial. There is not a simple one-to-one relationship between a given dietary component and the development of dental caries. The following section discusses some of the controversies surrounding tooth decay and nutrition.

It is very difficult to determine exact and specific effects of nutrients on the development of dental caries; a given nutrient may have a direct and primary effect as well as various indirect effects on the decay process. For instance, a nutrient imbalance occurring before tooth development can influence later tooth resistance to decay. A nutrient deficiency or excess occurring during development may influence tooth morphology or salivary gland function and hence may affect caries activity. After the tooth has erupted, the microflora in the saliva interact with the nutrient supply and affect the caries process. The nutritional status of the host also influences caries development.

It is difficult to describe the effects of all of these factors on the development of dental caries. However, it is possible to look at specific results of specific nutritional factors as they affect the development of caries at a given stage of tooth development.

PUBLIC HEALTH SIGNIFICANCE OF DENTAL CARIES[2]

In the United States and in many other industrialized nations, 98 per cent of the population have some dental problems related to tooth decay during their lifetimes. The Preschool Nutrition Survey noted an average of 2.6 decayed, missing, or filled (DMF) teeth in white children and 3.8 DMF in black children between the ages of 4 and 5 years.[3] The Ten-State Survey found an increase in dental caries with increasing age among children. Other studies have found that the average number of dental caries for children aged 5 to 6 was 3.7 for whites and 5.1 for blacks; by 10 years of age, 80 per cent of American children had caries affecting their permanent teeth.[5,6]

The Committee on Nutrition of the American Academy of Pediatrics suggested that dental caries was the most common disease found both among children and adults.[7] The public health significance of dental caries must be considered beyond that of the effect on teeth alone. For example, an untreated carious lesion may result in severely inflamed dental pulp, gingival inflammations, and dental calculus, all of which are severe in themselves. In addition, oral inflammations provide entry into the human internal systems for various invasive pathogens and other foreign and toxic compounds. The most severe consequence is that these processes may be lethal.[8]

ETIOLOGY OF CARIES DEVELOPMENT

Dental caries has been defined as an "infectious disease produced by certain microorganisms that live on the teeth and produce acids, chiefly lactic, from sugar and starches ingested as food and drink. The acid attacks the hard (enamel) surfaces of the teeth in specific areas of caries predilection, decalcifying and eventually destroying them."[9]

This description is a simplified outline of the development of dental caries. Actually the process is very complex. Various oral bacteria such as *Streptococcus mutans* are able, through enzymatic action, to convert sugars to long-chain, adhesive polymers that adhere to the teeth, entrap and hold bacterial growth, and accumulate masses of gelatinous material or dental plaque.

For this process to occur, suitable bacteria must be present in the oral cavity and be in close contact with the teeth. There must be available a suitable carbohydrate substrate to support microorganism growth, and the tooth must be susceptible to the caries development process. A vast amount of literature confirms that each of these conditions must be present if caries are to be produced.[8,9]

Two general factors determining the development of the caries process are (1) the length of time and the intensity of the adverse dietary components reacting with the teeth and (2) the resistance of the tooth to demineralization or dissolution. It is clear that the process is multifaceted and complex.[10-13]

The etiology of caries development can be considered in terms of the epidemiological triad of agent, host, and environment. Epidemiologists have traditionally considered disease to be the final result of the interaction between this triad of factors. This concept is useful in explaining the various interacting factors in the etiology of dental disease. The agent is the microbial agent; the host factors are those relating to the individual and include such characteristics as previous and present nutritional status, the presence of disease states, and genetic inheritance; the environment includes other factors influencing the availability of food and nutrients, the nutritional and health status of the host, and the intake of food.

Agent

A number of microbial agents can cause tooth decay. Carbohydrates enhance the caries production potential of these microorganisms. *S. mutans*, one of these microorganisms, has been the focus of considerable study because of the organism's ability to colonize tooth surfaces by producing dextran from sucrose.

Host

The individual and his or her teeth are variably susceptible to caries development. The chemical and histological nature of the tooth, as well as the amount and composition of the saliva, are important and reflect past and current nutritional and infectious influences.

The diet of the host influences tooth decay in three ways:[10]

1. By coming into contact with the tooth as food is eaten (local action).

2. By reacting with the tooth after absorption, as it may return to the mouth in the saliva (systemic-local action).

3. After absorption, by entering the tooth through circulating blood (systemic action).

Very little research data are available relative to the latter two routes; the main focus remains on the local action of food on the teeth.

Diet can affect the status of the host and hence influence the caries process either before the teeth erupt (e.g., maternal nutrition during pregnancy may affect the development and composition of the tooth or the oral environment) or after the teeth have erupted.

In humans, teeth begin to develop when the fetus is about 2 months old. Tooth mineralization begins in the fourth to the sixth month *in utero*; deciduous teeth start to erupt at about 5 months of age. By 1 year of age, the deciduous teeth are mineralized, and permanent teeth begin to come in around 6 years of age. Only the crown of permanent teeth are mineralized at the time of eruption; roots are not completely mineralized until about the age of 12. Tooth development, once it has occurred, is relatively set. Further, after development, the crown of the tooth is unlikely to be affected by systemic influences. In other words, teeth formed in a poor nutritional environment are not greatly changed in later years with an improved nutritional environment.

Few conclusive experimental results relate particular nutrients with preerupted tooth development. Available data are primarily from animal studies, and extrapolation to humans must be made with care. Because of dietary interactions of various foodstuffs, and the fact that a diet altered in one component (e.g., carbohydrate) is usually also modified in others (e.g., protein and fat), available data often yield inconclusive results.

However, it is known that normal tooth development requires vitamins A, C, D, calcium, and an appropriate calcium-to-phosphorous ratio, magnesium, and protein. Fluoride at a suitable level may enhance resistance to caries development.

When there is maximum caries development, the flow of saliva is decreased. Of interest in this regard is the fact that sweets tend to increase the flow of saliva. Saliva acts to protect the teeth by washing away substances that might come in contact with, and adhere to, the teeth. It also acts as a lubricant and as a buffer, counteracting the drop in pH associated with the microbial organism metabolism of carbohydrate in dental plaque. The chemical composition of saliva as well as its immunological characteristics are important determinants of caries development.[9]

Environment

The environment of the oral cavity is greatly related to caries development. Frequency of eating, the length of time that food is in contact with the teeth, and the composition of the food being ingested have been related to caries development. Caries-producing organisms require carbohydrate. Thus, individuals with a hereditary fructose intolerance, who must avoid all types of sweets to eliminate dietary fructose, have been found to have fewer caries than the average population.[13]

The length of time that cariogenic foods remain in contact with the tooth is a very important determinant of caries development. To illustrate this, Joseph suggested that if five cough drops are consumed in 15 minutes, resulting acid comes into contact with the tooth for approximately 35 minutes. If the same five cough drops are eaten 15 minutes apart, the tooth is exposed to acid for 100 minutes. The frequency of consumption of cariogenic foods may be a more important influence on caries development than the total quantity consumed.[10]

This concept may be the basis for the so-called "nursing-bottle syndrome," "baby-bottle caries," and "bottle-mouth syndrome." (See Figures 10-1 and 10-2). A child given a bottle of sugar-sweetened liquid at bedtime may fall asleep sucking. The liquid may pool in the mouth, the saliva flow ceases as the child falls asleep, and carbohydrates ferment. Caries development is thus enhanced, and this process can eventually destroy all of the upper deciduous teeth.

Cariostatic Foods

Various foodstuffs have been suggested as exerting protective effects on the teeth. Such foods are termed *cariostatic*. Fat appears to have anti-

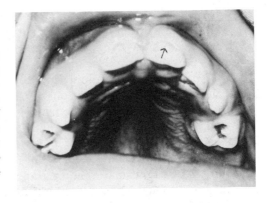

Figure 10-1. Nursing bottle caries affecting the maxillary anterior teeth and the first primary molars in an 18-month-old child. Note the extensive destruction of the labial surfaces of maxillary incisors (arrow) and the occlusal surfaces of the first primary molars. The lingual surfaces of the maxillary incisors (not shown) are also severely decayed.

microbial activity; it also reduces the retention of food to teeth, increases the flow of saliva, and produces a protective film on the teeth.[11] Other foods reported to be cariostatic include milk, casein, cocoa, and chocolate.[10]

Other environmental factors to be considered include social-economic factors, such as how much money is available to purchase various foodstuffs or what food choices are commonly made as a result of one's cultural background. Geography is also important, as fluoride concentrations are different in the water supplies of various locations.

PERIODONTAL DISEASE

Dental plaque has long been associated with the development of dental caries, but recent evidence suggests that plaque is also related to periodontal disease.[14]

Periodontal disease, the breakdown and decay of structures supporting the teeth, has a complex etiology that is not yet clearly understood. The oral environment, plaque, and calculus formation appear to be intimately related to causation. Gingivitis, thought to be the initial stage of periodontal breakdown, is also related to the accumulation of plaque. Nutritional factors may predispose an individual to periodontal disease or may modify the progression of the disease.

Figure 10-2. A typical example of a child affected with nursing bottle caries. Note the total destruction of the maxillary incisors. The first primary molars have required restoration with stainless steel crowns. In the early stages the lower teeth are relatively unaffected. (Figures 10-1 and 10-2 from Foman, S. J. and Wei, S. H. Y.: Prevention of dental caries, in Fomon, S. J. (ed.): *Nutritional Disorders of Children.* DHHS Publication no. (HSA) 77-5104)

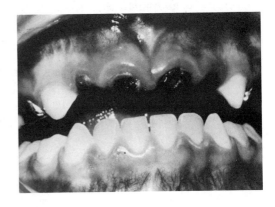

DENTAL PLAQUE

Dental plaque is the term used to refer to the white, gray, or yellow gelatinous adherent material that covers the teeth as a consequence of contact with food (notably sugar) and neglected oral hygiene habits. It is composed mainly of bacteria, but also of leukocytes and other cells combined and embedded in an organic matrix. The composition and metabolism of plaque may vary according to the specific site in the oral cavity.

Bacterial plaque is considered essential for caries development, but not all plaque results in caries formation. For example, N. Littleton and colleagues found considerable amounts of plaque in the mouths of a group of severely retarded children who had to be fed through a gastric tube; however, the incidence of caries in these children was low.[15]

ACQUIRED PELLICLE

The initial development in the process of dental decay involves the formation of the enamel pellicle. This is a protein film, derived from glycoproteins in the saliva, that is adsorbed onto the surface of tooth enamel. Acids formed by microbial metabolism may enhance glycogen deposition on the enamel; hence the acquired pellicle may be at least indirectly related to oral bacteria and sugar consumption. The pellicle is permeable to bacteria that form acids and also provides a medium on which oral bacteria can grow.[8]

EFFECT OF DIETARY CARBOHYDRATE

Dietary carbohydrates play an important role in the growth of microorganisms on enamel surfaces. When sugar is consumed, both sucrose and glucose are converted to lactic acid, the pH of the saliva falls, and the formation of intracellular polysaccharides takes place in bacteria. Bacteria then produce extracellular dextran, levan, and possibly glycogen.

A. T. Brown has suggested that four general aspects of dietary carbohydrate activities and use by oral bacteria are important to the role of bacteria in the formation of dental plaque and caries. These four important areas are:[16]

1. Dietary carbohydrate conversion to adhesive bacterial extracellular polymers.

2. Bacterial intracellular storage polysaccharides.

3. Bacterial extracellular storage polysaccharides.

4. Use of carbohydrates as fermentable energy (ATP) sources by plaque microorganisms.

This is illustrated in Figure 10–3. These four areas are discussed briefly.

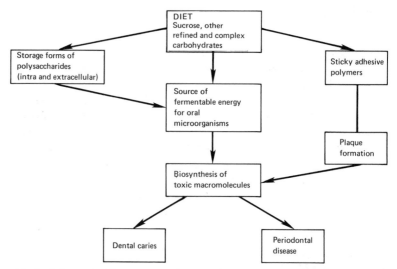

Figure 10–3. Schematic illustration of role of dietary carbohydrates in oral disease. (From A. T. Brown. The role of dietary carbohydrates in plaque formation and oral disease. *Nutr. Rev.* 33 (1975):353–361)

Production of Adhesive Bacterial Polymers

Dietary sucrose is converted to fructose and a glucose polymer by enzymes that are commonly present in the culture supernatants of streptococci. These sugars are then converted by bacterial action to the extracellular polysaccharides, the principal ones being levan and dextran. These may adhere to the enamel surface or aid in the cohesion of the streptococci.

Increased surcrose intake enhances the production of extracellular polysaccharides and results in increased plaque formation.[17] Conversely, it has been demonstrated that decreased sucrose intake may result in reduced plaque and caries formation.[18]

Intracellular and Extracellular Storage Polysaccharides

Dietary carbohydrates serve as substrates for the synthesis of intracellular and extracellular bacterial polysaccharides. They provide fermentable sources of energy within dental plaque, thus serving as reserve sources of energy in periods of nutritional stress.

The plaque matrix probably functions as the major nutrient source for plaque organisms. It is thought that sucrose has relatively easy passage into the deeper layers.[8]

Use of Carbohydrates As Fermentable Energy Sources by Plaque Microorganisms

One of the most important roles of dietary carbohydrates in plaque formation is their capacity to serve as fermentable energy sources for oral microorganisms. Most dietary carbohydrates can be metabolized and contribute to plaque formation by supporting the synthesis of toxic materials, of enzymes that produce adhesive polymers, or through the production of fermentation products from energy metabolism.

Direct Action on Enamel

Several investigators have suggested that sucrose may act to directly dissolve enamel and thus lead to the development of caries without the intervention of bacteria.[19,20] This work is controversial, and others have concluded that direct interaction of sucrose in enhancing caries development is unlikely.[21]

HUMAN POPULATION STUDIES

Differences in rates of prevalence of dental caries are on the order of at least sixtyfold. A. L. Russell suggested that such variations are related to remoteness in time and in location. For example, the ancient Egyptians rarely had caries. Modern-day populations exhibiting low prevalence rates of dental caries usually come from isolated areas of the world or from areas in which the habits and life-styles of the modern, industrialized populations have not intruded.[22]

Epidemiologically, a relationship between national sugar consumption and dental caries has been noted. For instance, A. L. Russell reported that 20-to-24-year-old-civilians living in countries in the Near East and the Far East who usually consumed approximately 6–19 kg of sugar per capita annually experienced a decay rate of 0.6–5.0 teeth. In contrast, among South American natives where the consumption of sugar varied from 23–44 kg per capita annually, the decay rates ranged from 8.4–12.6 teeth.[22]

A number of surveys have demonstrated significantly increased dental caries incidence in Eskimos and African tribesmen who changed from their traditional food habits (typically low in sugar) to diets containing modern refined foods and sugars. The natives in Tristan da Cunha have been cited as another example of the adverse effects of increased consumption of refined foodstuffs. In 1938, the diet there consisted of potatoes and fish, but no sugar. No decay in a first permanent molar was found in individuals under the age of 20. However, by 1962, when the average consumption of sugar in Tristan da Cunha was a pound per week per capita, the comparable age group demonstrated that 50 per cent of their first permanent molars were carious.[23]

Studies by the ICNND during the decade of the 1960s found no consistent relationship between caries and nutritional status, but they did report a relationship between national levels of sugar consumption and the incidence of dental caries.[22] However, there are evidences of dental caries among populations who have not used sugar.[24] Further, sugar added to typical diets of native Naurua children reportedly had little effect on the incidence of caries, which, over a generation, remained low.[25] On the other hand, some populations, such as those of Easter Island, evidence high caries prevalence rates though their diets are typically low in sugar and sweets.[26]

Clearly, the relationship between sugar and dental caries is complex and multifactorial. The food and refined sugar shortages that were characteristic of various populations during the two world wars provided a basis for investigating the relationship between decreased sugar consumption and dental caries. G. Toverud found that between-meal candy consumption almost disappeared in Norway during these periods.[27] The incidence of caries decreased during wartime, not only in Norway but also in Japan, England, and other countries. Although some have suggested that this was the result of the development of teeth with increased resistance to decay,[28] others attributed the effects to the reduction in sugar intake.[29] There is considerable agreement that the variable that determined the incidence of caries was the level of sugar used during the posteruptive teeth experiences.[30]

Numerous other studies have demonstrated the benefit of sensible eating habits on oral health. T. Grenby and G. Eikrem, for example, demonstrated that a low-calorie sweetener used in place of sucrose in tea and coffee and on breakfast cereals and the like was effective in reducing dental plaque and caries, as compared with the use of sucrose.[31]

A longer-term study was conducted on men in the Antarctic who lived in isolated areas where the dietary patterns could be controlled. A. Fry and T. Grenby reported results of a study of plaque formation in 19 men over two 14-week periods; one period involved the use of the usual diet containing sucrose; and the second period involved the use of a low-sucrose diet containing glucose syrup substituted for the sucrose. After 10 to 12 weeks on the latter diet, the plaque on teeth was significantly reduced over that on the ordinary sucrose diet.[18]

J. Hix and T. O'Leary studied the relationship between caries, oral hygiene status, and fermentable carbohydrate intake. Analysis of the dietary history information from a total of 244 subjects revealed a significant relationship between root surface caries and the number of fermentable carbohydrate exposures per week.[32]

Other investigators have studied the effect of a marked reduction in sugar intake on caries incidence. One such study under the direction of H. Becks at the University of California used dietary counseling with special diet plans and recommendations for groups of individuals with rampant caries. Progress was followed by studying changes in the *Lactobacillus acidophilus* counts. The general dietary recommendations consisted of restrictions of sugar, jam, jelly, syrup, honey, and the like, with substitutions of meat, eggs, vegetables, milk, and so on. For comparative purposes, a study was made on another group of subjects with rampant caries who did not receive the dietary counseling and restrictions. The counseled group had significantly reduced incidence of caries, which was maintained for periods of up to 10 years.[33]

A. Templeman, in an Australian study, noted that the use of a restricted carbohydrate diet resulted in improved dental health in 127 patients who were followed for a five-week period.[34] Many similar findings have been noted by clinicians in unpublished observations.

Other population studies have demonstrated that children living in institutions have lower caries rates than children of the same age living with their families.[27] The low incidence of caries among institutionalized children appears to occur among children receiving nutritionally adequate or inadequate diets. It has been suggested that this is related to the reduced intake of between-meal sweet snack foods.[27] Diabetic children also often have a low prevalence of caries. It is possible that this is related to their low sugar intake.[35]

To investigate the relationship between diet and dental caries, the Vipeholm Dental Caries Study was conducted in institutionalized children. The institutional diet offered little sugar and was of good nutritional quality; few between-meal snacks were allowed, except as allowed for in the experimental design. The incidence of caries in the children studied was low.

Over a period of five years, sugar was offered in bread, in solution, and in candy such as caramels, toffees, and chocolates. The bread was offered in meals and the candy was given between meals. Results of this study indicated that the sugar in bread and in solution at meals was not responsible for any significant increase in dental caries beyond that found in the control group but that candy, when fed between meals, caused appreciable increases in dental caries. The authors made a number of conclusions, among them the following:[36]

1. Sugar consumption can result in increased caries.

2. The risk of sugar increasing the development of caries is intensified if the sugar is sticky in form and if it is consumed between meals.

3. Sugar hazard to the teeth is great if the form of sugar eaten tends to be retained on teeth surfaces.

4. Individuals vary widely in their susceptibility to caries.

5. When the cariogenic foods are removed from the diet, the increased caries activity resulting from such foods also tends to disappear.

6. Caries may develop in the absence of natural sugars and total dietary carbohydrates.

In addition, the study suggested that there may be a threshold for sugar consumption as consumption below this level may not result in clinical evidence of caries. Such a threshold level varies tremendously among individuals.

The Vipeholm Dental Caries Study is not without its critics. M. Malm, for example, noted that the "sticky sweets" consumed by participants were composed not only of sucrose but of other sugars as well (i.e., maltose, monosaccharides and dextrins, and lactose). The actual amount of sucrose consumed was less than half of the total sugar. M. Malm suggested that the study design aimed to keep a combination of various sugars in contact with the teeth for a longer period of time than would be the case in ordinary candy consumption.[37]

A number of researchers have found positive relationships between dental caries and consumption of high sugar foods, whereas others have reported conflicting results, some of which are summarized in Table 10-1.[38-51]

Many explanations could be given for the variation in data. One factor could be that, with retrospective studies, dental caries prevalence (resulting from a lifetime of dietary influences as well as of other influences) might not necessarily demonstrate a significant relationship to specific dietary factors in the short time period of study.

Table 10-1

Studies Researching Relationship Between Sugar Consumption and Dental Caries

Population	Study Design	Results	Reference

958 Caucasian 3rd grade children from Minneapolis	Personal interviews for diet information. Analyzed and related to DMF:
	  1. Confection counting
	  2. Exposure counting
	  3. Oral retention
	  4. Estimate of "hidden sugars"
	  5. used 24 hour recall
		No significant relationship between sucrose containing food consumption and DMF teeth in both mealtime and between-meal period.	Bagramian et al., 1974[40]

143 adolescents	Studied relationship between frequency of eating various snack foods and increment in caries.	Negative correlation between increased DMF teeth and frequency of eating apples, fruit juice and sugarless gum; positive association between DMF teeth and chocolate candy.	Clancy et al., 1977[41]
Hawaiian school children	Studied relationship between plaque accumulation and diet.	Positive relation between plaque and foods of high sucrose content and high "stickiness." No relationship between plaque and dental caries.	Chung et al., 1977[42]
1266 secondary school children	Caries in children from schools serving sweets in canteens compared to caries in those attending schools where no sweets were available in canteens.	Children attending school with canteens where sweets were available had higher caries incidence than those in schools without canteens.	Fanning et al., 1969[43]
Children on Island of Lewis in Scotland (1937) with followup 30 years later	No significant difference in sugar intake during 30 years — increase in refined foods; decrease in fish; increase in meat.	Significant increase in dental caries in both urban and rural areas.	Hargreaves, 1972[44]
12-14 year old children	Sugar consumption related to caries incidence.	Only those consuming more than 8 ounces of sweets and chocolates weekly evidenced more caries than those who did not.	Mansebridge, 1960[45]
Croydon primary school children	Studied relation of food and drink consumed at bedtime to caries.	16% higher caries prevalence among those who snacked at bedtime.	Pulmer, 1971[46]
234 grade 1 and 223 grade 7 children	Evaluated relationship between diet, oral hygiene and caries.	No significant correlation between diet variables and caries or oral hygiene	Richardson et al., 1977[47]

Studies Researching Relationship Between Sugar Consumption and Dental Caries *(continued)*

Population	Study Design	Results	Reference
Greek children	Consumption of 5 sticks regular Wrigley's gum for 3 years related to oral health.	No significant harmful effects on oral health from such gum chewing.	Slack, 1972[48]
Lincoln Dental Caries study — 567 mentally subnormal patients of state school	12 oz of aciditated carbonated beverages consumed daily by children for 3 yrs.	No significant increase in caries except where incremental caries scores were analyzed by surfaces.	Steinberg et al., 1972[49]
783 children aged 4–5	1 day diet sample surveyed between-meal consumption of sweets.	Positive correlation between sugar sweetened snacks and dental caries.	Weiss and Tritnart, 1960[50]
200 Indianapolis children aged 5–13	Related total sugar & between-meal sugar intake to DMF scores. Analyzed a week's food intake.	Mean daily sugar intake was 141 g. Between-meal sugar was 47 g. Minimal correlation between DMF scores and total sugar, but high relation between DMF scores and between-meals sugar intake.	Zita et al., 1950[51]

A more valid study would be to follow subjects longitudinally and study the relationship of dental caries to diet. Another factor relates to the possibility that the diets of modern North American children may include refined carbohydrates to such a level that it would be almost impossible to identify individuals who have absolutely low intake. At the average high levels of sucrose intake, it may be very difficult to demonstrate differences in caries experience in a relatively homogeneous group as a function of sucrose consumption.

BREAKFAST CEREALS

Because of the recent increase in the production, availability, consumption, and advertising of presweetened cereals, there has been considerable interest in studying their cariogenicity. Investigations into the relationship between their consumption and dental decay in humans have not demonstrated any increase in caries from the consumption of presweetened, as opposed to nonsweetened, cereals.[52–54]

A significant positive relationship between cereals and dental caries has been reported in animals.[55] Thus, it has been suggested that the variations in experimental results may be influenced by the degree of exposure to the cereals. In the animals studied by J. H. Shaw, cereals constituted a significant part of their diet, whereas in the human studies, the cereals were fed at one meal daily, with milk.

Animal studies are not strictly applicable to humans, as there are significant differences. For example, there are differences in the composition of the saliva, in the shape and composition of the teeth, in tooth formation and development, as well as in diet composition and eating habits. All these factors must be considered in extrapolating the results of animal studies to humans.

Table 10-2 summarizes the salient features of three well-publicized studies investigating the relationship between the consumption of presweetened cereals and human dental caries. These reports have been subjected to severe criticism on the basis of their study design and the interpretation of results.[56,57] A closer look at the methodologies employed by these studies illustrates the weakness in experimental design and the resulting difficulty in accepting the conclusions of the researchers.

The study by S. Finn and J. Jamison is available only in abstract, thus making an interpretation of the study difficult.[52]

In the R. L. Glass and S. Fleisch study, mothers of participating children ordered types of cereals that were supplied by the Kellogg Company. Annual totals of the boxes of various types of cereals delivered to each family were divided by the number of family members to estimate the average consumption by type for each participant. There was a clear lack of knowledge about the type or amount of cereals that each individual subject consumed, although some attempt was made to ascertain food patterns through the use of the nutritional history of participants.[54]

On this admittedly somewhat weak data on food consumption, the au-

Table 10-2

Relationship between Consumption of Presweetened Cereals and Human Dental Caries

Population	Design	Results	Reference
600 children aged 6-13	Children divided into three groups; all ate basic breakfast plus one of following: sweetened cereal, raisins and juice, nonready-sweetened cereal with added buffer.	Under study conditions presweetened cereal did not produce greater caries incidence than other breakfasts.	(52)
375 adolescents	Permissive diet study including various cereals in self-selected diets. Other sources of sugar in diet not considered. Compared ready-to-eat cereal effects with noncereal effects.	No significant difference in caries with those reportedly eating presweetened cereals and those eating other breakfasts.	(53)
979 children aged 7-11	Different types of cereals ordered by children's mothers. Children given choice of presweetened or regular cereals or other types of breakfasts.	No significant difference, nor consistent pattern of variation between those eating various amounts of cereal, of either type, relative to caries.	(54)

thors of the study made assumptions about whether cereals were consumed in large or small amounts, and then related this to the incidence of dental caries. Other sources of sugar in the diet were not considered in the analysis of the results. Further, a control group used for comparison also had access to regular and presweetened cereals purchased at the store. The amounts of cereal consumption by the control group were not indicated in the report.

In the N. H. Rowe et al. study, cereals provided by General Mills were delivered to homes of participants who were "instructed that adherence to a rigid schedule for eating the study cereals was not required." On the basis of cereals delivered to participants, correlates with dental caries were made. Other dietary factors, and other cereals not supplied by the study, as well as the possibility that other family members may have eaten the study cereal, were not considered in the statistical analyses from which the conclusions were drawn. The authors acknowledged these weaknesses and suggested that telephone interviews with parents, as well as "good rapport" with the participants who were interrogated annually and the "candidness of children at this age," minimized errors in this regard.[53]

To clarify other factors involved in the cariogenicity of breakfast cereals, S. Katz et al. conducted a variety of studies in which they investigated the amount of sugar retained by teeth, the ability of cereals to induce plaque formation, the ability of cereals to induce acid formation, buffering capacity, and the ability of various cereals to induce caries formation on extracted teeth under mouth-simulation conditions. The results of the study indicated that various breakfast cereals differ markedly relative to the factors studied. Retention of sugar from cereals was not dependent upon cereal sugar content but upon other intrinsic factors that determined cereal adhesion to the teeth. The amount of plaque formation did not correlate with the sugar present in cereal, regardless of whether sugar was added during processing or before the test. Although all the cereals were similar in their ability to induce acid formation, they were markedly different in their ability to neutralize acids. The only factor that correlated directly with caries formation was the buffering capacity of the cereals.[58]

To further elucidate the relationship between sucrose consumption and dental caries, B. Bibby et al. studied 180 snack foods and beverages. They noted the following:[59]

1. The degree of enamel destroyed by fermenting foods was not directly related to sugar content or to the amount of fermentation acids produced.

2. There was an absence of relation between acid production and demineralization by acid candies and other fruit-flavored snack foods.

3. High-sugar-content foods were often more rapidly removed from the teeth and mouth than were those containing starch or other components, such as breads, cakes, cookies, or sticky candies.

4. Other, noncarbohydrate food components could either enhance or inhibit the development of dental caries.

RELATIVE CARIOGENICITY OF VARIOUS FOODSTUFFS[60]

We still lack knowledge about which foods are the most or the least cariogenic. Methods used to determine relative cariogenicity of various foodstuffs include

Caries production in animals.

Acid formed after fermentation in the mouth.

Demineralization enamel in saliva or bacterial culture.

Food retained on the teeth after food consumption.

In vivo softening of enamel with artificial plaque.

Evaluation of caries produced in an artificial mouth that resembles a human mouth.

Despite these various methods, none has gained the universal approval of all researchers. Each has its drawbacks, making it unlikely that one single method will provide acceptable information about the relative cariogenicity of various foods. Thus, until the relative importance of factors influencing caries production (i.e., acid production, demineralization, retention, and plaque acidity) can be determined, it is unlikely that we will have definite information about the relative cariogenicity of different foods.

Tables 10-3, 10-4, 10-5, and 10-6 and Figure 10-4 indicate the relative importance of various foodstuffs in the development of caries-producing factors according to different methods of assessment. As can be seen, the methods do not all agree. For example, the figures for acid production vary greatly from what might be expected on the basis of the sugar content of the foods. This is very obvious by noting that almost no acid is produced from a hard candy sucker that is 99 per cent carbohydrate, but the highest production results from potato chips, which contain 54 per cent soluble carbohydrate. Evaluating the cariogenicity on the basis of carbohydrate retention, we would most likely rate rock candy as low, but rye bread as high. These considerations demonstrate that, with the current state of knowledge, we must exert considerable caution when attempting to classify foods as high- or low-caries-producing foods.

SUMMARY — INFLUENCE OF DIETARY CARBOHYDRATES ON CARIES DEVELOPMENT

The following factors appear to play an important role in the development of caries, in addition to the actual amount of sugar consumed:[58]

1. Physical consistency of the food in which sugar is present. This then determines sugar retention on the tooth. Solid foods appear to be more cariogenic than liquid foods.

2. Circumstances under which foods are consumed. Ingestion of sugar at

Table 10–3
Acid Produced and Enamel Dissolved by Foods Fermented by Salivary Bacteria

Food	Fermentation Acid (ml 0.05M NaOH)	Enamel Dissolved (mg)
Lemon sucker	0	7.11
Raisins	1.95	2.06
Apple	0.78	1.03
Banana	2.62	0.92
Coca-Cola*	0.16	0.90
Rice pudding	1.26	0.78
White bread	1.35	0.74
Whole wheat bread	2.06	0.58
Potato chips	3.78	0.57
Chocolate cake	1.96	0.56
Chocolate coconut candy	1.88	0.48
Peanut brittle	1.61	0.42
Plain cracker	1.52	0.38
Milk	0.17	0.35
Caramel	0.88	0.33
Chocolate graham cracker	1.64	0.31
Jelly candy	0.37	0.29
Sugar breakfast cereal	1.40	0.26
Cream cookie	1.20	0.23
Plain breakfast cereal	2.07	0.18

*Calculated from control value for 2% sucrose = 1.
Source: E. A. Sweeney. *The Food That Stays: An Update on Nutrition, Diet, Sugar, and Caries.* New York: Medcom Inc., 1977.

Table 10–4
Carbohydrate Retained in Mouth 15 Minutes after Eating Various Foods

High Retention (mg CHO)		Low Retention (mg CHO)	
Plain cookie	14.21	Milk	3.66
Angel food cake	11.39	Sucker (cherry)	3.60
Bagel	11.08	Coca-Cola®	3.56
JuJube®	10.71	Chocolate graham crackers	3.43
Chocolate cake	10.63	Peanuts	3.29
Cracker (unsalted)	10.45	Orange juice	2.80
White bread	10.12	Rock candy	2.69
Rye bread	9.74	7 Up®	2.44
Clear mint candy	9.40	Sweetees® (USA, sorbitol)	2.40
Graham crackers	9.02	Trident® gum	2.00

Source: See Table 10–3.

mealtimes is believed to be less cariogenic than between-meal consumption of the same foods.

3. Frequency of eating. Consumption of a given amount of sugar food at one time is less cariogenic than consuming the same amount of food, or even less food, at various times throughout the day.

4. The ability of a sugary food to induce the formation of dental plaque.

Table 10–5

Length of Time of Acid Formation from Foods in Dental Plaque

Food	Food pH	pH Depression*
Angel food cake	5.15	4.48
Jelly candy	5.04	4.45
Orange sucker	2.92	4.30
Apple pie	4.10	4.17
Whole wheat bread	5.25	3.68
Chocolate graham cracker	7.13	3.66
Chocolate cake	8.20	3.66
Sugar breakfast cereal	4.85	3.35
Coca-Cola®	2.65	3.20
Banana	5.7	2.94
Plain cracker	7.65	2.87
Caramel	6.17	2.85
Stick chewing gum	6.08	2.55
Milk chocolate	6.27	2.35
Potato chips	6.15	2.04
Dark chocolate	5.55	1.98
Apple	4.55	1.80
Milk	6.6	0.75
Sugarless sucker	3.13	0.66
Peanuts	6.55	0.09
Sugarless stick gum	5.8	0.46

*As sum of pH depressions for 30 minutes.
Source: See Table 10–3.

Table 10–6

Comparative Depths of Carious Lesions Produced by Foods in Artificial Mouth (Orofax)*

Food	Proportionate Depth
Caramel	46.8
Fudge	45.0
Chocolate coconut bar	31.7
Potato chips	30.3
Graham cracker	28.6
White bread	26.7
Chocolate almond bar	26.2
Whole wheat bread	18.3
Plain breakfast cereal	18.3
Sugar breakfast cereal	18.2
Chocolate chip cookie	15.8
Dark chocolate	15.0
Sweet cookie	13.7
Ginger snaps	12.3
Fruit tart	11.2
Milk chocolate	7.5

*Proportionate values calculated from common control used in separate tests.
Source: See Table 10–3.

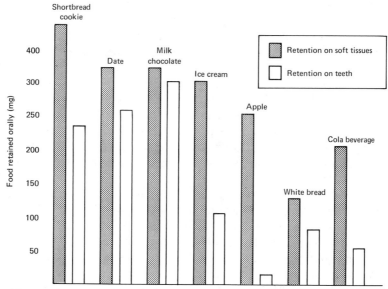

Figure 10-4. Comparison of retention of carbohydrate foods on teeth and soft tissues. (From E. A. Sweeney. *The Food That Stays: An Update on Nutrition, Diet, Sugars and Caries* New York: Medcom, Inc, 1977.)

5. The presence or absence of certain chemical factors within the sugar-containing foods. For instance, phosphates have been suggested to have cariostatic properties.

6. Genetic predisposition of the individual affects the development of dental caries.

The production of dental caries is the result of factors that can interact in varying degrees, in varying ways, and differently according to the individual host. Thus, it is very difficult to assign cariogenic characteristics to a given food.

OTHER DIETARY INFLUENCES ON DENTAL CARIES

Almost all dietary components, fats, protein, vitamins, and minerals have been studied in relation to the development of dental caries. Data from animals and from epidemiological studies suggest that maternal diets during lactation, or during gestation and lactation, that are greatly restricted in protein can affect the offspring by impairing optimal tooth development and the function of salivary glands, both of which enhance caries development.[61]

Similarly, vitamin A deficiency adversely affects tooth development and the salivary glands, whereas vitamin D deficiency or an abnormal calcium-phosphorous ratio may result in defective enamel mineralization. There appears to be a positive benefit resulting from diet supplementation with vitamin D, particularly in children under the age of 10 years. However, several studies have reported negative results with vitamin D supplementation in children over the age of 10.[62]

Some studies of individuals suffering from malnutrition, particularly pellagra, a vitamin B (niacin) deficiency disease, have found a lower than expected incidence of dental caries. Explanations that have been suggested for this decrease include the higher buffer capacity of saliva of malnourished individuals and the reduced consumption of highly refined carbohydrate foods by those who are malnourished. Thus, it is not possible to be certain if the reduced caries incidence is the result of a nutrient deficiency or of the general lack of highly cariogenic foods. Positive benefits from vitamin B_6 supplementation have been suggested but remain to be confirmed.[62]

Lack of vitamin C results in tooth demineralization in guinea pigs, whereas abnormal fluid accumulation in the pulp and abnormal dentin formation has been noted in vitamin C deficient adults. Vitamin E deficiency has produced edema and atrophy of the enamel tooth cellular layer and abnormal pigmentation of tooth enamel in rats, but its effect in humans has not been clarified.

There is considerable support for the value of specific phosphate supplements as an aid to reduce dental caries activity. However, not all phosphate salts are effective. A number of studies have added various phosphate supplements to flour, bread, sugar, chewing gum, and breakfast cereals. Although positive effects have been reported,[63,64] others have noted that the addition of phosphate to the diet did not prevent caries activity.[65]

G. Stanton has suggested that the calcium-to-phosphorous ratio associated with few or no caries was approximately 0.55.[66] G. V. Mann reexamined the data from the ICNND survey of Alaskan Eskimos. He noted that, in villages in which the populations did less trading with Western civilizations and in which caries development was low, the calcium-to-phosphorous ratio of the diet was approximately 0.55. However, in southern villages, in which Western eating habits had been more common and in which tooth decay was more prevalent, the calcium-to-phosphorous ratio was much higher.[67]

Low calcium-to-phosphorous ratios have been suggested as possible causes of the development of periodontal diseases in Western man.[68] These researchers suggest that periodontal disease is the result of a deficiency of dietary calcium and/or an excess of dietary phosphorous. To maintain adequate serum calcium levels in the presence of inadequate dietary calcium, a nutritional secondary hyperparathyroidism results in the release of calcium from the alveolar bone. This eventually results in a marked loss of bone structure.

I. Krook et al. support this theory by noting that most commonly consumed foods in the Western diet (with the possible exception of dairy foods) contain up to 20 times more phosphorous than calcium. Thus, many in the population either do not consume sufficient calcium, or their diets do not contain the recommended calcium-to-phosphorous ratio of 2 to 1.[68] Further, calcium therapy has been reported to be effective in the treatment of periodontal disease.[69] This hypothesis is still controversial.

Diets restricted in manganese and iron appear to result in abnormal tooth development and, ultimately, to an increased likelihood of caries in rats. However, R. Glass et al. related the mineral content of the water supply to caries development and suggested that higher levels of calcium, magnesium, molybdenum, and vanadium were inversely related to caries, whereas higher concentrations of copper, iron, and manganese were directly related to the incidence of caries.[70] Selenium has been termed a "caries-enhancing trace element."[10] Strontium has received great attention because of its hypothesized relation to dental caries.[71] Fluoride appears to be the nutrient whose presence during tooth growth and maturation exerts the most significant beneficial effect on later resistance to dental caries. The presence of fluoride in drinking water at a level of approximately one part per million (ppm) during as well as after tooth development has been found to retard dental caries, especially those on smooth tooth surfaces, by up to 65 per cent.[72]

Fluoride influences caries development through a variety of mechanisms. Enamel formed in a fluoride environment resists dissolution in acid mediums more than enamel formed without fluoride. Fluoride may promote remineralization of early carious areas, and may influence the type of extracellular polysaccharide produced by bacteria, as well as the synthesis of intracellular polysaccharide and the capacity of microorganisms to form acid from sugar.[72] Fluoride seems to exert its effect as it becomes incorporated into the hydroxyapatite crystal in the enamel. Before the teeth have erupted, fluoride is incorporated into bone as mineralization occurs. After the teeth have erupted, fluoride can be topically applied so it is absorbed whereby the fluoride content of the outer layers of enamel is increased. Thus, fluoride protects against the action of bacteria by impairing demineralization and enhancing remineralization.[73,74]

The fetus needs relatively little fluoride and does not profit from fluoride intake from the mother because fluoride does not cross the placenta in significant amounts.[73] At birth, fluoride is readily absorbed from the diet. The optimal time for fluoride ingestion, as it relates to tooth development, appears to be from birth to the age of 16.[11] Minute amounts of fluoride taken during the first 12 years of life (when dentition and enamel of permanent teeth are formed) may reduce dental caries by as much as 65 per cent.

Fluoride appears to be most beneficial when it is ingested at levels of 1.5 mg to 2.5 mg per day; intakes of 5 mg per day may result in mottled enamel. Fluoride ingestion may reduce caries development up to 60 per cent during tooth development, and topical application of fluoride can reduce the development of caries by about 20 per cent. Apparently, these benefits are additive.[11]

At present, fluoride is added to drinking water in many cities and communities in the United States to reduce dental caries. Many respected public health and medical organizations, including the American Medical Association, the American Dental Association, and the American Academy of Pediatrics recommend fluoridation of the water. The most beneficial level of fluoride is 0.7–1.2 ppm of drinking water. Fluoride in excess of 1.5 ppm may result in discoloring and mottling of enamel (fluorosis).[74-77]

The relationship between dental caries and the extent of fluorosis in different communities, relative to the fluoride content of the drinking water, is illustrated in Figure 10-5, which shows the results of a study of 7,000 children aged 12 to 19 years old. The average number of decayed, missing, and filled teeth went from 8 at low (0.1 ppm) fluoride concentrations to less than 3 at higher levels of fluoride.[2,77] Fluorosis remains minimal as fluoride in drinking water increases to 1.0 ppm, but with additional fluoride, fluorosis rapidly increases.

In 1975, about 177 million of the 213 million people in the United States used public drinking supplies, and about 105 million, or 59 per cent, of these people had access to fluoridated water supplies of at least 0.7 ppm fluoride.[2]

Many individuals who live in outlying or rural areas are not able to obtain fluoridated water supplies. Topical applications of fluoride may be effective in reducing the caries in these populations. Researchers are also investigating the use of single doses of fluoride, for example, in pills or drops, for populations that are not able to obtain fluoridated water.

Fluoride intakes of young infants may vary considerably because of the different fluoride concentrations in various milks and formulas. Although cow's and mother's milks are generally low in fluoride, often containing less than 0.02 ppm, formulas have a wide range of fluoride concentrations. It has been shown, that depending upon diet, an infant 1 to 4 weeks of age may take as much as 0.32 mg fluoride daily, a level that increases so that by the age of 6 months, the infant may be receiving 1.23 mg fluoride daily. Thus, some experts suggest that fluoride supplementation of infants be delayed until the age of 6 months.[60]

At present, it is not recommended that infants less than 6 months of age be given fluoride supplements. Between 6 and 18 months of age, the recommended daily dose of fluoride is 0.25 mg; between 18 and 36 months the recommended daily dose is 0.5 mg; and the maximum recommended daily dose between 3 and 6 years is 0.75 mg.[2]

The maximum recommended level of fluoride supplementation for those over age 6 is 1.0 mg per day.[2] Fluoride supplementation depends upon the fluoride content of the water supply. Table 10-7 summarizes the recommended fluoride supplementation for infants and children.

Figure 10-5. Relation between fluoride content of drinking water; average number of decayed, missing, and filled teeth; and index of fluorosis. triangles: cases of decayed, missing or filled teeth; circles; cases of fluorosis. (From H. C. Hodge and F. A. Smith: Some public health aspects of water fluoridation. J. H. Shaw, ed., *Fluoridation as a Public Health Measure.* Washington, D.C.: AAAS, 1954, p. 7)

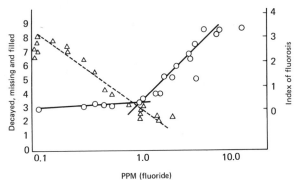

Table 10-7

Recommended Fluoride Supplementation

Fluoride Concentration of Water Supply (ppm)	Desirable Fluoride Supplementation (mg/day)				
	Age 0–6 Months	Age 6–18 Months	Age 18–36 Months	Age 3–6 Years	Age 6 Years
<0.2	0*	0.25	0.5	0.75	1.0
0.2–0.4	0*	0*	0.25	0.5	0.75
0.4–0.6	0*	0*	0	0.25	0.5
0.6–0.8	0*	0*	0	0	0.25
>0.8	0*	0*	0	0	0**

*0.25 for fully breastfed infants.
**In this age group, the hazard of fluorosis is low and some additional protection will probably be afforded by fluoride supplementation. However, fluoride supplementation is probably not desirable when drinking water provides more than 1.1 ppm.
Source: S. Foman. *Nutritional Disorders of Children: Prevention, Screening, and Follow-up*, Publ. No. (HSA) 77-5104. Rockville, Md.: U.S. Department of Health, Education, and Welfare, 1977 reprint.

CONCLUSION

The prevention of dental caries must logically involve an attack upon causative factors in all three components of the ecological triad. This involves the control of the agents producing caries, the increased host resistance, and the reduction of caries potential in the environment. The development of dental caries is the result of numerous different influences. Many unsolved questions relate to the etiology of dental caries, but current knowledge is sufficient to suggest that the methods available for attacking the problem of dental caries include the following:

1. Restrict sugar and sugar-rich foods between meals.
   a. If there is a choice between sweets in liquid or solid form, select the liquid.
   b. Restrict sweets that are sticky or will dissolve slowly.
   c. If sweets are consumed between meals, brush, floss, and rinse the teeth.
2. Add caries-inhibiting chemicals to food.
3. Make use of fluoride benefits that are available to the population.
4. Improve methods of dental hygiene.

REFERENCES

1. Clark, L. *Stay Young Longer*. New York: Pyramid Books, 1974.
2. Foman, S. *Nutritional Disorders of Children: Prevention, Screening, and Follow-up*, Publ. No. (HSA) 77-5104. Rockville, Md.: U.S. Department of Health, Education, and Welfare, 1977 reprint.

3. Owen, G. M., K. M. Kram, P. J. Garry, J. E. Lowe, and A. H. Lubin. A study of nutritional status of preschool children in the United States, 1968–1970. *Pediatrics* 53 (1974): 597.

4. U.S. Department of Health, Education, and Welfare. *Ten-State Nutrition Survey*, Publ. No. (HSM) 72-8134. Washington, D.C.: Government Printing Office, 1972.

5. Downer, M. C. Dental caries and periodontal disease in girls of different ethnic groups: A comparison in a London secondary school. *Brit. Dent. J.* 128 (1970): 379.

6. Federal Trade Commission. *FTC Staff Report on Television Advertising to Children.* Washington, D.C.: Government Printing Office, February 19, 1978.

7. American Academy of Pediatrics, Committee on Nutrition. Fluoride as a nutrient. *Pediatrics* 49 (1972): 456.

8. Makinen, K. K. Sugars and the formation of dental plaque, in H. L. Sipple and K. W. McNutt, eds., *Sugars in Nutrition.* New York: Academic Press, 1974, p. 645.

9. Finn, S. G., and R. B. Glass. Sugar and dental decay. *World Rev. Nutr. and Diet.* 22 (1975): 304.

10. Nutrition and oral health. *Dairy Council Digest* 49 (May–June 1978).

11. DePaola, D. P., and M. C. Alfano. Diet and oral health. *Nutr. Today* 12 (1977): 6.

12. Makinen, K. K. The role of sucrose and other sugars in the development of dental caries: A review. *Int. Dent. J.* 22 (1972): 363.

13. Newbrun, E. Sucrose, the arch criminal of dental caries. *J. Dent. Child* 36 (1969): 13–22.

14. Bahn, A. N. Microbial potential in the etiology of periodontal disease. *J. Periodont.* 41 (1970): 603–610.

15. Littleton, N. W., C. H. Carter, and R. T. Kelley. Studies of oral health in persons nourished by stomach tube. I. Changes in the pH of plaque material after the addition of sucrose. *J. Am. Dent. Assoc.* 74 (1967): 119–123.

16. Brown, A. T. The role of dietary carbohydrates in plaque formation and oral disease. *Nutr. Rev.* 33 (1975): 353–361.

17. Van Houte, J. Relationship between carbohydrate intake and polysaccharide-storing microorganisms in dental plaque. *Arch. Oral Biol.* 9 (1964): 91–93.

18. Fry, A. J., and T. H. Grenby. The effects of reduced sucrose intake on the formation and composition of dental plaque in a group of men in the Antarctic. *Arch. Oral Biol.* 17 (1972): 873.

19. Eggers-Lura, N. The Nonacid Complexing and Phosphorylating Theory of Dental Caries. New York: Holbaek, 1967.

20. Blackwell, R. Q., L. McMillan, and L. S. Fosdick. Sucrose retardation of acid etching in dental enamel: An electron-microscopic study. *J. Dent. Res.* 46 (1961): 16.

21. Jenkins, G. N. Enamel protective factors in food. *J. Dent. Res.* 49 (1970): suppl. to no. 6, 1318.

22. Russell, A. L. World epidemiology and oral health, in American Association for the Advancement of Science, *Environmental Variables in Oral Disease*, Publ. No. 81: 21–39. Washington, D.C., 1966.

23. Holloway, P. J., et al. Dental disease in Tristan da Cunha. *Brit. Dent. J.* 15 (1961): 19.

24. Anonymous. Discovery of prehistoric cemetery remains reveals Ohio Indians with arthritis and bad teeth. *J. Am. Dent. Assoc.* 77 (1968): 792–793.

25. Cadell, P. B. Dental conditions amongst native Nauruans. *Aust. Dent. J.* 4 (1959): 389–394.
26. Taylor, A. G. Dental conditions among the inhabitants of Easter Island. *J. Canad. Dent. Assoc.* 32 (1966): 286–290.
27. Toverud, G. *A survey of the Literature of Dental Caries*, Publ. No. 225. Washington, D.C.: National Academy of Sciences, 1952.
28. Sognnaes, R. F. Analysis of war-time reduction of dental caries in European children, with special regard to observations in Norway. *Am. J. Dis. Child.* 75 (1948): 792–821.
29. Schulerud, A. *Dental Caries and Nutrition during War-time in Norway.* Oslo: Fabritus and Sonners, 1950.
30. Toverud, G., L. Rubal, and D. G. Wiehl. The influence of war and postwar conditions on the teeth of Norwegian schoolchildren. *Milbank Mem. Fund Quart.* 39 (1961): 489–539.
31. Grenby, T. H., and G. Eikrem. Dental plaque formation in relation to type of carbohydrate. *Proc. Nutr. Soc.* 33 (1974): 24A.
32. Hix, J. O., and T. J. O'Leary. The relationship between cemental caries, oral hygiene status, and fermentable carbohydrate intake. *J. Periodontol.* 47 (1976): 398.
33. Becks, H. Carbohydrate restriction in the prevention of dental caries using the L.a. count as one index. *J. Cal. St. Dent. Assoc.* 26 (1950): 53.
34. Templeman, A. J. The dietary control of dental caries. *Aust. Dent. J.* 9 (1964): 163.
35. Bibby, B. G. Inferences from natural occurring variation in caries prevalence. *J. Dent. Res.* 49 (1970): suppl. to no. 6, 1194.
36. Gustafson, B. E., et al. The Vipeholm dental caries study: The effect of different levels of carbohydrate intake on dental caries in 436 individuals observed for five years. *Acta Odontol. Scand.* 11 (1954): 232.
37. Malm, M. The role of sugar in modern nutrition. Marabou Symposium (suppl. no. 91) Naringsforskning, argan 17, 1973, p. 28.
38. Harris, R. Biology of the children of Hopewood House, Bowral, Australia: Observations on dental caries experience extending five years (1957–1961). *J. Dent. Res.* 42 (1963): 1387.
39. Bagramian, R. A., and A. L. Russell. Epidemiologic study of dental caries experience and between-meal eating patterns. *J. Dent. Res.* 52 (1973): 342–347.
40. Bagramian, R. A., J. Jenny, P. J. Frazier, and J. M. Proshek. Diet patterns and dental caries in third-grade U.S. children. *Community Dent. Oral Epidemiol.* 2 (1974): 208–213.
41. Clancy, K. L., et al. Snack food intake of adolescents and caries development. *J. Dent. Res.* 56 (1977): 568.
42. Chung, C. S., et al. Dental plaque and dietary intakes in schoolchildren in Hawaii. *J. Dent. Res.* 56 (1977): 11.
43. Fanning, E., T. Gotjamanos, and N. J. Vowles. Dental caries in children related to availability of sweets at school canteens. *Med. J. Aust.* 1 (1969): 1131–1132.
44. Hargreaves, J. A. Changes in diet and dental health of children living in the Scottish island of Lewis. *Caries Res.* 6 (1972): 355–376.
45. Mansbridge, J. T. The effects of oral hygiene and sweet consumption on the prevalence of dental caries. *Brit. Dent. J.* 109 (1960): 343–348.
46. Palmer, J. D. Dietary habits at bedtime in relation to dental caries in children. *Brit. Dent. J.* 130 (1971): 288.
47. Richardson, A. S., M. A. Boyd, and R. F. Conry. A correlation study of diet, oral hygiene, and dental caries in 457 Canadian children. *Community Dent. Oral Epidemiol.* 5 (1977): 227.

48. Slack, G. I., et al. The effect of chewing gum on the incidence of dental diseases in Greek children. *Brit. Dent. J.* 133 (1972): 371–377.
49. Steinberg, A. D., S. O. Zimmerman, and M. L. Bramer. The Lincoln dental caries study. II. The effect of acidulated carbonated beverages on the incidence of dental caries. *J. Am. Dent. Assoc.* 85 (1972): 81.
50. Weiss, R. L., and A. H. Trithart. Between-meal eating habits and dental caries experience in preschool children. *Am. J. Publ. Health* 50 (1960): 1097–1104.
51. Zita, A. C., R. E. McDonald, and A. L. Andrews. Dietary habits and dental caries experience in 200 children. *J. Dent. Res.* 38 (1959): 860.
52. Finn, S. B., and J. Jamison. The relative effect of dental caries of three food supplements to the diet. *J. Dent. Res.* 48 (1969): 207 (special abstract issue).
53. Rowe, N. H., R. H. Anderson, and L. A. Wanninger. Effects of ready-to-eat breakfast cereals on dental caries experience in adolescent children: A three-year study. *J. Dent. Res.* 53 (1974): 33–36.
54. Glass, R. L., and S. Fleisch. Diet and dental caries: Dental caries incidence and the consumption of ready-to-eat cereals. *J. Am. Dent. Assoc.* 88 (1974): 807.
55. Shaw, J. H. Influence of cereal incorporation in a caries-producing diet on caries activity in rats. *J. Dent. Res.* 53 (1974): 397–401.
56. Horowitz, H. S. Caries and cereals: Letter to the editor. *J. Am. Dent. Assoc.* 89 (1974): 30–31.
57. Mellion, G. L. Presweetened cereals: Letter to the editor. *J. Am. Dent. Assoc.* 89 (1974): 767.
58. Katz, S., B. L. Olson, and C. Park. Factors related to the cariogenic potential of breakfast cereals. *Pharm. Therap. Dent.* 2 (1975): 109–131.
59. Bibby, B. G., and S. A. Mundorff. Enamel demineralization by snack foods. *J. Dent. Res.* 54 (1975): 461.
60. Sweeney, E. A. *The Food That Stays: An Update on Nutrition, Diet, Sugar, and Caries.* New York: Medcom Inc., 1977.
61. Kreitzman, S. N. Nutrition in the process of dental caries. *Dent. Clin. N. Am.* 20 (1976): 491.
62. Mandel, I. D. Effects of dietary modifications on caries in humans. *J. Dent. Res.* 49 (1970): suppl. to no. 6, 1201.
63. Carroll, R. A., G. K. Stookey, and J. C. Muhler. The clinical effectiveness of phosphate-enriched breakfast cereals on the incidence of dental caries in adults: Results after one year. *J. Am. Dent. Assoc.* 76 (1968): 564.
64. Brewer, H. E., G. K. Stookey, and J. C. Muhler. A clinical study concerning the anticariogenic effects on NaH_2PO_4-enriched breakfast cereals in institutionalized subjects: Results after two years. *J. Am. Dent. Assoc.* 80 (1970): 121.
65. Averill, H. M., and B. G. Bibby. A clinical test of additions of phospate to the diet of children. *J. Dent. Res.* 43 (1964): 1150.
66. Stanton, G. Diet and dental caries. *N. Y. St. Dent. J.* 35 (1969): 399–407.
67. Mann, G. V., et al. The health and nutritional status of Alaskan Eskimos: A survey of the Interdepartmental Committee on Nutrition for National Defense — 1958. *Am. J. Clin. Nutr.* 11 (1962): 31–76.
68. Krook, I., J. P. Whalen, G. V. Lesser, and L. Lubwak. Human periodontal disease and osteoporosis. *Cornell Vet.* 62 (1972): 371–391.
69. Alfano, M. C. Controversies, perspectives, and clinical implications of nutrition in periodontal disease. *Dent. Clin. N. Am.* 20 (1976): 519.
70. Glass, R. L., K. L. Rothman, et al. Prevalence of human dental caries and water-borne trace metals. *Arch. Oral Biol.* 18 (1973): 1099.

71. Strontium, other trace elements, and dental caries. *Nutr. Rev.* 36 (1978): 334.
72. Bowen, W. H. Dental caries. *Contem. Nutr.* 2 (1977).
73. DePaola, D. P., and M. M. Kuftinec. Nutrition in growth and development of oral tissues. *Dent. Clin. N. Am.* 20 (1976): 441.
74. Richmond, U. L. Health effects associated with water fluoridation. *J. Nutr. Educ.* 11 (1979): 63–64.
75. Dental Disease Prevention Activity, Center for Disease Control. Material cited in *Nutritional Disorders of Children: Prevention, Screening, and Follow-up*, Publ. No. (HSA) 77–5104. Rockville, Md.: U.S. Department of Health, Education, and Welfare, 1977.
76. American Dental Association. *Accepted Dental Therapeutics*, 36th ed. Chicago, 1975, p. 288.
77. Hodge, H. C., and F. A. Smith. Some public health aspects of water fluoridation, in J. H. Shaw, ed., *Fluoridation as a Public Health Measure*. Washington, D.C.: American Association for the Advancement of Science, 1954, p. 79.

11

Diet, nutrition, and other diseases (diabetes, hypertension, alcoholism)

Reader Objectives

After completing this chapter, the reader should be able to
1. List the public health significance of diabetes and hypertension.
2. Describe the possible role of dietary carbohydrates in the etiology of diabetes mellitus.
3. Describe the relationship between the development of hypertension and high sodium intakes.
4. List the dietary modifications recommended for preventing the development of diabetes and of hypertension.
5. Outline the general adverse effects of excess alcohol consumption.
6. Describe the fetal alcohol syndrome.

DIETARY INFLUENCES ON DIABETES WITH SPECIAL REFERENCE TO THE EFFECTS OF DIETARY CARBOHYDRATE

Public Health Significance

In 1974 diabetes was listed as the fifth most prominent cause of death from disease in the United States. Diabetes mellitus affects approximately 10 million individuals in the United States, 1.5 million of whom are juveniles. The prevalence of diabetes is increasing by 6 per cent annually; at this rate, a North American born today, living an average life span of 70 years, has more than a one-in-five chance of developing the disorder.[1,2] It is further estimated that by 1980 more than 10 per cent of the North American population will exhibit or have inherited the trait of diabetes.[2] In 1977 diabetes cost the nation about $6 billion in lost productivity and medical expenses — an average of $1,124 per diabetic — and this does not consider the cost of diabetic complications.[2]

Diabetics frequently experience greatly accelerated degeneration of blood vessels in many organs, which can lead to blindness, kidney failure, heart attack, stroke, gangrene in the extremities, and problems of the nervous system.[1]

Diabetics have twice the chance of succumbing to CHD than do nondiabetics. Diabetes is especially significant as a risk factor for occlusive peripheral artery disease. Female diabetics seem to be particularly vulnerable to the impact of diabetes on CHD. The processes by which diabetes exerts its effect on CHD is not firmly established. W. B. Kannel has suggested that the relationship is a function of the promotion of atherogenesis but noted that only 20–30 per cent of the impact of diabetes on cardiovascular disease can be attributed to atherogenic characteristics.[4,5]

Etiology of Diabetes

Diabetes cannot correctly be considered a single disease entity. At the least, a distinction between juvenile- and adult-onset diabetes must be made. The whole concept, etiology, and pathology of diabetes mellitus is extremely complex. It is impossible to postulate a simple cause-and-effect relationship between diet and the development of diabetes. As H. Keen has suggested, the issue is not does diet cause diabetes, but rather, is diet "one of the contributors to the heterogeneous entity that we understand as the clinical state of diabetes?"[6,7] The American Diabetes Association has suggested that improved nutritional practices in the United States could reduce the incidence of diabetes by 30 per cent.[8]

Current evidence relating nutritional factors to variations in the prevalence of juvenile diabetes is limited, but the possibility cannot be discounted. For example, as diets in Japan become more similar to those of the United States, significant increases in juvenile diabetes have occurred.

Many factors have been related to the etiology of diabetes, the most important of which include genetic factors and obesity. The degree and duration of adiposity have been most frequently and significantly related to the prevalence of adult-onset diabetes. Diabetes is rare in societies where obesity is uncommon. In addition, laboratory data support the notion that obesity is a potent risk factor in the development of diabetes. For example, excessive calorie intake and obesity are associated with insulin resistance. It has been estimated that about 75 per cent of American adult-onset diabetics are obese.[9]

It is well established that overweight adult diabetics who lose weight often enjoy improved blood glucose levels and glucose tolerances. Results of the Framingham study indicated that overweight adults were three times as prone as their normal-weight counterparts to develop diabetes, and adults who gained weight after the age of 25 had twice the probability of developing diabetes as did their normal-weight cohorts.[10]

Diabetes may also be caused by nutritional factors that damage the pancreas or impair glucose tolerance or the function of the beta cells. Such damage may result from protein deficiency, hemochromatosis (excessive iron absorption), or deficiencies of certain trace elements such as chromium, zinc, or iron. Peripheral vascular disease, high fat diets, elevated serum cholesterol levels, and high blood pressure have also been associated with diabetes.[9] Other nutritional factors currently being investigated as possible factors in the etiology of diabetes include

> intakes of sugar and refined carbohydrate products,
>
> complex carbohydrate consumption, and
>
> consumption of dietary fiber.

The following sections focus on the relationship between carbohydrate consumption and diabetes mellitus; special reference is made to dietary sugar consumption and dietary fiber consumption.

Epidemiological Studies

Epidemiological studies have suggested that dietary patterns are related to prevalence rates of diabetes. For example, Yemenite and Kurdish Jewish immigrants to Israel initially demonstrated very low prevalence rates of diabetes, but after a period of years following the usual Israeli diet, their prevalence rates significantly increased to rates approximating those of Western nations.[11] In searching for possible explanations, A. Cohen et al. noted that the diets of the immigrants contained very low levels of sucrose while they were in their native country, but, when they moved to Israel, the immigrants adopted diets that contained sugar at levels comparable to that consumed by Western populations. Thus, the relationship between sugar intake and the prevalence of diabetes was hypothesized.[11] G. D. Campbell, who reviewed dietary and diabetes prevalence data from South African Zulus, arrived at a similar conclusion.[12]

K. West et al., in studies of 13 populations in 11 countries, demonstrated a strong relationship between the prevalence of diabetes and nutritional variables.[13-16] However, there were several inconsistencies. For instance, diabetes prevalence rates in Costa Rica were similar to those in Malaysia, but sugar consumption in Costa Rica was approximately double that in Malaysia.

A review of available data on the past and current rates of diabetes in aboriginal populations of the New World (e.g., Indians, Eskimos, Polynesians, and Micronesians) also suggests that diet is strongly related to the risk of diabetes.[16] J. M. Reid et al. have noted that among Pima Indians, who have a high prevalence rate of diabetes, diabetics tended to consume less sugar than the nondiabetics.[17]

In Scotland, J. D. Baird found no relation between sugar consumption and diabetes.[18] H. Keen et al. and J. Himsworth also reported no relation between diabetes and sugar consumption in England.[6,19]

I. Prior studied the relationship between diabetes, diet, and related metabolic problems in the South Pacific. He found considerable variations in diabetes prevalence that were not adequately explained on the basis of differences in sugar consumption. Prior suggested that environmental factors play a key role in the variance of diabetes among population groups and that total calorie intake and degree of obesity may or may not be important factors.[20] Others report controversial data regarding the relationship between sugar intake and proneness to develop diabetes.[21-23]

There are a number of problems in interpreting the type of epidemiological data on which investigators such as J. Yudkin, T. L. Cleave, and others have suggested a relationship between diabetes and sugar consumption.[24,25] It is difficult to estimate national diabetes prevalence rates, and the criteria for diabetes diagnosis and prevalence estimations varies from place to place. In addition, diabetes prevalence rates may be different than the actual frequency because of variations in definitions, diagnostic criteria and screening procedures, and age distribution. Such research studies are hard to interpret because usually more than one dietary component is changed. An increase of fat, for example, may be at the expense of carbohydrate calories. Although the available evidence points to excess total caloric intake as the primary dietary factor related to diabetes risk, it does not address the question of the relative significance of nutrients, such as sugar and fat, either in influencing obesity or in inducing diabetes.

Fiber-depleted diets have also been suggested as important in the etiology of diabetes. This hypothesis has been advanced principally on the basis of epidemiological data suggesting that diabetes is rare in traditional, primitive cultures in which the population consumes diets that are high in less refined carbohydrate foods. Another piece of evidence used to advance this theory is the fact that mortality from diabetes in Britain fell during the world wars, when lower-extraction flour was consumed.[26]

However, as calories from refined foods are increased, or as the consumption of dietary fiber is increased, there are other accompanying changes in the diet, such as altered protein, fat, vitamin, and mineral intakes. Available studies indicate that, if diabetes is indeed related in some way to sugar, fat, or dietary fiber consumption, the relationship is very complex, not direct, and is probably mediated by a host of other environmental and individual variables.

Animal Studies

A number of animal studies have demonstrated that high intakes of sucrose as well as of fat result in an impairment of glucose tolerance, an increase in fasting blood insulin levels, and a reduced tissue sensitivity to insulin, all of which are characteristic of maturity-onset diabetes.[27,28]

A. Cohen et al. reported that mild diabetes without obesity was produced in rats through feeding of a high-sucrose diet.[29] However, diabetes has also been produced in animals (as has obesity) by high fat intakes, and in these cases the intake of sugar was often reduced.[9]

Human Experimental Evidence

As early as 1935, J. Himsworth demonstrated that a reduction of dietary carbohydrate without reducing calories resulted in impaired glucose tolerance in normal individuals.[19] Later studies have confirmed that, in normal individuals, high carbohydrate diets (but not necessarily high sugar diets) result in improved oral glucose tolerance.[30]

A number of investigators such as J. Brunzell et al. and J. Anderson et al. suggest that sugar is either harmless or perhaps even beneficial, relative to diabetes, when it replaces, but does not add to, other isocaloric amounts of food.[31,30]

There is, however, a lack of agreement in the literature, and other studies have noted that high sugar intakes resulted in:

> elevated serum insulin levels, [32]
>
> decreased insulin sensitivity, [32]
>
> impaired glucose tolerance,
>
> decreased blood glucose response,[30,33] and
>
> increased fasting serum insulin response.[32]

It has been suggested that the initial event in a synergistic cycle induced by sucrose feeding is hyperinsulinemia; this is followed by either hypertrophy of fat cells or reduced insulin sensitivity of peripheral tissue, which in turn aggravates the hyperinsulinemia and the cycle continues. These characteristics are usually associated with impaired glucose tolerance.[34]

It appears that certain individuals may have varying genetic sensitivity to high sucrose intake and, as a result, be more prone to develop high blood glucose values on high sugar diets than their normal counterparts who are not so predisposed. It is also possible that an individual who is genetically prone to develop diabetes may be prevented from doing so by avoiding the stimulation of a high-sucrose diet.

Recent human evidence has also suggested that the incorporation of sources of dietary fiber influences blood insulin and glucose levels.[35-38] In both insulin- independent and insulin-dependent subjects, increases in serum glucose have been found to be lower after eating a fiber-containing meal as compared with a meal without the added fiber.

Diabetic Complications

Various populations of diabetics also evidence significant variations in the frequency and severity of particular disease complications. For example, among diabetics in Japan, coronary disease and gangrene occur much less frequently than they do among United States diabetics. Among Asian, African, and Latin American diabetics, the low prevalance of atherosclerosis may be the result of diets that are usually lower in cholesterol and saturated fat and in total calories.

Prevention of Diabetes

Because the cause of diabetes is not definitely known, an appropriate strategy for prevention is uncertain. In July 1974, the passage of the National Diabetes Research and Education Act initiated Federal efforts to attack diabetes. Other national efforts to combat and prevent diabetes are undertaken by the American Diabetes Association, which emphasizes the importance of early detection programs and the control of the disease in an effort to minimize complications and arrest the progression of the disease.

The newest diet recommendations for the diabetic call for lower amounts of fat, saturated fat, and cholesterol as compared with the usual North American diet, as diabetics are most likely to die of coronary heart disease. This diet is higher in carbohydrate than the usual North American diet, but the carbohydrate should be chiefly complex carbohydrate, not sucrose or other simple sugars.

HYPERTENSION

Public Health Significance of Hypertension

Hypertension is the primary cause of an estimated 20,000 deaths in the United States annually.[39] According to data obtained by the Division of Health Interview Statistics, one in five individuals in the United States (20.6 per cent) aged 17 or older has been told by a physician that he or she has hypertension.[39] An estimated 23.4 million individuals in the United States have definite hypertension, that is, either systolic blood pressure of at least 160 mm Hg or diastolic blood pressure of at least 95 mm Hg.[40] This is an estimated one out of every seven American adults.

The prevalence of hypertension increases with age and is more prevalent among women (18.5 per cent) than among men (12.5 per cent). Approximately one third of hypertension in the United States is the result of a specific medical disorder such as a hormone aberration. The cause of the other two thirds of hypertension is not known; hypertension of unknown cause is termed essential hypertension.[41]

Proportionately more black than white individuals have hypertension. The highest proportion of hypertensive individuals is found in the South.[40] The prevalence of hypertension in the United States population is illustrated in Figure 11-1.

Early results of the Hypertension Detection and Follow-up Program suggest that the prevalence of hypertension is inversely related to education. As assessment of blood pressure measurements on 158,906 adults aged 30 to 69 in various areas of the United States was the basis for this conclusion. Hypertension was found to be 40 per cent less prevalent among those who had graduated from college than those who had less than ten years of formal education. Among blacks, the difference was particularly great. Many other variables influenced the factor of education. That is, race, social and economic status, and other environmental factors that influence education may have confounded the resulting correlation between education and hypertension. The effects of education

Figure 11-1. Incidence of hypertension in the United States, 1971-1974. (National Center for Health Statistics)

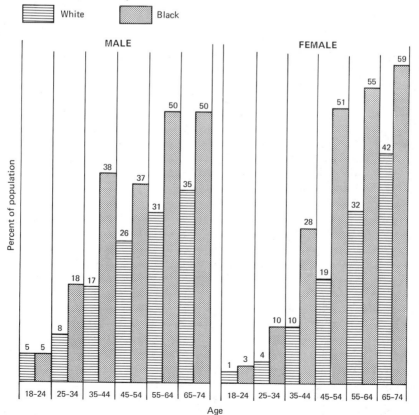

may also operate through factors such as diet (high salt intake, for example) and overweight. Overweight, which is associated with hypertension, is also associated with lower levels of education.[40]

Current data indicate that progress in achieving control of hypertension is being made. A survey of 14 communities identified individuals for a large clinical trial and found a large increase in awareness among those with hypertension, as well as a twofold increase in the number of controlled hypertensives as compared with previous national surveys.[42] Trends in the progress to control hypertension are illustrated in Fig. 11-2. Since the start of the National High Blood Pressure Campaign in the early 1970s, visits to physicians for hypertension treatment increased 48.5 per cent, compared with only a 5 per cent increase in visits to physicians for other reasons.[43]

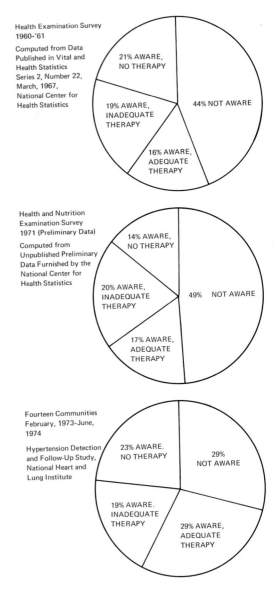

Figure 11-2. Percent of hypertensives aware, treated, and controlled: National Health Examination surveys, 1960-62 and 1971 and Hypertension Detection and Follow-Up Study, 1973-74. (HEW. National High Blood Pressure Education Program Fact Sheet. publication no. (NIH) 76-632. Washington, D.C., Government Printing Office, 1976)

Health Examination Survey 1960-'61

Computed from Data Published in Vital and Health Statistics Series 2, Number 22, March, 1967, National Center for Health Statistics

21% AWARE, NO THERAPY

44% NOT AWARE

19% AWARE, INADEQUATE THERAPY

16% AWARE, ADEQUATE THERAPY

Health and Nutrition Examination Survey 1971 (Preliminary Data)

Computed from Unpublished Preliminary Data Furnished by the National Center for Health Statistics

14% AWARE, NO THERAPY

49% NOT AWARE

20% AWARE, INADEQUATE THERAPY

17% AWARE, ADEQUATE THERAPY

Fourteen Communities February, 1973–June, 1974

Hypertension Detection and Follow-Up Study, National Heart and Lung Institute

23% AWARE, NO THERAPY

29% NOT AWARE

19% AWARE, INADEQUATE THERAPY

29% AWARE, ADEQUATE THERAPY

Adverse Effects of Hypertension

Elevated blood pressure, especially in individuals presenting other risk factors, is a powerful risk factor for the development of atherosclerotic heart disease. The International Atherosclerosis Project autopsy data demonstrated a high, statistically significant, relationship between hypertension and the incidence and severity of atherosclerosis.

The International Cooperative Study on the Epidemiology of Cardiovascular Disease demonstrated that hypertension was responsible, in part, for differences among populations in the incidence of CHD.[44] Other studies confirm the fact that high blood pressure is highly predictive for the development of CHD, at least for affluent population groups. The effect of hypertension appears to be independent of other risk factors, but it is also additive to the impact of factors such as elevated serum cholesterol levels and cigarette smoking.[45]

W. Kannel and T. Dawber in the Framingham study found hypertension to be the most significant contributor to cardiovascular morbidity and mortality. About 37 per cent of the males and 51 per cent of the females who died of heart disease had hypertension. If the incidences of borderline hypertension were included, the figures rose to 73 per cent of the males and 81 per cent of the females. Mortality from cardiovascular disease among hypertensives was almost three times that of the normotensives.[46]

In other reports from the Framingham study, hypertension was the dominant factor predisposing individuals to atherosclerotic brain infarction — the risk was proportional to the elevation in blood pressure.[47,48]

Conversely, the treatment and consequent reduction of blood pressure has been found to improve blood flow, myocardial function, and survival rates.[48] A four-year Swedish study of more than 1,000 hypertensive males, aged 47 to 54 revealed a significant reduction in the incidence of heart attacks among those treated, as compared with untreated controls.[49]

In a Veterans Administration study, researchers found that the control of hypertension could reduce the incidence of cerebral stroke. The population studied, however, was neither young enough nor large enough to conclusively establish the fact that the correction of hypertension can reduce coronary occlusion after it has been clinically identified.[50]

Here again, the findings are by no means clear. One report, for example, noted a randomized study in which antihypertensive therapy was provided to 452 stroke victims; the therapy was of little benefit in terms of survival rate or the rate of stroke reoccurrence over a period of three years.[51] Other reports have found no reduction in the frequency of coronary heart disease following hypertensive therapy.[52]

Hypertension and High Sodium Intakes*

A variety of evidence relates dietary sodium intakes to the etiology of hypertension. Animal studies have demonstrated that hypertension in rats could be produced by adding salt to the basic diet. In the groups of rats

---

*Although not the only source, salt is the main source of sodium in the United States diet. Table salt, NaCl, is about 39 per cent sodium.

studied by G. Meneely et al., salt was fed at varying and increasingly high levels. The elevated blood pressures were associated with sodium chloride intakes on a group basis, but there were individual variations, and some rats who did not follow the typical pattern.[53]

In another experiment, Meneely took three groups of older rats who had been raised on the basic ration diet; these rats were then fed high levels of salt. The animals responded with increased blood pressure but the elevation was less than that of young rats who had consumed high levels of salt early in life.[54]

L. K. Dahl found varying responses to high levels of salt in his animal studies; some rats developed hypertension on diets high in salt. He took two different groups of rats, one resistant (R) to the development of hypertension and the other sensitive (S) to the development of hypertension on the ingestion of high amounts of salt. Rats of later generations were inbred. Dahl found that Group S (sensitive) rats developed hypertension when their postweaning diets in the first year were high in salt, whereas the other group (R) developed no hypertension on the same high levels of salt.[55]

Dahl suggested that the salt intake during early childhood may be a critical factor in the development of later hypertension. To test this theory, he fed rats of the S strain commercially manufactured salted infant food — five of the seven rats studied developed hypertension, whereas none of the control rats that were fed a low salt diet developed hypertension.[56]

Dahl then studied human populations and tried to relate his findings from animal studies to man. One of his studies involved five population groups whose lifetime salt intakes ranged from 4–26 gm/day. He noted a positive relationship between the level of salt intake and the incidence of hypertension among these population groups.[57]

Once again it must be noted that, although associations can be demonstrated for population groups, the relationship of individual intakes and incidence of hypertension is not clearly established.[58,59] The Framingham study did not find a statistical correlation between salt intake and blood pressure; other studies have also failed to note a relationship between individual salt intakes and blood pressure. Dahl explains these individual variations by hypothesizing that some individuals are selectively bred to develop hypertension with the stimulus of a high salt diet. He suggested that a low salt diet may help to prevent hypertension in these individuals. Among those resistant to hypertension, Dahl suggested that high salt diets may have no effect as these individuals are somehow relatively protected against hypertension.[57]

Scientists and clinicians have long recognized that severe sodium restriction (at levels less than 500 mg/day) is helpful in reducing the blood pressure of hypertensive individuals. However, diets that take advantage of this idea, such as the Kempner Rice Diet,* have been criticized as being unpalatable and impractical for general use. During the late 1940s, with the advent of antihypertensive drug therapy, interest in using the diet,

---

*In the Kempner Rice Diet, the patient consumes 10 oz daily of dry rice, cooked without salt. An additional 900 to 1,000 kcal daily are supplied by sugar and fresh or preserved fruits. The diet is high in carbohydrates and supplies only about 100–150 mg of sodium a day.

particularly a low sodium diet, to treat hypertension declined. Recently, the use of a more moderate sodium restriction (between 1,500 and 2,000 mg/day) instead of drugs and medications to treat hypertension has again been advocated but has sparked considerable controversy.[60,61] Controlled clinical evidence suggests that moderate salt restriction can result in lowered blood pressure in hypertensive individuals.[61] Epidemiological evidence also suggests that mild essential hypertension can be prevented in a large part of the population by a diet limiting sodium consumption to less than 2,000 mg/day.[60,61]

Obesity and Hypertension

Available experimental data indicate a positive correlation between hypertension and increased weight for height in both children and adults. It has been estimated that weight differences account for about 10 per cent of the variations in blood pressure among the total population. However, it has not yet been determined whether or not elevated blood pressure relates to high body weight or to excess body fat. Further, it should be noted that many obese individuals are not hypertensive.[62]

Overweight adults tend to develop hypertension more frequently than do their nonobese controls; there is a definite relationship between the rate of weight gain and hypertension, as well as between obesity and an increased risk of developing hypertensive cardiovascular disease.

Hypertension in some overweight individuals can be significantly controlled simply through dieting. In one investigation, overweight patients with uncomplicated essential hypertension were studied for a six-month period. Patients in group I participated in a dietary program for weight reduction but received no antihypertensive drug therapy. Those in group II received regular but inadequate drug therapy, and half of this group also participated in the weight-reduction program. The salt intakes were in the usual range for both groups. Those who participated in the weight-reduction program lost at least 3 kg over the study period, and all but two of these patients achieved a reduction in blood pressure. The reductions in weight and blood pressure were highly significant in both sexes and at all age groups and were statistically related. Those who did not lose weight evidenced no significant changes in blood pressure. The authors concluded that weight reduction should be considered an important part of the treatment of any hypertensive patient who is above the ideal weight.[63]

However, few longitudinal studies have investigated the relationship between obesity and hypertension. Thus, it is difficult to make firm conclusions about the exact impact of obesity on hypertension.

Recommendations for Dietary Modification

The Committee on Nutrition of the American Academy of Pediatrics examined the effects of salt consumption on health and made the following statement:

> Because of the prevalence of essential hypertension in adults, there is a major public health concern with its causes. . . . These factors include race, family history, stress, variations in endocrine and kidney function, and body habitus. Salt has also

been cited as causing hypertension. There is no question that an increase in salt intake by most hypertensive patients will increase their blood pressure. The converse also is true. The question is whether salt intake induces hypertension and, in particular, whether salt consumption by the general population in this country is a risk.[64]

An estimated 20 per cent of American children are at risk for developing hypertension as adults. For this group, the academy suggested that there is "a reasonable possibility that a low salt intake begun early in life may protect, to some extent, persons at risk from developing hypertension."[64]

For the majority of the population not at risk, there is no firm indication that salt intakes in the present range are harmful.

The average salt intake for the North American public ranges from 6–18 gm daily.[65] The National Academy of Sciences, National Research Council, Food and Nutrition Board report that 1–3 gm of salt are sufficient to replace the sodium that is lost in moderate sweating. Individuals who are engaged in very heavy work or who live in hot climates may need as much as 20 gm of salt to replace the lost sodium.[66]

Other groups also suggest the advantages of low or moderate salt intake.[67]

The revised version of the *Dietary Goals for the United States* recommends a salt intake of no more than 5 gm daily. This intake may be adequate for the majority of Americans, but special circumstances, such as certain types of kidney disease, may require certain individuals to increase their sodium intake beyond this minimum.[68]

Although salt is one of the chief sources of sodium in the North American diet, many other commonly consumed foods are high in sodium. Sodium compounds are present in leavening agents, such as baking powder and baking soda; sodium phosphate is used in some cereals and cheese; monosodium glutamate is used to enhance the flavor of various foods; sodium alginate is present in ice cream and in some chocolate milks and drinks; sodium benzoate is used as a preservative; sodium hydroxide is used in food processing; sodium propionate is used to retard the growth of mold; and sodium sulfite is used in certain fruits as a preservative. Water may also be high in sodium, especially in areas where water "softening" treatment is used.[69]

Many natural foods, especially animal protein foods, such as milk, cheese, eggs, meat, poultry, and fish are fairly high in sodium. Certain vegetables such as beets, celery, carrots, kale, and spinach are often rich in natural sodium, containing 50–80 mg per serving.

With the increased intake of highly processed and heavily salted food products, the sodium content is significantly increased. Pastries, convenience foods, canned soups and casseroles, frozen dinners, and the like are usually very high in sodium. In the early 1970s the sodium content of baby foods was also high; however, in 1974 the Committee on Nutrition of the American Academy of Pediatrics suggested "actions that reduce or avoid increasing the present level of salt intake by children in the population at large" should be undertaken.[64] Since then, most baby food manufacturers have complied by reducing the sodium content of their products.

National High Blood Pressure Education Program (NHBPEP)

In 1973, the U.S. Department of Health, Education and Welfare launched the National High Blood Pressure Education Program, in cooperation with professional, voluntary, and public organizations. The NHBPEP aims to reduce the morbidity and mortality attributable to hypertension through public and professional education. The program is coordinated by the National Heart, Lung, and Blood Institute and is a collaborative government/private-sector effort. It involves federal and state health agencies as well as private and professional health associations, accrediting bodies, pharmaceutical companies, and labor, management, and insurance groups. These groups focus their attention on hypertension as a serious disease that can be detected, treated, and controlled. The specific areas of the program are education development and education services.[42]

Education Development

This effort attempts to "identify and promulgate state of the art concepts, guidelines, strategies and corresponding educational materials. It also endeavors to improve both the quality and extent of patient and practitioner involvement in high blood pressure management." The activities are designed to increase public and professional awareness and understanding, as well as to detect and control hypertension.[42]

Education Services

This program aids in public, professional, and community efforts to control hypertension. Communication media for the dissemination of hypertension information are emphasized.

The NHBPEP also coordinates a National High Blood Pressure Month each May, assesses educational materials, and conducts an education research program to investigate such issues as patient compliance, hypertension in various settings, and models for hypertension education.

ALCOHOL ABUSE AND RELATED DISORDERS

Alcohol is the only nutrient antinutrient. It is a food that causes a very special kind of malnutrition. It is pleasurable to the majority who do not become addicted to it, but poison to those who do.

— F. L. Iber[70]

Alcohol Consumption

It has been estimated, based on data similar to that obtained from the USDA food balance sheets, that the average annual consumption of absolute alcohol from beer, wine, and spirits among the drinking-age American public is 2.6 gallons per individual. The caloric value of this quantity of alcohol is approximately 210 calories daily per person. Alcoholic consumption is highly variable among individuals — many people do not consume any alcohol whereas many consume alcohol far in excess of the average. It is estimated, however, that on the average, adult females in the United States derive 10 per cent of their RDA calories from alcohol whereas males obtain 7.5 per cent.[68]

Alcohol Abuse

Alcoholism is one of the most common types of undernutrition in the adult North American population. Excessive alcohol consumption is the primary factor related to the development of cirrhosis of the liver, the ninth leading killer disease of the United States population.

Alcoholism in the United States has become a major social problem as well. It affects individuals at every socioeconomic level, as well as individuals in age groups from the adolescent to the elderly. An estimated 9.3–10.0 million U.S. adults, or 7 per cent of the U.S. adult population, are alcoholics or problem drinkers. In addition, there are approximately 3.3 million problem drinkers among teens and youth aged 14–17 years old — this represents 19 per cent of American youths. Alcohol-related deaths may reach as many as 205,000 annually; alcohol abuse in the United States cost almost $43 billion in 1975.[71]

Few of these alcoholics — only one in four — seek medical treatement. Nutritional consequences of alcoholism are significant public health considerations. F. Iber notes that 20,000 alcoholics yearly suffer nutrition-related illness, which necessitates their hospitalization.[70]

A variety of social pressures intensify the alcohol problem and lead to excessive alcohol use: business pressures, fear of ridicule at not accepting a drink, the urging of friends, the need to feel a part of a social affair, the attempt to overcome feelings of insecurity and shyness, seductive advertising appeals, and many similar pressures.

Effects of Alcohol Consumption

Alcohol, in different amounts for different individuals, is toxic. Excess alcohol consumption can lead to cirrhosis and even death, not only because of the accompanying effects of malnutriton but also because of the damage that alcohol inflicts on liver cells.[72] C. Lieber reports that an intake of 11–12 oz of 86-proof whiskey daily can lead to the development of a fatty liver, regardless of the rest of the diet.[73]

The American Medical Association reports that alcoholism is more dangerous to women than it is to men. A recent study at the University of Toronto found that the average time of hazardous drinking before the onset of an illness was shorter for women (14.1 years) than for men (20.2 years), and that alcoholic women had twice the incidence of cirrhosis of the liver.[74]

Malnutrition is common among alcoholics, in part because alcohol, which is very high in calories, replaces other foods in the diet. A gram of ethanol supplies 7.1 calories. Next to fat, alcohol is the most calorically dense item a person could consume. (One gram of carbohydrate supplies

4 calories; a gram of protein supplies 4 calories; and a gram of fat supplies 9 calories.) Twenty ounces of an 86-proof drink contains approximately 1,500 calories; this is equivalent to up to two thirds of the recommended dietary calorie allowance.[75]

R. Pirola and C. Lieber, however, suggest that the high calories from alcohol may not be fully utilized. They report that one of the possible metabolic pathways for ethanol metabolism is wasteful so that, in effect, some of the ethanol calories are wasted.[76] In spite of this fact, the caloric value of alcoholic beverages is significant. In addition, the calories are "empty" in that they contribute little other nutritional value. Furthermore, alcoholics frequently diminish their food intake — whether as a result of the appetite-suppressant effect of alcohol or the loneliness and poverty that are often associated with alcoholism — the vulnerability to malnutrition is set. Conditioned malnutrition* is also a factor.[77]

Alcohol causes inflammation of the stomach, pancreas, and intestines, thus interfering with normal digestion and metabolism, and leads to nutrient malabsorption and secondary malnutrition. Alcoholics often have a reduced capacity to absorb and utilize nutrients. Increased physiological requirements resulting from the body's adjustment to the oxidation of large quantities of alcohol compound the problems. Thus, alcoholics are vulnerable to a deficiency of protein, B vitamins, fats, fat-soluble vitamins, and minerals, such as potassium, magnesium, and zinc. In addition, alcohol adversely affects other physiological systems, such as protein-synthesizing cells, gastric mucosa, and the system producing red blood cells. Thus, for many reasons, alcoholics are especially prone to develop nutrition-deficiency disease.[72]

Lieber suggested that alcohol's toxicity in the liver occurs independently of an inadequate diet. He has demonstrated specific biochemical and structural changes in liver cells that result from alcohol consumption. Chronic alcoholism leads to the deposition of dietary fat in the liver, commonly known as *fatty liver*. This state of damage is then followed by alcoholic hepatitis, eventual decreased cell function and inflammation, cell destruction, and, occasionally, death. The final stage of liver disease is cirrhosis, characterized by fibrous scar tissue and permanent liver cell damage.[72,78] The complications from excessive alcohol consumption are illustrated in Figure 11–3.

Considerable evidence links alcoholism with cardiovascular consequences, not only in terms of alcoholic cardiomyopathy but also in terms of its role in hypertriglyceridemic hypercholesteremia and in terms of a tendency to elevated blood pressure.

There is also evidence to suggest that alcohol, contrary to widespread misconception, is a heart depressant and that chronic drinking can result in congestive heart failure. This seems to be an effect that is independent of dietary deficiencies. Thus, heart specialists often suggest that individuals with chronic congestive heart failure and severe heart damage should abstain from liquor intake. Other heart patients are counseled to limit their

---

*Conditioned malnutrition refers to secondary malnutrition — nutritional problems resulting from factors such as increased nutrient requirements, increased nutrient destruction, reduced nutrient utilization, and the like.

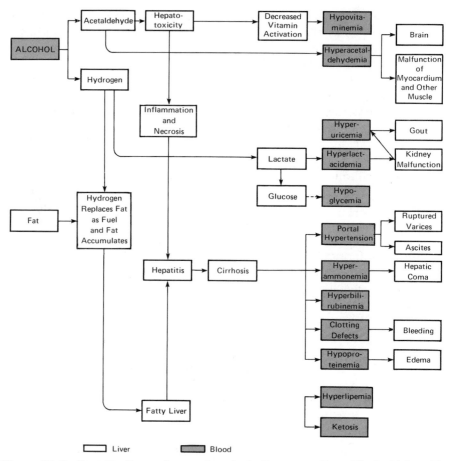

Figure 11-3. Complications of excessive alcohol consumption. (C. S. Lieber. The metabolism of alcohol. Sci. Am. 234 (1976): 33)

consumption of alcohol to 1.5 oz of whiskey, one can of beer, or a 6 oz glass of wine daily.[79] Alcohol consumption has also been associated with certain kinds of cancer. (See Chapter 8.)

Another severe consequence of alcoholism is the effect it may have on the offspring of a pregnant drinker. A study at the Boston City Hospital found that 32 per cent of the infants born to mothers who drank heavily had some type of abnormalities. A British study reported that 44 per cent of children born to alcoholic mothers had IQs below 80, as well as significantly higher rates of heart and joint abnormalities.[74]

There is increasing evidence that maternal alcohol consumption has teratogenic* effects on the developing fetus. Animal studies have confirmed observations made in humans, which suggest that the offspring of those who drink heavily exhibit a definite and specific pattern of developmental abnormalities.[80,81] The typical pattern, termed the *fetal alcohol syndrome,* is characterized by a delay in development and in psychomotor responses, by both pre- and postnatal growth retardation, retarded intellectual performance, and abnormalities in the development of crainofacial,

---

teratogenic — causing the production of physical defects in the developing embryo.

cardiac, and joint systems. It is also possible that infants born to moderate drinkers may exhibit some of these symptoms. These offsrping often display symptoms of trembling, touching of their faces, keeping their eyes open, and turning their heads to the left side and reduced arm and leg motion. The possible harm of small amounts of alcohol consumption during pregnancy is still being debated, but many authors suggest that alcohol should be considered to have teratogenic effects and that its use should be greatly restricted during pregnancy.[82]

Prevention and Treatment of Alcoholism

Although one out of every ten workers in the United States has a serious drinking problem, less than 10 per cent of these people seek medical or professional help. With treatment, up to 70 per cent of these problem drinkers can be helped to achieve significant recovery; without treatment the figure falls to 10 per cent.[83]

Strategies to prevent alcohol abuse are widely debated. Some recommend environmental control by the government, which would include increases in alcohol prices through increased taxation and extensive public education programs to inform and change the public's attitudes and behavior concerning alcohol.[84] Others, however, shy away from promoting stringent controls and suggest instead that individuals should take more self-responsibility in dealing with and providing for their own health needs.[85]

Federal involvement in the control and prevention of excessive alcohol use was initiated with the 1971 passage of the Comprehensive Alcohol Abuse and Alcoholism Prevention, Treatment, and Rehabilitation Act of 1970. This law authorizes state grants for the development of effective programs to control alcohol abuse and the consequent effects.[86]

Rehabilitation for Alcoholics

The past ten years have ushered in a significant change in attitudes toward problems of alcoholics and their treatment. Alcoholism is now gradually being viewed as an illness, requiring treatment, not only for the after effects of alcoholism but also for the disease itself.[87]

To meet the needs of the alcoholic, various types of detoxification centers have been established to offer specific types of care and rehabilitation. Such centers can generally be classified under four systems of care:[88]

1. Medical detoxification center — provides medical supervision. Registered nurses are able to give medications and deal with immediate patient problems.

2. Nonmedical detoxification center — minimal physician coverage and relatively few licensed health personnel are available. Medications are limited; this type of center must rely on hospitals and other medical services for back-up support.

3. Social detoxification center — fashioned after the halfway houses, it is a type of recovery residence. Drugs, licensed medical personnel, and medical care are not provided.

4. Outpatient detoxification center — established to provide medical attention and the use of specific medical detoxifying techniques.

Nutrition components of these rehabilitation centers are frequently provided. Many centers attempt to provide clients with at least one nutritious meal daily. Education is an integral part of the attempt to provide the alcoholic with a new way of life. Because of the previously mentioned close association between the effects of alcoholism and malnutrition, the role of nutrition in the general education of alcoholics is evident. Medical inpatient alcoholic units usually provide a balanced diet, which is often restricted in sodium to prevent fluid retention. The meals are often supplemented with multivitamins and minerals.

Alcoholics Anonymous (AA) is another support system available to rehabilitate the alcoholic. Established in 1935 by two "hopeless drunks," there are now 28,000 local groups in more than 90 countries.[89]

The only requirements for participation in AA are the desire and motivation to attempt to stop drinking. Local groups are self-supporting through contributions; there are no dues or other financial expenses. AA sponsors meetings at which alcoholics offer each other help and support and receive counseling and help to cope with their daily lives.

REFERENCES

1. Juvenile Diabetes Foundation. *1975 Fact Sheet.* New York, 1975.
2. U.S. Department of Health, Education, and Welfare. *Diabetes Data.* Bethesda, Md., 1978.
3. U.S. Senate Select Committee on Nutrition and Human Needs. *Sugar, Diet, Diabetes, and Heart Disease, Part 2.* Washington, D.C.: Government Printing Office, 1973, p. 146.
4. Kannel, W. B., M. Hjortland, and W. P. Castelli. Role of diabetes in congestive heart failure: The Framingham Study. *Am. J. Cardiol.* 34 (1974): 29.
5. Kannel, W. B. Status of coronary heart disease risk factors. *J. Nutr. Educ.* 10 (1978): 10.
6. Keen, H. Diabetes and sugar consumption. In S. S. Hildebrand, ed., *Is the Risk of Becoming Diabetic Affected by Sugar Consumption?* Bethesda, Md.: International Sugar Research Foundation, 1974, pp. 14–27.
7. Keen, H., R. J. Jarrett, and J. H. Fuller. Diet and glucose tolerance in man. *Diabetologia* 10 (1974): 372.
8. American Diabetes Association. *Annual Report 1974 — The Year of Momentum.* New York, 1974, p. 6.
9. West, K. M., E. L. Oakley, M. E. Sanders, and A. H. Rubenstein. Nutritional factors in the etiology of diabetes, in H. Keen, ed., *Epidemiology of Diabetes.* London: World Health Organization, 1977.
10. Kannel, W. B., G. Pearson, and P. M. McNamara. Obesity as a force of morbidity and mortality in adolescence, in F. P. Heald, ed., *Adolescent Nutrition and Growth.* New York: Appleton-Century-Crofts, 1969, pp. 51–71.
11. Cohen, A. M., S. Bavly, and R. Posnamski. Change of diet of Yemenite Jews in relation to diabetes and ischaemic heart disease. *Lancet* 2 (1961): 1399.

12. Campbell, G. D. Diabetes in Asians and Africans in and around Durban. *S. Afr. Med. J.* 37 (1963): 1195.
13. West, K. M., and J. M. Kalbfleisch. Diabetes in Central America. *Diabetes* 19 (1970): 656–663.
14. West, K. M., and J. M. Kalbfleisch. Influence of nutritional factors on prevalence of diabetes. *Diabetes* 20 (1971): 99–108.
15. West, K. M. Introduction. In S. S. Hildebrand, ed., *Is the Risk of Becoming Diabetic Affected by Sugar Consumption?* Bethesda, Md.: International Sugar Research Foundation, 1974, pp. 33–43.
16. West, K. M. Diabetes in American Indians and other native populations of the New World. *Diabetes* 23 (1974): 841–855.
17. Reid, J. M., S. D. Fullmer, K. D. Pettigrew, et al. Nutrient intake of Pima Indian women: Relationships to diabetes mellitus and gallbladder disease. *Am. J. Clin. Nutr.* 24 (1971): 1281.
18. Baird, J. D. Diet and the development of clinical diabetes. *Acta Diabetol. Lat.* 9 (1972): 621–637 (suppl.).
19. Aimsworth, J. P. The dietetic factor determining glucose tolerance and sensitivity to insulin of healthy men. *Clin. Sci.* 2 (1935): 67–94.
20. Prior, I. A. M. Diabetes in the South Pacific, in S. S. Hildebrand, ed., *Is the Risk of Becoming Diabetic Affected by Sugar Consumption?* Bethesda, Md.: International Sugar Research Foundation, 1974, pp. 4–13.
21. Reid, D. D., G. Z. Brett, P. Hamilton, R. J. Jarett, H. Keen, and G. A. Rose. Cardiorespiratory disease and diabetes among middle-age male civil servants: A study of screening and intervention. *Lancet* 1 (1974): 469.
22. Trowell, H. Diabetes mellitus death rates in England and Wales 1920–70 and food supplies. *Lancet* 2 (1974): 998–1002.
23. Walker, A. R. P. The epidemiological emergence of ischaemic arterial diseases: Editorial. *Am. Heart J.* 89 (1975): 113.
24. Yudkin, J. Sugar and disease. *Nature* 239 (1972): 197.
25. Cleave, T. L. *The Saccharine Disease.* Bristol, England: John Wright and Sons, 1974.
26. Trowell, H. C. Dietary-fiber hypothesis of the etiology of diabetes mellitus. *Diabetes* 24 (1975): 762–765.
27. Reiser, S., and J. Hallfrisch. Insulin sensitivity and adipose tissue weight of rats fed starch or sucrose diets *ad libitum* or in meals. *J. Nutr.* 107 (1977): 147–155.
28. Moser, P., and C. D. Berdanier. Effect of early sucrose feeding on the metabolic patterns of mature rats. *J. Nutr.* 104 (1974): 687.
29. Cohen, A. M., S. Briller, and E. Shafrir. Effect of long-term sucrose feeding on the activity of some enzymes regulating glycolysis, lipogenesis, and gluconeogenesis in rat liver and adipose tissue. *Biochim. Biophys. Acta* 279 (1972): 129.
30. Anderson, J. W., R. H. Herman, and D. Zakim. Effect of high glucose and high sucrose diets on glucose tolerance of normal men. *Am. J. Clin. Nutr.* 26 (1973): 660–607.
31. Brunzell, J. D., R. L. Lerner, D. Porte, and E. L. Bierman. Effect of a fat free, high carbohydrate diet on diabetic subjects with fasting hyperglycemia. *Diabetes* 23 (1974): 138–142.
32. Kelsay, J. L., K. M. Behall, J. M. Holden, and E. S. Prather. Diets high in glucose or sucrose and young women. *Am. J. Clin. Nutr.* 27 (1974): 926.
33. Palumbo, P. J., E. R. Briones, R. A. Nelson, and B. A. Kottke. Sucrose sensitivity of patients with coronary-artery disease. *Am. J. Clin. Nutr.* 30 (1977): 394–401.
34. Reiser, S. Metabolic effects of dietary carbohydrates — A review, in A.

Jeanes and J. Hodge, eds., *Physiological Effects of Food Carbohydrates.* Washington, D.C.: American Chemical Society Symposium Series 15, 1975, pp. 20–45.

35. Jenkins, D. J., D. V. Goff, A. R. Leeds, K. G. Alberti, T. M. Wolever, M. A. Gassull, and T. D. Hockaday. Unabsorbable carbohydrates and diabetes: Decreased postprandial hyperglycemia. *Lancet* 2 (1976): 172–174.

36. Jenkins, D. J., A. R. Leeds, M. A. Gassull, B. Cochet, and K. G. Alberti. Decrease in postprandial insulin and glucose concentrations by guar and pectin. *Ann. Int. Med.* 86 (1977): 20–23.

37. Miranda, P. M., and D. L. Horwitz. High-fiber diets in the treatment of diabetes mellitus. *Ann. Int. Med.* 88 (1978): 482–486.

38. Trowell, H. Diabetes mellitus and dietary fiber of starchy foods. *Am. J. Clin. Nutr.* 31 (1978): 553.

39. U.S. Department of Health, Education, and Welfare. *Blood Pressure of Persons 6–74 Years of Ages in the United States. Advance Data. Vital and Health Statistics of the National Center for Health Statistics.* Washington, D.C.: Government Printing Office, October 18, 1976.

40. U.S. Department of Health, Education, and Welfare. *Hypertension: United States, 1974. Advance Data. Vital and Health Statistics of the National Center for Health Statistics.* Washington, D.C.: Government Printing Office, November 8, 1976.

41. Cullen, R. W., A. Paulbitski, and S. Oace. Sodium, hypertension, and the U.S. dietary goals. *J. Nutr. Educ.* 10 (1978): 59.

42. U.S. Department of Health, Education, and Welfare. *National High Blood Pressure Education Program. Fact Sheet*, Publ. No. (NIH) 76–632. Washington, D.C.: Government Printing Office, 1976.

43. Colen, B. D. Deaths caused by strokes fall sharply in the U.S. *Washington Post*, February 25, 1979, p. A1.

44. Keys, A., ed. Coronary heart disease in seven countries. *Circulation* (1970): suppl. 1, 1.

45. Doyle, J. T., and W. B. Kannel. Coronary risk factors: Ten-year findings in 7,446 Americans. Paper presented to the VI World Congress of Cardiology, London, September, 1970.

46. Kannel, W. B., and T. R. Dawber. Hypertension as an ingredient of a cardiovascular risk profile. *Brit. J. Hosp. Med.* 11 (1974): 508–523.

47. Gordon, T., and W. B. Kannel. Predisposition to atherosclerosis in the head, heart, and legs: The Framingham Study. *J.A.M.A.* 221 (1972): 661–666.

48. Kannel, W. B., T. R. Dawber, P. Sorlie, and P. A. Wolf. Components of blood pressure and risk of atherothrombotic brain infarction: The Framingham Study. *Stroke* 7 (1976): 327–331.

49. Hypertension and the heart. *The New York Times*, January 29, 1978, p. 18E.

50. Veteran's Administration Cooperative Study Group on Antihypertensive Agents. Effects of treatment on morbidity in hypertension. *J.A.M.A.* 202 (1967): 1028–1034.

51. Hypertensive-Stroke Cooperative Study Group. Effect of antihypertensive treatment on stroke recurrence. *J.A.M.A.* 229 (1974): 409.

52. Moser, M., and A. G. Goldman. *Hypertensive Vascular Disease.* Philadelphia: J. Lippincott, 1967.

53. Meneely, G. R., R. G. Tucker, W. J. Darby, and S. H. Auerbach. Chronic sodium chloride toxicity in the albino rat: Occurrence of hypertension and of syndrome of edema and renal failure. *J. Exper. Med.* 98 (1953): 71.

54. Meneely, G. R., and C. O. T. Ball. Experimental epidemiology of chronic sodium chloride toxicity and the protective effect of potassium chloride. *Am. J. Med.* 25 (1958): 713.
55. Dahl, L. K. Effects of chronic excess salt feeding: Induction of self-sustaining hypertension in ràts. *J. Exper. Med.* 114 (1961): 231.
56. Dahl, L. K., M. Heine, and L. Tassinari. High salt content of Western infant's diet: Possible relationship to hypertension in the adult. *Nature* 98 (1963): 1204.
57. Dahl, L. K. Salt and hypertension. *Am. J. Clin. Nutr.* 25 (1972): 231.
58. Prior, I. A. M., J. G. Evans, H. P. Harvey, et al. Sodium intake and blood pressure in two Polynesian populations. *N. Eng. J. Med.* 279 (1968): 515.
59. Miall, W. E. Follow-up study of arterial pressure in the population of Welsh mining valley. *Brit. Med. J.* S 161 (1959): 1204.
60. Freis, E. D. Salt, volume, and the prevention of hypertension. *Circulation* 53 (1976): 589.
61. Morgan, T., W. Adam, A. Gillies, M. Wilson, G. Morgan, and S. Carney. Hypertension treated by salt restriction. *Lancet* 1 (1978): 227–230.
62. Lauer, R. M., L. J. Filer, M. A. Reiter, and W. R. Clarke. Blood pressure, salt preference, salt threshold, and relative weight. *Am. J. Dis. Child.* 130 (1976): 493.
63. Reisin, E., R. Abel, M. Modan, D. S. Silverberg, H. E. Eliahou, and B. Modan. Effect of weight loss without salt restriction on the reduction of blood pressure. *N. Eng. J. Med.* 298 (1978): 1.
64. American Academy of Pediatrics, Committee on Nutrition. Salt intake and eating patterns of infants and children in relation to blood pressure. Pediatrics 53 (1974): 115–121.
65. Dahl, L. K. Salt intake and salt need. *N. Eng. J. Med.* 258 (1958): 1152, 1205.
66. National Academy of Sciences, National Research Council, Food and Nutrition Board. *Recommended Dietary Allowances for the United States.* Washington, D.C., 1974.
67. National Heart, Lung, and Blood Institute's Task Force on Blood Pressure Control in Children. Report of the task force on blood pressure control in children. *Pediatrics* 59 (May 1977): 797–820 (suppl.).
68. U.S. Senate Select Committee on Nutrition and Human Needs. *Dietary Goals of the United States*, 2d ed. Washington, D.C.: Government Printing Office, 1977.
69. Krause, M. V., and L. K. Mahan. *Food, Nutrition, and Diet Therapy.* Philadelphia: W. B. Saunders, 1979.
70. Iber, F. L. In alcoholism, the liver sets the pace. *Nutr. Today* 6 (1971): 2–9.
71. U.S. Department of Health, Education, and Welfare. *The Third Special Report to the U.S. Congress on Alcohol and Health from the Secretary of HEW.* Preprint. Washington, D. C.: Government Printing Office, June 1978.
72. Lieber, C. S. The metabolism of alcohol. *Sci. Am.* 234 (1976): 25–30.
73. Lieber, C. S. The prolonged cocktail hour and liver disease. *J.A.M.A.* 185 (1963): 419.
74. Galton, L. Alcoholism in women: The hidden epidemic. *Parade*, February 5, 1978, p. 10.
75. Lieber, C. S. Alcohol and nutrition. *Nutr. News* 39 (1976): 1, 12.
76. Pirola, R. C., and C. S. Lieber. The energy cost of the metabolism of drugs, including ethanol. *Pharmacology* 7 (1972): 185.
77. Lieber, C. S. Alcohol and nutrition, in L. Hofmann, ed., *The Great Ameri-*

can Nutrition Hassle. Palo Alto, Calif.: Mayfield Publishing Co., 1978, pp. 238–241.

78. Lieber, C. S. Alcohol and malnutrition in the pathogenesis of liver disease. *J.A.M.A.* 233 (1975): 1077.
79. Horwitz, L. D. Alcohol and heart disease. *J.A.M.A.* 232 (1975): 959.
80. Chernoff, G. The fetal alcohol syndrome in mice: An animal model. *Teratology* 15 (1977): 223–229.
81. Jones, K., D. Smith, and J. Hanson. The fetal alcohol syndrome: Clinical delineation. Ann. N.Y. Acad. Sci. 273 (1976): 130.
82. Worthington, B. S. Nutritional considerations during pregnancy and lactation. *Fam. and Commun. Health* 1 (1978): 13–29.
83. Long, S. *News, Views, and Reviews from Rescue Mission Departments.* Rescue Mission Alliance, Fall 1976.
84. Terris, M. The epidemiologic revolution: National health insurance and the role of health departments. *Am. J. Publ. Health* 66 (1976): 1156–1158.
85. Vladeck, B. C., and R. J. Weiss. Policy alternatives for alcohol control. *Am. J. Publ. Health* 65 (1975): 1340.
86. U.S. Congress. The Comprehensive Alcohol Abuse and Alcoholism Prevention, Treatment, and Rehabilitation Act of 1970, P.L. 91–616.
87. Behnke, R. Recognition and management of alcohol withdrawal syndrome. *Hosp. Pract.* 11 (1976): 79–84.
88. Moore, R. Ten years of inpatient programs for alcoholic patients. *Am. J. Psychiatry* 134 (1977): 542.
89. Alcoholics Anonymous World Services. *A Brief Guide to Alcoholics Anonymous.* New York, 1972.

section three
END OF SECTION ACTIVITIES

1. Compare dietary recommendations for preventing heart disease, cancer, obesity, hypertension, dental caries, and diabetes. Are there any contradictions among these various sets of recommendations?

2. You are a nutritionist in an HMO. All clients who come to the HMO for a physical examination are routinely referred to you for preventive dietary counseling. John C. is a 35-year-old male. He has just had a complete physical examination and received a clean bill of health. He is 6 ft tall and weighs 185 lb. He is a former athlete and still remains very physically active and exercises frequently. All his life, John has eaten what he wanted to. His food preferences center around high-fat animal products (such as sausage, cold cuts, cheese, and eggs), fried foods, and high-calorie salty snacks. The only vegetable he likes is corn. He sees no need for a change in his eating habits because he has eaten this way all his life and continues to feel good. He says he would rather die younger and eat what he likes than greatly modify his food habits. How would you approach John in terms of nutritional counseling? What suggestions might you make?

3. Write an article for a lay magazine, such as *Good Housekeeping*, in which you explain the relationship between diet and heart disease. Conclude your article by suggesting dietary guidelines to be followed to

reduce the risk of heart disease. Did you experience any difficulty in explaining the relationship between diet and heart disease? How much information should the public be given about the subject, without danger of merely confusing them more? How close did your dietary guidelines come to those in *Dietary Goals for the United States?*

4. Assume that you are a pediatrician instructing a mother of a 2-year-old about the inclusion of certain foods in a nutritious diet. What would you suggest about the inclusion of foods moderate to high in fat and cholesterol, such as whole milk, dairy products, and ice cream?

5. Many Americans are so tired of hearing the possible carcinogenic effects of various foodstuffs that they "turn off" any messages regarding diet and cancer. Consider this, and write a pamphlet describing in lay terms the known relationships between diet and cancer. Suggest a prudent diet that might help to prevent cancer.

6. A diet camp for teenagers has engaged your services as a consultant dietitician. The camp has a well-standardized set of procedures and plans to continue current practices, but eligibility for a federal grant requires that they have a nutritionist on staff. The camp places each teenager on a very strict, 600 calorie-a-day diet and aims for a minimum weight loss of 5 lb a week. Large quantities of "diet" foods such as diet gelatin, diet soda, and the like are permitted freely and are greatly encouraged. Appetite depressants are prescribed for all campers. The exercise routine is strenuous and required. Behavior modification is not used as the director scoffs at such "psychological" techniques. A sample menu for the day suggests the following:

Breakfast: 1 poached egg
1 piece dry toast
1 cup black coffee or tea
1 multivitamin/mineral supplement

Lunch: tossed salad
½ cup green beans
2 oz tuna fish, packed in water
1 orange
diet gelatin

Supper: 3 oz chicken
tossed salad
½ cup broccoli
½ grapefruit
diet soda

The camp director refuses to change the policy from a 600-calorie diet and merely asks that you write nutritious menus within this limit. What would you suggest to the director? How would you jusfify your recommendations? What type of information would you collect to illustrate the disadvantages of the current program? Would you try to convince the director to take a different strategy?

7. In the near future, it may be possible to take a pill that will protect against tooth decay. Children might take the pill and be protected from dental caries for the rest of their lives. Consider what the effects of such a pill might be on eating habits. Would children then have the license to eat any kind of sticky sweet food? If this pill became available, how would you persuade children of the necessity to continue to view nutrition as an important aspect of good dental health?

8. The U.S. Department of Agriculture must make a policy statement regarding the inclusion of highly sugared food in the school lunch program. Develop a policy statement for the department. Support your statement with a literature review. Develop a strategy for the implementation of your policy. Would you allow the students to buy candy, cake, or cookies from a vending machine during lunchtime? How would you decide which foods would not be allowed? What about foods such as canned pears in sugar syrup that are currently a part of the school lunch meal? What about raisins? Many children may prefer to drink chocolate milk rather than white milk. Allowing chocolate milk in the lunch meal may increase the consumption of milk and also reduce the wastage of white milk. But the chocolate milk contains much more sugar than white milk. Would you allow it? How would you determine which foods were allowed and which were prohibited?

9. You are a nutritionist at a WIC clinic. Mary S., a 17-year-old, is 6 months pregnant. In a routine interview, Mary states that she and the group she spends a lot of time with have frequent parties and drink heavily. Mary has experienced a number of tensions during the pregnancy and feels the need to relax with a drink or two in the morning and often follows this with four or five more drinks throughout the day. Her diet is poor; she usually does not have an appetite for eating and sometimes the WIC package of foods goes unused. Mary knows she should stop drinking but says she cannot stop now because it is the only way she has to relieve her frustrations. She will make an effort to stop drinking after the baby is born and things "settle down" again. How would you counsel Mary without unduly alarming her? What referrals might you make? Would you scare her by telling her of the possible adverse effects of alcohol intake on the fetus?

10. On the basis of the current state of knowledge, support or refute the *Dietary Goals*. These goals have been criticized on the grounds that we have insufficient information relating diet to disease to make dietary recommendations geared to the public. Support or refute this criticism. Engage in a debate with others whose opinions differ from yours.

Nutrition education and health promotion

Section Objective

The general objective of this section is to review concepts and issues regarding the modification of food habits through nutrition education.

Section Overview

As preceding sections have pointed out, there is considerable evidence that many North Americans might improve their health by modifying their daily diets. This is much easier said than done. Food habits are the result of numerous personal factors that are deeply imbedded in inner layers of the human personality. They are also the result of influences of, for example, the existing food system, food industry activities, and advertising in the media, many of which are beyond the direct control of the consumer. Thus, nutrition education as a possible means of modifying food habits must be considered in the proper context. Given the multifactorial nature of food habits, what is the potential for modifying them through nutrition education? This section reviews definitions, concepts, and approaches to nutrition education and then considers current issues surrounding nutrition education in the United States.

## 12

Nutrition education in perspective -- influences on North American eating habits

Reader Objectives

After completing this chapter, the reader should be able to
1. Outline the factors affecting food habits that are under the control of the consumer.
2. Outline the factors affecting food habits that are largely beyond the control of the individual.
3. State the pros and cons of the food industry relative to North American food and nutritional status.
4. Describe nutrition education efforts of the food industry.
5. Describe the influence of mass media on food habits.

OVERVIEW

The modification of food habits presupposes an understanding of the factors that influence these habits. Food actually consumed depends upon available food supplies and the acceptability of these foods to the consumer. In other words, food supply and consumer demand are the two general influences on food consumption.

A number of researchers have attempted to explain what determines food habits and nutrition behavior. G. Pelto designed a comprehensive model suggesting that dietary intake and nutrition can, in large part, be conceptualized as the result of "life-style," which is defined as the "complex interaction of a large series of social, cultural and situational inputs." Life-style variables include household structural factors (i.e., number of people in household, age, sex, spacing between children, division of labor in household tasks, decision-making power within household, and so on); education, occupation, and employment of household members; attitudes toward health, families, childrearing, and the like; religious, social, and cultural traditions; migration history; geographical, social, and economic resources; place of residence (urban/rural); and health status.[1]

Life-style, in a broad sense, describes "the way in which people live." Pelto suggested that "life-style" represents an intermediate (or intervening) factor whereby the various environmental variables external to the household or family are integrated into and affect the relationship between food habits and other environmental factors.[1]

However, in most studies comparing various groups of people, broadly defined sociocultural variables account for a relatively small portion of the total variance in eating patterns. The degree to which the consumer can actually exert choice in food consumption is, in many aspects, beyond the consumer's control. Consider, for example, a very-low-income consumer whose limited mobility restricts his or her food buying to perhaps one retail outlet. Because of a lack of education, this consumer may not have the wisest selection of food. The limited income further restricts his or her food selection. The food supplies delivered to, or produced in, the area, the advertising of these food supplies and the price of food, all of which are largely beyond the consumer's control, actually determine a significant part of the selected diet.

Figure 12-1 illustrates the multiplicity of factors that influence food consumption. It is beyond the scope of this book to discuss all these factors. This chapter thus focuses on environmental factors that affect the food supply and North American eating habits and that are largely beyond the control of the individual consumer.

FOOD PRODUCTION

The foods that producers decide to grow or raise, such as vegetables, cereals, poultry, or livestock, will have a great effect on the types of food that become available for consumption. The food production framework is largely determined by consumer demand, as well as by import regulations, agricultural policy measures, farm price supports, and the resources available for production, such as land, water, energy, climate, technology, income, and capital.

Regulation of what kind of food, and how much will be produced and available to consumers, can be achieved in a variety of ways. Some of the ways that are currently used to some extent by the U.S. government encompass the following:

1. National programs for acreage to be planted in given crops. For example, the Food and Agriculture Act of 1977 allows the U.S. Department of Agriculture to implement a national program of acreage for wheat based upon the number of harvested acres determined to yield the amount of wheat that will be used domestically and for export during the marketing year. The USDA may thus limit the acreage

Figure 12-1. Factors influencing food consumption.

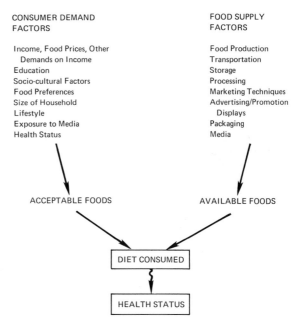

planted in a given crop and will pay producers to set aside this land, leaving it free of crops.

2. Price policies. Price policies are extremely important in determining food supply as well as consumer demand for food products. For most products, the demand rises as prices fall, and conversely, demand falls as prices rise. The degree to which demand reacts to price changes is influenced by a variety of factors, including the amount of price fluctuation, the money available for spending, and the specific food items.*

Thus, by intervening in food pricing, it is possible to modify consumer demand. Price policies include such things as:

— price negotiations between producer and the government; this may include import quotas on foods.

— price supports; prices of food commodities, such as milk, may be adjusted to reflect changes in the parity index.**

— government support loans to assist the farmer in the purchase of needed farm inputs.

— government purchase of commodities; surplus commodities are often purchased by the government and then offered to federal food programs. Such purchases stabilize producer prices and income.

— determination of a farmer's price floor as the basis for selling agricultural commodities to industrial nations.

3. Plant breeding and animal feeding and breeding measures designed to influence the nutritional value of production: for example, changing the ratio between fat and other nutrients in food, increasing the protein value of plant foods, and so on. Modifying the diet of an animal may result in a different composition of the milk or eggs or meat

---

*The range of food demand, sometimes termed *demand elasticity,* is used to measure the various factors that influence demand. Demand elasticity is composed of price elasticity, income elasticity, and cross elasticity:

Price elasticity is the percentage change in product demand when price changes by a percentage point. Price elasticity for food is usually less than zero; that is, the demand for a product falls as price rises.

Income elasticity is the percentage change in product demand when income changes by a percentage point. Elasticity for the majority of foods is greater than one; that is, the demand increases as income increases.

Cross elasticity is the percentage change (rise or fall) in consumption of a product as the price of another product varies by a percentage point.

Demand elasticities for foods tend to be low. In other words, moderate income and price fluctuations stimulate moderate variation in food demand. This tends to be a function of the fact that people must eat to satisfy basic needs; thus, food needs often take precedence over needs for other goods and services.

These remarks relate to food in general. Within and between food groups, however, the elasticity of demand varies considerably.

**Parity refers to the return that farmers obtain on their investments. Specifically, 100 per cent parity would mean that a unit of production, for example, a bushel of food grain, would buy now what it bought between 1910 and 1914, a time of farm prosperity. Thus, if the farmer could sell a bushel of grain in 1914 for the price of a pair of gloves, he or she should be able to do the same today, at 100 per cent parity. But, in reality, the price of a bushel of grain today would probably not cover half the price of the gloves.

(see pp. 266-267). Likewise, genetic breeding of particular plants, such as corn, has resulted in the development of a high-lysine corn product.

FOOD PROCESSING AND DISTRIBUTION WITH SPECIAL FOCUS ON THE U.S. FOOD INDUSTRY

The food industry in the United States plays a significant role in determining the quality of the food supply in this country. For this role, the food industry has been variously applauded and profoundly criticized. The following discussion looks at the contributions and the negative impacts of the food industry as they relate to the quality of the North American diet.

Contributions of the Food Industry

The food industry is a significant contributor to the U.S. economy. In 1970, food and food-related product manufacturers employed over 1.6 million workers at a total payroll cost of $11.7 billion; the value of these products exceeded $97.6 billion.[2]

Food preservation as such is not new; prehistoric men used methods of drying, salt, smoking, storage in root cellars and caves, fermentation, and the addition of sweetening agents to preserve foods. Chemical preservation dates back to the years around 1500 B.C. when preservatives, such as mustard, sulfur, and aromatic oils, were used.

Today's food industry processes foods, not only to preserve them but to add nutrients; modify the quality, color, shelf life, size, and flavor; make the foods better able to withstand travel over long distances; and cater to identified "consumer preferences."

The food supply available in the United States today is tremendous, and is characterized by a variety of foods of high quality. The North American consumer can go to the grocery store and find numerous different kinds of fresh fruit and vegetables throughout the year. For example, citrus fruits, tomatoes, cucumbers, and lettuce are available to the consumer in northern Maine in the middle of the winter, something that would not be possible without food technology.

We are fortunate to have a wide range of choice in our food supply. For example, the consumer can choose from fresh, canned sweetened, canned unsweetened, chunk, crushed, or sliced pineapple or pineapple juice. New food products can be found on the shelves almost every day. This is no small achievement. The development of many new products requires tremendous inputs of technology, knowledge, and skills, and we can choose among various food products. The consumer who prefers fresh vegetables can pass by the seasoned "vegetable thins" box of crackers, and can buy fresh Idaho potatoes and never succumb to the temptations of potato chips or of frozen, whipped, sliced, diced, hash browns, or the numerous other kinds of processed potatoes that are available. (See Figures 12-2 and 12-3.)

The food industry in the United States has significantly contributed to the alleviation of many vitamin and mineral deficiencies that once plagued

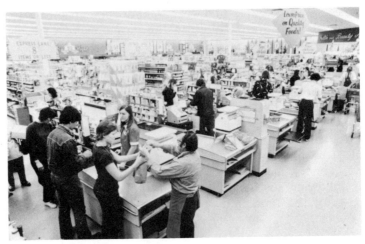

Figure 12-2. A wide variety of food products both natural and processed are now available to the American consumer. This trend may be associated with positive as well as negative influences in our nutritional status. (The Great Atlantic & Pacific Tea Company, Inc.)

many poor Americans at the turn of the century. Enrichment, fortification, and supplementation of the food supply are common food industry practices. Food technology added vitamin D to milk and helped to conquer rickets, and it added vitamin C to foods and helped to eliminate scurvy. Iodine in salt has virtually eliminated goiter. These are illustrations of steps that the food industry has taken to improve the American diet.

The food industry has also undertaken numerous nutrition-related activities, such as product advertising, product labeling, and providing product nutritional information. This can significantly heighten the public's awareness of nutrition. Product processing and production along with research and development can enhance the nutritional value of the food supply. The development of company research libraries and information data systems can offer a valuable information source on the food content that is available to the nation. Educational resources can

Figure 12-3. "Nowadays the harvest is bountiful all year long, in more ways than one. I wonder whether the average American's love affair with food is doing him in." — J. Stamler. (photo from *3 Times a Day*, prepared for Best Foods, a division of CPC International, by Medcom, Inc., New York)

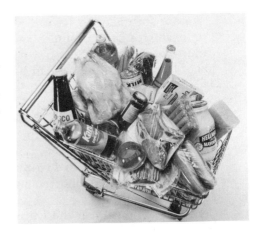

support research and nutrition-related activities of health professionals and universities.

Criticisms of the Food Industry

Many of the benefits of food industry activities are considered by many people to be hazards. For example, the abundant North American food supply is often cited as a critical concern in relation to the world's food, resource, and population crisis. In spite of the significant contribution the food industry in the United States has made to improve the national diet, food industry critics abound. The industry is frequently confronted by criticism from consumer advocates, nutrition and health professionals, and the public.

Increasing concern is being expressed by nutritionists, health professionals, government officials, and the general public over the role of the food industry relative to the nutrition and health status of the nation. Many people have contended that the food industry has not acted in a responsible way in providing nutritionally safe food products and has not taken an active role in health promotion or nutrition education.

Food processing has advantages, but it also poses a number of concerns from a nutritional point of view. Many nutrients may be lost or destroyed by large amounts of heating, peeling, cutting, milling, and refining. Although lost nutrients can be replaced by other processing techniques, such as enrichment, there is concern over the effectiveness of certain forms of added nutrients. There is also no certainty about what should be added to foods, and there is no assurance that, in the case of nutrients such as vitamins A and D, an individual who consumes large amounts of fortified products may not be in danger of consuming excess nutrients. The numerous chemicals that are added to food raise a serious question of food safety.

The trend toward highly processed foods dominates the food industry. In *Eat Your Heart Out*, J. Hightower describes what this means to the consumer: "Increasingly the cost of processing and packaging is greater than the cost of the food in the package." To illustrate this point, Hightower notes that a 53¢ package of Wheaties actually contains only about 2¢ worth of wheat. By adding some vitamins worth about ½¢ the industry can change the cereal name to Total and charge the consumer an additional 22¢.[3]

Highly processed foods often actually contain less nutritional value than their homemade counterparts. This point was made by the Consumers Union in tests of eight different brands of meat pies. Only three brands of chicken and turkey pot pies met the U.S. Department of Agriculture standards of 14 per cent cooked meat. The Consumers Union found the vegetable content of the pies to be only 6.5 per cent of pie weight.[4]

As the average American's diet becomes more reliant on processed and fabricated foods, dietary inadequacy may be more likely. We are not aware of all nutrients required for human health, as evidenced by the fact that almost every revision of the RDAs contains allowances for an additional nutrient. In addition, these allowances are revised as newer scientific knowledge becomes available. Thus, we cannot be sure that we have the scientific and technical knowledge to fabricate foods to meet human requirements. The individual who drinks instant breakfast in the morning, lunches on Granola bars and imitation fruit, and drinks and eats convenience meals and reconstituted foods for dinner may be at nutritional risk.

Another criticism that is frequently leveled against the food industry involves the industry's profit motive. Basic to any action by the food industry is competition; the assumption is that increased product lines will produce increased profits. Thus, more than $50 million is spent by the food industry each year in the development of novel food products, many of which are far from highly nutritious. This spending not only expands the number of food products that are available but also results in increased food prices for the consumer.[5]

Agribusiness

Agribusiness includes all the activities involved in producing, processing, and marketing farm produce. It includes concerns that supply machinery and farm inputs, farmers, transport and storage operators, food processors, wholesalers, and retailers. It encompasses all who are involved in producing and distributing the food from the farm, past the farm gate, to the table. It also includes organizations and institutions that regulate, control, and coordinate the activities of these various concerns such as government, farm and trade organizations, and futures.[6]

The entire food system, agribusiness, is often criticized for pursuing self-interests and profits to the neglect of sound nutritional objectives. The charge is frequently made that control over the food and nutrition industries is merely passed from hand to hand of representatives with the same interest vantage point. For example, J. Hightower in *Hard Tomatoes, Hard Times* suggests that the technological agricultural system is synonymous with agribusiness. He conceptualizes a conspiracy in which agricultural colleges are dominated by agribusiness in pursuit of profit-motivated interests.[7]

The close relationship between industry and the academic community and the scientific establishment has been brought under close scrutiny and increasing criticism in recent years. One widely publicized exposé accused university professors and food scientists of being advocates of the practices of the food industry. The report was issued by Rep. Benjamin Rosenthal (D., N.Y.) and the Center for Science in the Public Interest. Entitled "Feeding at the Company Trough," the report concluded that ". . . many professors are, quite frankly, on the take . . ."[8]

The report described the close ties that many food scientists and professors have developed with industry, such as offering consultation and advice, accepting large and long-term research grants, representing industry at congressional hearings, and serving on boards of directors and trade association committees. The authors of the report conducted a survey of nutrition and food science departments and suggested that "at most prominent universities, eminent nutritionists have traded their independence for the food industry's favors."[8]

Refuting the implications of the Rosenthal report, R. Deutsch provided another view of "Professors on the Take," suggesting that the report was not "very revealing." According to Deutsch most nutrition departments have received some support from the food industry but many who receive the support have remained unbiased and objective. J. Mayer, for example, who was listed in the Rosenthal report because of his association with Monsanto, a manufacturer of food additives, has called for a review of the federal regulations on food additives. The "lines continue to be drawn" and the need for a clear direction in seeking to separate fact from fiction in nutrition is more apparent than ever.[9]

Nutrition Education and the Food Industry

A basic question to be answered relative to nutrition education is whether or not the food industry can succeed in getting the nutritional message across in an unbiased fashion. Other efforts to do so have obviously failed. A first step in this direction was taken in September and October 1970, when the first Nutritional Awareness campaign was initiated by the food industry. The campaign was the result of recommendations made at the White House Conference on Food, Nutrition, and Health that a Food Council of America be established to conduct nutrition education campaigns.[10]

The Food Council, an intraindustry group made up of the chief staff officers of all the national food industry associations who chose to join, has a membership representing food chains, grocery manufacturers, convenience stores, wholesale grocers, canners, and numerous specific food institutes.

The first campaign selected the theme "Eat the Basic Four Foods Every Day." Each of the members of the Food Council pledged to volunteer its efforts and support for the 1970 campaign and to continue the program annually for at least five years. Campaign activities of 1970 included supermarket displays of the "Basic 4 Symbol," posters and displays advocating good nutrition, and newspaper and magazine advertisements promoting the theme of good nutrition. Since 1970, the program has been repeated and expanded.

In addition to the Food Council, the food industry has offered assistance to the USDA and to other agencies in the development of community teaching programs aimed at reaching all Americans, with special emphasis on reaching the poor. The food industry has cooperated in the training of paraprofessionals, has sponsored activities of professional nutritionists, and has helped to develop educational material to be distributed to developing nations.

Industry-sponsored education programs, which are offered in a variety of ways and through different channels, can help the food industry to meet the nutritional needs of the North American public. Many activities of the food industry have involved nutrition education. Nutrition resources developed and offered through the food industry include the following:[11]

1. American Institute of Baking (AIB) — a research and organizational group that represents baking and allied trade companies and conducts basic nutrition education as well as education in baking science and

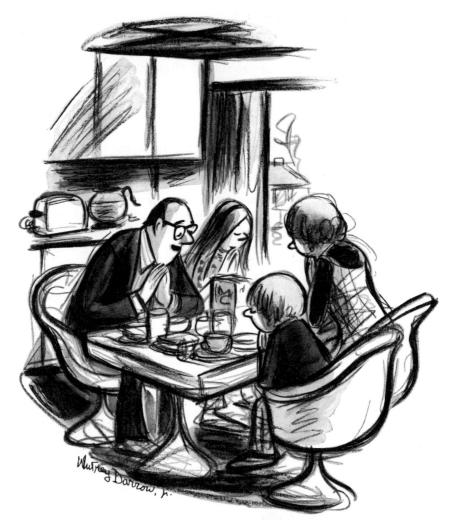

Figure 12–4. "We thank thee, Lord, for this instant coffee, this Redi-Quick Cocoa, this one-minute oatmeal, and the pop-up waffles. In haste, amen." (Drawing by Whitney Darrow, Jr., © 1973 The New Yorker Magazine, Inc.)

food technology. The AIB maintains a library of relevant materials and is engaged in preparing and disseminating sources of nutrition information.

2. The Cereal Institute — members have participated in a special program whereby product packages convey carefully designed and attractively presented nutrition information. The institute is also involved in the production and dissemination of educational resources such as film-strips, leaflets, and teaching guides available to professionals either free or at a minimal cost.

3. The National Dairy Council — is involved in designing nutrition educa-tion materials, developing learning objectives and activities to achieve stated objectives, and providing demonstrations and workshops for schools, health professionals, and the general public. The Dairy Council

has sponsored nutritional experiments as learning experiences for schoolchildren. Resources developed by the Dairy Council include a wide variety of pamphlets, filmstrips, games, slides and tapes, posters, and charts.

4. The National Livestock and Meat Board — supports nutrition research studies and promotes and educates about meats. The board has a Home Economics Department as well as a Nutrition Research Department and is in the process of developing an education department. *Food and Nutrition News* is a publication available to professional nutritionists.

5. The United Fresh Fruit and Vegetable Association — develops nutrition education materials available to the public. The association works with government agencies to develop regulations and maintain member awareness of government activities. It also conducts training sessions for member firms, promotes nutrition education and provides media releases, sets up trade meetings for member education and problem solving, and publishes other education materials.

6. Grocery Manufacturers of America, Inc. (GMA) — a national trade association of leading manufacturers of food and other grocery products. GMA works to maintain nutritional value of food products and to provide sound nutrition information to consumers on an organized basis. The association has prepared an annotated bibliography of consumer/educational information as well as other nutrition education materials. GMA has worked to help overcome local resistance to food stamps, has developed a comic book to explain nutrition to children, and has worked with the USDA and the USDHEW in a nutritional advertising campaign.

Although the interest in nutrition education by the food industry is clear, there has been much criticism of the bias in educational materials developed by the food industry:

> Though the Dairy Council (for example) deserves some credit for its interest in nutrition education, one wonders if its incomplete and biased program is, on the whole, worthwhile. Is nutrition education desirable when, in addition to teaching vitamins and minerals, it tells kids and parents that a diet rich in saturated fat and cholesterol is good for them?[12]

In addition to the previously-mentioned activities, the food industry has also worked jointly with the USDA in the development and distribution of some nutrition education materials. An example is "The Thing the Professor Forgot" a story book written in verse that was jointly prepared by the USDA and General Mills Corporation. This publication was the most popular publication distributed by the Consumer Information Center in fiscal year 1976. Over 1 million copies were received by children, parents, and teachers during the initial ten-month distribution period of this publication. Offers for the publication on cereal boxes further increased the distribution of the book.

A second successful example of a government/industry effort to disseminate nutrition information is "Food Is More than Just Something to

Eat." This illustrated booklet was jointly developed by the Grocery Manufacturers of America, the USDA, the USDHEW, and the National Academy of Sciences. Over 2 million copies of this booklet have been distributed nationwide. It is part of the Advertising Council's Campaign on Food, Nutrition, and Health, which also includes public service television spots and messages in the written media to encourage good nutrition. Although these efforts at nutrition education by the food industry may be commendable, they do not begin to approach what the industry could potentially do to improve nutrition.

A comprehensive survey of 28 major food industries demonstrated that food companies that are engaged in nutrition education efforts are merely promoting and advertising their own products. The survey found that:[13]

1. Nutrition is considered a way to encourage consumers to purchase a particular product rather than to maintain a healthy diet.

2. Food companies usually lack a general, stated nutritional policy.

3. Food companies that do attempt nutrition education believe that the message to be presented to consumers is the need to eat. Consideration of problems such as obesity and other health problems is not characteristic of advertising objectives.

4. Most nutrition education in the public schools by food industry groups promotes particular products rather than sound diet patterns.

The results of the survey were presented in testimony before the U.S. House of Representatives Nutrition Subcommittee in February 1978. The report indicated that, of the 13 food companies reporting nutrition education allocations, most spent less than $500,000. General Foods, the largest food company surveyed, spent only $836,000, or less than 1 per cent of its total $275 million advertising budget, for nutrition education.

Representative F. Richmond introduced the testimony and charged that the food industry's notion of nutrition education is "frequently nothing more than an excuse for such self-serving concepts as 'Breakfast Nutrition,' 'Snack Nutrition,' 'Dairy Nutrition,' or even 'Weiner Nutrition.' In the face of a rising incidence of obesity and other diet-related health problems, food company messages say "eat something of everything." Rarely is emphasis given to diet and health."[13]

> Food advertising as a whole has tended to blunt public awareness of the health significance of food choices and has encouraged patterns of consumption which are contributing to a decline in the nutritional status of major segments of the population.
>
> — Federal Trade Commission

> No amount of information about the nutritive or nonnutritive qualities of the foods advertised will compensate for the total imbalance in the nature of the foods advertised on television. The nature of the foods advertised is largely highly processed foods, many of them snack foods, highly sugared, highly salted. . . . We should have advertising of fruits and vegetables. There should be public service announcements selling people on those components of the diet which, in fact, they are not currently being sold on — dairy products, beans and rice and grains, and

other forms of protein foods. . . . And all these foods don't get sold because they do not have a high enough mark-up.

— Joan Gussow

INFLUENCE OF THE MEDIA ON FOOD HABITS

The media including television, radio, and printed publications, significantly affect the eating patterns of the American public. The potential of the mass media to influence nutrition behavior is tremendous.

The most commonly used of the mass media is television. An estimated 96 per cent of American homes have at least one television set. On the average, the television set is on more than 6 hours a day. When a child reaches the age of 3, he or she usually begins to view television frequently. This level of viewing remains relatively high until about the age of 12, when television viewing often begins to drop off. When young adults marry and begin to raise families, television viewing increases and then stabilizes. After middle age, viewing time again increases.[14]

Although the public has many sources of nutrition and health information, the media is often the most frequently used and, next to doctors, is often regarded as the most credible information source. A 1971 poll reported that almost 30 per cent of the American public gets most of its "information" on health from television advertising, as compared with 28 per cent from newspapers, 26 per cent from magazines, and 25 per cent from television documentaries.[15]

The media is a particularly "credible" information source for children. For example, one study found that 70 per cent of television health messages seen by fifth- and sixth-grade children were "believed"; this increased to 86 per cent among children from lower socioeconomic backgrounds.[16]

Television programming directed at children is greatly supported by food advertising. In 1975 an estimated $400 million was spent on television advertising to children alone, and more than 50 per cent of the commercials on programs directed to children were for food products.[17]

According to Broadcast Advertisers Reports, an industry source of advertising expenditures, the 1970 advertising expenditures in weekend daytime programming and for Captain Kangaroo totaled $81 million for television network time. If this amount is doubled to include local children's advertising, the total dollar figure comes to $162 million, which represents 5.8 per cent of all television advertising revenues in 1970 and 2.5 per cent of all national media expenditures in the United States.[18]

The top advertising priorities, however, often do not include nutrition. "A food industry axiom has it that people will not buy a product unless it looks and tastes good. Nutrition as a selling point, comes in a poor third."[19]

Tables 12-1 and 12-2 indicate food and beverage advertising expenditures in the United States for selected food products. The disproportionate amounts spent for snack foods, foods high in sugar and fat, and highly processed foods, as compared with natural foods containing essential nutrients, such as fresh fruit, vegetables, and unrefined grain products, are obvious.[20]

Table 12-1

Food and Beverage Advertising Expenditures in the United States, 1971

Type of Food	Amount (thousands of dollars)
Sugars, desserts, snacks, soft drinks	$283,547.2
Shortening, oil, fat, mayonnaise, sauces, dips	73,268.6
Milk, butter, eggs, cheese	41,529.2
Fruits, vegetables	36,239.5
Meat, poultry, fish	50,131.5
Breads, rolls, flour, baking mixes, cereals, pastas	183,334.0

Source: L. Masover. Unpublished thesis material. Evanston, Ill.: Northwestern University Medical School, 1976.

Table 12-2

Total Weekday Food Advertising by Food Groups

Group	Percentage of Time, Weekday	Percentage of Time, Weekend
Nonnutritive beverages	37.5%	51.7%
Grains	17.5	19.8
Sugars/sweets	10.3	12.9
Oil, fat, margarine	8.5	5.7
Food stores	7.0	0
Processed meat, fish, poultry	5.7	0.6
Snack foods	2.9	3.7
Dairy	3.1	2.0
Relishes, condiments	2.6	1.2
Vegetables	1.3	1.7
Fruit	1.7	0
Soup	1.1	0
Sugar substitutes	0.5	0.2
Nuts, nut products	0.3	0
Egg substitutes	0	0

Source: See Table 12-1.

Impact of Media on Children's Eating Habits

Television has had more impact on children's eating habits than has any other form of media. Children spend more time watching television than in any other single activity with the exception of sleeping. It is estimated that the average preschool child watches television about 26.3 hours a week and that children between the ages of 6 and 16 watch television 25 hours a week.[21]

In 1977 the average American child aged 2 to 11 viewed more than 20,000 television commercials, as well as an average of 3 ⅔ hours of television daily. Schoolchildren typically spent more time in front of the television set than they did in school. Further, the length of time children spend watching television has significantly increased since 1950.[22]

The concern with children's advertising goes beyond the amount of time children spend watching commercials.[23,24] J. G. Cooney, president of the Children's Television Workshop and the producer of the educational television shows "Sesame Street" and the "Electric Company," has stated that these programs make use of techniques used in commercials. This allows these shows to take advantage of the attention-gaining strategies that were developed by advertising professionals.[23] These strategies, according to K. G. O'Bryan, are so powerful that they "make the 30-second commercial the most effective teaching device yet invented for implanting any relatively simple idea in a child's mind — including the idea that a product is desirable."[25] (See Figure 12–5.)

Children are very easily led by the messages and ideas conveyed to them in commercials. An advertisement conveys a sense of urgency, almost a command to the child. The point is well illustrated by the case of Soupy Sales, who in 1965 suggested to his early morning young television audience that they take the wallets and purses of their sleeping parents and

Figure 12–5. Television advertising exerts an important and often counternutritional influence on the eating patterns of American children (from 3 Times a Day, prepared for Best Foods, a division of CPC International, by Medcom, Inc., New York)

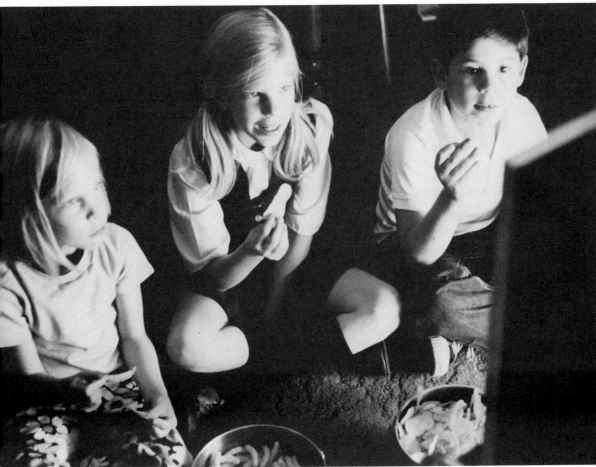

remove "some of those funny green pieces of paper with all those nice pictures of George Washington, Abraham Lincoln, and Alexander Hamilton, and send them along to your old pal, Soupy, care of WNEW, New York." Enough money was sent to Soupy to be "the biggest heist since the Boston Brink's robbery."[23]

Commercial advertising to children can be classified into at least four forms:[24]

Intentional — advertising using phraseology to appeal to a child for retail sales, possibly through a parent (for example, candy, gum, cereals, snacks, toys).

General — messages directed at all age groups (for example, toothpaste, movies, food).

Peripheral — messages for products typically used by adults, but directed to children's television in the hopes that the child will relay the message to the adult (for example, children's drugs, detergents).

Inadvertent — adult products advertised in an adult way to an audience not considered to have child members (for example, over-the-counter drugs, feminine hygiene products).

A variety of techniques used in children's television advertising are listed in Table 12–3. With these techniques, advertisers are able to create a direct learning experience for the child — the child learns to demand the product being advertised. In addition, the commercials may alter the way a child actually understands the message.[25]

No matter what the form of the commercial, the child is an active participant in the repercussions of these various advertisements. The parent may participate in the consequences by approving the purchase of re-

Table 12–3
Manipulative Techniques Used in Children's Advertising

---

1. Magical promises that a product will build strong muscles, "make you run faster," or otherwise improve performance.

2. The "chase or tug-of-war sequence in which one character tries to take a product away from another." This type of device stimulates the child to feel that the product must be very desirable and worth having.

3. The use of music, songs, dances, and animation.

4. The use of superheroes to stimulate children.

5. The voices of authority.

6. The voices of children agreeing with the announcer.

7. Depictions of children outperforming adults after eating a product.

8. Peer group acceptance appeals.

9. Selling by characters who also appear in programming.

Source: Federal Trade Commission. *FTC Staff Report on Television Advertising to Children*. Washington, D.C.: Government Printing Office, February 1978.

quested products, by offering money to the child to purchase the products, or by actually purchasing the products advertised. The child thus plays a central role in the process of food selection as mediated by advertisements.

A child who is exposed to such communication will respond to it in some way. The central question to be posed is, How do children receive and translate promotional messages for food products? Do the advertisement messages determine lifelong food and nutrition attitudes?

Studies that have analyzed the impact of television advertising on children have all observed different children's reactions, but all observed that children do respond to the advertising.[26-28]

R. B. Choate has summarized the effects of advertising as follows:

> The food industry seeks to influence children with its food advertisements, and they are affected. Children communicate their food desires and influence food selections as a result. By aiming certain products of dubious nutritional worth without nutritional information at young audiences, food companies seem to take advantage of their nutritional naïveté; the lack of nutritional information — including calories — in their advertisements compounds children's vulnerabilities. It is an unfair practice.[24]

Many critics of television advertising contend that it is virtually impossible for a child to select a nutritious diet from the foods advertised on television, and vitamin commercials compound the problem. There is an imbalance in the nutritional information offered through children's television advertising. Children receive a negative, antinutrition message when they are told that vitamins will "keep you growing right even if you don't eat right." As J. Gussow noted, "It is nonsense to say that the companies who advertise ingestible products to children do not or cannot give nutrition messages. They are doing so all the time and many of them are, at least by implication, lies."[29] The overwhelming message of children's food advertising is that high-sugar, high-calorie foods, either with meals or between, are normal parts of a good diet and that children eating them are healthy and happy.[22]

What is not said in commercials is, by implication, seen as not important by the children. Very little attention is devoted to vegetables, milk (except for sweet things to put into milk), eggs, meat, or cheese. Characteristics, such as "sweetness," "chocolateyness," "crunchiness," "honey taste," "marshmallow taste," being long-lasting in the mouth, chewiness, and stickiness, are desirable in food, according to commercials. The effect of these approaches on the child audience is portrayed in Figure 12-6.

Various critics of television advertising on children's programs contend that advertisers manipulate child consumers in such a way that the process becomes a deceptive hoax — that children are thus encouraged to desire certain products without questioning their real worth.[30]

Children respond to television advertisements for food in different ways. One of the significant factors relating to the response to advertising is age. Younger children (aged 5 to 10 years old) seem to be more attentive to commercials than are older children. Preschool children are particularly attracted to the commercials; kindergarten children often tend to mix the

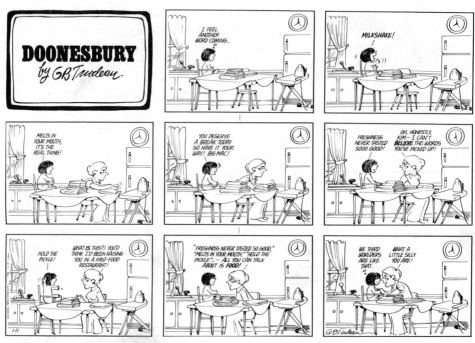

Figure 12-6. (Copyright 1976 G. B. Trudeau/Distributed by Universal Press Syndicate. Reprinted by permission)

commercial messa   with the program content. Older children are more
conscious of the r   ge and purpose of the commercial and begin to be
suspicious of certa   messages. Distrust of commercial messages increases
with age. Childrer   the second grade have been found to distrust commercials based on   ieir personal experiences with the products advertised
and children in the sixth grade have demonstrated a general distrust of
all commercials.[31]

Many studies have noted that children definitely influence their parents'
food-buying behavior as a result of watching television commercials. Commercials for food are the most likely to influence a child's demand for a
product, and mothers are more likely to respond to the child's request for
food than for other items.[31] A number of recent studies have focused on
the impact of television advertising of food products on children. Much
remains not understood, but certain salient facts, summarized in Table
12-4 seem apparent.[32,33]

Recommendations

To deal with these problems of food advertising, the Action for Children's
Television (ACT) was founded to allow parents, educators, and the concerned public to join forces to encourage and support good television for
children. ACT proposed at least a minimal amount of programming for
children of various age groups. Under this proposal, commercials would be
eliminated; programs would be underwritten through company name
announcements; toys, cereals, and candy would be advertised only on
adult programs.

As a result of the National Nutrition Policy Study, the Panel on Nutri-

Table 12–4

Facts Relating to the Impact of Children's Television of Food Products on Children

1. Children are attracted to television commercials before they enjoy other television viewing. It is not unusual for a very young child (less than the age of 2) to ignore television until the commercial comes on; then he or she will drop his or her play and stand, fixed to the television set.

2. Children seem to prefer and to use their influence to persuade their parents to buy the food products promoted to them on television.

3. Children are often successful in their attempts to have their parents buy the foods they request; parents often yield to their child's request for cereals, snack foods, and candy.

4. Television commercials are often misunderstood by the child who is watching them. Children may be unable to distinguish the television commercial from other programming; they may have limited understanding of the intent behind the commercial, that is, to promote a product; and children may put complete trust in the message of the commercial.

5. Children respond differently to food advertising depending on their age; younger children seem to express more acceptance of food product nutritional claims than do older children.

6. Studies have demonstrated shifts in children's beliefs about advertised foods after viewing specific commercial messages.

Sources: Federal Trade Commission. *FTC Staff Reports on Television Advertising to Children.* Washington, D.C.: Government Printing Office, February 1978. D. Yankelovich. *Mothers' Attitudes toward Children's Programs and Commercials.* Newton Center, Mass.: Action for Children's T.V., 1970. National Science Foundation. *Research on the Effects of Television Advertising on Children: A Review of the Literature and Recommendations for Future Research.* Bethesda, Md.: NSF Grant No. APR 75–10126, 1975.

tion and the Consumer drafted a proposed Children's Advertising Code that would:[34]

1. Prohibit the advertising of any edible product or beverage containing added sugar over 10 per cent by wet weight or 30 per cent by dry weight; or any product containing a nonnutritive sweetener.

2. Require that any commercial identifying or implying fruit or other characterizing ingredient or flavor in a product disclose its natural/artificial nature.

3. Prohibit any claim, directly or by implication, that any edible product or nutrient of itself produces, hastens, or enhances vigor, stamina, strength, energy, growth, or intellecutal performance.

4. Prohibit the advertising of vitamin or other supplements or over-the-counter drugs to children.

5. Prohibit more than 2 minutes of commercials for edible products during any clock hour of children's programming.

If this code were put into effect and these goals achieved, there would be a need for a continuing effort on the part of all concerned nutrition professionals and advocates as well as cooperation from the government and the food and media industry.

In view of their concern over children's advertising, the Federal Trade Commission (FTC) staff prepared a report recommending improvements in television advertising to eliminate the harm resulting from unfair and deceptive advertising. The report concluded that: "It is both unfair and deceptive . . . to address televised advertising for *any* product to young children who are still too young to understand the selling purpose of, or otherwise comprehend or evaluate, the advertising." R. Choate stated the idea as follows:

> Advertising to children much resembles a tug of war between 200-pound men and 60-pound youngsters. Whether called an unfair practice or thought subject to fairness doctrine interpretation, the fact remains that any communication that has a $1,000-per-commercial scriptwriter, actors, lighting technicians, sound effects specialists, electronic editors, psychological analysts, focus groups and motivational researchers with a $50,000 budget on one end and the 8-year-old mind (curious, spongelike, eager, gullible) with 50 cents on the other *inherently represents an unfair contest.*[35]

In view of the concern over the way television commercials "unfairly" and "deceptively" advertise to children, particularly sugared foods, the FTC staff proposed a rule to control such advertising. The FTC staff opinion suggested that the FTC has authority to regulate such commercials under current laws prohibiting unfair and deceptive advertising. The proposed rule contains the following provisions:

1. Banning all televised advertising directed at children who are not old enough to understand the purpose of advertising.

2. Banning televised advertising aimed at older children for high-sugar-content foods that are dangerous to dental health.

3. Requiring advertising for sugared products not included in the previous provision to be balanced with nutritional disclosures funded by the advertisers.

Although these proposals have been ridiculed by many, suggesting that the FTC is trying to act as a "nanny" for North American children, the ideas are not so foreign to those in many European nations. Table 12-5 summarizes advertising restrictions of some European countries.[36]

Early in 1979, the ABC network announced that the current 8.5 minutes of network advertising time per hour during Saturday and Sunday morning programming times, most of which is aimed at children, would be reduced by 20 per cent. This reduction would be accomplished in two stages beginning in January 1980. ABC also announced that "separaters" between children's advertising and the programs (short spots telling the viewer that the progamming has stopped and the advertising has begun, such as "Superman will be back after these commercial messages" and then "And, now, back to Superman") would be used.

These actions by ABC were described by an FTC official as follows:

Table 12-5

Restrictions on Children's Advertising — European Nations

Country	Restrictions
Britain	A voluntary code is under the supervision of Advertising Standards Authority of the British Director General of Fair Trading. The code bans appeals based on collecting coupons, wrappers, or labels; requires competition to be approved in advance by the authority; advertising not permitted to prey on child's credulity or sense of loyalty; use of cartoon characters to advertise children's products is banned; nature of products advertised at certain hours is restricted.
Germany	Commercial television is separated into 15-minute blocks, thus reducing involvement of children. Soft drink, candy, and gum commercials are aimed expressly at adults.
Austria	Numerous restrictions are placed on the use of children in advertisements. Children are not allowed to talk about a product or its benefits in commercials. Certain advertising, such as that of chewing gum and candy, is directed at adults, not at children.
Norway	Strict self-regulation by business is combined with protective consumer policy. Marketing codes for advertising are enforced by a consumer ombudsman. It is forbidden to "exploit the curiosity among children or their 'collection mania'."
France	The Bureau for the Verification of Advertising has established a list of industry recommendations. Advertising directed at children may not exploit their credulity or sense of loyalty; advertising is prohibited for "sugar products not forming part of normal nutrition, and which, with their carbohydrate base, cannot be consumed frequently between meals without causing inconvenience." Television stations are state-owned; advertising is handled by Regie Française de Publicité, which is able to reject advertising that does not comply with standards.
Italy	Industry self-regulation protects children aged 7 to 12. An advertising code states that "messages to children may contain nothing which will harm them psychically, morally or physically."
Spain	The Advertising Code of 1974 sets the standards for television advertising. Advertisements must comply with four requirements: comply with existing legislation, be truthful, distinguish advertising from news, and abide by principles of fair competition.

Source: Kidvid European style. *Nutr. Act.* (May 1978): 8-9.

The ABC action is the kind of incremental victory we expected from this inquiry (into children's advertising). We have hoped that there would be efforts by industry to regulate itself by placing some limitations on their children's advertising in an effort to head off government actions.[37]

CONCLUSION

The food supply in the United States is one of the most plentiful and varied in the world. But the trend toward increasingly greater processing and refinement of food; toward foods high in fat, cholesterol, refined sugars, and salt; and toward the use of many food additives and pesticides in production and processing now characterize much of the North American food supply. Because of the tremendous variety in available food, the consumer is faced with many difficult food choices for which nutrition knowledge is essential in making wise decisions.

Many factors seek to influence these decisions, a number of which could be termed counternutritional. Manipulative advertising techniques, for example, attempt to convince the consumer to desire certain kinds of food products, typically those high in sugar, fat, and calories, but low in dietary fiber. Thus, many influences on the food supply and consumer choice, which are largely beyond the control of the consumer, represent a significant barrier to nutrition education efforts. The discussion given in the following two chapters should be understood in this context.

REFERENCES

1. Pelto, G. Effects of family and life-style on nutrition and health. American Public Health Association Annual Meeting, Washington, D.C., 1977.
2. U.S. Bureau of Census. *Statistical Abstract of the U.S., 1972*, 93d ed. Washington, D.C.: Government Printing Office, 1972, pp. 708–709.
3. Hightower, J. *Eat Your Heart Out.* New York: Crown Publishers, 1975.
4. A (piece of) chicken in every pot (pie). Abstract from *Consumer Reports. CNI Week. Rep.* 5 (21 August 1975): 7.
5. Schreiber, M. J. Opening address nutrition and consumer session. Wisconsin Governor's Conference on Nutrition for Health, Madison, Wisconsin, April 4–5, 1975.
6. Editorial: The real loser. *Feedstuffs*, December 11, 1971, p. 10.
7. Hightower, J. *Hard Tomatoes, Hard Times.* Cambridge, Mass.: A. Schenhman Publishing, 1972.
8. Rosenthal, B., M. Jacobson, and M. Bohm. Professors on the take, in L. Hofmann, ed., *The Great American Nutrition Hassle.* Palo Alto, Calif.: Mayfield Publishing, 1978, pp. 379–391.
9. Deutsch, R. Another view of "professors on the take," in L. Hofmann, ed., *The Great American Nutrition Hassle.* Palo Alto, Calif.: Mayfield Publishing, 1978, pp. 391–393.
10. Mayer, J., ed. *U.S. Nutrition Policies in the Seventies.* San Francisco: W. H. Freeman, 1973.
11. Obert, J. *Community Nutrition.* New York: John Wiley, 1977.
12. Kilburn, E. The (nutrition education) gospel according to NDC. *Nutrition Action*, September 1978, p. 3.
13. Food firms hit on nutrition education. *CNI Week. Rep.* 7 (1978): 8.
14. U.S. Public Health Service, Surgeon General's Scientific Advisory Committee on Television and Social Behavior. *Television and Growing Up: The Impact of Televised Violence.* Washington, D.C.: Government Printing Office, 1972.
15. Blue Cross Association press release, Chicago, December 29, 1971, p. 16.
16. Lewis, C. E., and M. A. Lewis. The impact of television commercials on

health-related beliefs and behavior of children. *Pediatrics* 53 (1974): 431–435.

17. Charren, P. U.S. Senate Select Committee on Nutrition and Human Needs, Testimony before the Federal Trade Commission. *Edible T.V.: Your Child and Food Commercials.* Washington, D.C.: Government Printing Office, September 1977.
18. Banks, S. New products, new ideas: The case for advertising, in J. R. Moskin, ed., *Highlights of the Industry Presentation to the Federal Trade Commission.* New York: American Association of Advertising Agencies, 1973, pp. 57–63.
19. Advertising nutrition. *The New Republic.* March 6, 1971, pp. 7–8.
20. Masover, L. Unpublished thesis material. Evanston, Ill.: Northwestern University Medical School, 1976.
21. *Television, 1976.* North Brook, Ill.: A. C. Nielson, 1976.
22. Federal Trade Commission. *FTC Staff Report on Television Advertising to Children.* Washington, D.C.: Government Printing Office, February 1978.
23. Helitzer, M., et al. The youth market, its dimensions, influence, and opportunities for you, quoted in Federal Trade Commission, *FTC Staff Report on Television Advertising to Children.* Washington, D.C.: Government Printing Office, February 1978.
24. Choate, R. B. Federal Trade Commission testimony. Washington, D.C., Fall 1976.
25. O'Bryan, K. G. U.S. Senate Select Committee on Nutrition and Human Needs, Testimony before the Federal Trade Commission. *Edible T.V.: Your Child and Food Commercials.* Washington, D.C.: Government Printing Office, September 1977.
26. Atkin, C. K. The effects of television advertising on children: Parent-child communication, in *Supermarket Breakfast Cereal Selection,* Rept. No. 7. East Lansing: Michigan State University, June 1975.
27. Liebert, R. M., and R. Poulos. *Unintentional Negative Effects of Food Commercials on Children: A Case Study.* MARC, 1975.
28. Dussere, S., and T. Chen. The relationship between television advertising and children's eating habits. Paper presented at the American Public Health Association Annual Meeting, Washington, D.C., 1977.
29. Gussow, J. It makes even milk a dessert: A report on the counternutritional messages of children's television advertising. *Clin. Pediatr.* 12 (1973): 68–71.
30. U.S. Senate Select Committee on Nutrition and Human Needs, Council on Children Media and Merchandising. *Edible T.V.: Your Child and Food Commercials.* Washington, D.C.: Government Printing Office, September 1977.
31. Blatt, J., L. Spencer, and S. Ward. A cognitive developmental study of children's reactions to television advertising, in E. A. Rubinstein, C. A. Comstock, and J. P. Murray, eds., *Television and Social Behavior.* Vol. 4. *Television in Day-to-Day Life: Patterns of Use.* Washington, D.C.: Government Printing Office, 1972.
32. Yankelovich, D. *Mothers' Attitudes toward Children's Programs and Commercials.* Newton Center, Mass.: Action for Children's T.V., 1970.
33. National Science Foundation. *Research on the Effects of Television Advertising on Children: A Review of the Literature and Recommendations for Future Research.* Bethesda, Md., NSF Grant No. APR 75-10126, 1977.
34. U.S. Senate Select Committee on Nutrition and Human Needs, Panel on

Nutrition and the Consumer. *National Nutrition Policy Study.* Washington, D.C.: Government Printing Office, June 1974.

35. Choate, R. In Federal Trade Commission, *FTC Staff Report on Television Advertising to Children.* Washington, D.C.: Government Printing Office, February 1978, p. 30.

36. Kidvid European style. *Nutr. Act.* 5 (May 1978): 8–9. Reprinted from *Advertising Age,* February 27, 1978.

37. Krame, L. TV ads aimed at children are not a sugar-coated issue. *Washington Post,* February 20, 1979, p. A2.

## 13

Nutrition education–definitions and concepts

Reader Objectives

After completing this chapter the reader should be able to
1. Describe the process of nutrition education.
2. State five forces that signal an increased need for nutrition education in the United States.
3. List three strategies for approaching nutrition education.
4. List two nutrition education tools and state advantages and disadvantages of each.
5. List three modalities of any preventive health education program.
6. Define the "systems approach" to nutrition education.

[Nutrition] is the only field of human endeavor in which the population as a whole has regressed. We've forgotten the things we knew, and we've learned bad habits that are contributing to poor health in this country. When even doctors give as little attention to it as they do, we need a more effective and realistic nutrition education effort.
— C. Percy

As previously stated, there is great concern among many segments of the North American population about the effects of their diet and health status. Although some Americans are plagued by nutritional deficiencies, many others suffer the effects of overnutrition. There is much discussion among nutritionists, health professionals, policymakers, and program planners about what should be done to improve the national nutritional status. Perhaps the most frequently suggested solution is nutrition education. Nutrition education has been integrated into the regulations for many of the federal food programs. Nutrition education has been undertaken to some extent by the federal government, and is the focus of many community efforts to improve food habits. Nutrition education is the frequently suggested solution to all nutritional ills.

But, with all the nutrition education activity, food habits in the United States have not improved, and in fact appear to have worsened. Why is this so? Is it because nutrition education efforts have not reached those who are vulnerable to poor food habits? Would intensified nutrition education efforts improve the situation? What must effective nutrition education efforts consist of?

To answer these questions, we must look at what nutrition education is and examine the reasons behind nutrition efforts. We then need to consider approaches and strategies used to provide education in nutrition.

WHAT IS NUTRITION EDUCATION? DEFINITIONS AND CONCEPTS

Nutrition education refers to the planned use of any educational processes to modify food and nutrition behavior in the pursuit of improved health. The Joint Commission on Health Education terminology suggests that *health* education is a process with intellectual, psychological and social dimensions relating to activities which increase the abilities of people to make informed decisions affecting their personal, family and community well-being. This process based on scientific principles facilitates learning and behavioral change in both health personnel and consumers including children and youth.[1]

Nutrition is a very special subset of health education and should be considered within the same context.

According to the Task Force on Consumer Health Education of the National Conference on Preventive Medicine, the term *consumer health education* subsumes a set of activities that:[2]

1. Inform people about health, illness, disability, and ways in which they can improve and protect their own health, including a more efficient use of the delivery system.

2. Motivate people to want to change to more healthful practices.

3. Help them to learn the necessary skills to adopt and maintain healthful practices and life-styles.

4. Help other health professionals to acquire these teaching skills.

5. Advocate changes in the environment that facilitate healthful conditions and healthful behavior.

6. Add to knowledge via research and evaluation concerning the most effective ways to achieve these objectives.

Health promotion should involve all these measures. As the definition suggests, the purpose of education is to initiate behavioral changes in individuals, groups, and larger populations moving from behaviors presumed to be detrimental to behaviors that are thought to be conducive to present and future health.

Education should not only inform but should also motivate people to want to change and to enable them to adopt and maintain healthful practices. A key focus of health education is the "enhancement of skills to enable individuals to take matters into their own hands increasingly — to shape their own destinies, and to shape their environments to meet their needs."[3]

Nutrition education has been defined as:

the process by which beliefs, attitudes, environmental influences, and understanding about food lead to practices that are scientifically sound, practical, and consistent with individual needs and available food resources . . . nutrition education should be available to all individuals and families. The fundamental philosophy of nutrition education is that efforts should focus on the establishment and protection of nutritional health rather than on crisis intervention. It is needed, regardless of income, location, or cultural, social or economic practices, or level of education. Nutrition education must be a continuing process throughout the life cycle as new research brings additional knowledge.[4]

Nutrition education relates to learning the importance of foods and nutrients and their relationship to growth, development, health, and well-being. Food habits are determined by a host of environmental and personal factors. Thus, nutrition education must strike a balance between actual and advocated dietary patterns. As M. Mead noted, "To introduce adequate nutrition, it is important to bring about changes that are in keeping with the established food habits of the people, and are acceptable within the framework of their value system."[5]

The process of nutrition education requires expertise in making an educational diagnosis of nutritional needs relative to existing habits and of the environmental factors that influence them. The process also demands expertise in the subject matter of nutrition, in the art of planned behavior change, and in the subject matter of human needs, behavior, motivations, values, and cultures. It requires expertise in the ability to organize, direct, manipulate, and modify individual behaviors in the direction of desired change. Ideally it draws on a variety of strategies and selects the chosen strategy according to the needs and level of target audiences.[6]

The process involves much more than the dissemination of nutrition information, although this is an important aspect of nutrition education.

. . . our greatest bulwark against the interests that have helped to create the present problems is an informed public.

— P. Lee

WHY NUTRITION EDUCATION? ·

A number of forces have emerged to stimulate increased recognition of the need for a stronger, more comprehensive, and creative effort at nutrition education. These factors include:

1. Health concerns and the implication of nutrition and diet in the etiology of many of the leading causes of death in the United States.

Many serious as well as less serious health problems are the result of life-styles and personal habits, including habits of food consumption. Individual modifications in life-style may improve health status.

As previously discussed, analysis of the major causes of disease, disability, and death in the United States is leading health experts to the growing conviction that personal life-styles and environment are the principal culprits. It is becoming more and more apparent that future advances in disease control and health promotion must consider modification of personal life-style and control of environmental health hazards. The role that improved nutrition can play in this process has already been discussed. Nutrition constitutes perhaps the most readily improved environmental influence on health.

Further intensifying the need for nutrition information is the concern about the rising costs of health care and the seeming inability of the current health care system to provide adequate high-quality care to alleviate many major disease conditions, as well as the realization that public support of health promotion through nutrition is contingent upon sound information.

2. Changing food patterns. As previously discussed (Chapter 4), North American food habits have dramatically changed since the early 1900s and many of the changes have signaled concern about the quality of diet. In the mid-1800s, the typical family food consumption was limited to relatively few foods, such as meat, potatoes, fruits and vegetables, cheese, eggs, milk, coffee, tea, sugar, cereal, butter, and a few baking and seasoning ingredients.

The type and nature of the food supply has drastically changed in the past years. From traditional fresh fruits, vegetables, dairy and meat products, and cereals, we have switched to a wide range of processed and fabricated foods with added nutrients, stabilizers and preservatives, coloring agents, and other additives. One type of food item may be obtained in fresh, frozen, dried, concentrated, canned, fortified, powdered, or synthetic form. The typical family food fare of today includes TV dinners, carbonated or other sugar beverages, sugar-coated cereals, highly processed snack foods, and convenience baking mixes chosen from more than 10,000 grocery store selections.

These differing forms of food vary in nutritive value as well as in taste appeal. The average consumer is often mystified and unaware of how to make the wisest food choices from such a variety. Thus there is a great need for education to enable consumers to select wisely an appropriate diet from the vast supply of food available.

3. Life-styles are drastically different from those of the turn of the century. As the North American public becomes increasingly sedentary, nutritional needs change. The public must be knowledgeable about how to meet nutritional needs without overindulgence in foods. Other changes in life-style, such as the increasing number of working mothers and of single-family households, the increasing desire for convenience foods, and the trend toward increased eating out, all suggest the need for sound nutrition information to aid in selecting an appropriate diet.

4. Nutrition education is also necessary to aid the consumer to make economical food choices, that is, to save money while getting optimal nutrition. This is especially important for the low-income consumer. Nutrition information cannot take the place of financial resources, but it can aid the consumer to shop wisely and to make sound use of limited resources. The consumer needs sound food and nutrition information. The recent consumer movement has made it clear that consumers want to know and want to understand the nature of the forces that are affecting their lives and their health.

5. World food problems. On a global basis, there is a real possibility of food shortages. These shortages may be absolute, or they may involve shortages in specific foods which result in higher prices, making these foods unavailable to certain income groups. In any case, the consumer should know how to provide nutritional substitutes for unavailable food items. In addition, consumers should be knowledgeable about the effect their food patterns may have on ecological concerns or on scarce resources, such as energy.

Although a variety of strategies are available to policymakers for health promotion, in a democratic society health education is generally suggested as one of the most viable strategies. Education can enable individuals to take personal responsibility for improving their own health status and that of their families and, ultimately, that of their neighbors and their community. Health education can help people to skillfully and objectively *evaluate* the plethora of conflicting information relating to health and nutrition. It can also assist individuals in setting priorities for improving health, motivate them to positive health and nutrition actions, and enable them to use these skills to develop policies and formulate plans to improve the health and nutritional status of all. The goal of health and nutrition education is ". . . the educated consumer-citizen who adopts a health-promoting life-style, wisely selects and uses health care resources, products and services, and influences public policy and planning on health care issues and larger environmental matters that affect health."[7]

WHAT DO AMERICANS KNOW ABOUT FOOD AND NUTRITION?

Numerous studies suggest that there is a gap between nutrition knowledge and nutrition practices, and that many Americans have very limited knowledge of nutrition.

The USDA, in an attempt to find out more about the food and nutrition knowledge, attitudes, and practices of homemakers, conducted a probability sample of all private households in the United States (excluding Alaska and Hawaii). Data were collected from 2,545 households.[8]

Most respondents in the study said that they learned more about nutrition in high school courses than from any other source. Other information sources in order of importance include newspapers and magazines, mother or grandmother, grade school, college, own experience, and health professional.

About 40 per cent of the sample expressed interest in obtaining more nutrition information, 30 per cent were only slightly interested, and the remainder were not interested or not sure.

Most respondents felt that they knew how to handle and store foods properly but less than half of the sample understood the need for a varied diet according to life-cycle stage of the individuals in the household. About 60 per cent of all household members were reported to have had foods from all four basic food groups on the days that food recalls were taken. Most homemakers believed that their families were consuming adequate diets. However, when a comparison was made of those who believed that their families were well fed and those who recognized the need for improvement in certain members' diets, little difference in the quality of food choices was found. Thus, the belief that the diet is already nutritionally adequate is a factor confounding the introduction of nutrition education.[8]

In 1943–1973 and again in 1975, a national study was conducted by the Food and Drug Administration to determine consumer nutrition knowledge and self-reported food shopping behavior. Findings of the study suggested a particular need for education about iron, thiamine, riboflavin, and vitamins A and D. Nutrition knowledge was related to education, income, and prestigious occupations. The study found positive associations between nutrition knowledge, food beliefs, and reported shopping behavior.[9] Few consumers knew that beef and enriched bread were relatively unimportant for developing strong bones and teeth, and most were uncertain about substitute food sources, especially the foods that were similar in nutritive value to milk, tomatoes, and beef.[10]

Other FDA surveys have revealed myths held by food shoppers. A national probability survey by the FDA of 1,500 persons with primary responsibility for family food shopping found that:[11]

— Over half believed that food prepared from "scratch" was more nutritious than the same food bought canned or frozen (this is a half-truth as much depends on how food is kept or cooked).

— About 10 per cent believed that if a person knows little about nutrition, but eats a variety of foods, he or she will be well nourished (a random variety might contain carbohydrate but not enough of needed vitamins or minerals).

—About one shopper in five believed that if a person weighs what he or she should, that person is assured of proper nourishment.

—About 12 per cent believed that people can get enough nourishment by simply eating what they like.

In a nationwide survey designed to investigate health practices and opinions of North Americans, the Food and Drug Administration studied 2,839 adults. Some of the broad conclusions of the study include the following.[12]

1. Fallacious health beliefs are not systematic; there is no one general type of individual who is generally susceptible to all forms of health fads.

2. Most individuals cannot describe the underlying basis for their health beliefs; particular health practices are often not supported by logical health beliefs; many individuals participate in questionable health practices, not because they think that these practices will help, but because they feel that "anything is worth a try."

3. Many individuals acknowledge a relationship between diet and health; diet was considered to be the single most powerful factor to influence health; however, the relationship was often overemphasized. For example, almost 75 per cent of those studied agreed that if people are tired and run down, they probably need more vitamins and minerals.

4. Weight control was a concern, at some time, of more than 50 per cent of the respondents; women and individuals with more income and education were particularly concerned about weight control.

Considerable evidence suggests that health and nutrition concerns are changing the North American diet. As the public becomes more aware of the diet/health relationship, food habits change. To determine the extent of these changes, the Economic Research Service surveyed approximately 1,400 U.S. households in 1976. Almost 50 per cent of those households surveyed altered their diets as the result of health concerns, either to improve existing problems or to prevent additional ones. Diet modifications were most common in higher-income families. The foods that were most often avoided were sweets, snacks, fried foods, fatty red meat, ice cream, and soft drinks. Added food included low-fat milk, cheese, lean red meat, fish, fresh fruits, vegetables, poultry, and broiled and baked foods.[13] Approximately 40 per cent of the households reported using food labels to gain health information. About 25 per cent of the households read the labels in an effort to obtain information that was useful in preventing health problems.[13]

The evidence that North Americans are willing to modify their food habits in response to nutrition information is encouraging; the evidence suggesting the level of nutritional literacy of the U.S. public is much less encouraging.

A variety of forces point up the need for nutrition education. Many Americans are ignorant about what good nutritional practices entail, as well as how to achieve them. But many individuals who have been educated in nutrition and who know what food patterns have a positive effect on health, continue to eat diets that are high in calories, high in fat, and high in refined, processed foods, that is, diets that contribute to obesity and to other health problems. Does this suggest that nutrition education is not effective in modifying food habits? How can we design effective nutrition education? A look at different nutrition education strategies may help us answer these questions.

NUTRITION EDUCATION STRATEGIES

Food habits and nutritional practices have been the subjects of many research studies, reviews, and papers. People's food intake is motivated by learned and habitual taste preferences, visual and olfactory senses, psychological and cultural influences, socioeconomic and circumstantial situations, and physiological and emotional states. Eating habits are significantly affected by early food behavior patterns, cultural and social traditions, and attitudes. Food preferences result from food availability, climate, geographical conditions, and technological development as well as from social and personal factors.[14-17]

How one is fed as a child may have a greater impact on personality development than any other human experience. Eating and feeding are the most fundamental interpersonal actions between people; they are experiences that influence the way in which an individual perceives himself or herself, his or her family and work, and the individual's relationship to them. The implications of this for nutrition education are great. Suggestions that the way in which our dietary habits are formed and that we are not eating in the proper way can give rise to questions on the deepest level relative to our perceptions of ourselves and of those who fed us as children.

In view of the multifactorial influences on food habits, there is no one way to persuade people to change their food choices. Thus, nutrition education must use a variety of techniques that must be a part of total family and community environments.

Nutritional needs must be viewed in the context of the individual's total cultural, social, physical, and emotional needs. Regardless of nutrition-related needs, the individual's own perspective and values will be the principal determinants of food habit changes that are actually adopted. If these changes can be planned for in accord with cultural practices, the total culture and the total person will benefit.

In other words, nutrition education involves information exchange as well as techniques to motivate and reinforce improved food habits. Successful nutrition education must include endeavors to make beliefs, attitudes, values, environmental factors, and individual ideas about food conducive to nutritionally sound, practical, and acceptable dietary habits.

Attempts at nutrition education are difficult because achieving directed, significant, and sustained changes in habits is difficult. There is a vast body of literature — both research and theory — relating to the problem of changing habits. Theories of persuasion via communication as well as learning theory relate to the problem.

As far back as the time of Plato, who spoke of "the winning of men's minds by words," men were interested in persuading through communication. In more recent times, various educators have applied different learning theories and techniques to the modification of behavior. Selected principles of learning and motivation are summarized in Table 13-1.[18]

Nutrition education can be approached in various ways. What might be termed the *rational-empirical curriculum design* is the approach that is typically used by educators; it is logical and planned, and it involves behavioral objectives, activities that are designed to achieve objectives, and evaluation to determine the discrepancy between planned and achieved outcomes.

The idea of self-responsibility for health suggests the basic notion that the individual possesses a dignity, worth, and responsibility to maximize these characteristics. Self-responsibility assumes that the individual has the potential and the motivation to make wise judgments about factors that affect his or her health status. The assumption here is that the role of the educator is to provide the knowledge and the information, and to help make the conditions right for the individual to make wise choices.[19]

Another strategy has been termed the *travel* metaphor method. The idea is that there is a body of knowledge, facts, concepts, values, and beliefs that are known and understood by the educator. It is the educator's responsibility to lead the learner through this body of knowledge and beliefs and point out to the learner what is thought to be of importance. The educator is thus a travel guide whose job is to provide the student with a set of stimuli and the opportunity to take advantage and react positively. It then becomes the responsibility of the student to determine how he or she will make use of the contacts provided by the educator.[19]

Another design or approach is called the *garden* metaphor by G. Griffin, who explains that humans grow and develop and flower naturally in what might be called the garden of life. The educator has the opportunity to

Table 13-1

Principles Essential to Effective Educational Process

1. Meaningfulness. The subject materials must be relevant and meaningful to the learner. The student should be able to relate to content on a personal and a practical level. To achieve this, the teacher should attempt to develop the material in relation to past or current experiences of the learner; to the interests, values, and life-style of the learner; and to the goals or possible future activities of the student.

2. Prerequisites. The entry level knowledge and experience of the student is an important determinant of future learner success in the educational process. To determine the appropriate level of material, the teacher should analyze each learning task to determine those concepts that should be known beforehand and determine the entry level competencies of the learners.

3. Modeling. A student will be more receptive to the learning process if he or she can base learning activities on some sort of model or theoretical framework. The model should be fully explained to the student; all steps should be clearly delineated; and the student should be told about the strategy to be used, all decisions made, and their consequences.

4. Open communication. The most effective learning process occurs when students are able to actively participate in the process; communication between student and teacher should be two-way; the student should be informed of objectives for every unit; the student should be allowed to question, suggest, or discuss any material or learning activity that he or she engages in.

5. Novelty stimulates attention. Teachers should devise various methods of presenting materials. Audiovisual materials and media (such as tapes, films, slides) should be used, and all methods should be geared to the appropriate needs of the learner.

6. Active, appropriate practice. For effective learning to occur, the student must practice what is to be learned; problem solving, repetition, and application of learning material are essential to effective learning.

7. Distribute practice. It is often more helpful to allow the learner a period of time in which to gain competence in the subject matter rather than limiting him or her to short periods of time to learn extensive material. The student should be rested and should have an alert attitude for the most effective learning process.

8. Fading. Complex learning may require the teacher to prompt the student and to provide hints and suggestions. These aids should be decreased as the student becomes more adept.

9. Pleasant conditions and consequences. The best environment for learning is one in which tension and aversive stimuli are at a minimum. Feedback on student progress should always be immediate; rewards of student's efforts help to reinforce the learning progress. The student should not be ridiculed or humiliated for failing to accomplish a given task as desired by the teacher.

Source: G. Fargo. Summary of some selected principles of learning and motivation, in *Proceedings of Workshop I on Curriculum Development for Community Nutrition Training.* University of Hawaii, Honolulu, February 10-21, 1974, pp. 141-142.

nurture this environment so that the "child" has the most opportunity to mature and to learn.[19]

Another approach to health and nutrition education takes a strategy of *social manipulation.* The basic premise is that the matters affecting health are too urgent, too important, and beyond the individual's power to control on his or her own. Thus, the role of the health educator is seen as one of attempting to control behavior and to shape the desired responses. This approach is the one often employed by the mass media.[19]

The manipulative approach is more concerned with the behavior response patterns rather than the manner in which the individual reaches these patterns. The approach is an attempt to reach the desired behavior through a short-cut method and does not take the time to prepare the individual to make fully informed, wise choices. The method is thus in line with the current preference for a quick, technical approach to solving human problems and is thus often the preferred approach of politicians, social decision makers, and those eager to rapidly solve complex problems in a simplistic way. Although educators may in theory regard this approach as insensitive, in reality it is the approach often found not only in the classroom but also in public nutrition education efforts.

The most appropriate and effective strategy for stimulating improved food habits will depend upon the knowledge, background, personal characteristics, and motivation of the audience. It may also depend upon the size of the target group. Ideally the approach should be individualized to the target audience's needs, goals, objectives, and other characteristics. A mix of various approaches may be necessary.

To learn more about individual differences in food attitudes and possible educational emphases, P. Baird and H. Schutz investigated food attitudes that affected food behavior among Expanded Food and Nutrition Education Program (EFNEP) homemakers. Specifically, they studied 25 uses and attributes that they believed represented cognitive elements that affected people's food habits. These attributes included terms in which people think and talk about food as well as values such as health, status, money, and satiety that determine food choice.[20]

These authors identified 13 cognitive characteristics of "people types" that were considered to evidence "the different kinds of unrelated influences on the appropriateness judgments" for food and food uses. These psychological differences among the homemakers accounted for an average of over half the variation in the homemakers' levels of dietary adequacy. These findings led the authors to suggest possible educational approaches that might be helpful in working with various personality types. Table 13–2 summarizes the suggested educational emphases that might be used to reach these "people types." The successful approach depends upon an understanding of audience characteristics, motivations, and needs.[20]

WHAT NUTRITION INFORMATION DO CONSUMERS NEED?

The search for the right foods is very long. . . . We need to hear calm and thorough advice. We need to stop being told we are neurotic. We need more information and fewer evangelical cure-alls. We need to believe we ourselves can do the choosing.

— E. Kendall

It is very difficult to define the basic knowledge that should be conveyed to the public about nutrition. Much will depend upon what the learners already know, how they evaluate their present dietary habits and nutritional status, what their present eating habits actually are, how much they desire to know, and what changes they are willing, or can afford, to make.

Table 13-2

People Type	Possible Educational Emphasis
"Hostile"	Emphasize that good nutrition is necessary, that eating according to principles of good nutrition is what should be done every day. Give help with menu planning, recipe ideas, food budgeting, and preparation. Associate all these things with pleasant, familiar occasions, a positive self-image, acceptance by others. Reward progress and build self-confidence.
"Social Isolate"	Provide nutrition information and assistance with meal planning, recipe ideas, and food preparation. Associate these things with pleasant occasions, a positive self-image, acceptance by others. Reward progress and build self-confidence.
"Unhappy Eater"	Associate nutritious foods with pleasant occasions, a positive self-image, and acceptance by others. Reward progress and build self-confidence.
"Home Centered"	Present nutrition information and food preparation help in a context of pleasant occasions, a positive self-image, and acceptance by others. Raise consciousness of the importance of women in today's world. Reward progress and build self-confidence.
"Totally Negative"	Take a comprehensive approach. Begin with an effort to build trust and personal rapport, and help create a positive self-image. Then progress to nutrition information, menu planning. recipe ideas, food budgeting, and preparation.
"Escapist"	Emphasize nutritious menus that are convenient, quick, easy to prepare, and liked by everyone.
"Conservative"	Give special attention to food budgeting and to the selection of nutritious, economical foods. Give help with food preparation. Associate good nutrition with pleasant occasions.
"Pragmatist"	Take a straightforward, pragmatic approach. Provide nutrition information, help with menu planning, recipe ideas, preparation hints.
"Indigestion Problem"	Give help with menu planning and recipe ideas. Build self-confidence.
"Stuck in a Rut"	Emphasize the practical aspects of good nutrition. Expand food horizons with menu planning and new recipe ideas. Give help with food budgeting.
"Sociable"	Associate nutritious menus with social occasions; relate nutritional awareness to social approval.
"Confident Independent"	Take a low-key, nonauthoritarian approach. Indicate respect for knowledge and abilities already demonstrated. Teach nutrition in such a way that the individual is allowed to make discoveries for himself or herself.
"Good Cook and Enthusiastic Eater"	Use a low-key nonauthoritarian approach. Indicate appreciation of homemaker's individuality and creativity. Associate the use of nutritious foods with individuality, creativity, pleasant social occasions, and feelings of pride. Allow for self-expression in planning menus and designing new recipes.

Source: P. C. Baird and H. G. Schutz. The marketing concept applied to selling good nutrition. *J. Nutr. Educ.* 8 (1976): 13–17.

Some of the areas that are likely to be of concern include:

1. What constitutes an appropriate dietary pattern? How can this be achieved in terms of available, affordable, and acceptable foods?
2. What are the risk/benefit relationships between diet and health? What are the possible risks involved with adhering to certain dietary habits relative to the health benefits that may result from improved dietary practices?
3. What factors influence obesity and overeating? What are sound ways to reduce weight?
4. What is food safety? How can it be achieved? What ingredients in food or what aspects of food processing might affect food safety?
5. How does nutrition relate to health? Which groups are particularly vulnerable to malnutrition, and how can their special needs be met?
6. Who or what are qualified sources of nutrition information? What are suitable resources for increasing nutrition knowledge or for improving nutritional status?

What knowledge should the public be given to enable them to understand these concerns and to make wise use of existing food supplies? The following areas of nutrition-related knowledge have been recommended.

1. How the body uses food under normal as well as disease conditions. This should include a basic understanding of processes such as digestion, absorption, metabolism, and the uses and interrelationships of various nutrients within the body. It should also include a knowledge of the nutrient composition of various foods and how food contributes to good health.
2. How to select appropriate dietary patterns, and how to modify these patterns to meet special needs of various periods of the life span or during times of illness.
3. How to critically assess various sources of nutrition information, and how to determine ways to evaluate controversial nutrition issues.
4. How to understand and appreciate the social, cultural, emotional, or environmental influences on the food supply and dietary habits.

Because one of the basic objectives of nutrition education is to motivate people to adopt healthful nutrition practices, consumers must be provided with information about the current state of nutrition knowledge so that they will be able to make wise food choices. The public should be informed about the status of nutritional uncertainties that require further research. The public should be helped to realize the constant flux of nutritional knowledge and to appreciate the need to "keep current" and to constantly seek new knowledge and apply it to their nutrition behavior.[22]

A distinction between education and information in nutrition should be made. A wealth of information is available to various population groups from a great variety of sources: industry, health enthusiasts, medical professionals, and nutritionists all have been the source of writing and promotion on the subject of nutrition. But there has been "a surprisingly small amount of education in nutrition, if one defines education as the development of an understanding capable of producing intelligent decisions and actions." Education encompasses the dissemination and acquisition of knowledge, as well as the sound application of that knowledge to real life situations.[23]

A number of examples of nutrition education are available in which learner's nutrition knowledge improved but in which there was no noticeable improvement in food habits.[24,25] It is useful to consider why no behavioral differences were found. Very few individuals will be persuaded to improve their dietary habits on the basis of logic. As discussed previously, the dietary habits of most individuals are usually influenced by motivation, preferences, economic and circumstantial influences, and emotional, sociological, and cultural needs.

Early in the design of the nutrition education message, the educator needs to learn about the individual's current food habits, ideas, and attitudes toward nutrition and the available resources. By examining the actual factors that underlie the individual's present food habits, the educator is in a position to determine the existing positive characteristics of nutrition behavior. The education should then be adapted to build upon these positive factors.

The depth and extent of nutrition information to be provided will greatly depend upon the preliminary assessment. In certain instances, detailed information may be helpful. In other cases, it may be appropriate to limit the teaching to certain basic, relevant, and practical facts.

The Nutrition Education Project, developed by the Pennsylvania State University, represents a coordinated effort to "design and implement nutrition education programs with total impact." The project included plans to provide nutrition education to health professionals, the adult public, students from elementary school through college, and their teachers. A multidisciplinary team developed educational objectives for the curriculum. These objectives, termed Project Learner Objectives (PLO), were the base from which the curriculum was developed. A list of 87 initial PLOs was reduced and refined to 40.[26]

These 40 PLOs were then incorporated into a questionnaire distributed to 1,000 members of the Society for Nutrition Education (SNE). SNE members ranked the PLOs in terms of priority as a nutrition education objective. The results were used in a factor analysis design to determine factor association among the PLOs. These results are presented in Table 13-3.

As the table indicates, nutrition education experts feel that the principal focus of nutrition education efforts should be the topic of personal food choices for positive personal health. Upon the completion of a comprehensive nutrition education curriculum, a student should have the knowledge and skills to[27]:

1. Analyze his or her own food intake in relation to health needs and take corrective action if necessary.

Table 13-3
Item Summary Statistics by Factor (*n* = 599)

Factors and Numbered Item Questionnaire Item	Priority Mean	S.D.	Priority Rank	Factor Loading
1. Factor III — Relationship of nutrition and health				
27 Describe the relationship between nutrition and health.	6.33	1.07	2	.66
38 Be able to explain why the inclusion of a variety of foods in the diet is desirable.	6.21	0.99	3	.61
31 Identify the role of food and nutrients in different stages of the life cycle and problems common to these stages.	5.76	1.18	8	.56
32 Analyze one's own nutrition and food patterns, identify problems if any, and initiate action to correct these problems.	6.46	1.00	1	.52
2. Factor IV — Application of scientific and practical information in food choice decisions				
8 Critically evaluate food and nutrition claims on a logical and nutritionally informed basis.	6.11	1.14	4	.71
9 Apply principles of energy balance to plan a food and activity pattern which results in desirable weight.	5.75	1.24	9	.64
5 Plan an adequate daily diet based on nutrient/cost criteria, given food lists of nutrient composition and cost data.	5.71	1.32	10	.60
3. Factor II — Planning nutritionally adequate meals				
21 Plan and manage the preparation of meals for a specific living unit for a 3-day period.	4.77	1.68	24	.79
12 Prepare a meal, given certain food, time, and cost limitations.	5.01	1.64	21	.76
37 Prepare a nutritionally balanced diet for one week which includes a variety of foods.	5.53	1.59	13	.74
17 Prepare a market list as a basis for meal planning for a living unit, given time and cost constraints.	5.30	1.45	16	.71
11 Select an adequate diet for one week based on nutrient criteria, given limited food resources.	5.95	1.13	5	.54
33 Be able to store food to maintain the freshness and nutrient qualities.	5.51	1.43	15	.50
4. Factor VI — Solution of family and community nutrition-related problems				
28 Identify strategies useful in solving nutrition-related problems found in the community.	4.70	1.45	25	.68
20 Identify strategies useful in solving nutrition-related problems in families or living units.	4.94	1.43	22	.66
10 Utilize available resources in the community to prevent or solve nutrition problems of individuals.	5.06	1.41	20	.54
5. Factor VIII — Food, nutrients, and bodily functions				
35 Identify the biological processes involved in making nutrients available to the body.	4.64	1.49	26.5	.73
40 Describe the scientific methods used in the discipline of nutrition.	3.69	1.66	40	.70

Item Summary Statistics by Factor (*n* = 599) *(continued)*

Item	Factors and Numbered Questionnaire Item	Priority Mean	S.D.	Priority Rank	Factor Loading
29	Specify the role of food and nutrients in body functions.	5.81	1.25	6.5	.65

6. Factor I — Social and cultural aspects of food choice and use

Item	Factors and Numbered Questionnaire Item	Priority Mean	S.D.	Priority Rank	Factor Loading
14	List several ways in which food influences social interaction.	4.53	1.32	28	.80
7	Identify those situations in which food is used as an object of expressive behavior.	4.36	1.48	30	.70
18	Report which aesthetic and sensory qualities influence the selection of different foods by different individuals.	4.03	1.42	36.5	.64
25	Compare the eating patterns and habits of different families, and suggest possible factors which may be related to the differences.	4.64	1.26	26.5	.59

7. Factor V — Identification and solution of global nutrition-related problems

Item	Factors and Numbered Questionnaire Item	Priority Mean	S.D.	Priority Rank	Factor Loading
13	Identify the ways that inhabitants of this planet are interdependent on finite resources that include food.	4.48	1.57	29	.70
1	Specify several major nutrition problems in other areas of the world, and list some of the important factors that have a bearing upon the problems.	4.21	1.49	34	.69
		4.21	1.49	34	.69
34	Specify several ecological implications of the food distribution system.	4.20	1.38	35	.64

8. Factor VII — Nutrition as a career

Item	Factors and Numbered Questionnaire Item	Priority Mean	S.D.	Priority Rank	Factor Loading
6	List several career opportunities for individuals trained in nutrition.	3.98	1.57	38	.69
19	List the disciplines that contribute to knowledge of nutrition.	3.92	1.50	39	.60
4	Identify contributions of nutrition knowledge to other disciplines.	4.03	1.50	36.5	.57

9. Miscellaneous — Factor loadings less than 0.50

Item	Factors and Numbered Questionnaire Item	Priority Mean	S.D.	Priority Rank	Factor Loading
2	List the necessary steps to be taken to protect different specified foods from contamination in the household.	5.62	1.32	11	
3	Specify the changes in the quality and composition of food items from their points of origin to their presence on the plate.	4.22	1.34	33	
15	Identify major factors that affect cost, quality, availability, and variety of foods in the market place.	5.16	1.16	19	
16	Evaluate food products on the basis of the U.S. Recommended Dietary Allowances.	5.26	1.40	18	
22	Identify the nutritional and health risks associated with different food patterns.	5.81	1.11	6.5	
23	Specify ways to continue learning about food and nutrition beyond formal schooling.	5.52	1.32	14	
24	Select from a list of physical and environmental stresses those conditions which elevate energy and protein requirements.	4.88	1.32	23	

Item Summary Statistics by Factor (n = 599) *(continued)*

Item	Factors and Numbered Questionnaire Item	Priority Mean	S.D.	Priority Rank	Factor Loading
26	Enumerate the food distribution factors that influence the nutritional qualities of the diet of a population.	4.24	1.27	32	
30	Allocate food according to the needs of individuals in the family or living unit, given limited food resources.	5.29	1.32	17	
36	Compare the food practices of different communities and describe these differences in economic, cultural, social, and religious terms.	4.29	1.32	31	
39	Discuss major health problems in the U.S. today which are related to nutrition.	5.60	1.20	12	

Source: J. J. Barnette and M. Branca. Learner objectives for a nutrition education curriculum. II. Factor analysis. *J. Nutr. Educ.* 10 (1978): 65.

2. Describe how nutrition affects health.

3. Recognize the need for a variety of foods in the diet.

4. Recognize how nutrition needs change through life.

IMPORTANCE OF RISK ASSESSMENT IN DETERMINING AUDIENCES FOR SPECIALIZED NUTRITION EDUCATION

The public should be made aware of the relationship between positive dietary habits and good health, but the possible benefits from modifying current eating habits, such as decreasing the intake of excessive calories, sugar, saturated fat, and salt, must not be overstated. How much of the current controversies and uncertainty relating to nutrition should be translated for the public remains a problematic issue.

The public must be given information that will allow people to judge for themselves the benefits that can be gained by modifying their food habits. By providing the public with the knowledge available, by being open about the controversy, and by attempting to inform at an understandable level, we will be less likely to direct a change that will later be rejected by the public.

Some nutritional issues may never be totally resolved with certainty. The exact relationship between an individual's dietary intake and serum cholesterol levels, and the extent of the risk that this individual will later develop atherosclerosis and die from the complications, is a problem that will probably never be answerable for each individual, but the use of risk factors in assessing health status can be a helpful part of a total health education strategy. Adults as well as children should be helped to understand their individual health status and the possible benefits of modifying their life-styles, diets, or other factors in accordance with their individual status.

For example, an individual with a family history of coronary heart disease, who is overweight, consumes excessive calories, and has hypertension should be advised of the risk factors he or she presents. The individual should also be advised as to possible strategies for reducing such risk factors, thereby possibly reducing his or her chances of suffering morbidity or mortality from coronary heart disease. The concept of risk assessment has been discussed in previous chapters (see pp. 170–172).

The concept of risk assessment is especially important for young children. It seems likely that risk factors that increase the possibility of early morbidity or mortality from certain diseases in adulthood are detectable in youngsters. For example, there is increasing evidence to suggest that children who rank in the upper 5 per cent for their age group for blood pressure and for serum cholesterol levels may continue in this upper-risk level into adulthood.[28]

This points up the importance of identifying such high-risk children, advising their families as to possible beneficial changes, and then attempting to help the children to develop wise habits that will carry through into adulthood. This concept is the basis for the Early Periodic Screening Detection and Treatment (EPSDT) programs funded by Medicaid and implemented in most states.

NUTRITION EDUCATION TOOLS

Nutrition education should become an active force in the lives of the U.S. public. It should be available to consumers where they are and in forms that are appropriate and appealing to them and their nutritional needs.

Two nationally used classic tools are available to teach certain nutritional concepts, but both are in need of revision. The first, *Food for Fitness — A Daily Food Guide*, is the most widely used food guide in the United States. It was developed in 1956 by the USDA and was based on the 1953 RDA. The guide recognizes four food groups: milk, meat, vegetable/fruit, and bread/cereal. The guide specifies a minimum number of servings per food group to provide an adequate diet. The guide also recommends the addition of certain foods to meet energy needs and to satisfy the RDA for particular nutrients, such as vitamin A, vitamin C, and iron.

Another booklet, *The Basic Four*, offers a simple, practical, and easily understood approach to nutritional adequacy. It is a tool that can be used to help the lay person, who may have little knowledge of the functions and sources of various nutrients, plan an appropriate and nutritious diet. However, there are several disadvantages to the basic four food guide. The original guide stated that the guide was to serve only as a "foundation" diet and that additional foods might be needed to provide an adequate diet. However, many people now regard the guide as being able to suggest an adequate diet in and of itself. This misunderstanding may result in the planning of inadequate diets. Even if the individual realizes that quality foods must be added to the basic four, it is still possible to select a diet that satisfies the guide but lacks variety and is not nutritionally adequate. There is such a range of nutrient levels in foods within a given food group that food choices may provide inadequate nutrients. For example, the selection of corn and celery for vegetables, rather than of broccoli and green peppers, would provide considerably lower levels of vitamin A, ascorbic acid, and folic acid.

Because the basic four was originally based on the 1953 RDA, it does not supply 100 per cent of the current RDA. Since the 1953 RDA, the RDAs for calcium, vitamin A, ascorbic acid, and certain of the B vitamins have changed, and recommendations have been added for vitamin E, vitamin B_6, vitamin B_{12}, folic acid, iodine, magnesium, phosphorous, and zinc.

J. King et al. studied published sample diets based on the basic four and compared the nutritive content of these diets with the 1974 RDAs for 16 nutrients. The nutritive value of the sample diets was less than two thirds of the 1974 RDA for magnesium, iron, zinc, vitamin B_6 and vitamin E.[29]

Another major drawback is that the food guide does not address the problem of excessive consumption of fat, sugar, cholesterol, and calories and our flow fiber intake. Thus, it is not helpful in teaching people about the health hazards of overconsumption.

Another problem with the basic four food groups is that many popular ethnic foods, combination dishes (such as lasagna, macaroni and cheese, or soup) and fabricated foods (such as breakfast bars and many snack foods) cannot be easily classified into the basic four food groups.

King et al. have developed additional more refined subgroups of the original basic four. Their revised daily food recommendations for nonpregnant, pregnant, and lactating women, are shown in Table 13-4.

Another updated version of the basic four is shown in Table 13-5. Many educators agree that as a teaching tool, the basic four food groups have been, and are even more now, ineffective. Despite the widespread publicity afforded the four groups by the industry, the federal government, and nutrition educators, we remain a nation of nutritional illiterates.

The second tool, a conceptual approach to nutrition education, was developed by the Inter-Agency Committee on Nutrition Education in

Table 13-4
Revised Food Guide

	Servings Per Day		
Food Group	Nonpregnant Woman	Pregnant Woman	Lactating Woman
Protein foods			
Animal foods (2-oz serving)	2	2	2
Vegetable foods (should include			
at least one serving of legumes)	2	2	2
Milk and milk products	2	4	5
Breads and cereals (including whole-			
grain products)	4	4	4
Vitamin C-rich fruits and vegetables	1	1	1
Dark green vegetables	1	1	1
Other fruits and vegetables	1	1	1

Source: J. King, S. Cohenour, and C. Corruccini. In *Food Guides: Their Development, Use, and Specified Changes*. Sacramento: California Department of Health, June 1977.

Table 13-5
An Update of the Basic Four Food Groups

	Anytime	In Moderation	Now and Then
Group I Beans, grains, and nuts Four or more servings/day	Barley Beans Bread and rolls (whole grain) Bulghur Lentils Oatmeal Pasta Rice Whole grain cereal (except granola)	Granola cereals Nuts Peanut butter Soybeans White bread and cereals	
Group II Fruits and vegetables Four or more servings/day	All fruits and vegetables except those listed on right Unsweetened fruit juices Unsalted vegetable juices Potatoes, white or sweet	Avocado Fruits canned in syrup Salted vegetable juices Sweetened fruit juice Vegetables canned with salt	French fries Olives Pickles
Group III Milk products Children: three to four servings or equivalent Adult: two servings (Favor anytime column for additional servings)	Buttermilk Farmer or pot cheese Low-fat cottage cheese Low-fat milk with 1% milkfat Skim milk ricotta Skim milk	Frozen low-fat yogurt Ice milk Low-fat milk with 2% milkfat Low-fat (2%) yogurt, plain or sweetened Regular cottage cheese (4% milkfat)	Hard cheeses: blue, brick, camembert, cheddar, (note: part-skim mozarella and part-skim ricotta are preferable but still rich in fat) Ice cream Processed cheeses Whole milk Whole milk yogurt
Group IV Poultry, fish, egg, and meat products Two servings: (Favor anytime column for additional servings. If a vegetarian diet is desired, nutrients in these foods can be obtained by increasing servings from groups I and III.)	*Poultry* Chicken or turkey (no skin) *Fish* Cod Flounder Haddock Halibut Perch Pollock Rockfish Shellfish, except shrimp Sole Tuna, water-packed	*Fish* Herring Mackerel Salmon Sardines Shrimp Tuna, oil-packed *Red meats* Flank steak Ham* Leg of lamb* Loin of lamb* Plate beef* Round steak* Rump roast* Sirloin steak* Veal*	*Poultry and Fish* Deep fried and breaded fish or poultry *Red meats* Bacon Corned beef Ground beef Hot dogs Liver Liverwurst Pork: loin Pork: Boston butt Salami Sausage Spareribs Untrimmed meats

An Update of the Basic Four Food Groups *(continued)*

	Anytime	*In Moderation*	*Now and Then*
	Egg		Egg
	Egg whites		Egg yolk or whole egg
Miscellaneous	*Fats*	*Fats*	*Fats*
	None	Mayonnaise	Butter
		Salad oils	Cream
		Soft (tub) mar- garines	Cream cheese
			Lard
			Sour cream
Note: Snack foods should not be used freely, but the middle column suggests some of the better choices.	*Snack foods* None	*Snack foods* Angel food cake Animal crackers Fig bars Gingerbread Ginger snaps Graham crackers Popcorn (small amounts of fat and salt) Sherbet	*Snack foods* Chocolate Coconut Commercial pies, pastries, and doughnuts Potato chips Soda pop

*Trim all outside fat.

"Anytime" foods contain less than 30 per cent of calories from fat and are usually low in salt and sugar. Most of the "now and then" foods contain at least 50 per cent of calories from fat — *and* a large amount of saturated fat. Foods to eat "in moderation" have medium amounts of total fat and low to moderate amounts of saturated fat *or* large amounts of total fat that is mostly unsaturated. Foods meeting the standards for fat, but containing large amounts of salt or sugar, are usually moved into a more restricted category, as are refined cereal products. For example, pickles have little fat, but are so high in sodium that they fall in the "now and then" category.

Important:

To cut down on salt intake, choose varieties of the foods listed here that do not have added salt, such as no-salt cottage cheese, rather than the regular varieties. This guide is not appropriate for individuals needing very-low-salt diets.

Source: P. Hausman. Updating the basic four. *Nutr. Act.* (January 1979): 8-9.

1963. This approach is also currently the subject of discussion and review. It consists of four basic concepts that should form the basis for education in nutrition. These concepts are enumerated in Table 13-6.[31]

A variety of tools to replace current nutrition education tools have been suggested. One suggestion is that individual edible items could be given some sort of a nutritional rating, a number indicating their nutritional value. This value would then be included on labels and in any type of product advertising.[32]

The exact derivation of a nutritional rating has not been determined, but presumably it would be the sum of positive nutritional values minus the sum of the negative nutritional values. As an example, the optimal score for a food might be 100. If it is found that a given food, because of its wholesomeness and freshness and overall ingredient list is worth 80 points, but has certain negative qualities giving it a negative nutrient value of 30, then the overall nutritional score would be 50.[33]

Table 13–6
Basic Concepts for Nutrition Education

1. Nutrition is the food you eat and how the body uses it.

   We eat food to live, to grow, to keep healthy and well, and to get energy for work and play.

2. Food is made up of different nutrients needed for growth and health.

   All nutrients needed by the body are available through food.
   Many kinds and combinations of food can lead to a well-balanced diet.
   No food, by itself, has all the nutrients needed for full growth and health.
   Each nutrient has specific uses in the body.
   Most nutrients do their best work in the body when teamed with other nutrients.

3. All persons, throughout life, have need for the same nutrients, but in varying amounts.

   The amounts of nutrients needed are influenced by age, sex, size, activity, and state of health.
   Suggestions for the kinds and amounts of food needed are made by trained scientists.

4. The way food is handled influences the amount of nutrients in food, its safety, appearance, and taste.

   Handling means everything that happens to food while it is being grown, processed, stored, and prepared for eating.

Source: M. M. Hill. ICNE formulates some basic concepts in nutrition. *Nutr. Program News* (1964): 9-10.

The nutrient density concept, sometimes called the index of nutritional quality (INQ), is another possible way to rate foods. Nutrient density expresses the nutrient content of foods or a diet relative to calorie content. The nutrient density, or INQ, can be expressed as follows:

$$\text{Index of nutritional quality (INQ)} = \frac{\text{\% of standard requirement of a food}}{\text{\% of energy requirement}}$$

Thus, each nutrient in a food is considered and a profile of numbers can be determined to demonstrate the quality of a given food or diet. A diet that contains 100 per cent of the nutrient requirement and 100 per cent of the needed calories would be judged to be a perfect fit and a highly nutritious diet.[33] The INQ concept might be used to rate individual food items and thus indicate their nutritional quality. This could become a valuable tool for nutrition education of the public if used on food labels, in product promotion, or in other nutrition education strategies.

SYSTEMS APPROACH TO NUTRITION EDUCATION

Nutritional problems often have nonnutritional solutions. Thus, nutrition education is most effective when it is only one element of a total nutritional improvement strategy. In other words, to be successful, nutrition educators must be concerned with complete solutions. These solutions evolve from an analysis of environmental and individual factors that contribute to nutritional problems. Problems, not subjects, should be the basis of a nutrition education program.

The "systems" approach to nutrition education provides a useful and practical tool to aid the nutrition educator in deciding what should be taught and how it should be taught. Simply defined, the systems approach is a flow of steps needed to achieve the desired objective. The approach consists of input, process, and output.

A successful nutrition education effort must incorporate managerial elements that are crucial to the success of all program planning. These elements, which could be termed the input, are essential to an effective nutrition education process. They include needs assessment and identification of problems; study of available resources and alternative strategies of intervention; determination of objectives and goals; assignment of resources to implement program; staff development to implement program, and program monitoring and evaluation. Crucial to the entire process is a firm organization base and administrative and budgetary support for nutrition education efforts.

The development of an organized, coordinated nutrition education program requires a series of steps:

1. Consumer research is needed to determine consumer use of existing uses of information, consumer attitudes, knowledge, levels of awareness and concern; current nutrition practices; consumer perception of accuracy, usefulness, and reliability of current nutrition information; and type of education to which consumers would be most receptive.

2. Nutritional surveillance data are needed to determine the most important public nutrition problems; this knowledge is a prerequisite for determining reasonable objectives to be used in formulating the nutrition education.

3. It is important to determine the most appropriate target populations for nutrition education. Criteria of awareness, nutritional status, current knowledge, and receptivity to nutrition information should be used in this determination. The at-risk concept is very useful in setting priorities in terms of appropriate populations for specific nutrition education programs. (See Chapter 6.)

4. A nutrition education message should be designed that is appropriate for the needs of the selected population groups. A continuum of information is needed by the public, which ranges from very general nutrition information, such as the relation between good nutrition and good health, to more specific information, such as the role of various nutrients in promoting good health and appropriate food sources for these nutrients.

The information provided at various levels must, in sum, be consistent. Although every consumer cannot be knowledgeable about every aspect of nutrition, it is important that his or her knowledge be provided in a frame of reference that allows the consumer to practically apply his or her knowledge.

For example, the consumer must be aware of the importance of good nutrition before he or she will be interested in using labels to determine wise nutritional buys. But to wisely use food labels, the consumer must have a certain basic knowledge of the roles of various nutrients in contributing to an overall balanced diet.

Many of the currently available nutrition education messages are designed to educate the consumer of the need for a wide variety of many different kinds of foods. This concept really does not address the nutritional needs of the vast majority of Americans who are in the habit of overconsuming food. They need information how to select a diet to promote health.

5. The curricula for the nutrition education program must be well thought out and planned. At every step of the curriculum development, the learner and the educator should work together to develop goals, objectives, and appropriate activities and resources to meet these goals. The development process should also include health professionals or educators, or other individuals who will be involved at any point in the delivery or reinforcement of nutrition education. For example, if the curriculum is to be geared to the fourth-graders in all public schools in a particular county, the nutrition educator should meet with some representative fourth-graders, the teachers of the children, the school administrators, representatives from the PTA or interested parents, and those individuals who are responsible for the school lunch program offered to the children. A delegation of these individuals should work together to plan the curriculum. By involving these various individuals, the educator can learn from the learners, as well as others who will influence the learning process, of factors that may be essential to the success of the education effort.

A consideration of, and careful attention to these elements is crucial to the success of the educational process.

6. Basic to the design is the setting of criteria that will allow an evaluation of the progress (or output) of the process of education. Evaluation is crucial to any successful educational effort. A system for implementing the process should be combined with systematic attempts to monitor the effectiveness of the program and to obtain feedback for program revision and modification. Such monitoring also allows the educator to realize misconceptions, learner problems, and the like in the educational program.

Nutrition advocates face a serious policy dilemma in health promotion as it relates to nutrition education and nutrition programs. There is a newly awakened national interest in nutrition education, but we lack effective mechanisms of evaluation that might yield information on which to base policy development.

The methodology useful in evaluation is often very unsophisticated. Considerable work has been done on the development of standardized measures of behavioral outcomes, but educators and researchers are not yet able to arrive at a consensus relative to methods for the collection and evaluation of information. A commonly used way to evaluate nutrition education programs involves *outcome* evaluation, such as how many individuals participated in the program, how many questions were correctly answered in the posttest, changes in attitudes, or short-term changes in dietary or nutritional status. Numerous studies have demonstrated that nutrition education efforts can significantly improve nutrition *knowledge* and can result in more positive nutrition *attitudes* in the short run. However, there is a paucity of studies demonstrating long-term improvements in nutrition intake and in nutritional status as a result of education programs. We do not really know how to measure the process of education or how to determine in a practical way the impact of nutrition education on nutritional status. The evaluation of health and nutrition education is complicated by the many antecedent variables that act, interact, and combine to produce end results. As an example, consider a nutrition education program that is designed to accompany the WIC program. It would be very easy to give a written pretest and, after the education program, a posttest to measure the change in levels of knowledge. It would also be relatively simple to compare a food record kept by participants before and after the program to see if there was a significant improvement in reported dietary intake. We might also determine nutritional status in terms of certain blood values before and after the program and compare them to see if there was any change in nutritional status. But, if a considerable improvement were found in dietary and nutritional status, could this be the result of the nutrition education, or should it be attributed to the WIC food package? Other environmental factors may have influenced the change in nutritional status. How can we directly evaluate the nutrition education program? It is clear that our interest is not limited to knowledge gain but, rather, includes the effect of the program on nutritional status, which is extremely difficult to measure.

If nutrition policy is to be advanced in an effective, well-articulated manner, policymakers must have data on which to base their decisions. If nutrition educators are to learn more about the reasons for their effectiveness, or lack of effectiveness, they must know how successful their efforts really are. It is obvious that there is a need for improved methodologies in evaluating nutrition education. Until this is available, comparison of findings and data from different studies will be limited, and it will not be possible to generalize data from small studies to larger populations.

CONCLUSION

On a nationwide basis, nutrition education has been generally ineffective in improving nutritional intake and thus improving nutritional status. Nutrition education is vital for both the consumer and the provider of the food supply. The consumer who lacks a fundamental appreciation of the importance of diet in health promotion cannot be educated by distributing a few hastily designed pamphlets or by flashing a couple of pronutrition spots over the mass media.

In the past, nutrition education appears to have been "too little and too late." Basic nutrition information must transmit an attractive and motivating message and must be imparted to young children during their school years. Nutrition education efforts must be continuous as well as long term. The knowledge of the adult public must be constantly updated by various public information methods. The appropriate strategies should motivate the public to take personal responsibility for improving their own health through good nutrition. The message and the methods should motivate the consumer to make a responsible judgment about the value of an improved diet and to then make the required effort to take steps to improve the diet.

Successful nutrition education must be broad and community based; it should be integrated into other community health and education and food-related activities. Nutrition education must be a tool designed to help educators and health professionals reinforce the appreciation of the importance of good nutrition for the public. Nutrition education should stimulate providers of the food supply to modify various component parts to respond to the nutritional needs of the public. Nutrition education should offer stimulus to the government bureaucracy to take steps to respond to nutrition policy issues in such a way as to achieve the ultimate objective — to aid the public to attain good nutritional status. Because all these sectors — the health care system, the educational and governmental system, and the food system — are very influential in affecting the food behavior of the community, awareness and cooperation among them will significantly reinforce nutrition education efforts.

Table 13–7

Education Activities and Outcomes

Educational Input	Behavioral Outcome	Health or Administrative Benefit
1. Communications Component Demonstration of concern and interest in client needs	Comfort/satisfaction of client	Public support for program, increased compliance with suggested regimen, competitive with faddists or sources of "nonnutrition" information
Communication of facts and information	Increased client awareness, knowledge, changes in attitudes and beliefs, improved motivation	Improved compliance and better nutritional status
Innovative methods of education, such as entertainment, motive, appeal, and the like	Improved client interest and attention	Better chance of client participation and compliance
Inclusion of client's family in education	Improved family awareness, support, and interest	Support for client improvement, adoption of improved, preventive health behavior by others
Outreach activities	Public awareness, improved interest, support, and modified health-related behavior	Increased participation in health programs, increased utilization of available services
Mass communication	Increased public awareness, knowledge, understanding, and support	Increased support, participation in programs, decreased confusion about program offerings
Follow-up and evaluation	Reinforcement, ongoing patient interest and participation	Return visits to program, ongoing adoption and modification, and improvement of health-related behavior
2. Community Organization Activities	Resource coordination, improved community relations, support, social reinforcement for clients, increased participation in program	Service utilization, recruitment of clients, improved community health status
3. Staff Training and Development	Staff awareness, interest, support for program, increased staff referrals to program	Integrated health service delivery system, improved client satisfaction, improved service delivery efficiency

Source: L. W. Green. Methods available to evaluate the health education components of prevention health programs, in *Preventive Medicine, U.S.A.* New York: Prodist, 1976, Appendix M.

L. Green has outlined education activities and outcomes that are important for any preventive health program and that should be applied to the development and implementation of nutrition education programs. These are presented in Table 13-7.

What is the responsibility of the nutrition educator in this total process? The educator is responsible for a correct analysis of the nutritional needs and problems of the community, and for communicating nutrition information clearly, attractively, and correctly, and in a way that makes it important to the learner. The educator must play an active role in understanding the learner and the learner's needs, in setting priorities, and in helping the learner to act in a manner consistent with his or her own perceived best interests as they relate to diet and health. In short, the educator must help the learner to learn. The educator must not design programs as for white rats; rather, he or she should design a learning experience that is problem centered and learner centered, rather than message or curriculum centered. If the learning experience does not meet the needs of the learner, and does not consider the learner's world, problems, and unique situation, it is bound to fail. And, perhaps most important, the educator should develop a learning process that enables the learner to communicate personal ideas about diet, the meaning of food, the importance of nutrition, and difficulties in changing food habits and that builds on the positive food habits to help the learner share responsibility for learning about nutrition and for improving food habits in accordance with improved nutrition knowledge.

Finally, the nutrition educator must be able to influence the food suppliers, health professionals, educators, and public policymakers to consider how they might take an active role in improving the nutritional status of the U.S. public. The many issues involved in the process are the subject of the next chapter.

REFERENCES

1. Joint Committee on Health Education Terminology, 1972–1973. New definitions. *Health Educ. Mono.* 33 (1973): 63–69.
2. Task Force on Consumer Health Education. Definition of consumer health education, in *Preventive Medicine, U.S.A.* New York, Prodist, 1976, p. 3.
3. Simonds, S. K. Health education in the mid-1970s: State of the art, in *Preventive Medicine, U.S.A.* New York: Prodist, 1976, pp. 107–110.
4. American Dietetic Association. Position paper on nutrition education for the public. *J. Am. Diet. Assoc.* 62 (1973): 429.
5. Mead, M. *Cultural Patterns and Technical Change.* Paris: United Nations Educational, Scientific, and Cultural Organization, 1953.
6. Light, L. The role of the university in preparing nutrition educators for the future, in Conference on Education in Nutrition, *Looking Forward from the Past.* New York: Columbia University, Teachers College, February 26–27, 1974.
7. American Public Health Association. Health education and public health. *The Nation's Health*, September 1977, p. 12.
8. Walker, M. A., and M. M. Hill. *Homemakers' Food and Nutrition Knowl-*

edge, Practice, and Opinions, Home Econ. Res. Rep. No. 39. Washington, D.C.: U.S. Department of Agriculture, Agricultural Research Service, November 1975.

9. Fusillo, A. E., and A. M. Beloian. Consumer nutrition knowledge and self-reported food-shopping behavior. *Am. J. Publ. Health* 67 (1977): 846.

10. Fusillo, A. E. Testing consumers' food IQ. *FDA Consumer* 10 (1976): 28–30.

11. Fusillo, A. E. Food shoppers' beliefs — Myths and realities. *FDA Consumer* 8 (1974): 12–15.

12. Pearson, J. Nutrition-related health practices and opinions, in U.S. Department of Agriculture, *Nutrition Program News.* Washington, D.C., September–December 1972.

13. Jones, J. L. Are health concerns changing the American diet? *N.F.S.* 159 (March 1977): 27.

14. Lowenberg, M. E. The development of food patterns. *J. Am. Diet. Assoc.* 65 (1974): 263.

15. Ohlson, J. A., and L. J. Harper. Longitudinal studies of food intake and weight of women from ages 18 to 56 years. *J. Am. Diet. Assoc.* 69 (1976): 626.

16. Mills, E. R. Psychosocial aspects of food habits. *J. Nutr. Educ.* 9 (1977): 67–68.

17. Caliendo, M. A., and D. Sanjur. The dietary status of preschool children. *J. Nutr. Educ.* 10 (1978): 69–72.

18. Fargo, G. Summary of some selected principles of learning and motivation, in *Proceedings of Workshop I on Curriculum Development for Community Nutrition Training.* University of Hawaii, Honolulu, February 10–21, 1975, pp. 141–142.

19. Griffin, G. A. Strategies in curriculum development, in Conference on Education in Nutrition, *Looking Forward from the Past.* New York: Columbia University, Teachers College, February 26–27, 1974.

20. Baird, P. C., and H. G. Schutz. The marketing concept applied to selling good nutrition. *J. Nutr. Educ.* 8 (1976): 13–17.

21. Kendall, E. On food and the American psyche, in L. Hofmann, ed., *The Great American Nutrition Hassle.* Palo Alto, Calif.: Mayfield Publishing, 1978, pp. 419–433.

22. American Dietetic Association. Position paper on the scope and thrust of nutrition education. *J. Am. Diet. Assoc.* 72 (1978): 302.

23. Bosley, B. Panel discussion of making nutrition education effective, In Conference on Education in Nutrition, *Looking Forward from the Past.* New York: Columbia University, Teachers College, February 26–27, 1974.

24. Cosper, B. A., D. E. Hayslip, and S. B. Foree. The effect of nutrition education on dietary habits on fifth graders. *J. Sch. Health* 47 (1977): 475.

25. Baker, M. J. Influence of nutrition education on fourth and fifth graders. *J. Nutr. Educ.* 4 (1973): 55.

26. Sherman, A. R., K. J. Lewis, and H. A. Guthrie. Learner objectives for a nutrition education curriculum. I. Identification and priority ranking. *J. Nutr. Educ.* 10 (1978): 63.

27. Barnette, J. J., and M. Branca. Learner objectives for a nutrition education curriculum. II. Factor analysis. *J. Nutr. Educ.* 10 (1978): 65.

28. Lashof, J. C. In U.S. House of Representatives, Consumer Relations and Nutrition Committee on Agriculture, testimony before the Subcommittee on Domestic Marketing. Washington, D.C., October 6, 1977, p. 497.

29. King, J., S. Cohenour, and C. Corruccini. In *Food Guides: Their Develop-*

ment, Use, and Specified Changes. Sacramento: California Department of Health, June 1977.

30. Hausman, P. Updating the basic four. *Nutr. Act.* 6 (January 1979): 8–9.
31. Hill, M. M. ICNE formulates some basic concepts in nutrition. *Nutr. Program News* (1964): 9–10.
32. Neisheim, M. In U.S. House of Representatives, Consumer Relations and Nutrition of the Committee on Agriculture, testimony before the Subcommittee on Domestic Marketing, *Hearings on Nutrition Education.* Washington, D.C.: Government Printing Office, September 27, 1977, p. 126.
33. Hansen, R. G. An index of food quality. *Nutr. Rev.* 31 (1973): 1–17.
34. Green, L. W. Methods available to evaluate the health education components of prevention health programs, in *Preventive Medicine, U.S.A.* New York: Prodist, 1976, Appendix M.

14

Issues confronting nutrition education

Reader Objectives

After completing this chapter, the reader should be able to
1. Describe five general issues confronting nutrition educators.
2. Describe three general problems with federal involvement in nutrition education.
3. State three nutrition education measures to combat counternutrition education messages.
4. List three general ways to increase the effectiveness of nutrition education through mass media.
5. Describe the current state of nutrition education in the schools, in primary care settings and in medical schools.
6. State what we should expect from nutrition education in terms of the modification of food habits.

INTRODUCTION

Although nutrition education can be defined in theory, in practice, existing endeavors do not measure up to the current needs for such education. A variety of issues confront those engaged in nutrition education. This chapter discusses some of the following issues:

Federal Initiative in Nutrition Education

There is a lack of coordination between federal, industry, private, and professional sources of nutrition information, as well as a lack of coordination at various federal, state, and local levels. In spite of more than thirty federal programs involved in disseminating nutrition information, consumers still do not know where to look for reliable, practical information, or what to believe when they find such information. Few consumers are aware of the federal programs that exist, and they are usually ignorant of information disseminated by the federal government. Although channels such as the USDA Extension and the USDHEW Office of Consumer Affairs are designed to provide such information, the average consumer is unaware of the resources they provide.[1]

Channels for the Delivery of Nutrition Education to the Public

Nutrition information may not be accessible to the consumer when and where he or she needs it. The nutrition educator is often unaware of audience needs, concerns, characteristics, and problems, so that methods are frequently unrealistic and narrow. Nutrition education has often been presented as a set of facts to be learned and then applied to consumer and food behavior, whereas the needs, motivations, life-style, and habits of the learner were not considered when the education program was being developed. Further, nutrition is often presented to the public in such a dull and monotonous way as to "turn off" those who could profit from nutrition knowledge.

Consumers want nutrition information in the supermarket, in their children's classrooms, in the doctor's office, in places where food is served, and in the media. They are not able to get this information where they want it.[1]

Special target groups also lack access to needed information. For example, many food stamp recipients do not have adequate access to information that might guide them in economical food shopping habits. An estimated 40 per cent of adults 65 years of age and over and millions of middle-aged persons have been instructed to modify their diets to reduce fats, calories, sugar, and the like. Yet these individuals are often unable to get reliable information and help to modify their diets.[1]

The low-income consumer must try to reduce food costs. He or she is bombarded with the claims of advertisers from the food industry and is apt to fall prey to the appeals of the food faddist. Nutritionists try to counter these appeals by suggesting the elimination of junk food and other frills from the diet, but nutritionists often seem unaware of the very special difficulties as well as preferences and traditions that influence the food and nutrition behavior of consumers. Information offered in a vacuum is unlikely to be an effective or helpful guide.

Limited resources are available to allow nutrition educators to compete adequately with "counternutritional messages." The consumer is bombarded with claims from all sides. The food industry promotes highly processed, refined, high-fat, high-calorie, and high-sugar foods that are also highly fortified with vitamins and minerals. The "health foodists" preach the gospel of natural, health foods (see pages 454–460). Some health professionals warn about cholesterol and saturated fats whereas others praise the variation and large supply of food that is available, with the compliments of the food industry. The most effective message is often that which consumers hear the loudest and most frequently. Consumers are gullible and are looking for convenience, lower prices, and the quick, easy route to good health. Rarely do they find sound, reliable nutrition information appealing in the face of so many other attractive claims.[1]

Nutrition Education in the Schools

There is a lack of a universal, coordinated, systematic, or successful way to provide nutrition information throughout the public school curriculum. Education programs from nursery school through college offer an excellent opportunity for the integration of nutrition education, a resource that was largely untapped until the passage of the 1977 Child Nutrition legislation that provided states with $.50 per child for nutrition education programs. (See Chapter 17.) However, even with this support we lack a universal and systematic way to integrate nutrition education into the curricula. To launch a successful program of nutrition education in the schools, teachers and food service personnel must be adequately trained in nutrition and in nutrition education methods. Unfortunately, few teacher-preparation programs include training in nutrition. School administrators and parents also need to be convinced of the importance of the nutrition education program and be involved in its development and implementation.

Nutrition Education in Medical Schools and Health Care

There is a lack of universal concern for nutrition education in the medical school curriculum. Further, nutrition education in the medical care delivery system has focused almost exclusively on "diet counseling," that is, on instructing a patient about a modified diet designed to alleviate a given medical problem, rather than on nutrition as a way to promote health and prevent illness.

Nutrition education activities addressing these areas of concern are now discussed.

FEDERAL INITIATIVES IN NUTRITION EDUCATION

Food, nutrition, and health are not the sole concern of any single sector of society; rather, they should be viewed as a national concern. As with any major interest, what the government does, as well as what it does not do, significantly influence policy and practice. The lack of nutrition education effort received increasing attention during the mid-1970s. Responsibility for nutrition education falls into various categories, some of which are listed in Table 14-1.[2]

The Food and Agriculture Act of 1977 provided for the establishment of a national education program to be funded by the U.S. Department of Agriculture.[3] The Expanded Food and Nutrition Education Program is authorized to include nutrition education for low-income families. Despite this mandate and the impressive list of federal responsibilities in the area of nutrition education, many problems and issues surround federal nutrition education activities. The Congressional Research Service (CRS) survey of the nutrition education sponsored or provided by the federal government published in *The Role of the Federal Government in Nutrition Education* noted that nutrition education was the concern of 30 programs in 11 agencies of 2 departments (USDHEW, USDA) of the federal government. Two regulatory agencies also are concerned with nutrition education. However, of these, only 14 programs could identify the part of their budget that was actually devoted to nutrition education.[4] Federal nutrition education activities were classified into one of six categories:[4]

1. Specific nutrition education program.
2. A component or support service of a larger program.
3. Publications for the consumer, specific groups, or professionals in the health and nutrition fields.
4. Grants, educational courses, and training programs for people entering nutrition-related occupations and for professionals in the health and nutrition fields.
5. Funds for nutrition and nutrition education research.
6. Nutrition advertising and labeling.

Some programs, for example, the Expanded Food and Nutrition Education Program, had nutrition education as a primary mission. Other pro-

Table 14-1

Responsibility for Nutrition Education at the Federal Level

1. Provision of leadership — information, interpretation and methodology — for newly enacted congressional legislation — for the nation and to the states.

2. Provision of leadership for deserved federal legislation relative to food and nutrition.

3. Provision of an exchange of information on nutrition education for all population groups — agency to agency, state to state.

4. Maintenance of an inventory of present programs concerned with food nutrition.

5. Maintenance of an inventory of unmet needs of population groups related to food and nutrition; make recommendations to state governments, industry, research centers for educational programming, and for research studies.

6. Promotion of state, regional, national, and international workshops and seminars for purposes of delineating problems and outlining procedures for solution.

7. Provision of a national food and nutrition resource center — information resource personnel and materials.

8. Development of guidelines and plans for supervision for federally funded programs.

9. Continuous surveillance of nutritional status.

10. Special consideration of vulnerable groups.

11. Improvement of nutritive value of foods.

12. Provision of current nutrient food values, standards and tolerances, and so forth.

Source: U.S. Senate Select Committee on Nutrition and Human Needs. *Overview: The Federal Programs.* Washington, D.C.: Government Printing Office, December 6, 1977, p. 140.

grams provided nutrition education as a component of food assistance offerings; still other programs provided nutrition education as a small part of their general educational offerings (e.g., Office of Education programs). Some agencies provided money and funds for nutrition education and related research. The survey results are presented in Table 14-2, which illustrates the great variety and dispersion of federal nutrition education activities as they existed at the time of the Congressional Research Service study.[4]

F. Richmond noted some of the problems related to the role of the federal government in providing nutrition education:

> Duplication of effort and dispersion of severely limited funds point to a federal role in nutrition education that lacks clear goals, firm resolve or a workable strategy. A patchwork of isolated, independently conceived activities are performed to the extent that funding and agency or departmental jurisdictions allow. There is no unified federal policy with regard to the relation of food and nutrition to the consumer. Research . . . is conducted without a view of how this research may support policy or program planning. There is neither unity of purpose nor message in information programs for the consumer. Each agency and program has built its own network of distribution channels for its communications.[5]

Table 14-2
Federal Nutrition Education Activities Revealed by the Congressional Research Study

Program	Description, Background	Eligibility
	1. Department of Agriculture	
A. Extension Service		
1. Expanded Food and Nutrition Education Program* (A)	Mission is to aid poor families, especially those with small children, to achieve adequate nutrition. There are two general programs, one for adults, the other for youth in a 4-H type setting. Program aides, who are often indigenous local residents, assist in program operation	Low-income adults, youth aged 9–19
2. Extension Food and Nutrition Program (B, C)	Provides general nutrition information on topics such as money management, food procurement, food safety, storage, preparation, dietary management, and nutrition. Program works through clubs, with health professionals; provides printed publications, media coverage	General public
B. Agricultural Research Service (C, E)	Established to perform research in areas of plant and animal production, use of soil, water, and air, and marketing, use and effects of agricultural products	General public
1. Food and Nutrition Research Program (A, B, C, E)	Aims to improve consumer and professional with knowledge of nutrition. Provides education through publication of pamphlets and brochures. Publishes *Nutrition Program News* through Consumer and Food Economics Institute	General public
C. Food and Nutrition Service (A, B, C, D, E)	Established to alleviate poverty-related malnutrition in the United States. Administers food assistance programs	Nutritionally vulnerable groups
1. National Advisory Council on Child Nutrition (B)	Established to study child nutrition programs and make annual reports	Children
2. Food Stamp Program (B, C)	Mission is to help low-income people to increase their food buying power and achieve better nutrition	Households with low-income and few material assets
3. Child Nutrition Programs (A, B, D, E)	Programs include school lunch, school breakfast, special milk program	Children in institutions who participate in programs
4. Special Supplemental Food Program for Women, Infants, and Children (WIC) (B)	Provides food for pregnant and lactating women, infants and children up to age 5	Those pregnant, lactating mothers, infants, and children to age 5 determined to be at nutritional risk
5. Food and Nutrition Information Center (A, D, E)	Established to act as clearinghouse for instructional materials dealing with food and nutrition education, research, training and instruction and other materials related to Child Nutrition Programs, and to disseminate these resources to program participants and state educational agencies	General public; professionals, state agencies
D. Cooperative State Research Service (B, E)	Established to administer acts appropriating agricultural research funds to State Agricultural Experiment Stations (SAES)	
E. Office of Communication (B, E)	Mission is to disseminate results of agricultural research trends, consumer information, and educational materials. Mission is to coordinate information work, review all USDA materials published, and coordinate agricultural information on activities with those of other federal and state agencies	

II. Department of Health, Education and Welfare

Program	Description	Target population
A. Administration on Aging (B)*	Established by Older Americans Act of 1965, it is responsible for carrying out most of Older Americans Act programs, serving as clearinghouse for information on aging, and for coordinating federal programs related to aging	
1. Nutrition Program for the Elderly (B)	Goal is to provide inexpensive, nutritionally sound meals to older Americans	Adults over age 60 or the spouse of someone over age 60
B. Office of Child Development (B)	Established to serve Americans with special needs	
1. Head Start (B)	Mission is to provide low-income children with comprehensive social, educational, health, and nutritional services. Parents are to be intimately involved with program planning and operation	Preschool children aged 3 and up until school age whose family income meets Office of Child Development guidelines; 10 percent of those enrolled must be handicapped youngsters
C. Office of Consumer Affairs (A, C)	Established to deal with issues related to federal policies for consumer goods and services	General public
1. Food, Nutrition, and Health Campaign (A, C)	Developed in attempt to improve public knowledge and awareness about the importance of good nutrition for good health. Activities include television spots and publications.	General public
D. Office of Education (B, D)	Responsible for administration of programs offering financial assistance to education agencies, institutions, and organizations	
1. Consumer and Homemaking Education (B, D)	Offers educational programs for vocational home economic education to prepare individuals for homemaking	Preschoolers through elderly with special provision for economically disadvantaged
2. Follow Through (B)	Authorized to aid children of kindergarten and primary school age from low-income families. Main component is the Comprehensive Health Services program, which provides health screening, diagnostic, monitoring, treatment and immunization	Children in grades K–3 whose family income meets guidelines of Office of Management and Budget
Other programs within Office of Education that include components of nutrition education		
a. Library Services and Construction Act (B)	Assists in the development of public library services, prepares bibliographies on nutrition-related topics, identifies local resources on specific subject matter, serves as coordinating agency in community, and helps nutrition education agencies to plan for action and deal with community needs	Resource for communities
b. Basic grants, state vocational education programs, occupational home economics education (B, D)	Aims to prepare persons for jobs related to food production, management, and service; provides nutrition information as needed for occupation	Youth from seventh grade through elderly
c. Consumer's Education (B)	Provides consumer knowledge to general public in subject areas of food purchasing safety or human services	General public
d. Adult Education Program (B)	Assists adults aged 16 and over to complete secondary school education and to obtain job training. Nutrition training and education available where appropriate	Adults aged 16 and over

Federal Nutrition Education Activities Revealed by the Congressional Research Study *(continued)*

Program	Description, Background	Eligibility
e. School Health and Nutrition Services for Children from Low-income Families (B)	Aims to demonstrate methods for organizing comprehensive health and education services system	Children in grades K–8 from low-income families
f. Centers and Services for Deaf-Blind Children (B)	Nutrition curricula for deaf-blind children	Children aged 0–21
g. Severely Handicapped Children and Youth Program (B)	Offers special education to youths from birth to age 21 who are severely handicapped	Children aged 0–21
h. Handicapped Children's Early Education Program (D)	Develops model programs for meeting needs of handicapped children from birth to age 8. Nutrition components deal with meals, food habits, and parent education	Children aged 0–21
i. Migrant Program (B)	Aims to expand and improve educational programs to meet special needs of youngsters aged 5–17 who migrate with their families for agricultural or fish-related employment	Children aged 5–17 who migrate with families for agricultural or fish-related work
E. Health Services Administration	Aims to serve as national focus for programs and health services for the United States; is concerned with health care delivery systems	
1. Bureau of Community Health Services (B, C, D, E)	Administers programs to provide health services to underprivileged. Goals include leadership and technical assistance for the development of nutrition services, evaluation of nutrition programs, nutrition training programs, conducting nutrition education, and program evaluation studies	General public is eligible but special target groups include those with special health needs
2. Indian Health Service (B, C)	Provides medical services, programs in sanitation, dental and health education, ambulatory care, nutrition, maternal/child health, school health, medical-social services, family planning, public health nursing, and mental health; provides inservice training in nutrition for health professionals	American Indians and natives of Alaska
3. Bureau of Quality Assurance (B, D)	Responsible for assuring high-quality care in Medicare, Medicaid, and maternal and child health programs and to make expenditures more cost effective	Does not provide direct service
4. Bureau of Medical Services, Department of Hospitals and Clinics, U.S. Public Health Service Hospital (B, D)	Responsible for providing comprehensive medical care for specified federal beneficiaries and occupational health care and for developing and integrating emergency medical services systems. Nutrition-related activities focus on food service within systems	Merchant seamen; Coast Guard and U.S. Public Health Service Corps personnel and dependents; federal employees eligible for Federal Employee Compensation; retired military and dependents
F. National Institutes of Health (B, C, E)	Source of federal support for biomedical research; also conducts research directly	
1. National Heart, Lung, and Blood Institute (B, C, D, E)	Conducts research and training programs related to prevention, diagnosis, and treatment of cardiovascular and chronic lung disorders. Nutrition education is a component of programs	General public, persons with heart and lung-related disorders; research funding for academic institutions, professional and private groups

2. National Cancer Institute (B, C, E)	Responsible for implementation and coordination of National Cancer Program	General public, cancer victims, health professionals
a. Diet, Nutrition, and Cancer Program (B, C, E)	Begun to study and educate, it is concerned with nutrition programs for cancer patients and the relationship between nutrition and cancer	
b. Division of Cancer Control and Rehabilitation (B, E)	Responsible for coordination of cancer control activities in cooperation with state health departments and other health agencies. Activities include prevention, detection, and treatment and evaluation, rehabilitation, and ongoing care	
3. National Institute of Arthritis, Metabolism, and Digestive Diseases (B, C, D, E)	Has principal responsibility for medically oriented research that is federally supported. Provides nutrition education to disseminate research findings	General public, selected patients, health and nutrition scientists and professionals
G. Health Resources Administration (B, C, D, E)	Responsible for identifying and correcting imbalances and problems in distribution, supply, access to, utilization, and costs of health care resources and services	Does not provide direct service
H. Office of Public Affairs (B)	Reviews USDHEW publications of about three-fourths of department agencies. Is working to implement computerized tracking system of USDHEW publications	No direct service
I. Office of Health Information and Promotion (B, C)	Established to coordinate and develop health and nutrition policy and education programs	
J. Food and Drug Administration (C, D, E, F)	Provides nutrition education indirectly through labeling and advertising responsibilities	General public

III. Federal Trade Commission (F)

	Duties include preventing unfair methods of competition; compiling and investigating economic facts related to corporations engaged in interstate commerce; supervising export trade associations. Principal nutrition-related activities are concentrated on the Trade Regulation Rule on food advertising and children's television advertising	General public

*Letters indicate analysis by category.
A — Specific nutrition education program.
B — A component or support service of a larger program.
C — Publications in nutrition or related areas.
D — Grants, education, and training for professionals.
E — Funds for nutrition and nutrition education research.
F — Nutrition advertising and labeling.
Source: Congressional Research Service. *The Role of the Federal Government in Nutrition Education.* Washington, D.C.: Government Printing Office, March 1977.

Other problem areas relate to the gap between nutrition and federal dissemination of information. Most information provided by the federal government relies on the printed brochure, which is not the most effective technique of communication. These brochures often do not reach the majority of the population for whom they are intended. Many consumers do not know of their existence, or how to obtain them, whereas others are not able to read or understand them. Further, few of these materials have undergone any formal evaluation to determine their effectiveness.

The approach of many of these materials is the traditional one, often based on diet planning around the basic four food groups. The approach suggests the importance of including enough food from each of the groups. This material is not what many consumers want to know. Their concerns, rather, center around the relation between diet and health, the problems in obtaining wise, economical food buys, and the questions of food safety. The need for federal nutrition education activities has been well established.

The White House Conference on Food, Nutrition, and Health analyzed many nutrition issues and concerns and recommended actions to improve and strengthen nutrition education in the schools, at the professional level, in the community, and for the general public and disadvantaged groups.[6]

The 1971 White House Conference on Aging suggested that a significant part of the resources devoted to nutrition education activities should be "designated for nutrition education of all consumers, especially the aged."[7]

Hearings and testimony of the U.S. Senate Select Committee on Nutrition and Human Needs and the U.S. House Subcommittee on Domestic Marketing, Consumer Relations, and Nutrition have reiterated the need for nutrition education. Of particular concern to the Select Committee was ". . . the inadequacy of present federal efforts in nutrition education; the absence of nutrition education among the medical professions . . . and the present role of the private food industry through its advertising and labeling techniques."[8]

Distribution of Federal Nutrition Education Materials

The agencies of the USDA and USDHEW have the primary responsibility for the distribution of the nutrition education materials they prepare. The Government Printing Office (GPO) and the Consumer Information Center (CIC) distribute these materials. The GPO prints as well as distributes materials in GPO bookstores and through mail-order operations. Nutrition materials are listed in over 15 GPO subject bibliographies.

The CIC is responsible for encouraging the development of practical and relevant information by federal agencies, for increasing public awareness, and for providing public access to the information. The CIC publishes a quarterly catalog, "Consumer Information," that lists more than 200 items that can be obtained free or at low cost. It is not known how many nutrition-related materials are distributed by the CIC.

Because of the way in which printed materials are distributed, the same publication offered for sale by the GPO or the CIC may be obtained free of charge from the issuing agency. Another consequence of the current methods of dissemination is that there is no way of assuring that nutrition publications are actually meeting the needs of their intended audiences. There is no one central list of available nutrition information materials nor is there a central clearinghouse for obtaining these materials. Because the GPO and the CIC select materials on a "hit-and-miss" basis, the public cannot rely on them as a source of all federal publications on nutrition or even as a source of the most valuable publications on nutrition.[9]

Information about some of the key nutrition education information that is disseminated by the USDA and the USDHEW is presented in Table 14-3.

Since the publication of the 1976 CRS report, there have been significant improvements in the federal role of the federal government in nutrition education. Some of these improvements are particularly worth noting.[10] The U.S. Department of Agriculture has achieved:

— Recognition of its "poor past performance" and the importance of improvement in the areas of coordination and outreach.

— Increased emphasis on the quality of its nutrition materials in terms of design and content.

— Establishment of a Human Nutrition Policy Committee, a Human Nutrition Advisory Committee, and an Interagency Coordinating Committee.

— Increased use of mass media in the programs of extension, particularly in the EFNEP program, and increased federal review of state activities in the activities of extension.

— The awarding of a contract for a media project for nutrition education.

— Concentration of the *Agriculture Yearbook, 1979* on nutrition education for children aged 6-12.

— Development of new initiatives for nutrition education in the Food Stamp Program.

The U.S. Department of Health, Education and Welfare has provided:

— An advertising program for children sponsored by the Office of Consumer Affairs.

— A national conference on nutrition education.

— A joint endeavor between the National Institutes of Health and Giant Food Company to evaluate the point of purchase nutrition education.

— An extensive review by the FDA, in concert with USDA and FTC, of nutrition labeling.

— The development of a Consumer Nutrition Education Program by the FDA.

Initiatives for improving the role of the federal government in nutrition education have thus been undertaken. These improvements should

Table 14-3
Key Information on USDA/USDHEW Nutrition Materials Disseminated

Department/Agency	Number of Materials Disseminated	Predominant Central Themes of Materials (a)	Primary Intended Audience (b)	Primary Distribution Channels (d)
USDA				
Food and Nutrition Service	18	Basic nutrition, food selection, food service management, food buying, food preparation	Food assistance program participants	USDA, state
Agricultural Research Service	102	Food composition, food preparation, research on food practices, food selection, food preservation	Professionals, general public	GPO (c), USDA
Office of Communication	20	Consumer information, basic nutrition, food buying, food preservation	General public	USDA
Food Safety and Quality Service	61	Food buying, food safety	General public	USDA, GPO, CIC (d)
Extension Service	112	Basic nutrition, food selection, food preparation, federal program information	General public, professionals	USDA, state
HEW				
Office of Consumer Affairs	7	Consumer information, federal program information, basic nutrition	General public	USDHEW
National Institutes of Health	21	Diet and health, consumer information, basic nutrition	General public, special individuals	USDHEW, SPS
Administration on Children, Youth and Families	9	Basic nutrition, consumer information, food service management	Professionals	USDHEW
Administration on Aging	19	Federal program information, basic nutrition	Professionals, food assistance program participants	USDHEW, SPS, state
Food and Drug Administration	40	Food and nutrition labeling, basic nutrition, food and nutrition information	General public	USDHEW, CIC
Health Services Administration	5	Diet and health, food selection, federal program information	Professionals	USDHEW
Health Resources Administration	3	Diet and health, research on food practices	Professionals	USDHEW

a — Shows themes accounting for 10 per cent or more of materials from highest to lowest.
b — Accounts for at least 50 per cent of materials disseminated by the agency.
c — Government Printing Office.
d — Consumer Information Center.
Source: Congressional Research Service. *The Role of the Federal Government in Nutrition Education.* Washington, D.C.: Government Printing Office, March 1977.

form an ongoing endeavor to expand and broaden, as well as to improve federal nutrition education activities.[11]

NUTRITION EDUCATION — WHEN AND WHERE SHOULD IT BE CARRIED OUT?

Channels for the Delivery of Nutrition Education to the Public

Individuals throughout all stages of their lives have varying and unique nutritional needs. Similarly, on the continuum from illness to optimal health, the nutritional needs of individuals differ. For example, individuals of different sociocultural backgrounds experience different problems in meeting their nutritional needs. Thus, it is important that nutrition education efforts be continuous from and throughout early childhood to old age. Nutrition education should be provided at various stages of wellness and illness and should be targeted to meet individual needs in obtaining adequate nutrition. Because of the needs for nutrition education at all ages and for those from various backgrounds, nutrition education should "be provided in a variety of settings: in the home; in the school; in programs for senior citizens; in the workplace, in offices, institutions, and agencies where medical care is provided; in community civic and social organizations; and through mass media.[12] (See Figure 14-1.)

Some would describe anyone who influences what another eats as a nutrition educator. It is becoming increasingly clear that the nutrition educator is no longer limited to the dietitian and nutritionist. The practitioners of nutrition education include a variety of health professionals as well as paraprofessionals, educators in the classroom, family members, producers and sellers of food, advertisers, and members of the public in general.

Nutrition educators carry out a variety of activities in an attempt to help individuals become motivated to improve their food habits. They provide information about food and its relation to health and illness; they help people to acquire the knowledge and skills to improve their nutritional status; they aid in motivating individuals to practice healthier eating habits; and they assist health professionals, educators, public officials, and community leaders in becoming knowledgeable and skilled in the facets of good nutrition, and in helping these individuals to use their talents to improve the nutrition habits of others. Nutrition educators are also involved in program design, implementation, and planning as well as in evaluation and research efforts to improve the nutrition of individuals and communities. Examples of nutrition activities that are designed to disseminate nutrition education to the public are listed in Table 14-4.

As Table 14-4 illustrates, nutrition education for the public can be disseminated in a variety of ways. Some programs have been community based and have focused on low-income regions. For example, the Los Angeles King-Drew Consumer Health Education Services (CHES) implemented a multidisciplinary Preventive Health Education Team concept aimed at operating through existing community services in the Watts

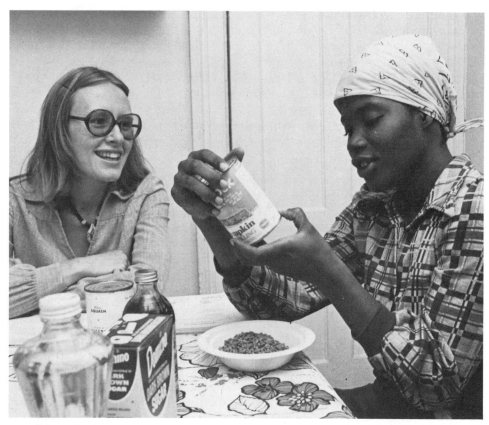

Figure 14.1 The involvement and nutritional education of the public is an important aspect of improving food habits. (from Food For Kids, U.S. Department of Agriculture, Food and Nutrition Service)

Table 14-4

Suggested Methods for the Dissemination of Nutrition Information to the Public

1. Training paraprofessional workers, aides, and volunteers to effectively relate to the people they will be teaching.
2. Family-life education programs based on group work methods and emphasizing nutrition and food.
3. Mobile nutrition units with staff and equipment to provide nutrition education to people of different backgrounds. Such units could also serve as a central base for food aides and community volunteers.
4. Food fairs that include cooking demonstrations, films, movies, or question-and-answer sessions. This would provide an opportunity to communicate nutrition concepts to the public in an entertaining way.
5. Television educational programs on nutrition and follow-up discussion of application and information with homemaker groups conducted by a paraprofessional worker.
6. Use of games or simulations for developing skills in selecting foods that provide good nutrition and family satisfaction for money spent.
7. Expansion of the nutrition education component of portable-meals programs and group-feeding programs for the elderly.

area. The health educators in the program included a nutritionist and a group of outreach workers to instruct the public in such areas as nutrition and maternal and infant care and the relation of food and nutrition to high blood pressure.[13]

A similar program, but one that is broader in scope and intended to reach people of all socioeconomic backgrounds, was developed in Pittsburgh. Under the aegis of the Health and Welfare Planning Association, an Interagency Council on Health Education and a Community Health Education and Information were developed to plan and direct the implementation of education programs.[13]

University extension services are examples of existing institutions that provide the impetus for nutrition education. A good illustration is Project HELP (Health Extension Learning Program), a jointly operated program of the Alabama Cooperative Extension Service of Auburn University, the Alabama Health Department, and the University of Alabama Birmingham Medical Center. Specially trained professionals are responsible for programs in broad geographical regions. Local community leaders participate in the program and are involved in various stages of the planning and implementation process.[13]

In most successful programs, nutrition education activities have been able to feed into existing networks — this type of "piggyback" arrangement has value for the nutrition component and for the other health care components. Nutrition education is only a single aspect of a total community nutrition improvement effort; other important components include nutritional assessment, surveillance, monitoring, referral, overall program planning, and coordination and evaluation. The educational component is often the most visible, but still only a part of the total structure of a public program. Thus, it is essential that the consumer education effort be integrated into every other aspect of the program and be well coordinated with all other concerned program components, resource, and personnel.

A variety of national health and nutrition organizations are providing nutrition education to the public. Such groups as the American Heart Association and the National March of Dimes provide nutrition literature including cookbooks, health records, pamphlets, and booklets to increase nutritional knowledge. Some organizations, such as the Planned Parenthood Federation of America, the Natural Childbirth Association, and La Leché League, provide nutrition information along with the promotion of the primary concerns of the organization.

Some groups, such as Weight Watchers, Tops, and Overeaters Anonymous, which are often run by formerly obese individuals, try to provide nutrition education along with motivation for specific target groups.

The National Health Council is the resource and "parent organization" for over 70 national and health-related groups that are interested in the promotion of health. Most of these groups provide some health guidance programs, and many of them incorporate nutrition education into their overall plan of work. The National Health Council is also developing an integrated framework for a national clearinghouse of health education.

The list of agencies and activities presented in Appendix IV describes further nutrition education activities of selected organizations.

NUTRITION EDUCATION TO COMBAT FOOD MISINFORMATION

Nutritionists and health professionals are in general agreement — we need to wipe out food faddism. But there is less general agreement about what food faddism really is. M. Jacobsen, for example, suggests that ". . . the guru of food faddism is not Adelle Davis, but Betty Crocker. The true food faddists are not those who eat raw broccoli, wheat germ, and yogurt, but those who start the day on Breakfast Squares, gulp down bottle after bottle of soda pop, and snack on candy and Twinkies."[14] Jacobsen has suggested that people who are hooked on a junk food diet, which is high in calories, saturated fat, and refined sugar, constitute the norm, whereas those who are truly concerned about nutrition and health, those who shop in health food stores, and those whose diets resemble the North American diet of the early 1900s are considered deviants or "food faddists." (See Figure 14-2.)

Many Americans avoid eating highly processed, packaged convenience foods and food filled with additives and chemical preservatives, the standard North American fare. Some people are truly fanatical in the quest for pure clean food — perhaps to the extent of mistrusting water from the faucet and carrying their own container of bottled water. Others merely prefer homegrown vegetables and fruits (grown without the aid of artificial or chemical fertilizers or pesticides) to the chemically altered "fresh" produce available in the supermarket.

Vegetarians are sometimes called "food faddists," although vegetarianism certainly is not a food fad; carefully planned vegetarian diets can be balanced, adequate, and can even offer nutritional benefits that are not characteristic of the typical North American diet. Vegetarian diets are usually lower in total saturated fat, calories, total fat, and cholesterol and are higher in dietary fiber. However, careful planning and nutrition knowledge to aid the vegetarian to include the variety and appropriate combinations of food is essential. The USDA has estimated that 5 per cent of the American population, or about 10 million people, consider themselves vegetarians.[15] Vegetarians have been classified into four groups according to the strictness of their dietary restrictions.[16]

1. Vegans or strict vegetarians — they consume no animal foods, fish, poultry, or dairy products.

2. Lactovegetarians — they eat no meat, poultry, fish, or eggs, but do eat milk and dairy products.

3. Lactovovegetarians — they eat only vegetables and dairy products and eggs (Seventh-Day Adventists belong to this group).

4. Fruitarians — they eat only raw and dried fruits and nuts.

A review of the literature on vegetarian and nearly-vegetarian diets concluded that "widely differing dietary practices appear among vegetarian and near-vegetarians. A reasonably chosen plant diet, supplemented with a fair amount of dairy products, with or without eggs, is apparently adequate for every nutritional requirement of all age groups."[17] The review

"Dear General Foods, Imitation this. Artificial that. Synthetic this. What's wrong with real food?"

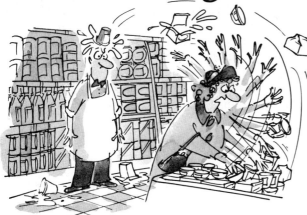

" *THERE MUST BE A REAL EGG HERE SOMEWHERE!* "

Actually, there's nothing wrong with "real" food. Or with any foods, natural or man-made, that you're likely to come across in the supermarket.

But there *is* some confusion regarding imitation eggs or artificial bacon, or any of those foods variously called synthetic or man-made. Now, the more you know about what you eat, the better. So toward that end, we'd like to clear up some of that confusion and provide a few explanations here.

Man-made foods: who needs them?

As with everything else you can buy, it's consumers who determine whether or not man-made foods exist. If people are willing to buy these foods, supermarkets will sell them. So when we're asked who wants these man-made foods, it isn't a glib answer to say that people do.

Okay. People need them. But why?

Because, for one reason, they can save you money. You actually spend less of your income on food than most people in other countries. Man-made foods are part of the reason. They usually cost less to produce, and therefore to buy, than many of the fresh foods they may replace.

Another reason for man-made foods

is simply that they taste good—not occasionally, but consistently. Since they can be made under conditions more controllable and predictable than the weather, man-made foods don't fluctuate in quality quite the way natural foods do. And, of course, they're produced and available year-round, winter *and* summer.

Then, too, most man-made foods store for a long time without spoiling and are usually easy to prepare—points so obvious we sometimes overlook them.

Finally—and maybe most important—man-made foods will help make sure the world has enough to eat. We're producing more and more people, and conserving less and less farmland to feed them. In a world with some 4 billion mouths to feed, man-made foods perform an important role now, and will perform an increasingly important one in the future.

How "imitation" butter became "real" margarine.

It's sometimes assumed that there are two kinds of food in the world: (1) real and (2) everything else. Actually, the distinction between "real" and man-made is nowhere near as sharp as it might seem.

Take margarine. It was invented over

a century ago as a sort of "imitation" butter. The margarine people couldn't have been very happy with the "imitation" label, suggesting, as it did, some inferior version. But over the years, margarine came to be known as something else: a good-tasting, long-lasting alternative that's especially useful for people concerned about animal fats and cholesterol. It's not "imitation" anything, anymore. It's genuine margarine. Not "imitation" butter, but certainly "real" food.

And that's the point: there are any number of man-made alternatives to natural foods in the supermarket, and these are no less "real" for being alternatives. In fact, the alternatives usually offer some benefit the original doesn't, or else there'd be no need for them.

Take our Dream Whip® Whipped Topping Mix. It isn't whipped cream. But it is a good-tasting alternative that's readily available, low-calorie, certainly long-lasting, and probably more dependable (it virtually always whips). Or take our Tang Instant Breakfast Drink. It's made with natural orange flavor. A 4-fluid-ounce serving gives you a full day's supply of Vitamin C, and not even an orange can give you better Vitamin C than Tang. It won't spoil quickly, and you can mix up as little or as much at a time as you want, without waste.

What's wrong with "real" food? Not a thing. It's just that today it comes in more varieties, and with more alternatives, than even the inventors of margarine ever dreamed.

For more information.

We hope this brief discussion of man-made foods has taken a little of the mystery out of why they're made.

If you have any questions about them, please feel free to ask. Just write to Miss Peggy Kohl, V.P., Consumer Affairs, G.F. Consumer Center, White Plains, N.Y. 10625.

Our reasons for telling you all this are a mixture of helpfulness and pride in our products. The more you understand about food, the better off you'll be. And the more you understand about our foods, the better off we'll be.

GF GENERAL FOODS

©1977 General Foods Corp.

Figure 14-2. Reprinted by permission of General Foods Corporation

noted that pure vegetarian diets that are generally nutritionally adequate contain foods such as unrefined grains, legumes, nuts, vegetables, and fruits. Inadequate diets generally include the following:

1. Vegan diets that may produce vitamin B_{12} deficiency in certain persons.

2. Grossly unbalanced nearly-vegetarian diets in which as high as 95 per cent of the calories come from low-protein, starchy foods.

3. Diets containing a high proportion of calories from refined cereals.

4. Diets in which total calorie intake is not adequate to meet nutritional needs.

In a well-balanced vegetarian diet, protein is rarely a problem. As D. M. Hegsted et al. have noted, for adults, "it is difficult to obtain a mixed vegetable diet which will produce an appreciable loss of body protein without resorting to high levels of sugar, jams, and jellies, and other essentially protein-free foods."[18] Many health benefits may be derived from vegetarian diets. For example, strict vegetarians have been found to average 20 lb less in body weight than nonvegetarians, who averaged 12 to 15 lb above their ideal weight.[19] The same study found that pure vegetarians had significantly lower serum cholesterol levels than did the lactovovegetarians or the nonvegetarians. Other studies have confirmed this finding.[20]

However, many possible nutrient deficiencies and nutritional problems may result from carelessly planned or overly strict vegetarian diets. The greatest risk is probably the reliance on a single or very limited food source, such at may be the case in the Zen macrobiotic diet. Plant sources of protein may not contain the proper mix and quantity of essential amino acids, or the appropriate quality, if an adult is not consuming sufficient calories to support normal weight from a wide variety of plant foods. Many vegetable and grain foods are low in essential amino acids such as lysine, methionine, threonine, and tryptophan. Thus failure to carefully plan a diet to supplement proteins can result in protein deficiency.*

Diets that are based primarily on whole grains are often lacking in vitamin A, vitamin D, and ascorbic acid; if milk is eliminated from the diet, the calcium intake may be very low.

A number of studies suggest that, in general, the risks of dietary inadequacy may be somewhat higher on vegan or on unplanned vegetarian diets than on nonvegetarian diets.[21-24] Noted adverse health effects of such diets in children include severe malnutrition and rickets in isolated instances as well as the more common deficits in size and in blood parameters such as hemoglobin and hematocrit.

A unique type of vegetarian diet that is the focus of much nutritional concern is the Zen macrobiotic diet. The word *macrobiotic* means the "way of long life", and Zen denotes the idea of meditation. The diet is thought to be a type of rejuvenation technique founded on a religious philosophy of the Far East that promotes the need for the balance of life forces (yin and yang). Yin is the passive element whereas yang is the active and more masculine element in the philosophy. Yin is female, cold, reticent, silent, and rich in potassium. Yang is loud, noisy, centipedal, and rich in sodium. Yin is thought to lead to silence and calm whereas yang results in heat, light, and action. George Ohsawa originally outlined a

---

*An excellent reference on complementarity of amino acids is Frances Moore Lappé, *Diet for a Small Planet*, revised edition. New York: Ballantine Books, 1975.

series of ten stages to the diet, each stage becoming increasingly more restricted. Table 14-5 illustrates these various levels.

Current followers of this diet have condensed these ten steps into seven. The basic dietary principles to be followed include

1. Eat no chemically refined white sugar or sugared foods.

2. Use only the minimum amount of water that will promote life and will enable urination limited to three times a day.

3. Use no animal products, especially in warm climates.

4. Avoid industrial foods or foods with chemicals and additives.

5. Eat no fruit.

6. Include 60–70 per cent of the diet as cereals and 25 per cent as well-cooked or baked vegetables.

7. Eat no potatoes, tomatoes, or eggplants.

8. Use salt to season food, and use vegetable oil in tropical climates.

9. Favor French, Chinese, or Indian food preparation methods.

10. Consume no vinegar.

11. Chew all food thoroughly; average about 30 chews per mouthful of food.

A common error of those who discuss the Zen macrobiotic diet as well as of some who adhere to it is to imply that regimen or stage 7 is the ultimate goal, the highest level, and that those who reach this level eat nothing but brown rice for the rest of their lives. Michel Abehsera, who received instruction about the diet directly from George Ohsawa, the guiding force behind the diet, stated the correct practice as follows (Table 14-5):

One begins with Number 7 . . . usually for ten days; one also goes back to Number 7 in case of illness. Numbers 6 and 3 should be where we spend most of our time.

Table 14-5
Zen Macrobiotic Diet

| | Per centage of the Diet in | | | Animal | Fruit/ | |
Stage	Cereals	Vegetables	Soup	Food	Salad	Dessert
7	100%	—	—	—	—	—
6	90	10%	—	—	—	—
5	80	20	—	—	—	—
4	70	20	10%	—	—	—
3	60	30	10	—	—	—
2	50	30	10	10%	—	—
1	40	30	10	20	—	—
-1	30	30	10	20	10%	—
-2	20	30	10	25	10	5%
-3	10	30	10	30	15	5

Source: R. T. Frankle and F. K. Heussenstamm. Food zealotry and youth. *Am. J. Publ. Health* 64 (1974): 11–18.

Those marked with minuses are slightly below the margin of safety, are resorted to occasionally in the search for variety, and are not recommended.[25]

The Council on Foods and Nutrition of the American Medical Association have spoken out against the Zen macrobiotic diet, suggesting that the diet created among its followers a major health problem by inducing scurvy, hypoproteinemia, anemia, hypocalcemia, and the emaciation of starvation with a concomitant loss of kidney function.[26] Those who seem to be particularly vulnerable to the adverse effects of the diet are pregnant and lactating mothers and their young children. Mothers who adhere to the Zen macrobiotic diet during their pregnancy often tire easily, contract infectious diseases, lose body fat as well as muscle, and present severe anemia. Their infants often gain weight at a very slow rate.[27]

A possible nutritional consequence of long-term consumption of this diet is vitamin B_{12} deficiency. Vitamin B_{12} is primarily found in animal foods. Since there is no known plant source, vegans should supplement their diet with vitamin B_{12}. The symptoms of B_{12} deficiency include soreness of the tongue, pernicious anemia, "vegan back" (i.e., irreversible spinal cord degeneration), and menstrual irregularity. Other possible problems include lowered intake quantity and quality of protein, riboflavin, calcium, and zinc.

Those who prefer the so-called health foods are often labeled as food faddists. Among these foods are the unrefined ones, such as granola, whole-grain products, nuts, legumes, foods free from chemical additives, and organic foods grown with the aid of organic rather than chemical fertilizers and free from preservatives, hormones, or antibiotics. These individuals prefer "health" foods for a variety of reasons. They may feel that the highly processed foods are unsafe and are detrimental to their health or that the production of these foods imposes serious strains on an environment already overtaxed by pollution and resource exploitation. Various authors and researchers have attempted to determine which people use "health foods," and what are the attitudes and beliefs of these individuals. Many users of health foods are extreme in their search for clean, healthful, and uncontaminated food. Examples of these health food users are those who adhere to extreme forms of the Zen macrobiotic diet, those who consume huge quantities of vitamin/mineral supplements, those who depend on large amounts of "body-building" high-protein supplements, and those who subsist on only a few foods. However, recent research suggests that "food faddists" (defined as those with extreme practices) may not be the primary users of health foods — many young people, students, concerned mothers, and homemakers favor the use of health foods, and their diets may in fact be much "healthier" than those of the average North American.[28,29]

R. Wolff suggests that these individuals should be described not as food faddists but as "health foodists." The term *health foodist* refers not to the long-haired, scrungy radical but to those who have realistic ideas about nutrition and are seriously concerned about promoting health through eating good food.[28]

Why would an individual choose to eat health foods? A number of health foods are more costly than comparable items available in the supermarket. Further, users of health foods usually restrict their diets and limit their consumption of many things that the average American considers "good" to eat. Why would anyone want to adhere to a diet that is expensive and also limited to nonprocessed foods? Research suggests that many of today's health food users are concerned about food and the effect of its means of production and processing on the ecology and environment. They are also concerned about the safety and quality of their food, and they are knowledgeable and concerned about the existing food supply and nutritional problems in the United States. Many health food users are merely trying to use their food and nutrition knowledge to practice what seems to be a sincere and long-term effort to improve their food selection.[29]

However, the eagerness of health food users to translate nutrition knowledge into a healthful diet may backfire, as, for example, when misunderstanding or misinformation is translated into extremely limited food choices, especially in the case of planning diets for young children. In their study of the nutrition knowledge of Hawaiian health food users, M. Anderson and B. Standal noted individuals who avoided meat because "too much meat protein causes the body to become too acidic" or who avoided animal fats because they "cannot be digested."[29] If this reasoning led these health food users to feed a strict vegetarian diet to young growing children, and if care was not taken to balance the protein content of the diet, the children would be at risk of developing nutritional deficiencies. Anderson and Standal found that the eagerness of the health food users to find nutritional information led them to look for such information in the most readily available places — the health food store or in lay literature. Thus, they were vulnerable to questionable nutrition information that was often offered from these sources. It is easy to see, then, why food misinformation might easily be accepted by many health food users. They should not be faulted for their search for nutrition information. Rather, nutritionists may be at fault for failing to provide useful and meaningful nutrition information to those who seek it.

We have only to look around us to see the numerous sources of nutrition information available to the public — mass media advertisements, interesting and intriguing writings of authors such as Adelle Davis, suggestions and recommendations of health professionals (more often than not untrained in nutrition), and the counsel of friends and relatives. Such sources not only inform but also reinforce food beliefs. But where can the average consumer go to find scientifically valid and yet practical and useful information? Nutrition scientists are trained to phrase their recommendations in often nebulous and ambiguous terms. Frequently, the conclusions of research studies that investigate what a good diet should contain are that "no definite conclusion can be stated at this time — more research is needed to determine . . .". This conclusion, which is actually not a conclusion, is of no use to lay consumers and may likely "turn them off." Can nutritionists blame the so-called "food faddist" for seeking alternative sources of information on which to base their food choices?

As R. Wolff points out, food attitudes and beliefs will not be maintained unless they are part of a larger set of attitudes and ideas, and unless they are frequently reinforced. Health faddists find this reinforcement by talking with individuals who hold similar beliefs, by reading information available in health food stores, by finding more of their preferred foods available in the local grocery store, and by seeing more people adopt their food practices. They find comfort in sharing not only their food beliefs but other beliefs about health, ecology, international food problems, and society and its possible fate. Food ideology is of interest to them, often because it is a real way to express their dissatisfaction with a manipulative world, an artificial world controlled by seemingly uncontrollable technology. Adherents to health food diets are seeking ways to reduce the risk of contamination of the food supply, they are seeking a simpler diet similar to that of their ancestors, and they are seeking a diet they believe will make them feel better.[28]

Nutritionists must be concerned with the individual who quickly latches on to a new idea, unsupported by scientific evidence, or who refuses to admit a fact, despite significant scientific evidence, and who then bases an entire diet on such limited or unfounded claims. How are nutritionists to deal with these individuals? Perhaps the single most important aspect of counseling adherents to food misinformation is to *listen* to them and to determine the message that the individual is trying to convey through his or her food practices. Is the individual seeking a quick magical cure? trying to express himself or herself in a unique and different way? trying to control his or her own environment and hence rejecting dependence on others? trying to win the acceptance of peers? trying to attain health through natural means rather than through drugs and medicines? or seeking stability in an unsure and threatening world? By listening to the message conveyed, we may quickly realize the extent to which a rational, scientific approach will be accepted by the person to dispel the erroneous notions and the extent to which an alternative approach may be required.

The nutrition counselor must understand the basic ideas and premises of the misinformation and then determine exactly how the erroneous ideas are actually affecting the individual's food habits. Is the effect severe? If it is minimal, no change in behavior may be needed. It is also important to emphasize the positive aspects of the individual's eating habits and to build on the positive, suggesting small, perhaps minimal, changes in those habits in a very gradual way. Can the individual relate any personal experiences, such as a feeling of tiredness, a weight loss, or some other negative influence on health that might possibly be related to the diet? If this information can be gained, it may suggest a starting point for further counseling. Above all, the nutrition counselor should not preach and should not expect the rational, scientific approach to work wonders; it may do more harm than good.

D. Erhard, after vast experience with counterculture groups in the San Francisco Bay Area, noted that the traditional methods of nutrition education were rarely effective. To be successful in nutrition education efforts with groups such as the Zen macrobiotics, Erhard suggested the need to define the beliefs and practices of the deviant behavior, determine the reasons for the beliefs, and then work within the given value system to produce necessary change.[27,30]

What Is Being Done to Combat Food Misinformation?

The National Academy of Sciences has taken steps to act against food misinformation. The academy has appointed a Committee on Nutritional Misinformation whose mission is to prepare short, straightforward, and nontechnical statements on food and nutrition issues in an attempt to refute inaccurate or misleading information that might adversely affect the health of the North American public. These statements are to be released to journals, magazines, newspapers, and the like, where a sizable proportion of the public might be reached. An example of these statements is "Dietary Supplementation with Vitamin E." Other statements deal with possible hazards of high intakes of vitamin A and D, the danger of depriving athletes of water, and the dangers of vegetarian diets and unsound reducing diets. These statements are probably most useful to professionals rather than to general readers.[31]

Other professional organizations attempt to combat food misinformation. The American Academy of Pediatrics Committee on Drugs and on Nutrition has issued statements on controversial nutrition information, as has the American Medical Association. And the American Dietetic Association has taken a variety of routes to inform the public about hazardous food misinformation.

An effective example of such activity was undertaken by the Executive Board of the Illinois Dietetic Association, which used five 90-second spots per week on public service radio time to refute misinformation that was being promoted on a sponsored radio program. The spots were called, "Nutrition I.Q." and used a question-and-answer format. These spots were so successful that the program that was originally responsible for disseminating the wrong information was forced off the air because it was unable to find a sponsor.[31]

Reliable Sources of Information

A problematic issue for the consumer is where to go for reliable and understandable sources of nutrition information. There is no single easy way to determine with certainty whether information and materials are accurate and truthful. There are a variety of reasons for this:[32]

1. There is often only limited or inconclusive information available pertaining to some aspects of nutrition.

2. Controversy and conflict often surround the nature of available data.

3. A number of self-styled experts abound with a wealth of information to divulge to the public. The zeal and the conviction of these so-called authorities make it difficult for the public to discount their messages. "The health quack often talks a brand of gobbledygook that sounds technical and may use perfectly valid terms."

Even with these difficulties, a variety of reputable nutrition information sources are available for the public. Scientists, educators, federal, state, and local government agencies, and professional and voluntary nutrition organizations can often refer the inquiring consumer to a source of sound information. The U.S. Department of Agriculture publishes numerous consumer information reports, and the U.S. Department of Health, Education, and Welfare also issues printed materials informing the public about programs and services available. The Extension Service of the U.S. Department of Agriculture is usually a good source of consumer information. Societies such as the American Dietetic Association, both nationally and locally, can direct the consumer to a source of sound information. Other reliable sources of nutrition-related information include the Food and Nutrition Board, the Federal Trade Commission, the Nutrition Foundation, and the American Medical Association. In many cities in the United States, "Dial-a-Dietitian" services answer questions on food and nutrition. This service is sponsored by local American Dietetic Association groups. Table 14-6 lists guidelines that are helpful in determining the validity of health information that can easily be extended to include nutrition information.[32]

On the other hand, the dispenser of nutrition misinformation, sometimes referred to as a quack, must be recognized for what he or she is, and the information that he or she provides must be relegated to the realm of misleading or false information. Table 14-7 presents some guidelines that may be useful for recognizing this type of individual.[32,33]

Nutrition education, which is geared toward preventive medicine and prevention of nutrition-related health problems before their inception, could eventually decrease the prevalence and the severity of many of the major "killer diseases" in the United States and also improve national

Table 14-6
Guidelines to Help in Determining the Validity of Nutrition Information

1. What is the purpose of the book, magazine, presentation, or statement? Is it to sell something and, hence, to make money? Or is it designed to present factual information or to make some type of a professional contribution?

2. What is the style and the procedure of presentation? Is it educational or scientific? Are propaganda techniques, such as misleading statements, ambiguous claims, or gross exaggerations, used?

3. What are the qualifications of the individual or organization disseminating the information? Is the individual or organization perceived as reputable by professional nutrition organizations? Is the group or individual listed in reputable biographic or information sources, such as *American Men and Women of Science*?

4. Are the data based on actual research experiments or on the opinions of one or two individuals? Is the tone of the message one of appeal and emotion, or of scientific logic?

5. Has the information been previously published in scientific or professional journals? If so, what is the reaction of nutrition or medical authorities about the information?

6. Where there is conflict surrounding the information, is the proponent able to summon up scientific support to defend his or her stance? Are the claims made the result of sound research or single, perhaps coincidental, incidents?

Source: H. J. Cornacchia. *Consumer Health.* St. Louis, Mo.: C. V. Mosby, 1976, pp. 216-251.

Table 14-7
Characteristics of the Dispenser of Nutrition Misinformation

1. He or she suggests that you buy something out of the ordinary and asserts that this purchase will provide a magic result, a quick cure for an illness, or have some other type of amazing effect on your health. For example, "Lose 10 pounds in only 5 days and keep it off with . . . ".

2. He or she is promoted as being an expert, the president of an unfamiliar organization, such as the society for concerned nutrition advocates, or the holder of an advanced degree from an unknown university.

3. He or she supports his or her claims with testimonials from people who supposedly experienced marvelous results with his or her products, or he or she asserts that famous people, such as athletes or television personalities, got where they are today because of the fantastic benefits from the product he promotes. For example, "I was always overweight. As a child I was 50 pounds overweight. All my life I suffered the pain and misery of being obese until I discovered product X. After only 3 weeks on the product, my life changed . . . ".

4. He or she suggests that an improved diet can work miracles, can give you newfound energy, a new lease on life, extra years of rich living, or a similar phenomenal feat. On the other hand, he or she claims that poor health, fatigue, tiredness, depression, anxiety, and so forth are attributable to a poor diet.

5. He or she tells you not to worry about a poor diet; a single serving of product X, or a particular combination of vitamins and minerals, can reverse the adverse consequences of a poor diet.

6. He or she overenthusiastically supports one of the following claims:
   — organically grown foods, that is, those grown without the use of chemicals, and processed without chemicals or additives, are nutritionally superior to foods grown with the aid of chemical fertilizers.
   — "health" foods are needed to sustain health and good nutrition.
   — vitamin/mineral supplements should be taken by everyone to ensure good nutrition.
   — natural vitamins are superior to synthetic vitamins.

Source: H. J. Cornacchia. *Consumer Health,* St. Louis, Mo.: C. V. Mosby, 1976, pp. 216–251. V. Herbert. The health hustlers, in L. Hofmann, ed., *The Great American Nutrition Hassle.* Palo Alto, Calif.: Mayfield Publishing, 1978, pp. 303–319.

health status by diminishing the prevalence of certain chronic diseases.

However, such an educational campaign will require time, thought, resources, and commitment. To date, neither the medical establishment nor the government have "been interested in such an effort":

> To illustrate, the Center for Disease Control, the federal agency charged with the largest responsibility for preventive public health education, spent $113 million to fulfill its mission in 1974. The money spent on advertising (1974) by Pepsi Cola and Coca Cola together was larger than CDC's entire disease prevention and control budget. In fact, in the same year, 19 major corporations spent 1.06 billion dollars on advertising. This was nearly three times the amount spent by our entire federal government for all of its disease prevention and control efforts.[34]

One way to rectify this situation is for nutrition advocates, concerned consumers, medical establishment, and nutrition experts to allocate resources into "Madison Avenue" advertising to "bring to the public, in a creative, vigorous, and continuous way, a new message designed to promote prevention of disease and health maintenance through healthful eating habits.[34]

Some suggest that advertising the nutritional values of food would be too complex or boring. This contention can be countered by a consideration of pet food commercials, many of which are filled with nutritional information. "If pets could understand television, they would have greater access to nutrition education than most of the population."[35]

Numerous studies on commercial advertising techniques as applied to educational media provide evidence that the way the commercial is presented is more critical to the formation of learning concepts than the actual message of the commercial. Available evidence indicates that the more a child likes a particular advertisement, the more likely he or she is to like the product being promoted. This suggests that commercial advertising techniques could be equally effective in promoting nutritionally sound concepts, provided that there are sufficient resources of talent, time, and funds.[36]

Media experts believe that there is a need to develop a "nutritional" figure or character, such as has been done with Ronald McDonald or the Trix rabbit. It is thought that if the character were attractive to the children's television audience, and if the children were able to identify with it, they might be able to get and retain information provided by this character. This idea has been considered by the American Dietetic Association in its promotion of the character, "Nutribird," which is illustrated in Figure 14-3.

It has been also suggested that some type of graphic that displays four points of nutrition information be used to accompany all food advertisements on television. The graphic should communicate the following facts.[35]

1. A food contains calories that can be measured or counted.

2. Many foods contain protein; the protein content of the advertised food should be noted.

3. Many foods contain vitamins; the vitamin content of food should demonstrate the food's nutritional worth.

4. Many foods contain minerals; the mineral content should be noted for a given food.

A graphic of this type is illustrated in Figure 14-4.

R. Choate noted that there should be stated standards for the conspicuousness with which the nutritional graphic display would be shown:

> The advertisement should include a nutritional graphic display, not less than five seconds in length or 16 per cent of the commercial's length, whichever is longer. The left side portion of the screen would present the graphic which is to be at least one-fourth the size of the total video picture. The setting of the graphic should emphasize the message of the graphic.[35]

Figure 14-3. The American Dietitic Association "Nutribird," (American Dietetic Association)

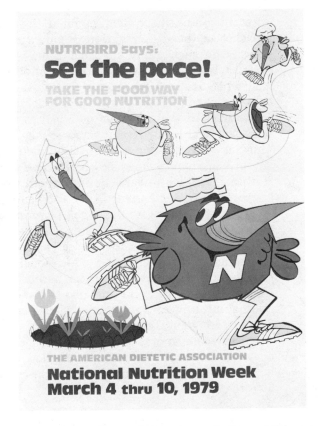

N. Feshbach et al. conducted a study to determine whether children could remember the information contained in television commercials, could interpret it, could evaluate foods on the basis of graphic representations, and could consider more than one dimension in the evaluation of foods. Eighty-eight children ranging in age from 4 to 10 were studied. The treatment variables looked at were the method of presenting calorie data on the Nutrition Computer graphic and the presence or absence of an orientation session. The results of the study showed that young children could learn and utilize nutritional information that was graphically communicated to them. Data suggested a developmental trend — the child's age was related to his or her ability to report and reproduce the information. However, the study showed that "children at all age levels . . . were able to learn, to comprehend the complex relationship of calories and nutrients and use both these dimensions in evaluating foods."[37]

Figure 14-4. Graphic illustration of calories, protein, vitamins, and minerals in one ounce of cereal

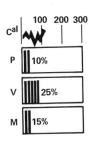

Recent studies have demonstrated the effectiveness of mass media approaches in the dissemination of nutrition information to various audiences. One such study involved a mass media campaign of prime-time radio, television spots, and spot announcements through which local media personalities provided nutrition facts. The campaign was aimed at teenagers, and follow-up nutrition brochures were distributed to schools. The results of the campaign demonstrated that a large percentage of the teenagers heard and remembered seeing both radio and television spots. Thus, it appears that an appealing media campaign, with which target groups can identify, may be an effective approach to nutrition education. However, further research is important to determine the effects of the improved nutrition knowledge on food and nutrition habits.[38]

To further investigate the type of communication techniques that might be effectively used in informing children about positive nutrition, the USDA initiated an awareness campaign, incorporating various media, marketing, promotional, and educational techniques. Nutrition messages provided through television, radio, and printed media are intended to reinforce nutrition education provided to the children in the classroom. Evaluation and follow-up are intended to determine the most effective methods for nutrition education via the media.

An alternate approach to developing explicit nutritional messages for television is the development of implicit messages that can make the public more aware of the nutritional status and nutrition-related health problems that are currently facing them:

> There is nothing to stop nutritionists from going to the writers and producers of soap operas, family shows, situation comedies, and even variety shows and giving them ideas for working incidental (but appropriate) food and nutrition messages into their programs. Nothing appears to be more effective on the TV screen than modeling possible behaviors and the consequences of those behaviors — making what people ought to do look feasible and attractive.[39]

It is also important to use the positive benefits of advertising to promote sound nutrition. For example, cereal advertisers, in promoting their product, often suggest the need for a well-balanced breakfast. Orange growers promote the consumption of citrus fruits that are high in vitamin C. These efforts should be backed by, and used for, the advantage of nutrition advocates.

Of great help are advertising experts who can help develop the message that will effectively reach the intended audiences. "Tell them what to say, but let them show us how to say it."[40]

The local media is one of the potentially most influencial resources for nutrition education. The following section summarizes some important considerations in working with the local media.

Tips on Working with the Media[41]

The local media can be the source of nutrition education. Before going too far ahead with plans, it is often helpful to consult the media in the area. This can save time and help in the definition of the materials and resources that are needed. A variety of questions might be asked to clarify the most appropriate approach and content of media messages:

What is the preferred format for news releases and announcements?

What is the preferred form for television: film, videotape, audio, or written copy to accompany slides?

What is the length and form for the announcements?

How many announcement copies are requested?

Could local feature stories be used? If so, what is the preferred content?

Could a nutrition expert be used as a speaker for a local talk show?

Can public service announcements be used?

Can material for editorials be used?

To whom should the material be sent?

What are the material and information deadlines?

Are there existing films or documentaries that can be localized and adapted?

In addition to representatives from the local media, other helpful communication experts that might be consulted include executives from local advertising groups or public relations firms, representatives from minority media or public broadcasting stations, and others who have had previous communication and public awareness experiences through work with campaigns such as United Way and the American Red Cross.

Television

Although television is glamorous and has a wide audience, it may also present certain problems. Television is frequently very expensive and the right effect may require professional expertise and know-how beyond what is available. It is wise to investigate the possibility that a television station or agency might sponsor nutrition messages as a public service.

Radio

Radio is underutilized as a health and nutrition education medium. Radio stations often devote more time per hour to public service announcements than do television stations. Radio stations often adopt a "community" improvement theme for a week or a month and have very creative ways of involving the local audiences. In addition, radio stations often have such features as the "Community Bulletin Board," "Call for Action," or some other services that might be used for announcements of nutrition programs.

Some considerations related to the development of radio messages include the following:

1. Talk to the station before developing the message. Stations often appeal to specific audiences and, hence, prefer specific message formats.

2. If possible, involve the whole station in promoting the program.

3. Radio spots for airing are often given more time than television spots; this means that more care will need to be taken to assure that the message does not become too repetitive.

Printed Media

The following approaches may be used to become involved with local printed communication channels:

1. Public service advertisements are used by a few newspapers but are more frequently used by magazines or local shoppers' guides.

2. News is always important. If the program content and description can be communicated as a newsworthy item, it is more likely to get coverage. Many program activities, such as participation of local agencies and personnel, program activities, and program attendance can be promoted in news feature stories.

3. Feature stories also provide an interesting slant. A public interest story about an individual who lost weight through participation in a nutrition education program and is now able to enjoy an expanded life, or another such local angle, is usually well received.

4. Editorials are a useful means of communication if the publication editors can be convinced of the importance and the health significance of improving nutrition. Editorials are helpful in communicating program efforts and are also a useful way to enlist support of local community organizations.

5. Photographs of program activities and participants, especially if they have an unusual angle, are a good way to get newspaper coverage.

Other Opportunities

In addition to these traditional media opportunities, other opportunities can be used in communicating and promoting nutrition programs and activities. Local bulletin boards, billboards, the outsides of transit vehicles, the inside advertising cards of buses or subways, college or business publications, or neighborhood newsletters, health department notices, organization bulletin boards, and dormitory ride lists, all provide sources of promoting programs and activities. Fliers included in direct mailings from business or hospitals, and classroom educational materials are other possible routes. Local businesses may be interested in sponsoring the messages or in helping with the advertising costs; if the businesses are given credit, their returns in public recognition may compensate them for the expense.

Message promotion can be viewed as advertising; the basic principles of advertising should be considered in developing the message:

1. Is it interesting? Can it attract and hold attention?

2. Is it easy to understand and simple enough not to be confused?

3. Does the message reinforce the content to be conveyed? Do words detract from the basic message?

4. Is the message suitable for the medium? For example, if the medium is radio, can the message be understood without any visuals?

For the development of any successful nutrition education activity, community participation at every step of the way is essential. Planning should involve the felt needs and the local expertise of the community. Respected leaders and community figures should be relied upon to help map out the appropriate program strategy and promotion methods. Local community organizations may be able to offer help in the form of volunteers, from addressing and sealing mail all the way through participating as aides in the program.

Another important benefit to be gained from involving the community in nutrition education is that of local political endorsement. Programs will have a much better chance to be successful if they are backed and supported by members and constituents of local organizations. The media is sometimes more responsive to messages sponsored by local organizations.

Another advantage of involving the local community is that participants can provide helpful information about how the program is going, once it has been implemented, and can often offer helpful suggestions about new methods, approaches, and activities.

NUTRITION EDUCATION IN THE SCHOOLS

The importance of beginning nutrition education in the early school years if it is to achieve maximum impact cannot be overstated:

> The school, as a social structure, provides an educational setting in which the total health of the child during the impressionable years is of primary concern. No other community setting even approximates the magnitude of the grades K–12 school educational enterprise, with an enrollment in 1973–74 of 45.5 million in nearly 17,000 school districts comprising more than 115,000 schools with some 2.1 million teachers. . . . Additionally, more than 40 percent of children aged three to five are enrolled in early childhood education programs. Thus, it seems that the school should be regarded as a social unit providing a focal point to which health planning for all other community settings should relate.[42]

Historical Perspective

R. Emerson was credited with the origin and development of the first "nutrition class" in Boston in 1908. Emerson believed that the "under-par" children he worked with needed to learn what to eat and that they needed continued supervision and encouragement in the formation of improved habits of eating, rest, exercise, and sleep. Emerson's work with 15 poorly nourished children resulted in improved food habits and weight gain. Thus, as early as 1910, there was evidence in the literature that nutrition education can produce beneficial results.

Emerson's work was soon expanded; in 1918, he conducted a nutrition class in a New York City public school. His methods were modified for the school situation and several conclusions soon become evident:

(1) Subject matter and methods could be developed by such teachers as those in home economics, biology, general science, and school lunch management; (2) methods of parent cooperation other than weekly attendance at the class were needed; and (3) nutrition should be fitted into the whole health program of the school and made available to every child.[43]

Nutrition education programs continued to develop and expand in scope, depth, and intensity as interest and knowledge advanced.

In 1944 the first longitudinal work in the United States was initiated in Ascension Parish, Louisiana, to determine effective methods of teaching nutrition. The work was founded on the premise "that the effectiveness of teaching nutrition would be manifested not only in measurable changes in nutritional status but also in measurable changes of behavior."[44]

The study methodology involved data collection concerning dietary practices and dental information; the gathering of these data was intended to help evaluate the program as well as to stimulate in the children an interest and an awareness of the importance of good nutrition in dental health. Results of the study indicated highly significant changes in food habits.[44]

The second half of the twentieth century witnessed a proliferation of work that was aimed at determining which classroom methods and techniques of nutrition education were most effective. Workers began to realize that education must not be confined to the school classroom, but should be prevention oriented and directed at the public. Work also began to suggest that nutrition education programs should be much more than information-giving techniques and that careful program planning, implementation, and evaluation were essential if long-term results were to be sustained.

Despite the evidence for successful nutrition education efforts, little has yet been done to implement effective nutrition education into either the primary or secondary school curriculums. Even diagnosed and obvious medical problems, such as diabetes, are often ignored from an educational point of view.

In general, health and nutrition education programs in the schools are limited in three main ways: "(a) a tradition of low visibility and low priority; (b) a narrow definition of the appropriate content and jurisdiction for health education efforts; and (c) a shortage of adequately trained health educators."[45]

A large responsibility has been charged to American teachers for providing nutrition education that would be useful to the students. But teachers are faced with a very poor nutrition education preparation themselves and consequently, the "level of understanding of nutrition by a majority of America's teachers is low." As the Panel on Nutrition and Government of the U.S. Senate Select Committee on Nutrition and Human Needs noted:

Current nutrition education and teaching programs during the formal learning experiences from kindergarten through college are largely ineffective or nonexistent. Frequently what is taught is misleading or unsound. . . . The lack of sound, well-prepared, challenging educational materials and failure to commit school time to nutrition education have limited the health benefits derivable from our abundant wholesome food supply.[45]

F. E. Whitehead conducted an extensive literature review of nutrition education studies from 1900 to 1970, noting that "there is evidence that nutrition education which purports to improve dietary habits can be expected to do so within carefully defined limitations."[43] Factors of length of time, method and technique of education, age, interest, and personal background of the learner are all important determinants of the impact of nutrition education.

Based on her literature survey, Whitehead formulated the characteristics of effective school nutrition education programs. These characteristics are listed in Table 14-8. Unfortunately, because of a variety of reasons, such as lack of funding and resources, lack of appreciation by teachers and school boards of the importance of nutrition education, and lack of administrative support, school nutrition programs often lack these components.

If an integrated program of nutrition education is to be effectively implemented, it must have the support of all administrative personnel involved in primary, secondary, and upper levels of education.

If professionals such as primary or secondary school teachers are to effectively teach nutrition, they must be trained in nutrition basics as well as in educational techniques. Thus, colleges should offer nutrition-related courses, which should be required for teaching credentials for all pro-

Table 14-8
Characteristics of a Successful School Nutrition Education Program

1. It is planned, developed, and evaluated by nutritionists, teachers, pupils, parents, and other community leaders.

2. It does not begin *after* a survey of food habits is made but rather with the *planning* for that survey.

3. It is based on children's needs as determined by an appraisal of food habits.

4. It is guided by leadership from school personnel and a qualified nutritionist.

5. It is not limited to individual children or to a few courses of study.

6. It is a part of the regular school program centered upon needs, interests, and age level of groups of children.

7. It is a program in which classroom teachers are responsible for instruction and guidance of their own pupils, both in classrooms and in lunchrooms.

8. It is a program in which classroom teachers and nutritionists together determine nutrition education problems and guide groups in the solution of those problems.

9. It is a program that contributes to the in-service training of teachers in the science of nutrition.

Source: F. E. Whitehead. *Nutrition Education Research Project: Report of Feasibility Study.* Iowa City: October 20, 1970.

fessionals. Provisions for continuing education, such as workshops or night courses, should also be made.

Teaching guides and tools and materials have been prepared for some teachers. Many states have prepared booklets that outline concepts and learning experiences that can be developed and applied at various grade levels. An example of a model curriculum for nutrition education in schools is presented in Table 14-9. The National Dairy Council has also developed nutrition teaching guides, objectives, materials, and media to teach the essentials of good nutrition in an interesting, practical, and meaningful way.

Table 14-9
Model Curriculum for Nutrition Education in Schools

First cycle (Grades 1, 2, 3)
> Various types of food — regional and ethnic foods.
> Descriptions of plants and animals that are used as food.
> Where milk comes from, how butter is made.
>
> Rapport with families, stores — wheat growing and milling, fishing.
> Discovery of corn and potatoes.

Second cycle (Grades 4, 5, 6)
> The human body, with special attention to how food is used: chewing, the role of the stomach, intestine, liver. How food and oxygen are brought to all cells in the body. Taste and olfaction.

Third cycle (Grades 7, 8, 9)
> The nutrients: carbohydrates, fat, protein, vitamins.
> Calories.
> Calories in foods, caloric expenditures — nutritional labeling.
> Ingredient labeling.

Fourth cycle (Grades 10, 11, 12)
> Weight control. How to calculate your diet.
> Proteins and amino acids: animal and vegetable sources.
> The identification of vitamins ("natural" and synthetic vitamins).
>
> Fads and fallacies.
> Nutrition and athletics.
> Nutrition and the prevention of disease.

Throughout: Recipes and ingredients in the school lunch program will be emphasized. From the seventh grade on all foods presented in the school lunchroom will be labeled both in terms of nutritional labeling and ingredient labeling.

The federal government should assist state education departments in establishing and supporting a required course on human biology to be given sometime in the last two years of high school; this course would include as one of its components the physiological and health aspects of nutrition.

Source: J. Mayer. Testimony before U.S. Senate Select Committee on Nutrition and Human Needs. Washington, D.C., 1977.

The legislation for many federal food assistance programs mandates that nutrition education be a component of the program operation. The 1970 Child Nutrition Act, which liberalized the school lunch program, called for nutrition as a part of the schoolchild's development. (See Chapter 17.) It set the tone for a national goal of providing for nutrition education along with free or reduced cost lunches to all schoolchildren.

The Nutrition Education and Training Program was created by PL-95-165, the 1977 Child Nutrition legislation. The law provides $.50 per child enrolled in a school or institution entitlement funding through 1979. Each state is to receive at least $75,000; some states may receive much more than this amount because of the number of school-age children in its population. The money is to be used for the following.[47]

Figure 14-5. The legislation of the school lunch program mandates that nutrition education be an integral program component. (from *Food for Kids*, U.S.Department of Agriculture, Food and Nutrition Service)

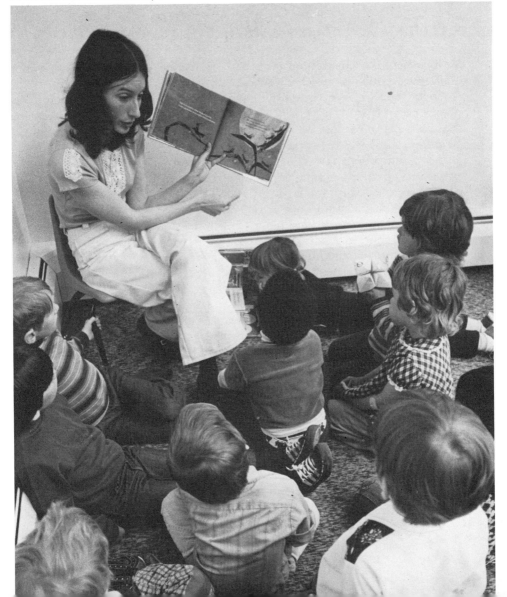

1. Nutrition education and training for school educators and food service personnel.

2. Food service management of school food service personnel.

3. Nutrition education resources and activities for children in schools and child care institutions.

Federal money is given to state agencies to hire a state nutrition coordinator, to implement a state needs assessment for nutrition education, to develop a state plan to address identified needs, and to implement the plan. The program is to be coordinated with other nutrition activities conducted with federal and state funds; it may not be used to replace existing nutrition education programs. States are currently in the process of implementing activities in areas of teacher education, the education of school food service personnel, and the integration of nutritional subject matter into the general school curriculum. The impact of these activities remains to be seen.

PATIENT EDUCATION IN HOSPITALS OR PRIMARY CARE SETTINGS

Most patients or clientele of a clinical facility have recognized some sort of medical problem and have turned to the medical profession for help. As such, they invest a certain amount of time, and usually of money, to obtain corrective therapy for their problem. It is to be expected, then, that such people would be responsive to therapeutic regimens and would be willing audiences for education.

This assumption, however, seems to be contradicted by recent studies of patient compliance with therapeutic treatments. In other words, there is often a gap between medical orders and what the patient actually does.

For example, a study by T. Williams of diabetics' compliance with therapeutic measures regarding medication, diet, foot care, and blood/urine found that, in general, fewer than 10 per cent of the patients studied carried out even a minimally acceptable regimen in all of the areas of daily diabetic management.[48] Reasons for patient noncompliance are complex and varied. Some of the causes of noncompliance are summarized in Table 14-10.[49] A recent workshop on compliance with therapeutic regimens concluded that about 50 per cent of patients (with a large variance) comply with prescribed medications for the treatment of different medical problems; approximately 33 per cent always comply, the same percentage never comply, and the other third are variable in their degree of compliance.[13,50]

Another study that examined patients with congestive heart failure (CHF) concluded that patient compliance with prescribed medication is related to the patient's understanding of the disease process. Individuals who did not understand their illness felt that they did not receive an adequate explanation from their physician. Thus, communications were an important difficulty. These problems appear to be a function of education. In the study, 20 out of 27 patients (74 per cent) who had an eighth-grade education or more took digitalis as often as prescribed; this was

Table 14-10
Causes of Noncompliance

Cause	Characteristics	Comments Regarding Research on Compliance
Patient	Sociodemographic traits	Inconsistent results; often contradictory association between specific variable and observed compliance
	Personality traits, such as self-esteem, anxiety level, dependency, impulsivity, and the like	Inconsistent results
	Effect of knowledge, health education	Many studies indicate positive relationship between knowledge and compliance, although others indicate no relationship
Physician	Simplicity of approach; convenience of access; degree of pressure applied to patient to adhere; ability of physician to obtain negative patient feedback; clear and specific instructions; short duration of treatment; confidence inspired in treatment	All characteristics linked to increased patient compliance
Patient perceptions of treatment	General health motivation: value of reducing threat of given illness; perceived probability that compliant behavior will be threat	Behavior and health compliance related to these categories
Professional/ patient interaction	Structured, rigid, authoritarian approach; relationship satisfactory to both; two-way communication; professional monitoring of compliance; eliciting fact of noncompliance by professional; increased professional approachability; description of treatment rationale	May result in improved compliance

Source: R. N. Podell. Physician's guide to compliance in hypertension, in *Preventive Medicine, U.S.A.* New York: Prodist, 1976, Appendix V.

compared with only 13 of 33 patients (39 per cent) who had less education.[13,51]

The implications of this finding for nutritional counseling and guidance of hospital patients are self-evident. Because eating habits are the result of numerous personal, social, and cultural factors, and are a firmly entrenched part of an individual's life-style, they are very difficult to change.

Dietary prescriptions are probably less complied with than are other types of medical regime.

What can be done to improve patient compliance with prescribed dietary modification? The first step requires effective counseling and education that in turn motivate the patient's desire to change. Effective diet counseling must recognize that long-term change of dietary habits requires:[52]

1. Active client participation in all phases of nutritional change strategies: planning, execution, and evaluation.

2. Continuity of care over a long period of time; however, the client should be guided to ultimate independence and self-responsibility for his or her own health as much as possible.

3. Intervention strategies designed to meet the individual needs of the client.

4. Mutual respect between client and professional.

These components must form the minimum groundwork for the effective modification of dietary habits. Within this context, some points may prove helpful in designing, implementing, and sustaining a program of successful planned change.

Basic to any successful program is a realistic assessment of the problem and factors related to the program. This includes an understanding of the dietary patterns of the individual and the emotional and material factors that affect these patterns. This assessment should then direct the development of a patient care plan. The plan should follow carefully developed client objectives formulated by the client in concert with the counselor. The client must understand that the responsibility for modifying food habits rests with him or her, and not with the health professional. The client must realize that his or her full cooperation is needed and that he or she must agree to participate in the counseling process under these provisions. With these considerations in mind the following guidelines are suggested as helpful in promoting lasting nutritional change.[52]

1. The client should notice and record his or her daily eating habits; he or she should record the type of food and the quantity of food eaten, the time of day this food was eaten, and circumstances related to the eating experience. Asking the client to carefully observe and write down these diet patterns actively engages the client in his or her own "change process." Events or locations associated with eating may often serve as helpful leverage points in designing a change strategy. For example, if an individual tends to eat when the television is on, he or she can be alerted to this and can resolve to restrict his or her eating to the kitchen, while seated at the table.

2. The counselor should promote the accurate recording of all dietary information. Keeping a food diary is often a helpful way to base suggestions for change and to evaluate progress over a period of time. These food records might then form the basis for discussion in the counseling sessions. By reviewing the diary, the client, with the aid of the counselor,

can recognize ways in which his or her immediate environment should be changed to facilitate a modification of food habits.

3. Plan for small, gradual changes in food habits. The planned changes should be designed to promote a slow but steady trend toward improved dietary patterns. Use the immediate past client performance as a benchmark from which to gauge future planned change. Eating habits, which are usually the result of a lifetime of eating, will be resistant to broad, sweeping, and unrealistic modifications. If the objectives are too general, the client's failure to meet them will reinforce his or her feelings of not being able to change.

4. Encourage the client to expect a realistic level of success, and make it very clear that there will be times when the client does not succeed; this is to be expected and should not signal discontinuation of efforts; provide support when the client does not meet his or her goals, and assure the client that, over time, continued efforts will be rewarded with success.

5. Be ready to offer sustained and extended support. Although it may be difficult to schedule counseling sessions on a basis of more than once or twice a month, the client should understand that frequent contact with the counselor, by mail or by phone, is encouraged. The client should be especially encouraged to seek support if he or she experiences special problems with dietary modification. This is particularly important during the early phases of counseling. The counselor should also seek the support and encouragement of family members or close acquaintances of the client. This cooperation will provide support when the counselor is unavailable. If possible, the family should be included in the counseling meetings.

6. Evaluation of client progress should be determined by observing the client's behavior. Evaluating adherence to a particular dietary regimen by weekly weigh-ins, or measurements of parameters, such as serum cholesterol levels, may only frustrate the client. These measurements are subject to variability and may be slow to respond to actual dietary modification. Thus, the counselor's efforts should be focused on the specific dietary changes and behavior patterns of the client. If these patterns follow a trend in the hoped-for direction, the client's physiological parameters should begin to change over time.

These guidelines suggest that the client-counselor relationship should be an active and dynamic one; both parties should follow the general behavior-based, problem-solving approach to modifying food habits. Individual problems will vary, and it is difficult to state broad approaches to every individual problem. Rather, the problems should suggest possible techniques to be used in overcoming them. In the long run, lasting change is most likely to occur when the client takes the responsibility for improving his or her own dietary patterns. These guidelines will help the counselor to facilitate this process.[52]

In attempting to modify an individual's food habits, the nutrition educator should make a number of options available to the client. Behavioral principles that might aid in suggesting promising options have been previously discussed in Chapter 9.

Recent studies have confirmed the importance of including the family as part of specific efforts to modify problematic food habits. K. Brownell, in a study in which three groups of ten obese persons each were treated, used behavioral modification techniques. In one group the patients attended ten weekly sessions. Their spouses came to the sessions with them and participated in certain specified activities designed to help the obese to lose weight. In the second group, the spouse was willing to come and participate but was informed by the therapist that, in the interest of time, this would not be possible. In the third group, the spouse was not willing to participate.[54]

After the end of the ten-week period, weight loss was measured, and it was measured again three and six months later. Results of the study indicated that those patients whose spouse participated lost significantly more weight (a mean difference of 13.5 kg per patient) after the ten-week period. This positive result continued through the six-month period. The weight loss of those in the two groups in which the spouses did not participate were similar and were significantly less than the first group.[54]

J. Witschi et al. report the results of a short-term study in which families participated in a dietary study with the objective of reducing serum cholesterol levels. Dietary modification included the reduction of dietary cholesterol and saturated fats, and sunflower oil and margarine were added to provide polyunsaturated fat. After a period of ten days, an average reduction in serum cholesterol of about 10 per cent was attained. This result persisted for a three-week study period. The researchers suggested that the high level of cooperation among the free-living families who participated in the study had positive implications for enlisting family participation in future attempts to improve health and nutrition behavior.[55]

Part of the difficulty in patient nutrition education relates to the lack of nutrition knowledge of medical professionals. For example, nurses in public health agencies and in school or industrial settings are often left with the responsibility of providing a significant part of the nutrition education. If such an educational process is to be effective, the nurse must perceive herself or himself as playing this role of health and nutrition educator and must also have the basic framework of theory and knowledge in nutrition.

Nurses have widely varying levels of experience and expertise in nutrition. H. Gifft et al. have suggested that nurses who have a baccalaureate degree typically have a better grasp of nutritional concepts than do those who have come through a traditional three-year hospital nursing degree program.[56]

Many nurses seem to have negative feelings about the subject of nutrition. Their experiences with nutrition in nursing school are often negative, and consequently they do not advocate the need for nutrition education in their nursing practice.

J. Vickstrom and H. Fox studied the nutrition knowledge of nurses and found that older nurses typically had less knowledge of nutrition than did their younger colleagues but that they usually had more positive attitudes and were more receptive to nutrition education. The researchers, in studying nutrition knowledge, found that nurses' knowledge of normal and therapeutic nutrition tended to be accurate about 50 per cent of the time but that the nurses were often unsure about their knowledge and, hence, hesitated to apply it.[57] Perhaps the most serious lack of nutrition knowledge among health professionals involves physicians.

NUTRITION EDUCATION IN MEDICAL SCHOOLS

Clinical nutrition is not even taught in most medical schools. . . . Of course the matter goes deeper than a mere question of deficiencies in the medical school curricula. It involves the way the medical profession approaches the whole subject of preventing disease.

— *R. T. Williams*

One of the main problems resulting from the lack of nutrition training in the nation's medical schools is that however much individual physicians in the federal or state planning agencies may protest their interest, nutrition almost invariably ends up being left out as a component of health care delivery systems.

— *J. Mayer*

The physician occupies a pivotal role in the delivery of any type of health information or service. Most people perceive the physician to be an almost infallible source of information on health-related subjects. L. Baric has written about the role of the physician in health education and notes that the individual decision to comply with a suggested treatment or preventive action is related to the individual's knowledge but also to the way the person perceives his or her health state. If an individual views himself or herself as ill or at least in a very vulnerable position, he or she is more likely to take the prescribed actions. Thus, Baric believes that the medical profession has a serious responsibility to make the "at-risk role" a legitimate state deserving of medical or health care. Because the "at-risk" state is very loosely defined, individuals need the physician's support if they are to comply with preventive behavior changes over a long period of time.[58] However, this posture is not the traditional one for the doctor. Baric suggests that if the physician is to serve in this role, a variety of changes will be needed in the orientation and focus of medical school training, in the physicians' own self-perception, in the scientific legitimacy of preventive as well as therapeutic measures, and in procedures to identify and screen out at-risk populations. Furthermore, the prestige status of preventive approaches must improve relative to that of crisis intervention and sickness care.[59]

Although many groups influence the nutrition education of the general public, the physician is often credited by the public with having expert special knowledge of this subject. If the doctor is called on to give nutritional advice, is he or she likely to have the necessary knowledge to make sound recommendations? Moreover, a physician who obtains a laboratory report of a serum cholesterol level of 300 mg/100 ml and is unable to direct the patient to nutritional therapy or to provide this information to the patient may indeed be guilty of the equivalent of medical negligence. The lack of nutrition education in most medical schools is a significant contribution to such incompetence.[60,61]

The inadequacy of nutrition in medical school education has recently received much attention. That improvements in this area of medical school education are forthcoming is indicated by the burgeoning interest in the subject as well as by the increasing concern of medical students with the social and preventive aspects of medicine. This concern is frequently greater than that of the faculties of medical schools.[62] The recent attention being paid to the wide prevalence of "hospital malnutrition" and the health implications of this is another indication that physicians are becoming increasingly open to receiving more medical education.[63-65]

Nutrition, as a formal subject in the curriculum of medical schools, has been largely neglected. A realization of this gap in medical education prompted the Council of Foods and Nutrition of the American Medical Association (AMA) and the Nutrition Foundation to jointly sponsor a national conference to discuss the teaching of nutrition in medical schools. The Chicopee Conference, held in 1962, was attended by 47 individuals, many of them practicing physicians, as well as educators and scientists. The proceedings of the conference emphasized the importance of nutrition as an integral component of medicine, which plays a role in diagnosis, treatment, rehabilitation, and prevention. Participants stated that "It is the responsibility of the faculty of each medical school to assure the student an opportunity to learn the modern concepts of nutrition and to obtain some supervised experience in the application of nutrition to clinical (and public health) problems."[66]

Recommendations from the conference related to the delegation of duties for the development, implementation, and evaluation of programs; the establishment of standards for nutritional components of internships and residencies; offerings in continuing education for physicians; resources and support for nutritional activities; and nutrition research.[67] Participants called for the implementation of "meaningful opportunities through required and/or elective courses in nutrition for medical and other health personnel to learn the modern concepts of nutrition and to obtain supervised experience in the application of nutrition to clinical (and public health) problems." Ten years later, a follow-up conference, jointly sponsored by the AMA and the Nutrition Foundation, with the assistance of 13 other institutions, was held in Williamsburg, Virginia. This conference, attended by 87 participants, reiterated the principles that were previously voiced in Chicopee.[68]

The latter conference noted that, whereas limited progress had occurred in certain schools, the "teaching of nutrition has not generally been integrated into the curriculum of the medical student, the training of the house staff or teaching of the allied health professionals. Where medical students' awareness of nutrition has become evident, it often has stemmed from factors or influences outside of the schools.[68]

The 1972 Conference on Guidelines for Nutrition Education Programs suggested the following essential nutritional principles that every physician should master:

1. Science of nutrition. "The physician should have a scientific understanding of digestion, absorption, metabolism and metabolic balance; nutrient requirements for growth and maintenance; the dietary management of metabolic and other diseases; and the diseases of malnutrition including deficiency diseases, undernutrition, overnutrition, and abnormal nutritional needs. This basic knowledge is best obtained during medical school training and perfected in postdoctoral education."

2. The sociology of nutrition. "Understanding of the role of nutrition in medicine includes an awareness by the physician of its sociologic aspects. He should be able to serve as a consumer-advisor to his patients, understand food within the context of the family and cultural setting, and be aware of available sources of nutritional information."[69]

The Conference suggested that an effective medical school training program in nutrition require three things.[69]

1. Nutrition advocates who are interested and skilled in program administration.

2. Agreement on the appropriate nutrition curriculum and its integration into the medical school curriculum.

3. Necessary financial support. A fund allotment was suggested. First, medical schools or schools of public health that were interested in nutrition should receive financial commitments for the endowment of chairs in nutrition. Second, funds should be provided for the development and expansion of teaching programs and methods to aid clinical nutrition programs. Third, a financial commitment to the career development of "future leaders" in clinical nutrition was indicated.

To achieve these recommended goals, a task force should explore ways in which nutrition might be better identified as a medical specialty and in which continuing education could be provided.

The Conference further suggested that "nutrition centers of excellence" be developed to "expand the availability of nutrition training beyond the confines of present medical schools." These centers might be places in community hospitals or in health centers of other community settings. The mission of these centers should be the development of potential nutrition program directors and the provision of a variety of nutrition services and educational opportunities. By giving physicians the chance to specialize in nutrition, these centers have the potential to be the training grounds where students could blend didactic nutrition knowledge with the appropriate application of nutrition to real-life community situations.

More recent conferences continue to encourage medical schools to establish programs, resources, and faculty to include nutrition education in the medical curriculum. In April 1976, the American Society for Clinical Nutrition and the American Institute of Nutrition cooperated to sponsor a conference, Teaching Nutrition in Medical Schools, in Anaheim, California.[70] The Society for Nutrition Education, in July 1976, sponsored a special session on the subject in Kansas City.[71] The American

Medical Association published a Summary of Nutrition Curricula in Medical Education in 1976.[72]

The federal government has also become involved in the concern for improved nutrition education. The Bureau of Health Manpower of the USDHEW-HRA supported a study of nutrition education in nine selected medical schools. Federal funding is beginning to become available for projects that are designed to increase the emphasis on the awareness of education and research in nutrition.[67]

Much additional evidence supports the conclusion that nutrition does not receive adequate attention in the preparation of health professionals.

C. Wen et al. conducted a survey of the nutrition education status in medical schools in the United States through catalog descriptions and types of questions on licensure examinations.[73] In catalog descriptions, nutritional topics were usually included in biochemistry courses but rarely as components of clinical courses. Wen noted that, of the 94 medical school catalogs evaluated, 50 per cent did not mention nutrition in any course description. Paralleling this was the lack of nutritional questions in review books for medical licensure examinations. Generally, the questions judged to be nutritional were emphasized in the basic medical sciences (e.g., biochemistry), which related to the catalog descriptions. In some clinical specialty examinations, a small number of questions were related to nutrition, whereas in others (e.g., obstetrics or surgery) few or none of the questions concerned nutrition. Wen et al. concluded that students are motivated to learn only those aspects of nutrition that are emphasized in qualifying examinations.[73]

To illustrate the lack of formal nutrition instruction in medical schools, J. Coombs reported the results of an evaluation of nutrition teaching in New York City-area medical schools. Coombs concluded that senior medical students, although they had more nutritional knowledge than did first-year students, had less understanding of most basic nutrition concepts than graduate students. Major deficiencies were identified in the areas of applied and community nutrition and in the sociological and psychological aspects of nutrition.[74]

In a recent survey, the Nutrition Foundation found that, of approximately 80 medical schools studied, 23 reported significant required education in nutrition. Seventy-three of the 80 institutions offered elective nutrition courses.[67]

C. Cyborski surveyed the teaching of nutrition at 114 medical schools in the United States. Of the 102 schools responding, 19 offered a required course in nutrition; 72 schools offered electives in nutrition, and 94 offered nutrition as part of the content of other subject areas. Twenty-seven schools offered clinical nutrition clerkships, 81 offered research opportunities in nutrition, and 30 offered postgraduate or continuing education in the area of nutrition. Although the report allowed for only quantitative analysis, the author noted that about 75 per cent of the medical education institutions have demonstrated an increasing awareness of the long neglect of nutrition.[75]

E. Nelson, reporting on the results of a 1976 survey of 60 medical schools, found that only about 10 per cent of the schools appeared to give adequate training in nutrition.[76]

According to the results of a 1978 survey by the American Medical Association of 124 accredited medical schools in the United States, 25 per cent offered required nutrition courses, 70 per cent offered elective courses, 97 per cent incorporated nutrition teaching into other courses, and 37 per cent had clinical nutrition clerkships. Eighty-five per cent of the schools provided research opportunities for students, and 50 per cent offered postdoctoral nutrition training or medical education courses. Thus, there has been a recent improvement in the required nutrition courses, in postgraduate studies, research opportunities, and clerkships in nutrition.[77]

The problem of teaching nutrition to medical students raises the question of appropriate methods. Should nutrition be integrated into already existing courses or should it be made into a separate course? In 1968 a nutrition teaching program was developed by the faculty of the Nutrition Division of the Department of Community Medicine at the Mount Sinai School of Medicine of the City University of New York. One of the major issues at that time was whether the school would adopt a "block time" or "integrated curriculum" approach. A balance was struck that provided for the integration of biology with clinical medicine, the social sciences, and community medicine.[61] In this context, nutrition seems to have the unique characteristics that could link the basic and clinical sciences and could possibly act as a curricular model of a "bridging" discipline.

The development of an elective nutrition course at the Mount Sinai School of Medicine has proven to be a success. The course, entitled "Nutrition Problems: U.S.A.," encompasses problems of obesity, malnutrition, coronary heart disease, hypertension, and nutrition in drug rehabilitation.[78] The course consists of class lectures; student participation in grand rounds in which the physician and the student discuss nutrition principles, diagnosis, therapy, and preventive medicine; and case studies that permit the student to make home visits. The major contributing factors to the success of the program have been the presence of faculty conducting clinical and community research in nutrition, the presence of a division entitled "Nutrition" (thus making the existence of nutrition obvious), the fact that Mount Sinai is a relatively new medical school, and the presence of a chairman of the Department of Community Medicine who recognizes the clinical and community medical aspects of nutrition.[78] A number of other models for nutrition education in medical schools have been developed.[79-84]

The Nutrition Foundation has assumed a very active role in supporting and promoting the inclusion of nutrition education in the medical school curriculum. The foundation has assisted in the planning, implementation, and evaluation of particular programs and has participated in national meetings and seminars designed to further the cause of medical school nutrition education. Financial grants from the foundation have supported the career development of promising individuals who are interested in teaching nutrition. The foundation sponsored and published an example of a model curriculum, "Nutrition Education in the Medical School: A Curriculum Design," which offers units at three different levels.[85]

1. Science of nutrition, with problem-oriented clinical applications.
2. Sociology of nutrition, including community situations and family medicine.
3. Application of the science and sociology of medicine in the clinical scene.

Each unit includes behavioral and learning objectives, activities, and suggestions for evaluation.

The Nutrition Foundation also published an annotated bibliography, "Education in Nutrition for Physicians and Dentists," which summarized 60 journal articles, as well as conference proceedings and congressional hearings dealing with nutrition education in medicine.[86]

Continuing Education in Nutrition

Innovative physician education offerings in nutrition have been developed as part of the activities of the continuing education program for physicians on infant nutrition, in cooperation with Health Learning Systems. The latter organization provides expertise and help in the areas of medical communications. Since 1971, Health Learning Systems has used funding available from the pharmaceutical industry to support continuing education activities in subject areas of nutrition, hypertension, contraception, and ulcer management. The organization provides expertise in communications and education and acts as a third party to translate the knowledge and practice of medicine into skillful communication.[87]

In 1976 the idea for providing continuing education to physicians in the area of infant nutrition was conceived. As a result, a course was developed to extend over a two-year period. The first part consisted of a live, three-hour symposium that was telecast to a national physician audience in 23 major cities of the United States and Canada. The initial telecast was followed by 40-minute films, monographs with text and illustrations, and question-and-answer newsletters.

The overall purpose of the program was to identify sound infant nutrition principles and to resolve, to the degree possible, those controversies in nutrition that confront the practicing pediatrician.

A total of 5,053 physicians returned the self-administered, preassessment test, which they perceived to be difficult. The physicians recognized their poor test performance; the mean pretest score was 67 per cent. Follow-up evaluation of the program consisted of a participant critique; the results indicated that the participating physicians were generally pleased with the program and rated it highly.[87]

Summary: Nutrition Education of the Medical Student

There are various patterns and approaches to the successful inclusion of nutrition education in the medical school curriculum. Nutrition may be included in the offerings of a variety of different departments, ranging from medicine, pediatrics, surgery, preventive medicine, community health, biochemistry, physiology, or dietetics.

Experiences and approaches to nutrition education are also varied. Some curricula emphasize academic and lecture preparation, whereas others include laboratory research, clinical activities, or community experience. The most successful approaches provide a forum for the incorporation of nutritional concepts into the practical application of medical and health care.

Although it is difficult for medical schools to develop a broad model that includes courses in nutrition science, clinical nutrition, and the sociology of nutrition, schools can start to integrate nutrition into existing programs and courses. This approach can provide basic nutrition knowledge as part of existing courses. Another approach has been to introduce the medical students to nutrition through seminars organized by the dietary departments.

There are many problems in setting up an adequate nutrition program for training medical students to respond to the nutritional needs of their clients. Convincing curriculum committees to introduce nutrition courses is one of the major initial hurdles. Aside from this, another major problem involves the development of a core faculty able to teach basic, clinical, and community nutrition and to conduct research in these areas.

J. Vitale and R. Hodges, summarizing information on the successful implementation of nutrition education in medical schools, suggested that two minimal steps should be followed.[88]

1. Senior faculty should be designated to be responsible for the nutrition program.
2. Curricular time should be allotted for nutrition education.

The President's Biomedical Research Panel Report suggested that, in view of the current neglect of nutrition at most medical schools, the greatest immediate need is to develop new programs in schools providing close interactions of such subjects as biochemistry, analytical chemistry, genetics, and physiology. In such an environment it is possible to develop new techniques and research essential for a strong and nutrition component of medical education.[89]

However, medical schools must be provided an incentive for setting up a nutrition program. Practically speaking, an external financial stimulus is probably required. Suggested stimuli include the provision of independently funded nutrition chairs for designated individuals or institutions, which would allow independent salary and research support for a given time period. Funds are also needed for the initial education of nutrition faculty. This support might come from annual postdoctoral fellowships specifically for nutrition, nutrition training grants, and postgraduate training grants for physicians. The establishment of broad-based nutrition centers emphasizing nutrition research and training would also stimulate the development of nutrition education in medical schools.

CONCLUSION

What Should We Expect from Nutrition Education?[90-92]

Nutrition education cannot be hailed as the only link between individuals and an improved diet. Nutrition education is only one strategy that nutritionists might use to improve the nutrient intake of individuals. Consumers must have available to them a supply of food from which they can select their diets, but education should aid people in making sound and informed choices about their food intake. Such education should enable people to recognize that different eating patterns can result in adequate nutrition, and it should aid people in recognizing that there is no one right diet — there are many "gray" areas or uncertainties as to what constitutes an optimum diet and what foods can safely be eaten. Nutrition education should also give people a perspective in planning for improved nutritional status of the community and of those who are economically unable to purchase adequate nutrition. In addition, such education should give people a perspective on planning for future food problems, including those related to world food problems, the environment, ecology, and the energy/resource crisis.

Where Do We Go From Here?

Many recommendations have been made to improve nutrition education efforts. A summary of these recommendations appears in Table 14-11. A study of these guidelines reveals that they are as relevant today as they were when they were first developed. We have yet to agree that nutrition education is the right of all consumers. National policy statements on nutrition education are needed. These policies should emphasize the need for the coordination of all nutrition education activities and resources.

A basic priority of a national policy dealing with education and nutrition should stress "universal nutrition literacy." Such literacy should help individuals to apply nutrition knowledge to their food choices to promote good health; the changing food supply should be a consideration in this education. Nutrition education should be integrated into the curricula of preschool, primary, and secondary school levels to facilitate the development of sound nutrition practices early in life.[91]

A number of measures to enable the implementation of these recommendations are clearly needed. Some of the primary strategies for action include the following:[92]

1. Third-party reimbursement plans of public and private health insurers should specifically include nutrition education and counseling as mandatory and as reimbursable services in health care programs.

2. Nutrition education and counseling should be included in all services provided in either public or private settings.

3. Public health agencies at the federal, state, and local level should receive financial support to expand and strengthen nutrition education components of health care delivery systems.

Table 14-11
Recommendations for Improving Nutrition Education Address the Following Issues[90]

1. Need for the fullest participation of consumers in planning and implementation of nutrition education programs.
2. Greater stress on the problems of excessive or unbalanced consumption associated with chronic disease and less on dietary inadequacies that are increasingly rare in our population.
3. Attention to motivation of the public as well as providing factual information.
4. Reporting and evaluating requirements for all nutrition education programs for which federal funds are authorized.
5. More flexibility and innovativeness in approaches to nutrition education, both at the community and national levels.
6. Improved coordination and cooperation among nutrition education programs, federal, voluntary, or privately sponsored.
7. Positioning of nutrition information and education programs in accessible and identifiable places in communities to improve public access (e.g., the point of purchase, the home television screen, the daily or Sunday newspaper).
8. Emphasis on "outreach," especially for groups hard to reach, such as the poor, the elderly, the working wife and mother, single adults, and teenagers.
9. Pretesting and field testing of all communication and information materials to assure high levels of comprehensibility, acceptability, and practical usefulness.
10. Development of Centers of Excellence at leading universities to conduct research and demonstration activities vital to improvement of national efforts in nutrition education.
11. Support for the education and training of food and consumer leaders, health professionals, teachers, and others pivotal in counseling the public about food, diet, and health.
12. Widespread and creative use of mass media, with special emphasis on television.
13. Consumer and market research to identify high-priority nutrition issues and opportunities for motivating public use of federal nutrition education programs.
14. Extending nutrition education to food and health writers, food marketers, radio and television commentators, and others in direct contact with large segments of the public.
15. Development of food selection guidance material appropriate for the diversity of food life-styles now apparent in our population (e.g., the "snacker," the one- or two-meal eater, the dieter, the vegetarian).
16. Use of campaign approaches to reach specific groups or population segments known to be in need of diet improvement.

Source: L. Light. Nutrition education: policies and programs. *Nutr. Program News,* January–April 1978, pp. 1–12.

4. The efforts of all health care delivery systems should be organized and coordinated so that those individuals who are particularly vulnerable to nutritional problems (such as pregnant and lactating mothers, infants, children, and the elderly) can be reached with appropriate nutrition education.

5. Nutritional surveillance should be the foundation on which nutrition education efforts are developed, and ongoing monitoring should constantly evaluate nutrition education efforts.

6. Demonstration projects should be supported to determine costs and other important factors essential to nutrition education effectiveness.

Nutrition education cannot succeed in isolation. Knowledge alone, or passive transfer of information, is not sufficient to motivate changes in life-style or in eating habits. To confirm this we have only to look at the numerous nutritionists whose diets conflict with their knowledge of sound nutrition or at the many health professionals who realize the hazards of smoking and continue to smoke. Thus, to be successful, information transfer must be coupled with other strategies designed to improve food habits. One possibility is for nutrition educators to work through social organizations. Group acceptance and awareness of the need to improve food habits may often reinforce individual decisions to change.

Nutrition education should be coupled with broad incentives designed to motivate improved nutrition. As was pointed out in Chapter 12, many of the influences on the North American food system are beyond the control of the consumer. Thus, strategies designed to modify some of these factors that negatively impact on eating patterns in the United States should be coupled with nutrition education. Subsidies, grants, price policies, and other incentives designed to reverse the declining consumption of fresh fruit, vegetables, and whole grain as well as to reverse the rising consumption of high-fat, high-sugar, high-salt, and highly processed foods should be considered. It is clear that we cannot expect nutrition education to "do it all." A total strategy supported by public, private, and industrial efforts is the only practical or realistic approach.

REFERENCES

1. Richmond, F. W. The role of the federal government in nutrition education. *J. Nutr. Educ.* 9 (1977): 150.
2. U.S. Senate Select Committee on Nutrition and Human Needs. *Overview: The Federal Programs.* Washington, D.C.: Government Printing Office, December 6, 1972, p. 140.
3. U.S. Congress. Food and Agriculture Act of 1977, PL-95-133. September 1977.
4. Congressional Research Service. *The Role of the Federal Government in Nutrition Education.* Washington, D.C.: Government Printing Office, March 1977.
5. Richmond, F. In Congressional Research Service, *The Role of the Federal Government in Nutrition Education.* Washington, D.C.: Government Printing Office, March 1977.
6. White House Conference on Food, Nutrition, and Health. Washington, D.C., 1969.
7. White House Conference on the Aging. *Section Recommendations on Nutrition.* Washington, D.C.: Government Printing Office, 1971.
8. U.S. Senate Select Committee on Nutrition and Human Needs, Hearings on Nutrition Education. *Overview: Consultants' Recommendations, Part 1.* Washington, D.C.: Government Printing Office, 1973.
9. Comptroller General, Report to the Congress. *Informing the Public about Nutrition: Federal Agencies Should Do Better.* Washington, D.C.: Government Printing Office, March 22, 1978.
10. U.S. House of Representatives, Subcommittee on Domestic Marketing,

Consumer Relations, and Nutrition. Subcommittee memo on improvements in the federal role since publication of the 1976 report and subcommittee hearings, unpublished. Washington, D.C., February 1979.

11. Richmond, F. In U.S. House of Representatives, *The National Consumer Nutrition Information Act.* Washington, D.C.: Government Printing Office, March 1978.

12. American Public Health Association. Health education and public health. *The Nation's Health*, September 1977, p. 12.

13. John E. Fogarty International Center for Advanced Study in the Health Sciences et al. *Preventive Medicine, U.S.A.* New York: Prodist, 1976.

14. Jacobsen, M. Stamp out food faddism. *Nutr. Action* 2 (1975): 1.

15. Grotta-Kurska, D. Before you say baloney . . . here's what you should know about vegetarianism. *Today's Health* 52 (1974): 18–21.

16. Frankle, R. T., and F. K. Heussenstamm. Food zealotry and youth. *Am. J. Publ. Health* 64 (1974): 11–18.

17. Hardinge, M. G., and H. Crooks. Nonflesh dietaries. III. Adequate and inadequate. *J. Am. Diet. Assoc.* 45 (1964): 537.

18. Hegsted, D. M., M. F. Trulson, H. S. White, P. L. White, E. Vinas, E. Alvistur, C. Diaz, J. Vasquez, A. Loo, A. Roca, C. Collazos, and A. Ruiz. Lysine and methionine supplementation of all-vegetable diets for human adults. *J. Nutr.* 56 (1955): 555

19. Hardinge, M. G., and F. J. Stare. Nutritional studies of vegetarians. I. Nutritional, physical, and laboratory studies. *J. Clin. Nutr.* 22 (1954): 73.

20. West, R. O., and O. B. Hayes. Diet and serum cholesterol levels: A comparison between vegetarians and nonvegetarians in a Seventh-Day Adventist group. *Am. J. Clin. Nutr.* 21 (1968): 853.

21. Robson, J. R. K., J. E. Konlande, F. A. Larkin, P. H. O'Conner, and H. -Y. Liu. Zen macrobiotic dietary problems in infancy. *Pediatrics* 53 (1974): 326.

22. Brown, P. T., and J. G. Bergan. The dietary status of "new" vegetarians. *J. Am. Diet. Assoc.* 67 (1975): 455.

23. Trahms, C. M. Dietary patterns of vegan, vegetarian, and nonvegetarian preschool children. Abstract presented at Society for Nutrition Education Annual Meeting, San Diego, 1974.

24. Nagy, M. J. Teenage vegan. *J.A.M.A.* 211 (1970): 306.

25. Abehsera, M. *Zen Macrobiotic Cooking: Book of Oriental and Traditional Recipes.* New York: University Books, 1968, p. 4.

26. Council on Foods and Nutrition. Zen macrobiotic diets. *J.A.M.A.* 218 (1971): 397.

27. Erhard, D. The new vegetarians. I. Vegetarianism and its medical consequences. *Nutr. Today* 8 (1973): 4–12.

28. Wolff, R. J. Who eats for health? *Am. J. Clin. Nutr.* 2 (1975): 116.

29. Anderson, M. A., and B. R. Standal. Nutritional knowledge of health food users in Oahu, Hawaii. *J. Am. Diet. Assoc.* 67 (1975): 116.

30. Erhard, D. Nutrition education for the "now" generation. *J. Nutr. Educ.* 2 (1971): 135.

31. Henderson, L. M. Programs to combat nutritional quackery. *J. Am. Diet. Assoc.* 64 (1974): 372.

32. Cornacchia, H. J. *Consumer Health.* St. Louis, Mo.: C. V. Mosby, 1976, pp. 216–251.

33. Herbert, V. The health hustlers, in L. Hofmann, ed., *The Great American Nutrition Hassle.* Palo Alto, Calif.: Mayfield Publishing, 1978, pp. 303–319.

34. Evans, T. E. Madison Avenue vs. the medical establishment. *Nutr. Today* 12 (1977): 41.

35. Choate, R. Testimony before the Federal Trade Commission. Washington, D.C., 1976.

36. O'Bryan, T. Testimony before the Federal Trade Commission. Washington, D.C., November 1976.

37. Feshbach, N. D., T. S. Jordon, and A. S. Dillman. A report on a developmental study on the use of graphics in conveying nutritional information, in U.S. Senate Select Committee on Nutrition and Human Needs, *Edible T.V.: Your Child and Food Commercials.* Washington, D.C.: Government Printing Office, September 1977.

38. Axelson, J. M., and D. S. Del Campo. Improving teenagers' nutrition knowledge through the mass media. *J. Nutr. Educ.* 10 (1978): 30.

39. Gussow, J. Is anyone fat in videoland? *CNI Week. Rep.* 8 (5 January 1978): 4-5.

40. Guthrie, H. A. Is education not enough? *J. Nutr. Educ.* 10 (1978): 57-58.

41. U.S. Department of Health, Education, and Welfare, National High Blood Pressure Education Program. *The 120/80 Notebook for Consumer Education on High Blood Pressure*, Publ. No. (NIH) 75-745. Washington, D.C.: Government Printing Office.

42. American Public Health Association. Resolutions and position papers: Education for health in the school community setting. *Am. J. Publ. Health* 65 (1975): 201.

43. Whitehead, F. E. *Nutrition Education Research Project: Report of Feasibility Study.* Iowa City: University of Iowa, October 20, 1970.

44. Whitehead, F. E. Research in nutrition education. *J. Am. Diet. Assoc.* 23 (1947): 310.

45. U.S. Senate Select Committee on Nutrition and Human Needs, Panel on Nutrition and Government. *Report of the National Nutrition Policy Hearings.* Washington, D.C.: Government Printing Office, June 21, 1974.

46. Mayer, J. Testimony before U.S. Senate Select Committee on Nutrition and Human Needs. Washington, D.C., 1977.

47. National School Lunch Act and Child Nutrition Act, P. L. 95-166, Part 227. Nutrition Education and Training Program, 1977.

48. Williams, T. F. Health education in the primary care setting, in *Preventive Medicine, U.S.A.* New York: Prodist, 1976, Appendix E.

49. Podell, R. N. Physician's guide to compliance in hypertension, in *Preventive Medicine, U.S.A., op. cit.*, Appendix V.

50. Sackett, D. L., chairman. *A Workshop Symposium: Compliance with Therapeutic Regimens.* Hamilton, Ont.: McMaster University Medical Center, May 1974, p. 3.

51. Marsh, W. W., and L. V. Perlman. Understanding congestive heart failure and self-administration of digoxin, In A. I. Wertheimer and M. C. Smith, eds., *Pharmacy Practice: Social and Behavioral Aspects.* Baltimore, Md.: University Park Press, 1974, pp. 202-203.

52. Zifferblatt, S. M., and C. S. Wilber. Dietary counseling: Some expectations and guidelines. *J. Am. Diet. Assoc.* 70 (1977): 591.

53. Mahoney, M. J., and A. W. Caggiula. Applying behavioral methods to nutritional counseling. *J. Am. Diet. Assoc.* 72 (1978): 372.

54. Brownell, K. D. Couples training and spouse cooperativeness in the behavioral treatment of obesity. Unpublished Ph.D. thesis. New Brunswick. N.J.: Rutgers University, 1977.

55. Witschi, J., M. Singer, M. Wu-Lee, and F. Stare. Family cooperation and effectiveness in a cholesterol-lowering diet. *J. Am. Diet. Assoc.* 72 (1978): 384.

56. Gifft, H., M. Washbon, and G. Harrison. *Nutrition, Behavior, and Change.* Englewood Cliffs, N.J.: Prentice-Hall, 1972.

57. Vickstrom, J. A., and H. M. Fox. Nutritional knowledge and attitudes of registered nurses. *J. Am. Diet. Assoc.* 68 (1976): 453.

58. Baric, L. Recognition of the "at-risk" role — A means to influence health behavior. *Int. J. Health Educ.* 12 (1969): 453.

59. Baric, L. Health education practice in the years ahead . . . could physicians be more effective in health education? *Int. J. Health Educ.* 13 (1970): 43.

60. Christakis, G., R. Frankle, R. Brown, et al. Nutrition teaching at the Mount Sinai School of Medicine: A three-year experience. *Am. J. Clin. Nutr.* 25 (1972): 997.

61. Frankle, R. T. Nutrition education in the medical school curriculum: An analysis of planning, a description of practices, and a proposal for action. Unpublished Ph.D. thesis. New York: Columbia University, Teachers College, 1975.

62. Nutritional Sciences Training Committee, National Institute of General Medical Sciences, N. I. H. Status of research in nutritional sciences. *Am. J. Clin. Nutr.* 23 (1970): 196.

63. Yates, B. E., S. Jackson, and I. Alfredo Lopez. Prevalence of malnutrition in a large hospital. *Fed. Proc.* 36 (1977): 1093 (abst. 4343).

64. Bistrian, B. R., G. L. Blackburn, J. Vitale, et al. Prevalence of malnutrition in general medical patients. *J.A.M.A.* 235 (1976): 1567.

65. Merritt, R. J., and R. M. Suskind. Nutritional survey of hospitalized pediatric patients. *Am. J. Clin. Nutr.* 32 (1979): 1320.

66. Council on Foods and Nutrition. Nutrition teaching in medical schools. *J.A.M.A.* 183 (1963): 955–957.

67. Darby, W. J. The renaissance of nutrition education. *Nutr. Rev.* 35 (1977): 33.

68. Conference on Guidelines for Nutrition Education Programs, P. L. White, L. K. Mahan, and M. E. Moore, eds. New York: The Nutrition Foundation, 1972.

69. Conference on Guidelines for Nutrition Education Programs. Williamsburg, Va., June 25–27, 1972.

70. American Institute of Nutrition and American Society for Clinical Nutrition. *Teaching Nutrition in Medical Schools.* Anaheim, Calif. April 12, 1976.

71. *Revitalization, Re-evaluation, Redirection.* Ninth Annual Meeting of the Society for Nutrition Education. Kansas City, Mo., July 11–14, 1976.

72. Cyborski, C. *Summary of Nutrition Curricula in Medical Education Survey.* Chicago: American Medical Association, Department of Foods and Nutrition, 1976.

73. Wen, C. P., H. D. Weerasinghe, and J. T. Dwyer. Nutrition education in U.S. medical schools. *J. Am. Diet. Assoc.* 63 (1973): 408.

74. Coombs, J. B. *The Role of Nutrition Education in Medical Schools. I. Review of Curriculum.* New York: Cornell University Medical School, Fall 1970.

75. Cyborski, C. Nutrition content in medical curricula. *J. Nutr. Educ.* 9 (1977): 17.

76. Nelson, E. S. Nutrition instruction in medical schools. *J.A.M.A.* 236 (1976): 2534.

77. Medical schools giving more nutrition training. *Am. Med. News* (13 October 1978): 14.

78. Frankle, R. T., E. R. Williams, and G. Christakis. Nutrition education in the medical school: Experience with an elective course for first-year medical students. *Am. J. Clin. Nutr.* 25 (1972): 709.

79. Graham, R., and J. Royer, eds. *A Handbook for Change Recommendations*

of the Joint Commission on Medical Education. Philadelphia: William F.
Fell, 1973.

80. Agency for International Development. *Report of Conference on Nutrition in Schools of Medicine and Schools of Public Health in Latin America.* Washington, D.C., September 19–22, 1966.

81. Baumslag, N., K. Gatins, D. Watson, and A. Englund. Interdisciplinary nutrition education. *J. Med. Educ.* 51 (1976): 64.

82. Young, E. A., and E. Weser. Integration of nutrition in medical education. *J. Nutr. Educ.* 7 (1975): 112.

83. Flynn, M., D. Keithly, and J. Colwill. Nutrition in the education of the family physician. *J. Am. Diet. Assoc.* 65 (1974): 269.

84. Cooperman, J. M. Nutrition education in the medical school. *Urban Health* 6 (1977): 31.

85. Frankle, R. T. *Nutrition Education in the Medical School: A Curriculum Design.* Washington, D.C.: The Nutrition Foundation, 1976.

86. *Education in Nutrition for Physicians and Dentists. An Annotated Bibliography.* Washington, D.C.: The Nutrition Foundation, 1976.

87. Filer, L. J., and E. F. Calesa. Multimedia education about infant nutrition for physicians. *J. Am. Diet. Assoc.* 72 (1978): 404.

88. Vitale, J. J., and R. E. Hodges. Symposium on teaching nutrition in medical schools. *Am. J. Clin. Nutr.* 30 (1977): 791.

89. Conclusion of the *Nutrition Cluster Report of the President's Biomedical Research Panel. Nutr. Today* 12 (1977): 14–17.

90. Light, L. Nutrition education: Policies and programs. *Nutr. Program News* (January–April 1978): 1–12.

91. Conference on Education in Nutrition. *Looking Forward from the Past.* New York: Columbia University, Teachers College, February 26–27, 1974.

92. American Dietetic Association. Position paper on the scope and thrust of nutrition education. *J. Am. Diet. Assoc.* 72 (1978): 302.

section four
END OF SECTION ACTIVITIES

1. Consider your own diet and the factors that influence it. Why do you eat the way you do? Is your diet as nutritious as it should be? Is it in line with the concept of nutrition and health promotion? Should it be changed? How difficult would it be for you to change? Would nutrition education help you to change? What techniques might be effective in helping you to improve your eating habits?

2. In its efforts to combat the deceptive advertising aimed at children, the FTC has been referred to as the "nation's Nanny." Should the FTC take it upon itself to monitor children's advertising? If not, should another group? Debate the pros and cons of the FTC proposal. Is this proposal likely to be accepted in total? Do certain parts of the proposal have a better chance of being accepted? Can you propose other means to limit the counternutritional messages that are often conveyed through mass media advertising?

3. Watch 1 to 2 hours of children's television on a Saturday morning. Keep a record of the commercials shown during this period.

What products are advertised?

What are the products notably not advertised?

To whom are the advertisements directed?

What techniques are used to promote the products?

Are the commercials effective in conveying their messages?

What are the overwhelming messages conveyed by food advertisements?

What moods, thoughts, or desires are conveyed to you by the commercials for food?

What types of nutrition advertisements might be effective in combating counternutritional messages of advertising?

Create an advertisement to promote a nutritious food. What types of images, techniques, and messages have you used?

Could your advertisement counteract any of the non-nutritional messages you viewed?

What other techniques might be effective in combating counternutritional television advertising?

4. In general, would you consider yourself a staunch supporter or a critic of the food industy? Support your position. Engage in a debate with those who disagree with you. Consider both the contributions and the harm resulting from food industry activities.

5. Many forces that are largely beyond the control of the consumer determine the American food supply. Thus, some have suggested that the American consumer really does not have freedom of choice in selecting a nutritious diet. How much freedom do you have in selecting your diet? How are your food choices restricted? Many people, because of health or economic reasons, may be much more limited in their food choices. Give an example of such an individual or a population group. Should the American public have more freedom in determining their food habits and diet? How might more freedom be achieved?

6. The food industry has been severely criticized for much of its nutrition education efforts. For example, read The (nutrition education) gospel according to NDC, by Eric Kilburn, *Nutr. Action,* September 1978, pp. 3-7, about the nutrition education endeavors of the National Dairy Council. Do you agree or disagree? How reliable is nutrition education material developed by the food industry? How biased is it? Should such material be used in nutrition education of the public, or in the schools?

7. In the past, nutrition education efforts have often failed to result in sustained changes in food habits. Why do you think this is so? Does nutrition education have a chance as a way to improve nutrition and food habits? How can the effectiveness of nutrition education be improved?

8. Collect educational resource materials used by schoolteachers involved in nutrition education. Assess the materials in terms of the following:

What is the source of the materials?

Is the information valid and reliable? Is it complete?

Is the material presented in such a way as to catch and hold a student's interest?

Does the material attempt to promote a given industry interest?

Suggest ways to improve materials.

Are the teachers who use the material pleased with it? Do their students enjoy learning about nutrition from the materials?

Develop your own resource that might be used by schoolteachers in nutrition education. Develop objectives for the use of the material. How might the material be evaluated?

Nutritional programs and policies

Section Objective

The general objective of this section is to discuss nutrition programs and the policies and institutions that influence them and to review ways in which nutrition advocates can become effectively involved in the policy-making and program development process.

Section Overview

A brief consideration of current federal nutrition efforts supports the idea that the United States does not lack nutrition programs or a nutrition policy. What seems clear, however, is that there is a lack of agreed upon policy direction and of program coordination. If we are to influence the formation of food and nutrition policy, we must understand the mechanics of the legislative and regulatory processes. We must be familiar with the agencies involved in nutrition activities and must understand the operation of, and be able to evaluate, the effectiveness of current food and nutrition programs. These considerations lead logically into an assessment of the current state of national nutrition policy in the United States. Do we need a unified national nutrition policy? Is it realistic to expect such a policy? Is it wise to organize efforts and work to this end? This section considers these issues.

15

The legislative and regulatory processes

Reader Objectives

After completing this chapter, the reader should be able to
1. Outline the federal policy-making process.
2. Describe the legislative process and the regulatory process.
3. State how nutrition advocates should become involved in the policy-making process at the federal, state, and local levels.

The time is now to capitalize on the interest in nutrition and develop nutrition education legislation. . . . There are many legislators and others who need to know what nutrition education is before legislation can be passed. . . . It is not possible to legislate the motivation of the individual nor to ensure that the educational process takes place. It is possible to develop lines of communication to provide information that is adequate and motivational. It is also possible to identify those areas such as the school, community, health care delivery systems, mass media, and food supply sources which have regulatory and informational resources through which nutrition education is either established as an entity or incorporated into the social programs developed for target areas.

— H. D. Ullrich

INTRODUCTION

Convincing the public to accept the application of the nutrition/preventive health care relationship requires a conviction by national leaders of the validity, universal applicability, practicality, and effectiveness of improving nutritional status in the United States.

Stimulating such conviction among top political decision makers should be the responsibility of the academic, health, industrially trained, and governmental professional nutrition leaders. This can be accomplished in a variety of ways, including the following:

1. Presenting scientifically founded diet-health relationships at public meetings, hearings, and the like to legislators and government executives.

2. Educating the public to appreciate the importance of positive nutritional habits on health status through mass media and nutrition education programs.

3. Joining with consumer and other advocacy groups to lobby for the passage of nutrition legislation by Congress.

4. Enlisting the support of other health professionals and persuading them to use their influence on behalf of the promotion of nutrition.

These strategies imply that nutritionists must become key players in the entire nutrition planning and policy-making process. One of the important channels to this end involves active participation in the legislative and regulatory processes.

Thus, it is important to have some knowledge of policy development to appreciate the appropriate actions that might be taken to influence the legislative and the regulatory processes.

FEDERAL POLICY PROCESS

The government policy-making process can be thought of as a circular process in which the relationships and interactions between the executive, judicial, and legislative branches of the government are related to various interest groups. These interest groups exert influence and affect governmental decision and policy making as they identify problems, make recommendations, and participate in the election process.

All three government branches, the Congress, the president, and the courts make decisions that determine national policy. The Congress is involved in decision making primarily through its actions on specific programs as it legislates, makes financial appropriations, or fails to act on particular issues. These actions then provide general direction for executive agencies that are responsible for program development, implementation, and enforcement of regulations.

Interest groups are involved in every aspect of the total process: they affect decision making and are in turn affected by program decisions. The judicial branch typically becomes involved only in matters of disagreement or dispute among other participants. In recent years the role of the judiciary branch has significantly increased to the point at which the courts now make decisions in cases in which legislation is ambiguous and confusing. This process is illustrated in Figure 15-1.[2]

Frequently there is conflict at different points in the process. The conflict may be between the various branches, between interest groups and the legislative or executive branch, or within a given branch. It is particularly important that the legislative process be better understood to fully appreciate the process of program and policy development.

LEGISLATIVE PROCESS

Congress and the executive branch are the focal points for the legislative process. Nutrition-related legislation may originate in the Congress, the executive branch, or through the relevant federal agency. Often the staff of a legislator draws up the initial proposal for legislation. Congress initially receives suggestions, proposals, and input from various interest groups and individuals; from other government agencies, such as the USDA and the USDHEW; from testimony submitted at congressional hearings; from papers and reports; and from a variety of other similar sources.

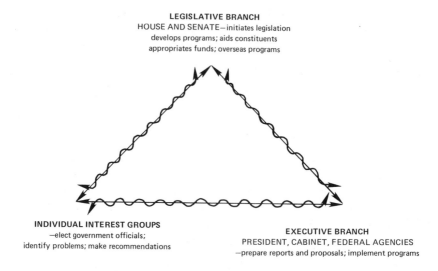

LEGISLATIVE BRANCH
HOUSE AND SENATE—initiates legislation
develops programs; aids constituents
appropriates funds; overseas programs

INDIVIDUAL INTEREST GROUPS
—elect government officials;
identify problems; make recommendations

EXECUTIVE BRANCH
PRESIDENT, CABINET, FEDERAL AGENCIES
—prepare reports and proposals; implement programs

JUDICIAL ARBITRATION AS NECESSARY

Figure 15-1. Components of the federal policy-making machinery.

The proposed bill or resolution is introduced to either the House or the Senate by a representative or a senator and is then given a number. Laws are numbered according to the number of the Congress in which they are passed, and according to order. For example, P.L. 96-231 means Public Law 231, 96th Congress. The proposed bill is then passed on to the committee that is engaged in the particular issues involved, such as the House and Senate Agriculture committees. Individual committees review, consider, and react to initial proposals and eventually decide upon specific action to be taken for a given bill. These committees then interact with various interest groups, other agencies, or individuals in the development of legislation. The importance of congressional committees is significant in that ". . . the power to frame the question is often the power to determine the answer."[3] Committees are frequently the places where bills originate and where bills may be ratified. House and Senate Committees are listed in Table 15-1.[4]

Congressional strength and influence in the development of policy depend upon an ability to gain a unified bloc to back a given proposal. The nutrition bloc is generally not strong in Congress; so that nutrition legislation usually stands a chance of being passed only if nutrition advocates are able to gain the support and consensus of other influential groups. Frequently nutrition legislation is "tacked on" to a given agricultural bill. As an example, the Food and Agriculture Act of 1977 focused on numerous agricultural issues, but also included changes in food stamp legislation, mandates for the reorganization of parts of USDA dealing with food and nutrition, and nutrition research and education.[5]

If the committee believes it necessary, public hearings are conducted in subcommittee on proposed legislation. Testimony is evaluated, generally in executive session, and the recommendations are made to accept

Table 15–1

Congressional Committees of Interest to Nutritionists (standing committees)

House of Representatives	Senate

Agriculture
  Subcommittee: Domestic Marketing,
               Consumer Relations,
               and Nutrition
	Agriculture, Nutrition, and Forestry
	  Subcommittee: Nutrition

Appropriations
  Subcommittee: Labor, Health, Educa-
             tion, and Welfare
	Appropriations
	  Subcommittee: Labor, Health, Educa-
	             tion, and Welfare

Banking, Finance, and Urban Affairs
  Subcommittee: Consumer Affairs
	Commerce, Science, and Transportation
	  Subcommittee: Consumer Affairs

Education and Labor
  Subcommittee: Compensation, Health,
             and Safety Select Ed-
             ucation
	Finance
	  Subcommittee: Health

Interior and Insular Affairs
  Subcommittee: Indian Affairs and Pub-
             lic Lands
	Human Resources
	  Subcommittees: Aging
	                 Children and Human
	                    Development
	                 Health and Scientific
	                    Research

Interstate and Foreign Commerce
  Subcommittee: Health and the Environ-
             ment
	Veterans' Affairs
	  Subcommittee: Health and Readjust-
	             ment

Ways and Means Subcommittee: Health	

the proposed bill as it exists, to modify the bill, to reject the bill, or to table it. The subcommittee then gives its report to the standing committee to review and act upon. The standing committee may accept or reject the report of the subcommittee.

If the bill is to go forward, the bill is assigned a calendar number that indicates the order in which it will be reported to the full House or Senate. Standing committees are usually called in alphabetical order — each committee then calls up any bill it reported on that is pending on the calendar. After the House debates a bill, it votes on its passage.

The Senate is then given a copy of the bill in the form in which it passed the House. The bill is again referred to the appropriate committee where it is considered and reported on. The procedures are similar in the House and in the Senate, but specific rules vary.

After the bill, with any amendments, has been passed by the Senate, it is returned to the House, with a request that it be accepted. If it is accepted, the bill is then ready to be enrolled for presentation to the president.

Similar bills are often presented in both the House and the Senate. When this happens, both bills are sent to a conference committee where the two bills are developed into one, which then must be passed by the House and Senate. After the House and Senate both pass the bill, it goes to the president, who may sign the bill, veto it, or take no action. In the latter case, the bill becomes law after ten days if the Congress is still in session. If Congress is not in session, the president's failure to take action results in a veto, called a pocket veto.

After the bill becomes law, it is referred to an appropriate federal agency that will be responsible for its enforcement. The agency is required to write regulations for operationalizing the congressional mandate. This process is illustrated and described in Figure 15-2, in which an

Figure 15-2. How a bill becomes a law. Courtesy of American School Foodservice Association. Copyright by School Foodservice Journal, January 1973.

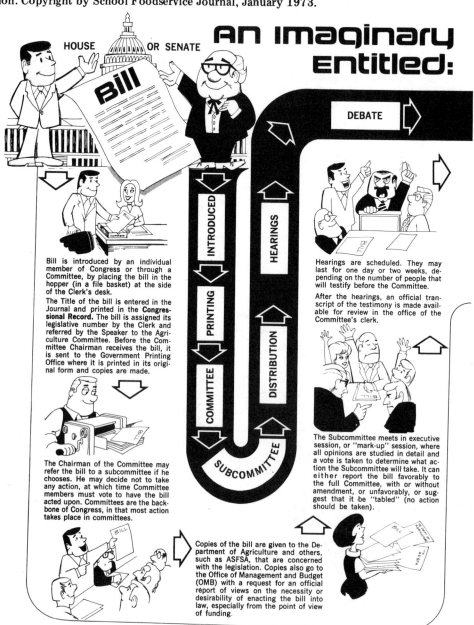

AN IMAGINARY Entitled:

HOUSE OR SENATE

Bill

DEBATE

INTRODUCED

HEARINGS

PRINTING

COMMITTEE

DISTRIBUTION

SUBCOMMITTEE

Bill is introduced by an individual member of Congress or through a Committee, by placing the bill in the hopper (in a file basket) at the side of the Clerk's desk.

The Title of the bill is entered in the Journal and printed in the **Congressional Record.** The bill is assigned its legislative number by the Clerk and referred by the Speaker to the Agriculture Committee. Before the Committee Chairman receives the bill, it is sent to the Government Printing Office where it is printed in its original form and copies are made.

The Chairman of the Committee may refer the bill to a subcommittee if he chooses. He may decide not to take any action, at which time Committee members must vote to have the bill acted upon. Committees are the backbone of Congress, in that most action takes place in committees.

Hearings are scheduled. They may last for one day or two weeks, depending on the number of people that will testify before the Committee.

After the hearings, an official transcript of the testimony is made available for review in the office of the Committee's clerk.

The Subcommittee meets in executive session, or "mark-up" session, where all opinions are studied in detail and a vote is taken to determine what action the Subcommittee will take. It can either report the bill favorably to the full Committee, with or without amendment, or unfavorably, or suggest that it be "tabled" (no action should be taken).

Copies of the bill are given to the Department of Agriculture and others, such as ASFSA, that are concerned with the legislation. Copies also go to the Office of Management and Budget (OMB) with a request for an official report of views on the necessity or desirability of enacting the bill into law, especially from the point of view of funding.

imaginary bill is traced through Congress, passed, enacted into law, and then implemented as a child feeding program.

The law usually includes the authorization needed to obtain money for accomplishing its mandate. However, the Congress must appropriate funds after the bill's passage. Because of congressional budgetary constraints, the authorized amount may not be fully appropriated. Figure 15–3 illustrates the budgetary process.[6]

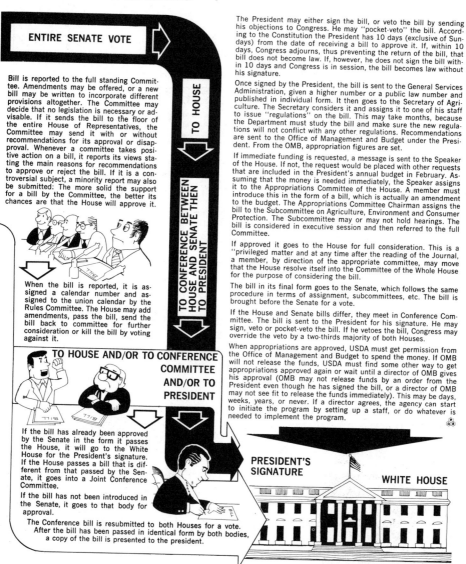

Bill, numbered - HR 0000

A BILL TO INSURE EVERY CHILD A FREE BREAKFAST FUNDED THROUGH SUPPLEMENTAL APPROPRIATIONS.

ENTIRE SENATE VOTE

Bill is reported to the full standing Committee. Amendments may be offered, or a new bill may be written to incorporate different provisions altogether. The Committee may decide that no legislation is necessary or advisable. If it sends the bill to the floor of the entire House of Representatives, the Committee may send it with or without recommendations for its approval or disapproval. Whenever a committee takes positive action on a bill, it reports its views stating the main reasons for recommendations to approve or reject the bill. If it is a controversial subject, a minority report may also be submitted: The more solid the support for a bill by the Committee, the better its chances are that the House will approve it.

When the bill is reported, it is assigned a calendar number and assigned to the union calendar by the Rules Committee. The House may add amendments, pass the bill, send the bill back to committee for further consideration or kill the bill by voting against it.

TO HOUSE

TO CONFERENCE BETWEEN HOUSE AND SENATE THEN TO PRESIDENT

TO HOUSE AND/OR TO CONFERENCE COMMITTEE AND/OR TO PRESIDENT

If the bill has already been approved by the Senate in the form it passes the House, it will go to the White House for the President's signature. If the House passes a bill that is different from that passed by the Senate, it goes into a Joint Conference Committee.

If the bill has not been introduced in the Senate, it goes to that body for approval.

The Conference bill is resubmitted to both Houses for a vote. After the bill has been passed in identical form by both bodies, a copy of the bill is presented to the president.

The President may either sign the bill, or veto the bill by sending his objections to Congress. He may "pocket-veto" the bill. According to the Constitution the President has 10 days (exclusive of Sundays) from the date of receiving a bill to approve it. If, within 10 days, Congress adjourns, thus preventing the return of the bill, that bill does not become law. If, however, he does not sign the bill within 10 days and Congress is in session, the bill becomes law without his signature.

Once signed by the President, the bill is sent to the General Services Administration, given a higher number or a public law number and published in individual form. It then goes to the Secretary of Agriculture. The Secretary considers it and assigns it to one of his staff to issue "regulations" on the bill. This may take months, because the Department must study the bill and make sure the new regulations will not conflict with any other regulations. Recommendations are sent to the Office of Management and Budget under the President. From the OMB, appropriation figures are set.

If immediate funding is requested, a message is sent to the Speaker of the House. If not, the request would be placed with other requests that are included in the President's annual budget in February. Assuming that the money is needed immediately, the Speaker assigns it to the Appropriations Committee of the House. A member must introduce this in the form of a bill, which is actually an amendment to the budget. The Appropriations Committee Chairman assigns the bill to the Subcommittee on Agriculture, Environment and Consumer Protection. The Subcommittee may or may not hold hearings. The bill is considered in executive session and then referred to the full Committee.

If approved it goes to the House for full consideration. This is a "privileged matter and at any time after the reading of the Journal, a member, by direction of the appropriate committee, may move that the House resolve itself into the Committee of the Whole House for the purpose of considering the bill.

The bill in its final form goes to the Senate, which follows the same procedure in terms of assignment, subcommittees, etc. The bill is brought before the Senate for a vote.

If the House and Senate bills differ, they meet in Conference Committee. The bill is sent to the President for his signature. He may sign, veto or pocket-veto the bill. If he vetoes the bill, Congress may override the veto by a two-thirds majority of both Houses.

When appropriations are approved, USDA must get permission from the Office of Management and Budget to spend the money. If OMB will not release the funds, USDA must find some other way to get appropriations approved again or wait until a director of OMB gives his approval (OMB may not release funds by an order from the President even though he has signed the bill, or a director of OMB may not see fit to release the funds immediately). This may be days, weeks, years, or never. If a director agrees, the agency can start to initiate the program by setting up a staff, or do whatever is needed to implement the program.

PRESIDENT'S SIGNATURE

WHITE HOUSE

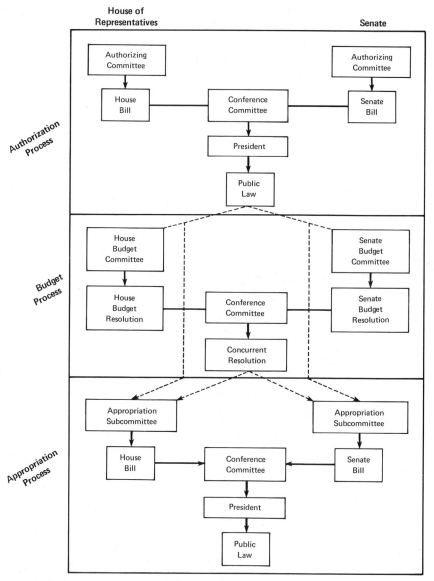

Figure 15-3. Congressional funding process.

The *Congressional Record*, issued in Washington on a daily basis while Congress is in session, reports on the proceedings of congressional hearings and actions as they occur.

Major Factors Shaping Federal Nutrition Legislation[6,7]

Many factors influence federal nutrition legislation. Often the personal judgment and values of as few as six to ten congressmen and their staff may determine the fate of a given bill. Although a given bill may have many issues, each issue is often determined and resolved by only a handful of influential individuals. This resolution is then typically ratified by the House and Senate. The personal experiences, values, and judgments of these few influential people thus may determine the shape that a given piece of legislation will take. For example, Congressman F. Richmond was very personally concerned with his health, diet, and physical fitness, which led him to the broader concerns of nutrition education. Because of his position on the House Subcommittee on Domestic Marketing, Consumer Relations, and Nutrition and his contacts with key nutrition educators, Congressman Richmond did much to advance the current state of nutrition education at the federal level.

Another important factor shaping nutrition legislation is the various assumptions about the budget and the economy. A member of Congress may be greatly swayed in creating new programs and policies by what he or she senses to be economic needs and priorities. This is an area in which hard, strong facts about a given program can be used to influence thought. A nutritionist at the local level who has developed a model nutrition program or a demonstration nutrition project, and who can provide real information about costs outcomes in terms of specific nutritional status indicators, can be of real value in influencing the legislative process by providing such information to the appropriate staff member or legislator.

Public opinion and the mass media also influence federal nutrition legislation. If the Congress believes that the public is likely to be very supportive of a given idea, this will greatly shape their attitudes and support of the idea. A legislator seldom supports ideas for which there is little public sympathy. Many legislators shape their notions about sound nutrition by reading popular lay nutrition books and materials, rather than professional journals. The people who are most intimately involved with a given issue do keep informed and up to date through specialized newsletters or professional journals.

Of utmost importance are the strong views and the activities of major lobbying and interest groups. Although the nutrition lobby is not one of the strongest in Washington, many who oppose efforts by the nutrition lobby, such as certain representatives of the food industry or mass media, often have great power and can exert tremendous influence, even in the face of what seems to be a majority of consumer opposition. An example is the battle over competitive foods, in which public comment was 80 per cent against the sale of competitive foods, but the candy and soft drink industry was successful in forcing USDA to rescind the proposed regulations against the sale of competitive food products. (See Chap. 17.) On the other hand, the nutrition lobby, including groups such as the Food Research and Action Group, the Community Nutrition Institute, the Children's Foundation, and representatives from professional associations, such as the Society of Nutrition Education and the American Dietetic Association, were very influential in achieving passage of Child Nutrition legislation in 1978.

Information about existing programs, at the local, state, or national level will help to determine what legislators come to expect from such programs. This information may be transmitted to them through federal and state agencies or through local practitioners who keep abreast of issues and respond with information about their program when it is likely to be influential. Congressional hearings may be the setting for sharing important information that may help to shape ideas about nutrition legislation, programs, and policies. Witnesses who testify at these hearings may frequently not be completely candid in the on-the-record sessions, so that field hearings may be more important in determining action.

Reports from the General Accounting Office and the Office of Technical Assistance or other independent reports about programs may influence a congressman in favor of, or against, a given program. Because the General Accounting Office and the Congressional Research Service are key investigative bodies for the legislative branch, their reports often have great credibility.

Formal research studies and reports are often too lengthy and full of academic jargon and statistics and may thus frequently go unread. These studies often come up with conclusions that provide little helpful direction to the legislator: "More research is needed"; or "We don't have enough information at this point to make a decision on the issue."

By being aware of these various factors that influence federal nutrition legislation, and by considering them, the nutrition advocate can be very influential in taking action to influence the legislative process.

REGULATORY PROCESS

There is often a series of gaps and discrepancies between the drafting of legislation for a federal program and the translation of the legislation into practice at the local level. For example, the Congress may pass legislation for a nutrition program and then direct the USDA to draft regulations. This agency is then responsible for drafting and publishing regulations to implement the legislation. These regulations typically include definitions, timetables for action, criteria for translation of legislative intent into reality, and methods by which the regulations will be evaluated.

There is much concern among many groups about the way in which some executive agencies respond to legislation with regulations. Critics of a given agency frequently suggest that legislative intent is ignored while concerns of the regulating agency are foremost. "Congressional intent" is often unclear. On very difficult issues, congressional language is the result of difficult compromise. Thus, language is written in such a way so that the bill will be most assured of passage. When an executive agency later has to regulate this and interpret it, there may be considerable difficulty.

Once written, the regulations must be implemented by the state, regional, or local agency mandated to do so. Where the local department is overburdened, overworked, understaffed, and has limited available resources, the regulations may be impossible to comply with. Local officials may not be clear on what is directed.

Thus, the net effect is that a program, which was thoughtfully and carefully conceived and which might have provided effective nutritional services to needy clients, may actually have little if any impact in the immediate future. Its potential may never be reached.

Regulations issued for the Food and Agricultural Act of 1977 pertaining to the Food Stamp Program illustrate some of the controversy and dissatisfaction that frequently result from a given agency's stance. The USDA issued the first package of proposed regulations in early May 1978. The original timetable called for the USDA to propose regulations in the fall of 1977. This delay, in itself, raised serious questions about the willingness of the department to ensure that implementation of the new food stamp law would actually begin within a reasonable time.[8,9]

Critics have suggested that a second package of regulations, including provisions on staffing standards, outreach, location and hours of certification and issuance places, regulations on Indian lands, and the development of joint Supplemental Security Income/Food Stamp Program (SSI/FSP) applications should be issued immediately following the first set of regulations, that is, in May 1978. The U.S. Department of Agriculture was also criticized for not providing regulations for meaningful public participation in the planning and implementation process and for not adequately improving access and outreach provisions.

Other criticisms were directed at the complexity of regulations regarding income determination of certain households and to the emergency issuance regulations.[8]

The final regulations were published in October 1978. Antihunger advocates again criticized the regulations on the grounds that they lacked provisions for ongoing outreach, staffing standards, and points and hours of office operation, and that there was a lack of a strong stance on potential state administrative problems and inadequate standards for public training sessions.[9]

In March 1978 a presidential directive ordered federal agencies to take steps to make all federal regulations more understandable to the public, to identify significant agency actions, and to establish "decision calendars" about upcoming rule making.

In late 1978, the USDA published procedures for complying with this directive. These rules require all USDA agencies "to actively solicit public comment and other inputs" and, before most agency actions, to develop "public participation plans . . . tailored to the agencies programs (stimulating) the broadest possible range of public input at each significant stage."[10]

USDA agencies are to use various means to facilitate "broad, meaningful public input," such as financial aid for citizen participants, public meetings, outreach and training of citizen participants, and organized follow-up of citizen comments.[10]

The *Federal Register*, published daily, provides information to the public about federal regulations as well as about executive branch documents.

SUMMARY: LEGISLATIVE AND REGULATORY PROCESSES

Federal laws affecting nutrition policy are made and regulated by hundreds of individuals who are often unaware of what others are doing. The birth of a program is a long, tedious, complicated, and often painful drama in many acts. Some of the scenes in the drama are summarized in Table 15-2.

Table 15-2

The Birth of a Program — A Drama in Six Acts

Act I — The Idea

Scene 1 — A problem is identified and a need is noted
Scene 2 — Data are gathered
Scene 3 — Discussions ensue
Scene 4 — A new policy direction is formulated

Act II — Informal Discussions

Scene 1 — Discussion with department or agency or congressional staff is held
Scene 2 — Support for bill is gathered
Scene 3 — Specifications are written
Scene 4 — Steps are taken to reach agreement

Act III — Writing Legislation

Scene 1 — Legislative support is gathered
Scene 2 — Legislative language is written
Scene 3 — Bill is introduced in Congress

Act IV — Congress Acts

Scene 1 — Hearings: Committee reports are held in one house
Scene 2 — Bill passes one house
Scene 3 — The other house has hearings, reports, and votes
Scene 4 — Other house passes different bill
Scene 5 — Conference report is developed
Scene 6 — Finally, a bill emerges
Scene 7 — President signs bill

Act V — Implementation

Scene 1 — Budget justification is developed
Scene 2 — President's budget is developed
Scene 3 — Congressional action. Final appropriations are made
Scene 4 — Rules and regulations by appropriate agency are issued
Scene 5 — Comments on rules and regulations are received
Scene 6 — Grants are awarded
Scene 7 — Regulations are evaluated and possibly revised
Scene 8 — Evaluation of regulations in final form is conducted

---

Source: Institute for Educational Leadership. *Washington Policy Seminar.* Washington, D.C.: George Washington University, October 1978.

INFLUENCING THE POLICY-MAKING PROCESS

Before considering ways in which the nutrition advocate can actively influence nutrition policy, a few basics that are often overlooked must be discussed; four points are of particular note.

1. In nutrition program design and policy making, the stakes, other than personal and political, are usually relatively small. They are frequently only marginal to the more central concerns of agricultural policy,

industry, and the like. In contrast, the legislative stakes outside nutrition may be multibillion dollar in nature. They may affect entire agricultural sectors or industries, posing "life or death" consequences. These concerns and industrial institutions are able to voice their contentions through the aid of professionally designed public relations campaigns, expensive law firms, and powerful lobbying groups. The result is that nutrition politics appear even more unimportant. In addition, many federal laws that have a significant impact on nutrition were passed for other reasons, typically with little consideration as to how nutrition objectives might be affected. Acts relating to agricultural production, consumer protection, and welfare programs are only a few examples.

2. Authorization politics are significantly different from appropriations politics. In other words, politics behind actions to legislate new bills are not the same as actions that are designed to appropriate funds. Legislative committees that grant program authorizations are rarely under real disciplinary pressure to limit the power of legislation. On the other hand, committees that are responsible for appropriating funds are under the constraint of never having enough real dollars to cover all needs. Members of these committees are well aware that they will never please everybody, and hence they may not even try. As one well-known lobbyist has stated, "appropriations members like to say that they give dollars only to 'proven' programs while they accuse their counterparts on authorizing committees of 'ignoring the facts,' or 'trying to please everybody' or never terminating 'bad programs,' and of generally creating false and unreasonable expectations about what can, in fact, be funded."[11]

The implications of these varying political roles and the differing congressional uses of information should thus be understood and appreciated. The type of information desired by the authorizing legislator may be radically different from that to which an appropriating congressman might respond.

3. A given committee member often works on legislating preconceived programs or policies. Thus, information in the congressional decision-making arena is rarely sought for its own sake, or even as an aid to general policy making. Rather, information is sought to serve a preconceived point of view. If given data can help to advance an already held point of view, this data will be used repeatedly. Conversely, "harmful" data are not wanted and are generally ignored.[11]

This does not mean that Congress is inherently "biased" or that "facts mean nothing." Rather, information must be carefully collected, cogently presented in "dejargonized" terms, and stated compellingly in language that can be understood and appreciated by the legislators. As. S. Halperin suggests, the "seedbed of values and judgments of our elected representatives must first be prepared before the seeds of information may truly germinate."[11] And this too is part of the role of the health professional.

4. Nothing in a democratic system of decision making and legislation is simple, clear-cut, or neat. There is no single department or ministry of nutrition; rather, those responsible for nutrition policy include hundreds of sponsors and actors in both the private and the public sector. Similarly, there is no coherent federal policy on nutrition and food. Single agencies

are limited in the control or authority that they can exert over others. With these ideas in mind, let us consider ways in which the health professional may be able to influence the policy-making process.

Participation in the Legislative and Policy-Making Process at the State and Local Levels

The nutrition advocate may play a variety of roles in promoting nutrition legislation. At the local or community level, the nutritionist may help to organize needed public support, plan the community statement of the need for legislation, and promote other activities that facilitate needed change. A significant local activity involves the development of innovative projects that can serve as models for broader nutrition programs. The following is an example of such local activity.

In Greenburgh, New York, a group of concerned parents, in response to what they perceived as wasted school lunches, low-quality food, and unsatisfactory meal service, decided to form a committee to evaluate and monitor the school lunches that were being served to the children. The parents found little variety in the food, poor menu planning, and unmet minimal government standards. The result was the formation of an ongoing monitoring committee.[12]

The committee was able to assist the food service manager in planning appealing and nutritious foods and to offer a wide variety of foods. But, beyond these activities, the group created an outreach project to provide lectures, consultations with school and community groups, publication of a pamphlet on ways to improve school lunch programs, and participation in conferences related to improving nutrition. The committee produced a 12-minute, 16-mm motion picture as an educational tool.

Another project sponsored by the Greenburgh group is the school-community farm located on the high school campus, which is made available to residents of the community for farming. Provisions are made to allow the handicapped and elderly to garden by using specially raised plots. All who farm are required to return 10 per cent of their produce to the district for use in senior citizen programs. This example illustrates that local action can help not only to improve existing programs but also to raise the awareness levels of the public and stimulate new ideas and strategies for improving nutrition in the community.

Individuals can help to shape legislation in other ways, as well. It is important to establish links with state and local agencies at the proper time to "have a say" about plans of operation, outreach, standards, educational and training programs, and the overall implementation of legislation. The Food Research and Action Center suggests a number of ways in which interested parties can become involved at the state and local levels.[13]

1. Identify important actors in state government. How do they function? What is the planning process? Where does the real power lie? How are decisions influenced? How can that influence be modified? Who are the resource people and consultants for the decision makers?

2. After you have identified "who's who," meet these individuals. Initiate a dialogue with them about your concerns and how you might effect action.

3. Build up a coalition of interests that can back up your concerns and can effectively influence the decision makers and planners. Inform people; gather support; get commitments of help, time, and money; and "use that political clout to muscle your way into the state planning process."

4. For given pieces of legislation, decide which issues are important for your state or locale. Identify important problems and how they might be alleviated through planning and implementation. Discuss your findings with those involved. When possible, provide the policymaker with hard data to support your position. This is usually more readily accepted than an emotional appeal.

5. Implement ways for your coalition to become involved in the planning and decision-making process. If necessary, arrange to hold public hearings on controversial interests, and make sure that your point of view is adequately supported. "Make sure there are *real* avenues for ongoing input."

Participation in the Legislative and Policy-Making Process at the National Level

The most important prerequisite for effective participation in the legislative arena at the national level is to be informed, not only about the facts and the pros and cons of a particular policy issue but also about the entire legislative machinery and about significant influences on federal legislation.

If a bill is being prepared by a congressman or by an agency, such as the USDA, one who is viewed as being very knowledgeable about the specific area of legislation may be consulted by the staff of the congressman or by staff of the agency about what should be in the legislation. A nutritionist who has worked at the local level and who is familiar with how federal legislative machinery works can be quite influential at this stage. It is not, however, necessary to wait to be consulted. An individual who has relevant information on a given issue should make that information available to the appropriate staff. Any data that can provide insights into the issue at hand are generally well received.

Participation in congressional hearings is another important way to communicate effectively with legislators. The individual testifying at a congressional hearing should be aware of the various factors that may determine whether the testimony is effective or merely ignored. Of utmost importance is the reliance on hard, sound data to back up a given position. Legislators are interested in tangible results — they are interested, for example, in the effect of an implemented program on nutritional status, rather than in a theory about what *might* work. Table 15-3 details other factors of importance in presenting effective congressional testimony.

Another means of influencing legislation is through the support of congressional candidates who are sympathetic to nutrition concerns. By voting for a candidate who is known to be interested in promoting health and nutrition, the nutrition advocate may be taking a basic step toward improving the chances of passage of favorable nutrition legislation at a future date.

Lobbying is difficult for those who are not familiar with the legislative

Table 15–3.

Pointers on Effective Congressional Testimony

1. Prepare your statement far enough in advance that copies are delivered to both majority and minority staff at least 24 hours in advance of the scheduled hearing. It is simply impossible to absorb the facts and details of a statement during a hearing. There are too many other distractions — phones, visitors, staff, bells, votes, and so on. Your statement will have much greater impact and the questions will be much more specific and helpful if they are seen ahead of time.

2. Prior to the hearing, call the appropriate staff on both sides of the aisle to ask what concerns may be expressed during the hearing and what points should be covered in the written statement.

3. In preparing for questions at the hearing, check all recent correspondence files to find out what issues the committee members or their constituents have written about. Be prepared to deal with these issues during the hearing, even if they are only marginally related to the issues at hand.

4. Know something about the district and personal background of the committee members. It will assist you both in anticipating questions and in understanding the member's frame of reference when a question is asked.

5. Regardless of the length of the written statement, do not read it. Summarize and paraphrase it, but take no more than 20 minutes. Be prepared to be quite brief if the hearing is running late. Don't feel offended when the chairman tells you that your carefully honed statement will be inserted in the record without having been read to the committee. Your statement *will* be seen and read by the people who are interested and will make the decisions.

6. If there are other points not in your statement that you feel need to be elaborated upon, ask a friendly staffer or member if you can suggest an area of inquiry. (Note for executive branch types: This is a good way to get material into the record that you can't get cleared through the Office of Management and Budget).

7. Use graphics — tables, charts, and the like — wherever possible. Always have letter-sized copies of any large charts available for the members and staff, and distribute them before they try and copy the chart you have. Use devices like slides and overhead projectors sparingly.

8. Don't use a hearing to spring a surprise upon a committee or the unsuspecting public unless you have given the chairman and ranking minority member advance notice.

9. Do work through the appropriate staff people. If you contact a member outside the presence of the staff person without telling the staff person in advance, do inform the staff person after the fact about your conversation and any commitment that was made.

10. When coming to testify, don't bring an army of associates or aides. A cabinet officer or agency head should have no more than two or three other people at the witness table. Other supporting staff should be kept to an absolute minimum.

11. Before the hearing starts, if at all possible, go up to the dias and introduce yourself and your colleagues to the committee members and staff.

12. If, when a question is asked, you don't have the necessary information, offer to supply it for the record and then attempt to do so within 24 hours. Be certain that both majority and minority staff have copies of the answer and the question.

Pointers on Effective Congressional Testimony *(continued)*

13. Don't argue with committee members. They will always have the last word. If you disagree with a member, say so, state your case, and leave it at that. If you think of additional rebuttal material after the hearing (known as the "I wish I'd thought of that syndrome"), write the appropriate member a note and see that other interested parties receive a copy.

14. Do not interrupt a member when he or she is taking a question or making a statement. If that member's time for questioning expires before you can respond, ask the chairman for a minute or two to respond.

15. Never assume that what happens in one legislative body is known in the other, and do not attempt to play the policies or members of one house against the other. Each body is constitutionally separate and does not want to acknowledge the existence of the other until the stage of conference is reached.

16. When you are supplied with a transcript to edit after a hearing, do it quickly and do not attempt to alter the facts or fundamental direction of oral testimony.

17. Keep your answers brief and to the point. In many cases they can be expanded in the written transcript.

Additional Comments on the Effective Executive/Legislative Relations

1. The administration can have impact on legislation beyond the committee stage in several ways: (a) letter to the speaker when a bill reaches the floor, (b) taking positions on points of difference and talking with members and staff of conference committee, and (c) use (and misuse) of the threat of veto.

2. Relations with congressional members and staff can be significantly enhanced by (a) not waiting until a crisis comes to forewarn them of a potential problem and (b) inviting key members and staff to politically and symbolically significant events, such as bill signings and swearings in.

3. Know when and how to ask the secretary (or even the president) to intervene and use personal influence.

4. The top person (secretary, commissioner, assistant secretary, and so on) should be sufficiently briefed on the major issues so that, when a member of congress meets that person informally, the department officer will know enough to respond. One example: A recent secretary of HEW was asked, by a member, a major policy question about a major issue in a pending bill. Two days later, an assistant secretary telephoned the staff person saying that "the secretary did not understand anything that Mr. X was talking about and can you explain?"

Source: C. Cross. In Institute for Educational Leadership, *Washington Policy Seminar.* Washington, D.C.: George Washington University, October 1978.

process or those who are involved in it, but it is a highly important activity. Lobbying involves various activities designed to influence the passage of particular legislation, such as finding sponsors for a bill and seeing that the bill is properly written, introduced, and finally passed. Although lobbying is often thought of as coming from large and organized interest groups working directly with legislators, it may also involve activities such as calling, visiting, or writing to key legislators or staff to guarantee their support for the bill. It entails attending meetings and supplying information at the appropriate time. It is often useful to engage in letter-writing campaigns. Writing an effective letter to a legislator demands practice and skill. Some tips on writing to legislators are summarized in Table 15-4.[15]

The importance of lobbying cannot be overstated. Lobbying should be conducted at every stage in the legislative as well as during the regulatory process. The lobbying may be influential in the development of the initial bill all the way through the process until the bill is passed, implemented as a program, and the program is then evaluated.

The timing of various activities is extremely important. In Congress all

Table 15-4
Tips on Writing to Legislators

1. Be specific in the opening paragraph about the bill or issue you are writing about. "I am writing about the Food Stamp bill . . . "

2. Pay attention to the timing of your letter. Don't wait until the bill has passed through the committee. Make sure you give the congressman enough time to carry out his or her work.

3. Write to your own representative or senator. Letters from outside the district are often ignored as organized mail.

4. Be brief; come to the point; use cogent facts to back up your points.

5. State your own views; don't copy someone else's. It is much more effective to write your own letter; don't use a form letter or merely add your signature to a petition.

6. State your reasons for taking a stand on a given issue. For example, "I'm a community nutritionist and realize from personal experience that H.R. 100 will . . . "; this is much more effective than statements such as "Vote against H.R. 100; I am bitterly opposed to it.

7. Be constructive. If you feel that the wrong approach is being taken, suggest what you feel the right approach is.

8. Share your expert knowledge with your representative. It will be welcome.

9. When a job has been well done, compliment your representative on it; congressmen are human and appreciate a compliment from individuals who believe they have taken the right course of action.

10. Don't make threats or promises; they will rarely change the minds of members of Congress.

11. Don't berate your congressmen; you won't persuade them by name calling or vindictive language.

12. Don't pretend to have great political influence you do not have. Write to your representatives as an individual, not as a self-appointed spokesperson from a community group. Unsupported claims to fame will cast doubt on your position and views.

13. Don't demand a definite commitment before the facts are in. Understand that bills are long and complex and often frequently amended before a final vote is taken. You have a right to know your representative's stand on an issue, but give him or her sufficient time to make up his or her mind.

Source: M. K. Udall. A congressman on writing to Congress, reprinted from the *Washington Spectator*, mimeo. Washington, D.C.: Society for Nutrition Education, 1978.

bills, regardless of their status or order, die automatically at the close of a session; to be reconsidered, they must be reintroduced in a later congressional session. One way to kill a bill involves stalling action so that it will not be ready for a vote. Often interest in the bill will wane, and there will be less chance of its passage at the beginning of the next session.

Lobbying should be viewed as a never-ending process — even if lobbying efforts to secure passage of a certain bill fails, lobbying must continue. Then the effort may be to try to rescind a bill that has a negative impact on a given program or to modify a bill to weaken its impact. If lobbying efforts are successful in securing passage, the efforts must continue to support the concept of the bill and to secure the development of sound regulations as well as effective program implementation. At this point, opponents will continue to lobby against the intent of the legislation, so that lobbying for the legislation must continue.

Thus, there is an important role for the nutrition advocate to play at every stage of the process. Activities designed to strengthen and promote interest and support for the bill may be influential in initiating it, in speeding up the passage of the bill, in effecting sound regulations, or in modifying the impact of an undesirable bill.

Many professional associations are active in the legislative process and offer the nutritionist a channel for influencing legislation. For example, the American Dietetic Association (ADA) has a representative who works in Washington, testifies in relevant legislative hearings, and informs membership of current legislative happenings through a special section in the *Journal of the American Dietetic Association*, the "Legislative Highlights." The ADA also offers guidance to members and state and local chapters regarding ways in which to be influential in the legislative process.

The Society for Nutrition Education (SNE) has developed a legislative organization to aid in the effective dissemination of legislative information. A Washington Legislative Liaison and Washington-based Legislative Network Committee provide leadership for this organization. The country has been divided into five regions; each member of the SNE Network Subcommittee is responsible for coordinating communications within a given region. Members of SNE periodically receive "Legislative Alerts" that explain current issues in nutrition and suggest ways that individual members can express their feelings on these issues to key federal legislators and administrators.

Other types of consumer advocacy groups who also have strong Washington lobbies include the Food Research Action Center (FRAC), the Children's Foundation, and the Community Nutrition Institute (CNI).

PARTICIPATION IN THE REGULATORY PROCESS

The process of developing regulations for specific nutrition legislation also requires the participation of health and nutrition advocates. Because of the frequent problems associated with the way in which federal agencies draft regulations, nutrition advocates should work to be included as consultants to these agencies before the regulations are established. As expert and committed as most federal officials may be, their expertise is usually in the general administration of programs; they cannot be expected to be experts in the management of a given nutrition program. Thus, nutritionists should expect federal officials to offer instruction in the goals and applications for funding. But they must not be allowed to instruct professionals in the standards of nutrition programs or in the shaping of nutrition policy. That should be the nutritionist's contribution to the development of nutrition policy.

After an agency or department, such as the USDA, proposes regulations for a specific piece of legislation, interested parties are allowed a comment period in which to respond to and make suggestions about the regulations. It is important that interested individuals exercise their right to respond because frequently there is organized opposition to the regulations.

State officials, powerful lobbying groups, politicians, and others with vested interests in specific legislation make efforts to become actively involved and to comment or take other action to affect the legislation or final regulations. Thus, it is very important that nutrition advocates also participate in a similar manner so that their interests are considered. Both positive and negative comments can be directed to the agency. It is also helpful to address comments to members of Congress and to the leaders of the particular House or Senate committees from which the legislation originated. Such comments may help to negate the political pressures that are exerted by powerful lobbying and political groups.

As noted previously, there is often conflict and disagreement over the promulgation of regulations and considerable possibilities for influencing their development. As an example, consider the issue of establishing guidelines for competitive foods (foods that compete with the meals sold in the school lunchroom). These foods may be sold from a vending machine or in an à la carte line. They may not necessarily be sweets or empty calorie foods, but many of them can be categorized as such. Consumer advocates are generally opposed to the sale of competitive foods because of their high-sugar and -calorie content. In regulations issued in April 1977, the U.S. Department of Agriculture tried to ban the so-called "junk foods" such as candy, soft drinks, frozen desserts, and gum until the end of the last school lunch period.[16] But the candy company representatives and many food industry people were adamantly opposed to such a ban. The USDA received 2,100 comments; 82 per cent were for the regulation, and 40 per cent of these believed that the regulations should be even more strict — that is, that the regulations should be extended to the entire school day, not just until after the last lunch period.[17]

The food industry engaged in heavy lobbying efforts intended to kill the proposed regulations. Because of the power of the candy and other food producing and processing industries, who threatened to take the USDA to court for banning their products, the USDA was forced to rescind the ban. The food industries maintained that candy may contain as many nutrients as other foods whose sale may be allowed in the school lunchroom. "On a 100-calorie basis, Mr. Goodbar is superior to Del Monte canned pears in protein, thiamine, niacin and calcium content" stated lawyers for the Hershey Food Corporation.[18] Their concern clearly was not with the high-calorie, -fat, or -sugar content of their products. Actually at issue was whether or not the secretary of Agriculture should have regulatory power to set standards for what is to be sold in the school lunchroom. Consumer groups contended that children's health and nutritional status would suffer if they substituted candy and soft drinks for the type A lunch.

Regulations issued in 1979 based the rationale for banning or not banning certain foods on a standard employing the index of nutritional quality concept. As of this writing the competitive food decision still lies with the USDA. But it is conceivable that, because of the lobbying power of the food industry, Congress could rescind the regulatory authority of the USDA in this regard.

The issues extend far beyond that of regulatory sale of competitive foods and concern issues of nutrition education, health, and food habits. The School Lunch Program is designed to be a model program teaching children, through example, education, and food service, about the selection of a wise diet. Overconsumption of food, fat, sugar, and calories — major concerns among many North Americans — comes into play if the school lunchroom is to be the setting for the sale of foods that reinforce these trends in the eating habits of children. It is clear that there is much

Table 15-5
"Regulations" for Dealing with Federal Regulation

1. Never accept any regulation as final. It is final only if we content ourselves with it. There is no such thing as a final regulation. Comments on existing regulations may be submitted at any time. If we find that given regulations impose undue or unnecessary difficulties, it may be our fault for failing to document these difficulties and suggesting practical and appropriate changes to the legislative body concerned.

2. We must do our homework. If we do not know what we are complaining about, we have no right to complain. Unless we are able to pinpoint the exact offending regulation language and illustrate how it surpasses or misinterprets the language of the law, document the imposed burdens, and suggest alternatives, we deserve to be ignored.

3. We should give the federal officials the benefit of our expertise, whether they ask for it or not. We should not hesitate to make our case on the assumption that they are more fully aware of the issues at stake. Federal actors may know more about legislative language and the law, but they cannot possibly know as much about how those laws and regulations shape given programs. Thus, do not rely on the wisdom of federal officials unless the regulations make sense to you. Make it your responsibility to read and comment on proposed regulations and on the potential impact of given legislation.

4. Double the effectiveness of your voice by making use of your professional association. Alert the association to a specific problem, offer your data in support of your position, and help to generalize about the given issue from a broader perspective. If your associations fail to aid you, it may be because you failed to alert them and ask for their assistance.

5. We must work harder to identify, articulate, and maintain the highest standards of professional conduct and competence. If we fall down on the job, we have little case for complaining when different standards are established or when federal agencies fail to seek out our expertise.

Source: C. B. Saunders. Is regulation strangulation? *College Board Rev.* 100 (Summer 1976): 2–5.

at stake, to be gained or lost, by participating in the regulatory process whereby decisions of this nature are made. C. B. Saunders suggests some "proposed regulations for dealing with Federal regulations." These are listed in Table 15-5.[19]

CONCLUSION

Congress needs a complete and operational data base from which to make decisions. These data include facts relating to:

What programs should be eliminated? What new programs should be instituted?

What are possible areas of shared programs between institutions or agencies?

What institutions are producing better or more effective outcomes in the given program area?

What are innovative and perhaps cheaper ways to provide nutrition and food programs?

With the appropriate dialogue, and with respectful understanding of mutual problems, health professionals and legislators can aid each other in responding to current health and nutrition needs. Both sides must recognize the limited resources available. Neither side should stereotype the other. There should be an attempt to define common ground on which to join and work together.

Legislators and health professionals both possess expertise that can aid the other in achieving the mutual goal of improving the health and nutritional status of the public. Health professionals are skilled in determining what is needed from a health and nutrition standpoint. Legislators have the skill to make political processes respond to these needs. In sum, health professionals and legislators should not simply coexist but should work together to see that the health care delivery system and the political system are most responsive to today's needs.

It is clear that we need to change in significant ways to increase our involvement not only in the legislative but also in the regulatory process. If we fail to change, we may never be able to influence these processes. As Saunders suggests, "one day we may interrupt our criticisms of the bureaucracy long enough to reflect like Pogo that we have met the enemy, and he is us."[19]

Communication with Members of Congress

Letters to members of the Senate or the House of Representatives can be addressed as follows:

The Honorable ————
U.S. Senate
Washington, D.C. 20510

Dear Senator ————:

The Honorable _____
U.S. House of Representatives
Washington, D.C. 20510

Dear Mr. _____ :

Although members of Congress have telephone numbers by which they can be reached, it is usually difficult to make direct telephone contact with them. However, each senator and representative has one or more administrative assistants or legislative assistants who are much more accessible and who are often the ideal first contact to work with.

Obtaining Copy of Legislation

Specific bills or public laws may be obtained from the appropriate house:

H.R. Bills from the U.S. House Document Room
Washington, D.C. 20510

S. Bills from the U.S. Senate Document Room
Washington, D.C., 20510

Bills should be ordered by specific number: for House bills, H.R. _____ ; for Senate bills, S. _____ ; and for public laws, P.L. _____ .

REFERENCES

1. Ullrich, H. D. Editorial. *J. Nutr. Educ.* 5 (1973): 224.
2. Stucker, T. A., J. B. Penn, and R. D. Knutson. Agricultural food policy making: Process and participants, in *Agricultural Food Policy Review*, Rept. No. AFPR-1. Washington, D.C.: U.S. Department of Agriculture, January 1977.
3. Barone, M., G. Ujifusa, and D. Matthews. *The Almanac of American Politics.* New York: E. P. Dutton, 1975.
4. American Dietetic Association. *Legislative Handbook.* Chicago, Illinois, 1977.
5. Food and Agriculture Act of 1977, P.L. 94-113, September 1977.
6. Institute for Educational Leadership. *Washington Policy Seminar.* Washington, D.C.: George Washington University, October 1978.
7. Andriga, R. C. Major factors influencing federal education legislation, In Institute for Educational Leadership, *Washington Policy Seminar, op. cit.*
8. Hart, R., J. Lipner, and B. Moore. *Memo to Food Stamp Advocates.* Washington, D.C.: Food Research Action Center, May 3, 1978.
9. First package of food stamp regs due for publication. *CNI Week. Rep.* 8 (1978): 1-2.
10. USDA sets guidelines for citizen participation. *CNI Week. Rep.* 8 (1978): 4.
11. Halperin, S. Congress and information: A commentary, In Institute for Educational Leadership, *Washington Policy Seminar, op. cit.*
12. Dwyer, J. . . . At school. *Food Monitor* 2 (1977): 17.
13. Food Research Action Center. Comments needed on food stamp regs. *CNI Week. Rep.* 8 (1978): 5.
14. Cross, C. Pointers on effective Congressional testimony, In Institute for Educational Leadership, *op. cit.*
15. Udall, M. K. A congressman on writing to Congress, reprinted from the

Washington Spectator, mimeo. Washington, D.C.: Society for Nutrition Education, 1978.

16. *Federal Register*, 43 Fed. Reg. 17476, April 25, 1978.
17. Food Research Action. *USDA Wants to Hear How You Feel about Competitive Foods*. Washington, D.C., March 1979.
18. Milius, P. Sweet talking seeks to save school candy. *Washington Post*, April 9, 1979, pp. A1–A2.
19. Saunders, C. B. Is regulation strangulation? *College Board Rev.* 100 (Summer 1976): 2–5.

16

Agencies dealing with nutrition-related issues

Reader Objectives

After completing this chapter, the reader should be able to
1. State the major purposes and activities of the following:
   USDA agencies: Human Nutrition Center, Science and Education Administration, Extension, Food and Nutrition Service.
   USDHEW agencies: Public Health Service, Health Services Administration, National Institutes of Health, Health Resources Administration, Center for Disease Control, Food and Drug Administration.
2. State the nutrition concerns and activities of the Federal Trade Commission, the U.S. Department of Commerce, the U.S. State Department, the Community Services Administration.
3. List two quasi-government agencies involved in nutrition-related activities.
4. List three private foundations concerned with nutrition issues.
5. List three private agencies concerned with nutrition issues.
6. State the general activities of the state and local health departments as they relate to nutrition.

OVERVIEW

Nutrition-related activities are the concern of governmental agencies at the federal, state, and local level. Quasi-government agencies, as well as numerous private and professional agencies and organizations, are also concerned with nutritional issues and programs.

The primary federal agencies responsible for nutrition activities are the U.S. Department of Agriculture and the U.S. Department of Health, Education, and Welfare. Other agencies charged with the responsibility for nutritional activities include the Federal Trade Commission, the U.S. Department of Commerce, the Veterans Administration, the U.S. Department of Defense, the Community Services Administration, and the U.S. Department of State. The organization of the agencies of the federal government is illustrated in Figure 16–1. In addition there are many state and local agencies engaged in nutrition-related activities.

This chapter reviews the structure and some of the divisions within these agencies that are responsible for food- and nutrition-related activities. Some of the specific nutrition and food programs administered by these agencies are discussed in Chapter 17.

It should be noted that in government, being what it is, organizations and agencies are frequently reorganized. Information on the organizational structure of the programs that may be accurate today may be out of date tomorrow. This chapter is thus based on the most current information available at this time, but the reader should be aware that changes frequently occur.

THE GOVERNMENT OF THE UNITED STATES

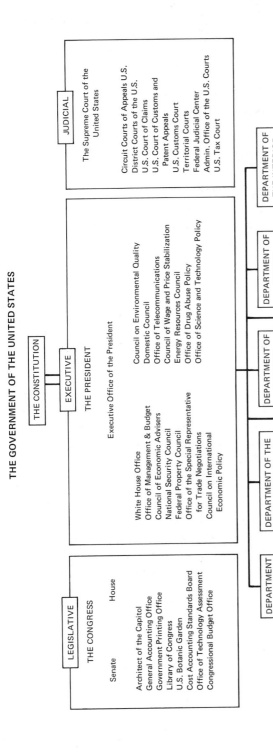
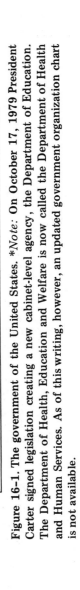

Figure 16-1. The government of the United States. *Note:* **On October 17, 1979 President Carter signed legislation creating a new cabinet-level agency, the Department of Education. The Department of Health, Education and Welfare is now called the Department of Health and Human Services. As of this writing, however, an updated government organization chart is not available.**

U.S. DEPARTMENT OF AGRICULTURE (USDA)

The mission of the USDA is to improve farm income, agriculture, and food production and to develop markets for agricultural production; to assure consumers of an adequate food supply at reasonable cost; and to curb poverty, hunger, and malnutrition. Activities of the department include:[1]

— Provision of food assistance programs to help improve the diets of those in need.
— Efforts to enhance food production, on the one hand, and reduce surplus on the other.
— Research and education in food and related areas.
— Efforts to ensure food quality and safety regulation through the inspection of meat and poultry at the processing and slaughtering sites and of meat and poultry that enter interstate commerce.
— Grading varieties of meats, vegetables, fruits, bread, and dairy products according to eating quality, safety, and wholesomeness.

Figure 16–2 illustrates the various agencies within the USDA.

The USDA was created in 1862. The department works closely with the land-grant colleges, which were also established in 1862 by the Morrill Act. This act established the system of the land-grant colleges in the United States by donating 11 million acres of public lands to the states and territories to offer colleges to provide the support needed for agricultural activities. There are now 71 land-grant colleges and universities in the 50 states, as well as in Puerto Rico, Guam, the Virgin Islands, and the District of Columbia. Each state also has an authorized agricultural experiment station. The experiment stations, the land-grant colleges, and the USDA work together to maximize the quality and productiveness of the United States food supply.[2]

Science and Education Administration (SEA)

In 1977 a major reorganization of the USDA was undertaken, in compliance with the mandate of the 1977 Food and Agriculture Act, to "increase cooperation of coordination in the performance of agricultural research."[3] A new Food and Agricultural Science and Education Administration (SEA) was created to provide a uniform focus to the previously fragmented and piecemeal nutrition and agriculture research and education activities of the USDA.

SEA is to carry out the lead agency responsibilities of the USDA in the food and agricultural sciences. The scope of food and agricultural sciences is defined in PL 95–113 as including "sciences relating to food and agriculture in the broadest sense, including the social, economic, and political considerations of —

(A) agriculture, including soil and water conservation and use, the use of organic waste materials to improve soil tilth and fertility, plant and animal production and protection, and plant and animal health;

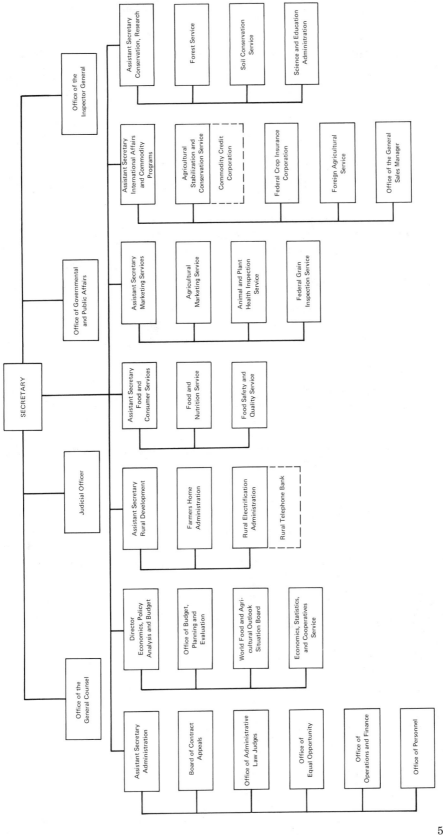

U.S. DEPARTMENT OF AGRICULTURE

Figure 16-2. Organization of the Department of Agriculture.

Table 16-1

Functions and Responsibilities of Science and Education Administration

---

1. Provide support for and coordination and planning of food and agricultural research, extension, and teaching efforts responsive to local, state, regional, and national goals.

2. Promote and support the identification of high-priority national objectives in the food and agricultural sciences and initiate special projects to meet those objectives.

3. Support programs and activities responsive to world food and agricultural needs.

4. Develop and provide information and expertise needed by policy, regulatory, and action agencies of the department and other federal agencies.

5. Build on present partnership and cooperative arrangements and develop with all performers and supporters of food and agricultural research, extension, and teaching activities, whatever their source of funding, improved cooperation and coordination in the planning and execution of such programs and activities.

6. Conduct federal research programs in the food and agricultural sciences.

7. Assure that the results of agricultural research are effectively communicated and demonstrated to farmers, processors, handlers, consumers, and other users.

8. Support and promote information systems and libraries in the food and agricultural sciences and encourage their effective use in coordinating, planning, and implementing research, extension, and teaching programs.

The new agency will provide a centralized organization to further the congressional mandate under PL 95-113 for establishing USDA as the lead agency in the food and agricultural sciences. It is designed to increase cooperation and coordination of food and agricultural research, extension, and teaching by federal departments and agencies, the states, state agricultural experiment stations, colleges, universities, and other private and public institutions.

The agency also is designed to achieve the president's reorganization goals to improve management, reduce overlapping and duplication of effort, and provide better service to the American people. Functions and responsibilities of the agency include the new thrusts required under PL 95-113, plus those previously carried out by the Agricultural Research Service (ARS), Cooperative State Research Service (CSRS), Extension Service (ES), and the National Agricultural Library (NAL). The agency also will perform a coordinating role for research performed in the Forest Service (FS) and the Economic Research Service (ERS).

Source: U.S. Department of Agriculture. The organization of S.E.A. (internal communication). Washington, D.C., December 15, 1977.

(B) the processing, distributing, marketing, and utilization of food and agricultural products;

(C) forestry, including range management, production of forest and range products, multiple use of forest and range lands, and urban forestry;

(D) aquaculture;

(E) home economics, human nutrition, and family life; and

(F) rural and community development."[3]

Table 16-1 details the functions and responsibilities of the agency.[4] Figure 16-3 illustrates the organization of SEA. SEA activities include

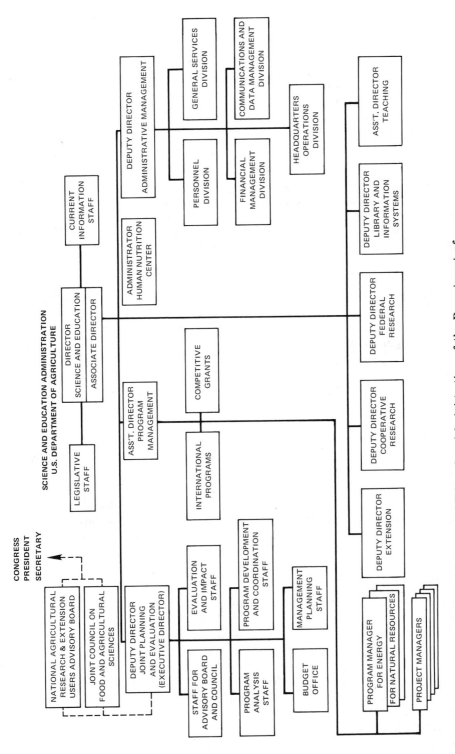

Figure 16–3. Organization of Science and Education Administration of the Department of Agriculture.

those of the Human Nutrition Center, Federal Research, Extension, Cooperative Research, and Technical Information Service.

Human Nutrition Center

The purpose of the Human Nutrition Center is to foster programs concerning the role of nutrition in human health. This is done by administering human nutrition research within the USDA, coordinating USDA nutrition activities, and cooperating with other federal agencies.[5]

The Nutrition Center is responsible for planning, directing, and coordinating human nutrition research delegated to SEA and is involved in cooperative research with universities throughout the country. In carrying out these research activities, the Nutrition Center is expected to work closely with the Joint Council on Food and Agricultural Sciences, the National Agricultural Research and Extension Users Advisory Board, the director of Science and Education, and the directors of other divisions of SEA. The major research organizations that make up the Nutrition Center are listed and described in Table 16–2.

Agricultural Research

Agricultural Research, formerly the Agricultural Research Service, is responsible for conducting basic and developmental research on animal production; plant production; the use and improvement of soil, water, and air; marketing; and the use and effects of various agricultural products. The research applies to a wide range of areas: commodities; natural resources; science; and geographic, climatic, and environmental conditions. The research is categorized into approximately 300 research activities.[6]

Cooperative Research

The principal function of Cooperative Research is to administer congressional acts authorizing federal appropriations for agricultural research carried out by the state agricultural experiment stations, approved forestry schools, and nonprofit institutions. Cooperative Research is responsible for reviewing research proposals submitted by institutions, disbursing funds, and maintaining ongoing review and evaluation of the programs and expenditures.[9]

Technical Information Service: The National Agricultural Library (NAL)

NAL, located in Beltsville, Maryland, contains more than 1.5 million books on food, agriculture, nutrition, and related subjects. The library gathers material from all areas of the world and extends services to other libraries, institutions, and the public. Library information is disseminated through loans, photographs, microfilm, and reference service.

The Food and Nutrition Information and Educational Resources Center (FNIERC) is designed to gather and disseminate resource materials for those who implement USDA's Special Food Service Program for Children.

FNIERC resources related to food service and nutrition education include books, journal articles, pamphlets, government documents, special reports, proceedings, bibliographies, and the like, as well as a collection

Table 16-2
Research Directed by the Human Nutrition Center

Research Organization	Description
Nutrition Institute Beltsville, Md.	Conducts research on carbohydrates, lipids, proteins, vitamins, minerals, and nutrient composition of foods. The mission of the institute is "to identify the requirements of nutrients for optimal health and to recommend foods and dietary patterns that meet these requirements. . . . The program is also concerned with the changes in dietary habits of our population as they have occurred in this century and as they can be projected to continue in the future. . . . " (see ref. 7).
Consumer and Food Economics Institute Hyattsville, Md.	Conducts research on food consumption and use, develops nutritional guidelines, evaluates dietary habits, and develops procedures for the use of food in homes or institutions. Primary activities emanate from these organizations (see ref. 8):
	—Nutrient Data Research Center (NDRC) is responsible for maintaining current data on nutrient composition of foods. Activities have included publication of *Agricultural Handbook No. 8* and the *Nutritive Value of Foods*. Current thrust involves revising food composition data into National Nutrient Data Bank (NNDB), which will include food composition data from industry, land-grant colleges, and special contractors.
	—Food Consumption Research Group is responsible for the national surveys of household food consumption.
	—Food and Diet Appraisal Group is concerned with nutrition education and publishes literature for the public such as food guides, recipes, canning, safe public guidance, and food plans for various income-level households.
	—Interpretation of Research for Applied Programs develops dietary guidance materials based on research findings, such as the *Daily Food Guide* used to aid consumers in selecting food for health.
	—Consumer Use of Foods Section conducts research on food storage, preparation, and quality. Publishes research results.
	—Nutrition Programs Service applies nutrition research to education programs. A bimonthly publication, *Nutrition Program News,* provides for an exchange of nutrition education information among those who work in nutrition.
Human Nutrition Laboratory on Trace Elements Grand Forks. N.D.	Conducts research related to human requirements for trace elements such as zinc, cadmium, nickel, and copper.
Human Nutrition Laboratory on Aging Tufts University, Boston, Mass.	Carries out research on nutrition and physiological and biochemical factors related to the aging process.
The Children's Nutrition Laboratory In cooperation with Baylor College of Medicine and the Texas Children's Hospital Waco, Tex.	Develops the scientific basis for standards of nutrient intake and nutritional assessment for infants and children and will study the relationships between nutrition and the physical and mental development of children from prenatal through adolescent years.

of nonprint media in the form of films, filmstrips, slides, games, charts, audiotapes, and video cassettes.

Sponsors who may be interested in borrowing resource material from FNIERC may obtain a current catalog from:

Head, Food and Nutrition Information and Educational Resources Center
Room 304
National Agricultural Library
Beltsville, Maryland 20705
Phone: (301) 344-3719

FNIERC is a joint venture by the National Agricultural Library and the Food and Nutrition Service of the USDA. FNIERC provides users access to the total resources of the National Agricultural Library.

Extension

Extension, formerly the Cooperative Extension Service, was established in 1914 and represented a novel system of education. Designed to take nutrition directly to rural people in the United States, the system was founded on the belief that human progress would be greatly enhanced if research findings could be translated into lay language and made available to, and practical for, rural Americans.

One of the keys to the success of Extension has been its unique structure as a partnership of all levels of government and its contribution to the people it is designed to serve. There is much flexibility in the system as well as a framework for providing problem-solving education that is applicable to a broad range on emerging and dynamic national, state, and local needs.[10,11]

Several Extension functions are directly aimed at effecting improvements in the nutritional status of Americans. Extension personnel conduct ongoing educational activities in which public issues are addressed in a variety of forums, such as 4-H youth groups, extension homemaker clubs, agricultural producers, special interest groups, and local community decision-makers. Extension program activities are categorized and detailed in Table 16–3.[10]

Table 16–3
Activities of Extension

Target Group	Direct Method	Indirect Method	Current Program and Program Effectiveness
General Audience	Group meetings, workshops, self-instruction packets, public demonstrations.	Training volunteers to conduct programs; newsletters, multimedia instruction, computer instruction, audiovisual programs for the use of volunteers; use of mass media; work with other federal agencies to design nutrition education materials for their target audiences.	General food and nutrition education program; in 1978 approximately 11 million Americans (5 per cent of population) were reached through Extension.
Low Income	One-to-one and small group teaching by trained paraprofessionals through the Expanded Food and Nutrition Education Program (EFNEP).	In some areas EFNEP participants receive newsletters reinforcing material covered by the paraprofessionals.	In FY 1978 approximately 9 per cent of low-income families in the United States were reached through current EFNEP funding levels. During that year, approximately 6,500 paraprofessional aides reached approximately 440,000 families. Since 1968 well over 1 million families (more than 6 million individual members) and approximately 3 million youths (through 4-H EFNEP) have been reached.

Source: J. Nielson. Testimony before the U.S. House Subcommittee on Domestic Marketing, Consumer Relations, and Nutrition. Washington, D.C.: Government Printing Office, October 1977.

A unique feature of Extension is that its educational activities are programmed in response to needs and problems identified at the local level. Extension can also serve as a neutral agency and thus can provide a forum for debate, at the local level, of food and nutrition issues; in short, Extension functions as an objective, nonpolitical education and information system in cooperation with other government agencies.

An important program of Extension is the Expanded Food and Nutrition Education Program (EFNEP). The EFNEP is designed to teach low-income families, particularly those with small children, the skills needed to develop and consume an adequate, varied, and balanced diet. A target group for the service are families who receive food stamps. In the EFNEP program, nutrition education programs are conducted in the homes of low-income homemakers by trained paraprofessional nutrition aides, who are often members of the local community and are able to work well on a one-to-one basis with the homemakers. The program includes the identification of nutrition-related needs, the educational component, and ongoing monitoring of progress and evaluation.

Other divisions of USDA are also highly relevant to nutrition activities. Summary descriptions of the Food and Nutrition Service, the Food Safety and Quality Service (Food and Consumer Services), and the Economics, Statistics, and Cooperative Service (Economics, Policy Analysis, and Budget) follow:

Food and Consumer Services

Food and Nutrition Service (FNS).

President Nixon's message on hunger of May 1969, in which he committed his administration to undertake a massive effort to eliminate hunger and malnutrition in the United States, resulted in the creation of a Food and Nutrition Service. Since its inception in August 1969, FNS has had the primary responsibility for federal administration of feeding assistance programs and the development of a strong and effective system for actual program operations at federal, state, and local levels.

The efforts of the Food and Nutrition Service of the USDA are primarily directed at eliminating poverty-caused hunger and malnutrition in this country. Educational efforts are carried out cooperatively with state and local governments. The Food and Nutrition Service has the principal responsibility for the delivery of federal food and nutrition programs including the Special Supplemental Food Program for Women, Infants, and Children; child food programs (such as the school lunch, school breakfast, special food service programs); and the food stamp program. These food assistance programs are intended to provide access to a nutritionally adequate diet for families and individuals with low incomes and to encourage better eating patterns among the nation's children. These programs are discussed in greater detail in Chapter 17.

Food Safety and Quality Service (FSQS).

The FSQS works to assure the wholesomeness of the food supply by inspecting meat, poultry, eggs, and related products; it also aids trade in foodstuffs and assists consumers in choosing the quality of product through grading. The FSQS, established in March 1977, administers the Federal Meat Inspection Act and the Poultry Products Inspection Act, providing uniform federal-state inspection programs, and may actually implement inspection where state programs do not meet federal requirements. The FSQS also develops and sets standards of identity or content for meat and poultry foodstuffs.[2]

Economics, Policy Analysis, and Budget

Economics, Statistics, and Cooperative Services (ESCS)

The Economics, Statistics, and Cooperatives Service (ESCS) was created by the merger of the Economic Research Service, the Statistical Reporting Service, and the Farmer Cooperative Service.

The functions of the agency include the provision of economic analysis on factors influencing agricultural demand and supply; on nutrition and food labeling; on the production, marketing, and distribution of agricultural produce; and on the status of rural population groups. The agency also conducts research and offers technical assistance on the various economic and marketing issues involved in cooperatives.[12]

USDA In-House Policy Agencies Dealing with Nutrition Concerns

Joint Council on Food and Agricultural Sciences.

The council was established through the Food and Agriculture Act of 1977. Membership is composed of representatives from the USDA, the Office of Science and Technology Policy, land-grant colleges, state agricultural experiment stations and extension services, and other public and private groups or individuals who are interested in and able to contribute to the development of national food and agricultural policy.

The primary mission of the Joint Council is to "foster coordination of the agricultural research, extension, and teaching activities of the federal government, the states, colleges and universities, and other public and private institutions and persons interested in the food and agricultural sciences."[3]

Responsibilities of the Joint Council are to:

— provide a forum for information on interchanges among various agencies, thus increasing awareness about food and agricultural matters.

— analyze and evaluate effects of research, teaching, and extension, and determine needs, priorities, and appropriate research areas.

— develop a system for the compilation, maintenance, and dissemination of research related to nutrition, food, and agricultural research and extension.

— provide a forum able to interpret and evaluate research findings and promote understanding among various agencies.

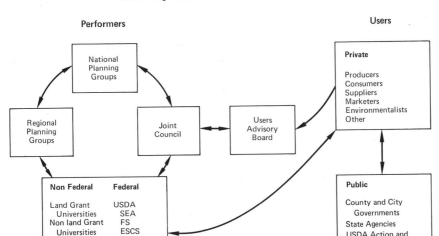

Figure 16-4. Food and agriculture science and education system.

National Agricultural Research and Extension Users Advisory Board.

Established within the USDA, this board was authorized by the Food and Agriculture Act of 1977. The board was given the "general responsibility for preparing independent advisory opinions on the food and agricultural sciences."[3] Other responsibilities include reviewing, consulting, assessing, evaluating, and making recommendations about matters involving food and agricultural sciences, research, education, and extension. The relationship between the Joint Council and the Advisory Board is illustrated in Figure 16-4.

Human Nutrition Policy Committee.

Created in 1978, the committee is jointly led by the assistant secretary for conservation, research, and education and the assistant secretary for food and consumer services. The charge of the committee is to oversee food assistance, food safety, and quality, research, and education. The committee is to "provide a mechanism for continuing coordination on matters related to human nutrition policy which concern various agencies of the Department" and to "maintain liaison with other government agencies or departments concerned with human nutrition" and related issues.[13]

Office of Governmental and Public Affairs.

Responsible for the development of policy and control of all department printed matter, the office has the authority to approve or disapprove department publications. However, each individual agency within USDA is solely responsible for the nutrition materials that it develops.[14]

U.S. DEPARTMENT OF HEALTH, EDUCATION, AND WELFARE (USDHEW)*

The nutrition policy goal of the Department of Health, Education, and Welfare is to "improve the quality of life by enabling all Americans to reap the health benefits of sound nutrition."[14] Under the mandate to improve the health of the American public, the USDHEW has a wide span of nutrition-related activities.

The primary responsibility for these activities rests with seven agencies in the USDHEW:

> Administration on Aging (AOA)
>
> Administration on Children, Youth, and Families (AOCYF)
>
> Food and Drug Administration (FDA)
>
> Health Resources Administration (HRA)
>
> National Institutes of Health (NIH)
>
> Health Services Administration (HSA)
>
> Office of Consumer Affairs (OCA)

Also within HEW, the Office of Health Information, Health Promotion, and Physical Fitness and Sports Medicine, formally called the Office of Health Information and Health Promotion, is mandated to coordinate public and private efforts for health promotion, preventive health services, and health information. Nutrition is identified as a high priority by the office.

The missions of these seven agencies, as well as the activities of other USDHEW agencies that are more indirectly related to improving the nutrition status of Americans, is summarized in the following sections. The way these agencies relate to each other is illustrated in the organization chart, Figure 16–5.

Office of Human Development Services (OHDS)[15]

This office is responsible for administering broad-based human development programs that are targeted to the needs of special subgroups of the population, such as children, the handicapped, older people, and native Americans. Most (about 80 per cent) of OHDS funds are grants-in-aid to states that use the money to operate their programs, such as the Head Start preschool program and the nutrition program for the elderly. The agencies most directly concerned with nutrition-related activities within the Office of Human Development Services include the Administration on Aging, the Administration on Children, Youth, and Families, and the Administration on Native Americans.

Administration on Aging (AOA) (Office of Human Development Services)

AOA is the federal coordination point for meeting the needs and interests of elderly individuals; one of its primary functions is the administration of

*In 1979 Congress created a separate Department of Education, but an updated organizational chart of the new department is not yet available.

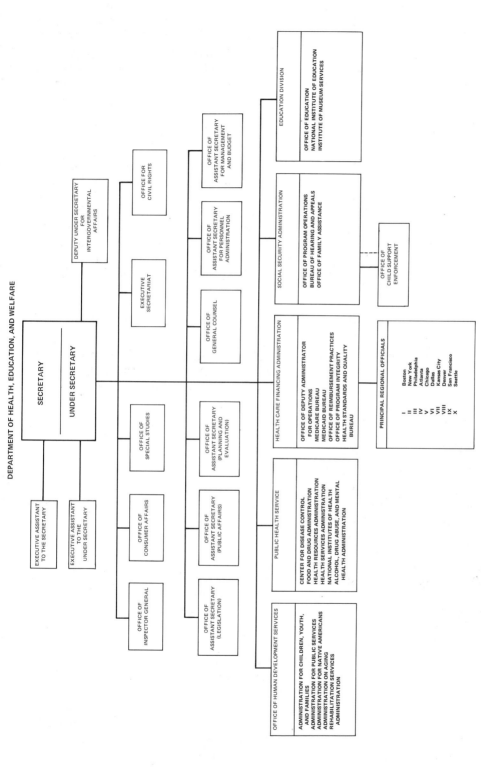

Figure 16–5. Organization of the Department of Health, Education, and Welfare. On October 17, 1979 President Carter signed legislation creating a new cabinet-level agency, the Department of Education. The former Department of Health, Education and Welfare is now the Department of Health and Human Services. As of this writing, however, organization charts of these two new agencies are unavailable. The principal change is that the Education Division shown here now constitutes the new Department of Education.

programs of the Older Americans Act. AOA administers the National Nutrition Program for the Elderly, a program designed to provide low-cost nutritious meals to older Americans. (See Chapter 17.) AOA also administers a research, demonstration, and training program designed to improve the effectiveness of services that are available to older persons and to train manpower to meet the needs of the aging. AOA has a National Clearinghouse on Aging and has staff to serve on the Federal Council on Aging.

Administration on Children, Youth, and Families (AOCYF) (Office of Human Development Services)

This administration, which was formerly the Office of Child Development and Office of Youth Development, offers services and activities that impact on the development of children and youth, such as Head Start. The agency is responsible for developing innovative programs for children and parents; for serving to coordinate federal programs for children, youth, and families; for removing the barriers to youth development; and for acting as an advocate for American children by informing the government and the public of their needs. The AOCYF also awards research and demonstration grants in the areas of children, youth, and families.

Administration of Native Americans (Office of Human Development Services — ANA)

This agency aids native American Indians in achieving their economic and social potential; it provides direct funding for programs authorized under the Native American Programs Act of 1974 to native American tribes, Alaskan communities, agencies working for native Hawaiians, as well as other organizations serving native Americans.

Health Care Financing Administration (HCFA)

The Health Care Financing Administration (HCFA), established in 1977, oversees the Medicare and the Medicaid programs, both of which are designed to provide access to comprehensive health care for elderly, disabled, or impoverished Americans.[15]

The enabling legislation for both Medicare and Medicaid is the Social Security Act. Title XIX established Medicaid whereas Title XVIII established Medicare. Medicare provides low-cost health insurance to elderly and disabled Social Security beneficiaries; Medicaid is jointly funded by federal and state governments and offers health insurance coverage for the poor who are unable to afford other types of health insurance.

The HCFA, in addition to overseeing these two programs, is responsible for developing and enforcing standards to promote high-quality health care delivery and services that are supported through federal funds.

Of current concern to nutrition advocates is the fact that nutrition services or other medical services provided in comprehensive health centers or comprehensive mental health centers are not usually reimbursable. Clearly the scope of nutritional services could be significantly broadened if this regulation were changed. The American Dietetic Association has been active in advocating a change in this aspect of the Medicaid regulations.

Medicare covers part of hospital or extended care facility costs, as well as home health care, physicians' or other services, certain prescriptions, and other medical equipment. According to Medicare regulations, only that care that is "reasonable and necessary" is covered and reimbursable. Bills have been introduced to amend Medicare legislation so that services of nurse practitioners and physician extenders at rural health clinics might be reimbursed without the on-site supervision of physicians. Registered dietitians have been suggested to be included under the term "physician-extenders"[16]

Social Security Administration (SSA)

The national Social Security program is the responsibility of the SSA. Through this program, covered employees and their employers contribute part of their earnings while they are working. Upon retirement or disability, these employees receive a monthly payment based upon their lifetime earnings. Cash benefits may also be paid to survivors in the event of the death of the employee.

The SSA is also responsible for administering the Supplemental Security Income (SSI) program, which pays benefits to the elderly, blind, or disabled who have limited incomes. The Aid to Families with Dependent Children (AFCD) is another program adminstered by SSA.

Office of Consumer Affairs (OCA)

The Office of Consumer Affairs is responsible for advising the secretary of HEW and the presidential special assistant for consumer affairs about federal consumer-type programs and positions. This office is engaged in policy analysis and in the analysis of federal legislation and regulations related to consumers, and it helps to develop consumer programs. The office is also an advocate for consumer education and responds to consumer inquiries and complaints.

Public Health Service (PHS)

The Public Health Service of the Department of Health, Education, and Welfare is the agency responsible for promoting optimal health for the U.S. population. The principal functions of the PHS are:

> To stimulate and assist States and communities with the development of local health resources and to further development of education for the health professions; to assist with the improvement of the delivery of health services to all Americans; to conduct and support research in the medical and related sciences and to disseminate scientific information; to protect the health of the Nation against impure and unsafe foods . . . [1]

The PHS is also responsible for providing leadership in the promotion of health and the prevention of disease, as well as for other public health functions. Within the PHS, the following are involved with food and nutrition activities:

Alcohol, Drug Abuse, and Mental Health Administration

Health Services Administration

National Institutes of Health

Health Resources Administration

Center for Disease Control

Food and Drug Administration

The following discussion elaborates on the functions of these agencies in greater detail.

Alcohol, Drug Abuse, and Mental Health Administration (ADAMHA).

The National Institute of Drug Abuse (NIDA) is engaged in supporting nutrition-related research and demonstration projects to improve the health, nutritional, and social status of addicts and drug abusers. Some of these projects include nutrition education. Other projects research the relationship of alcohol intake to nutritional deficiencies.

The National Institute on Alcohol Abuse and Alcoholism (NIAAA) works to increase high-quality treatment and rehabilitation devices for victims of alcoholism at the community level. The institute also funds training and education programs designed to prevent and control alcohol abuse. The institute maintains a data collection and information dissemination facility, the National Clearinghouse for Alcohol Information, and a National Center for Alcohol Education.

Health Services Administration (HSA)

The Health Services Administration centers its activities around five basic missions:[17]

1. To build primary health care capacity in underserved areas.

2. To maintain primary health care capacity in circumstances where it cannot become self-sustaining.

3. To improve the organization and efficiency of health care delivery.

4. To promote effective and equitable public health and preventive services.

5. To assure the quality of federally financed health services.

These goals are accomplished through HSA-administered grant and contract programs designed to improve the distribution, organization, and effectiveness of health services, with emphasis on demonstrating leadership in innovative health programming through its direct health service delivery programs.

Within HSA are the Bureau of Community Health Services, the Bureau of Indian Health Services, the Bureau of Quality Assurance, and the Bureau of Medical Services.

1. *Bureau of Community Health Services (BCHS).* A variety of activities in the Bureau of Community Health Services are designed to help local communities provide health care and nutritional services to the poor, the disadvantaged, and the underserved, especially members of minority groups, the young, and others who are most in need of such services.

Nutrition services form an integral part of BCHS programs. Nutritional components include:[18]

1. Nutritional status assessment and surveillance; diagnosis and follow-up of problems.

2. Nutritional education and counseling for the sick as well as the healthy.

3. Nutrition education for health professionals, the families of individual patients, and for the general public.

4. Nutrition training programs for nutrition personnel and other members of the health care team who are involved in public health, and in maternal and child nutrition.

The Bureau of Community Health Services administers various health services programs, many of which provide funding for nutrition programs and projects in urban and rural areas. These programs include:

— Maternal and Child Health program (MCH), mandated by Title V of the Social Security Act, offers health care services to mothers and children through formula grants to State Maternal and Child Health and Crippled Children's agencies.

— Community Health Centers (CHC) program, originally developed for community-based urban projects, now operates in conjunction with Rural Health Initiative Program to serve rural areas also. Grant funds are available to support supplemental health services to meet the needs of the community. The regulations include nutritional assessment and referral as part of the minimum set of services to be provided for preventive health. Supplemental health services incude nutrition education.

— Rural Health Initiative (RHI) provides grants to aid in the development of comprehensive health care services for the underserved in rural areas.

— Appalachian Health Program, administered by the Appalachian Regional Commission and the Public Health Service, is designed to provide Appalachian communities with assistance to improve health and nutrition services.

— Family Health Centers, modeled after the projects of CHC, use a prepaid, per capita system of finance. They offer a prescribed package of benefits to people in medically underserved areas.

— Migrant Health (MH) program provides funds for projects designed to promote health services for migrant and seasonal farm workers and their families. Nutritional services are part of the preventive health services in the primary health service package; they may also be part of the supplemental health services.

— Family Planning Program (Title X, Public Health Service Act) provides support to assist individuals to have a free choice in planning their families; services in the program include education, counseling, medical, and social services. Nutrition is part of the total package of services.

— Comprehensive Public Health Services provides financial assistance to aid states to determine and implement appropriate community, mental, and environmental health services.

— National Health Service Corps (NHSC) provides for the training and laboratory assignments of health professionals to rural, medically underserved areas. The Corps now includes nutritionists among the ranks of health professionals who will be trained and assigned to medically underserved areas.

2. *Bureau of Indian Health Service (BIHS).* The Indian Health Service is responsible for planning and implementing total health programs for American Indians, including environmental, health, health education, maternal and child health, and well-child clinics. The BIHS also works in training Indians for health professional and paraprofessional programs.

3. *Bureau of Quality Assurance (BQA).* The Bureau of Quality Assurance works to ensure the quality of the HSA's activities; it also works with the SSA and the HCFA to develop standards and policies for these agencies. BQA is also responsible for the Professional Standards Review Organization Program (PSRO), which requires physicians to form and operate local PSRO to review the health care services provided by their fellow peers.

4. *Bureau of Medical Services (BMS).* The Bureau of Medical Services operates Public Health Service hospitals and clinics, conducts basic and clinical research and training to health professionals, and works to improve national emergency medical services.

National Institutes of Health (NIH)

Most of the nutrition research activities of the U.S. Department of Health, Education, and Welfare come from the National Institutes of Health. The mission of NIH is to improve the health of the American population through the support of biomedical research into etiology, prevention, and cure of conditions such as cancer, heart and lung diseases, allergies, tooth decay, and neurological problems. The research is conducted in the laboratories and clinics of the National Institutes in Bethesda, Maryland, and in various universities and medical centers throughout the nation. Studies are also conducted overseas in areas where malnutrition is present in large population groups.

NIH research can be classified as related to normal nutrition, nutritional disorders, and nutrition in disease.[19]

Normal nutrition — research projects deal with such topics as digestion and absorption of nutrients; hunger, satiety, and food intake; appetite regulation; biochemistry and metabolism of nutrients; interrelationships of various nutrients; nutritional requirements; and the functions of nutrients such as fiber, vitamins, carbohydrates, fats, trace elements, proteins, and amino acids.

Nutritional disorders — topics studied include malnutrition, nutrition deficiency disease, and obesity.

Nutrition in disease — this research studies the relationship of nutrition to specific disease states such as diabetes, hypertension, cancer, heart disease, endocrine problems, and inborn errors of metabolism. Also studied is the role of diet modification in the treatment of particular diseases.

In addition to these kinds of research, the NIH also conducts research into the development of improved research methods and techniques for the assay of specific nutrients and for the determination of nutritional status.

Training programs are also sponsored by NIH. The Institutes aim to train research manpower in nutrition so that skilled investigators can then follow careers in health science academic and research environments. Research training grants and fellowship awards support these training activities.

The NIH feels a strong responsibility to communicate new research findings to the scientific community and to the public. To this end, nutrition education efforts are undertaken. Publications such as "Facts about Nutrition," "How a Mother Affects Her Unborn Baby," "Malnutrition and Learning," and "Nutrition and Society" are available for the public. An example of a professional publication is the handbook on the dietary management of the hyperlipidemias; more than 2 million copies have been distributed to educate nutritionists, physicians, and patients.

Health Resources Administration (HRA)

The mission of the HRA is to offer leadership in the standards for, and the distribution of, health resources and manpower. The HRA plans to place increased emphasis on human nutrition in medical education through support designed to improve and broaden the scope and effectiveness of training in primary care.

HRA is engaged in the training and education of community health workers, such as those in public health nutrition, health education, and health administration and planning. Training in dietetics is supported through the encouragement of coordinated integrated programs at the undergraduate level.

The National Center for Health Statistics of the HRA implements programs designed to gather needed health statistics and data. Data are collected, analyzed, and disseminated to reflect the health and nutritional status, needs, and resources of the population. The first national survey of nutritional status (HANES I) and the follow-up (HANES II) are the responsibility of this division of HRA.

Health planning is a major mission of HRA, through the Bureau of Health Planning and the Bureau of Health Facilities Financing, Compliance, and Conversion (BHFFCC). The HRA is working to develop a national network of state and local health planning agencies to plan and identify health services needed by individual communities in the United States.

Center for Disease Control (CDC)

The Center for Disease Control is charged with protecting public health by providing guidance in the prevention and control of disease and the promotion of health. The CDC administers programs to this end, provides consultation and aid in improving the standards of clinical laboratories and research, and administers a national program of research and education in health. The CDC has supported and worked with the Health Resources Administration's (HRA) HANES projects by providing the principal health laboratory and analyzing much of the data. The nutrition surveillance activities of CDC are described on page 127.

Food and Drug Administration (FDA)

The Food and Drug Administration is a regulatory body designed to assist and ensure citizen compliance with federal legislation. The FDA administers parts of the Public Health Service Act; the Federal Food, Drug, and Cosmetic Act; the Fair Packaging and Labeling Act; the Federal Hazardous Substances Act; the Import Milk Act; the Filled Milk Act; the Federal Caustic Poison Act; and the Flammable Fabric Acts.

There is a broad variety of functions and responsibilities charged to the FDA. Some are:[20]

1. Clear new drugs for safety and effectiveness before they are marketed.
2. Establish safety tolerances for food additives, pesticide residues, and color additives.
3. Establish standards of identity, quality, and container fill for food products.
4. Inspect factories, warehouses, and distributors.
5. Sample and examine interstate and imported shipments.
6. Conduct research.
7. Assist in the interchange of scientific information.
8. Work with state and local agencies on consumer protection matters.
9. Conduct consumer education and information programs.
10. Prevent the use of unfair or deceptive methods of packaging or labeling.
11. Work with industry to promote voluntary compliance.
12. Test drugs and food chemical additives before they are sold.
13. Evaluate labeling and safety of household products containing hazardous substances and prevent the sale of items that are too hazardous for home use.
14. Evaluate state shellfish sanitation programs.
15. Review the design of sanitary systems for new interstate conveyances and support facilities.
16. Provide educational dissemination of scientific information to public health professionals, educational institutions, and other government agencies.
17. Oversee food and nutrition labeling program.

These functions are performed to advance three goals:[21]

1. Assure that the North American public is able to benefit from sound technology.

2. Work with other public and private agencies to increase the quality, safety, and nutritional content of the food supply.

3. Stimulate public awareness of the need for good nutrition and determine how nutritional information can be most appropriately conveyed to the American public.

The FDA is the primary agency responsible for regulating the nutritional safety of the nation's food supply. More than 50 regulations directly affecting the safety and quality of the food supply have been promulgated by the FDA. These regulations have dealt with such topics as the standards of identity for enriched flour and bread, the addition of vitamin A to margarine, and special diet foods. Some of the rules and regulations promulgated by the FDA include:[22]

1. Filth guidelines that define the levels of natural filth allowed in foods marketed in interstate commerce.

2. Pesticide guidelines defining allowed levels in foods.

3. Heavy metal and other environmental contaminant guidelines.

4. Aflatoxin guidelines.

5. Standards of identity guidelines that define a standardized food product in terms of how it can be produced and what is allowed in it.

6. Packaging guidelines defining the type, size, and labeling information required on food packages.

7. Guidelines to ensure safe thermal food processing.

8. Good manufacturing practice guidelines defining methods to be used in food processing to ensure food safety and wholesomeness.

9. Hazard analysis and critical control point rules developed to assure a safe product. The procedure involves process analysis to identify those critical points at which pathogen contamination could occur.

10. Nutritional guidelines to define what should be on food product labels relative to the nutritive value of the food.

11. Recall procedures, that is, guidelines designed to help retrieve food from the market channels if it is in violation of the Food, Drug, and Cosmetic Act.

12. Common or usual name regulations that provide that the producer use a product name that accurately describes the product; and that pictures on package labels not be misleading.

The FDA, in the past decade, has greatly expanded its nutrition education activities. Nutritional labeling, based on the FDA-originated U.S. recommended daily allowance (USRDA) method, is one technique that has been used to disseminate nutrition information. The FDA has been involved in conducting consumer education relative to the use of food labeling through public service announcements and other educational systems.

The FDA has ten regional offices; there are 19 district offices and 97 resident inspection stations in the United States. Consumers can take an active part in the regulatory activities of FDA by reporting a food that is believed to be mislabeled, unsanitary, or harmful. The address and telephone number of the closest FDA office can be found in the telephone directory under the heading "U.S. Government, Department of Health, Education, and Welfare, Food and Drug Administration."

U.S. Office of Education (OE)[23]

Two programs are administered by the U.S. Office of Education that include nutritional components: (1) Vocational Education (Part F, Consumer and Homemaking Education and Follow Through) and (2) Demonstration Projects to Improve School Health and Nutrition Services for Children from Low-Income Families. The latter has been consolidated in Elementary and Secondary Education Act (ESEA), Title IV.

Title IV of the Elementary and Secondary Education Act is a consolidated program that provides grants to state departments of education according to state populations of children aged 5 to 17.

Under this program, nutrition education is provided for the following:[23]

— Libraries, learning resources, media, materials, counseling, and evaluation; funds are provided to local education agencies on a formula basis; local agencies then decide how the money will be used.

— Supplementary educational centers and services designed to provide needed educational services and to aid in the development of school programs.

— Supporting demonstration projects to improve nutrition and health services in schools serving large numbers of disadvantaged families.

— strengthening the state and local educational leadership resources and helping these groups to improve programs designed to meet state and local school district educational needs.

The projects under Title IV are demonstration projects of a developmental nature and have the potential for greatly improving the nutritional knowledge and food habits of schoolchildren. A case in point is an elementary school in Hamilton, Ohio, which had the lowest attendance rate of any school in the school district, a high incidence of problems such as dental caries, and very low test scores, as compared with other schools in the district.

School administrators developed a broad and comprehensive approach to health education, with a focus on nutrition in the school. By working with students as well as with parents and community, the educators found that they could increase nutrition knowledge and also implement a program of sound nutrition. The program was an integrated one, relating breakfast and health programs to the health curriculum to bolster the health services and the physical fitness program.

Support included not only funds from Title IV but also school breakfast and lunch, technical assistance from the USDHEW, and local industry support. One academic year after the start of the program, the school went from the lowest quintile in attendance in the district to the highest quintile. Test scores were also greatly improved. The administration attributed the program's success to the nutritional program and the relationship that it had to the comprehensive school health and physical fitness program.[23]

Other programs in the OE provide for nutrition- and health-related activities. Among them are: Consumer Education, Community Education, Environmental Education, Career Education, and Right to Read. The possibility of local emphasis on nutrition in its various programs exists. Thus far, the concern with nutrition has been minimal because nutrition is not viewed as a top priority, and hence resources have not been available to offer leadership in nutrition education at the federal level. There is currently no coordination point within the OE to organize, monitor, and advocate nutrition-related programs.

FEDERAL TRADE COMMISSION (FTC)

The Federal Trade Commission (FTC) was established by Congress in 1914 as an independent administrative agency, its purpose being to foster effective consumer protection in cooperation with local, state, and other federal agencies. The FTC also conducts educational programs and provides assistance to other agencies in developing education programs to prevent deceptive advertising, foster compliance, and prevent unfair business practices.

The original 1914 law, the Federal Trade Commission Act, was enacted to preserve competition in industry. The FTC, as first created, was to act as a source of information and advice to business and as a source of bad publicity on the effects of trusts and monopolies. In 1938 the Wheeler-Tea Amendment gave the FTC power to move against "deceptive" business practices, thus protecting consumers from false advertising.[1] Other congressional and court decisions have given the FTC more power and control in the area of consumer protection.[24-26]

The goal of the FTC is to help consumers to make informed choices. The principal activities of the FTC, relative to food and nutrition, include:

— The promotion of free and fair competition in interstate commerce.

— The prevention of false or deceptive advertisements of consumer products including food.

— The prevention of discriminations in price.

— The regulation of packaging and labeling on consumer commodities within the preview of the Fair Packaging and Labeling Act to prevent deception and fraud.

— Formal litigation resulting in orders against offenders.

Of great current interest are the FTC efforts to restrict deceptive television advertising to children. This is discussed in greater detail in Chapter 12.

U.S. DEPARTMENT OF COMMERCE (DOC)

The National Marine Fisheries Service is engaged in a program to develop and provide basic and applied information on the use of fish as human food. This research program includes studies on seafood processing into nutritious and acceptable food, studies on nutrient content and composition of seafood products, and studies on how seafood can be used to provide nutrition and eating pleasure in the diet.

Much research is being undertaken to determine practical and efficient ways to obtain high-protein products or concentrate from fish and then to use these in acceptable food products.

VETERANS ADMINISTRATION (VA)

Human nutrition research has been a component of the VA Department of Medicine and Surgery programs. The scope, purpose, and goals of VA-supported nutritional research is expressed in the following general statement of VA objectives:

> The mission of the Department of Medicine and Surgery of the VA is to provide quality medical care to eligible veterans. Research within the Department aims to improve the care by increasing, directly or indirectly, the capacity to deliver such care. The VA thus supports research by its professional staff that is directly applicable to patient care and research that is more basic, indirectly improves medical care, and supports the work of the professional staff.[27]

The VA also includes a service function in terms of the VA hospitals. The nutrition component of the VA hospitals is normally a very active one, being involved in patient assessment, counseling, and education as well as in research and food service.

U.S. DEPARTMENT OF DEFENSE (DOD)

The role of the DOD in human nutrition is summarized by the following quotation:

> The United States Government, through its various branches, has contributed much of value to the science of nutrition. The War Department and the Navy Department, in their efforts to secure the most satisfactory diet for the soldiers and the sailors, have collected a great deal of information and conducted many investigations which have to do with the subject of dietetics.[28]

The DOD supports human nutrition research projects, primarily in the areas of nutrition requirements, diet, and disease, and food composition studies.

Community Services Administration (CSA)

The Community Services Administration, originally the Office of Economic Opportunity, administers the Community Food and Nutrition

Program (CFNP). Nutrition programs are funded through community action agencies, other community groups, Indian tribal councils, and so on. The CFNP attempts to provide effective and relevant nutrition education to low-income populations at the community level.

The CFNP is designed to:

> provide, on an emergency basis, directly or by delegation of authority . . . financial assistance for the provisions of such supplies and services, nutritional foodstuffs, and related services as may be necessary to counteract conditions of starvation or malnutrition among the poor. Such assistance may be provided by way of supplement to such other assistance as may be extended under the provisions of other Federal programs, and may be used to extend and broaden such programs to serve economically disadvantaged individuals and families where such services are not now provided . . . [29]

The focus is on linking the needy with opportunities to improve their nutritional status. The CSA is an advocate for needed changes to improve the use of existing nutrition programs and provides funds for outreach, education, and counseling that are relevant to participation in federally funded nutrition programs. The CSA also tries to represent the interests of the low-income poor in matters related to public policy.

A suggested way to meet the nutritional needs of the poor is through Community Action Agencies (CAAs), which are an urban-rural network of community-based agencies concerned with meeting the needs of the low-income poor in such areas as housing, food, jobs, education, social service, and early childhood development. CAAs have demonstrated their effectiveness in dealing with these needs and are thus appropriate channels to provide nutritional services to meet the needs of low-income populations on a national basis.[30]

U.S. DEPARTMENT OF STATE — AGENCY FOR INTERNATIONAL DEVELOPMENT (AID)

AID is responsible for carrying out U.S. programs of assistance to underdeveloped nations. The Office of Nutrition and Technical Assistance, acts as a source of information, technical assistance, and resources for other divisions of AID in the design, implementation, and evaluation of nutrition program activities in developing nations.

AID emphasizes development assistance for areas where critical problems affect the majority of the population. Areas of focus include food and nutrition, agricultural research, population planning and health, education and human resources development, and Food for Peace (the U.S. food aid program under PL 480 that attempts to combat hunger and malnutrition).

Food and nutrition activities aim to "alleviate starvation, hunger, and malnutrition by means of agriculture, nutrition, and rural development programs, to provide basic services for poor people by enhancing their capacity for self-help, and to increase agricultural production in those countries with the lowest per capita income. . . . "[1] Other activities attempt to assist the productivity and income of rural poor by promoting labor-intensive, small-scale agriculture and by supporting marketing, financial, and development institutions.

OTHER FEDERAL GROUPS DEALING WITH NUTRITION INFORMATION

The *Federal Information Center (FIC) Program*, a branch of the General Services Administration, operates 37 centers in major metropolitan areas; it provides toll-free telephone linkages to 37 other cities.

The mission of this program is to encourage and help the public to identify the federal agency that is best able to resolve a problem or answer a question dealing with federal services. The FIC centers are also to provide information about certain local, state, and regional activities.[1]

The *Federal Intercommunications in Nutrition Group (FICIN)* is an informal group of people in "responsible positions" who are committed to nutrition-related activities. The objective of the FICIN is to provide a forum for mutual information exchange on programs and to plan for future work, research, and coordination. FICIN representatives include the National Institutes of Health, the Health Resources Administration, the Food and Drug Administration, Agricultural Research, the Agency for International Development, and the Federal Trade Commission.

SOME QUASI-GOVERNMENT AGENCIES[31]

A number of quasi-governmental agencies are concerned with nutrition-related activities. A quasi-governmental agency is a nongovernmental agency that, because of its work and activity, appears to be a governmental agency. Such agencies have charters from the government, often perform specific, officially mandated government activities, and may receive support from private as well as federal sources.

National Research Council (NRC)

One of the most significant quasi-governmental agencies relative to nutrition is the National Research Council, a branch of the National Academy of Sciences. NRC was established in 1863 under President Lincoln for the purpose of serving as a federal governmental advisor for science, technology, research, and reporting.

The National Research Council seeks to stimulate and support efforts of individual scientists and to coordinate studies of broad-based national and international problems. To this end, the NRC is involved in arranging conferences, technical committees, surveys, and scientific data collection and analysis; sponsoring scientific and technical publications and research organizations; and administering funds for research and education.

Food and Nutrition Board (FNB).

A branch of the NRC, the FNB was organized in 1940 to advise in the areas of nutritional needs. FNB activities include the preparation of Recommended Dietary Allowances (RDAs). The initial RDAs were developed in

1941 and are revised about every five years. The Food and Nutrition Board is composed of 15 members who are prominent in the area of nutrition. The board evaluates nutritional research, promotes wise food habits among the U.S. public, evaluates food safety and dietary standards, and recommends maternal and infant nutrition.[32]

American National Red Cross (ARC).

The Red Cross is another quasi-governmental agency operated under a federal charter for the purpose of providing voluntary relief and communication between the North American people and the armed forces and for providing national and international emergency relief services.

Although the ARC is primarily associated with disaster and emergency services, it is also engaged in various activities designed to promote health and to prevent diseases. Programs are developed with a view toward local community needs and resources and include community preparedness, emergency health, and rehabilitation aid.

Activities of particular interest to those in the nutrition field are quantity food service under emergency conditions and the provision of public education and advice in food and nutrition.[1]

SOME FOUNDATIONS[31]

According to *The Foundation Directory*, a foundation is defined as

a nongovernmental, nonprofit organization, with funds and program managed by its own trustees or directors, and established to maintain or aid social, educational, charitable, religious, or other activities, serving the common welfare, primarily through the making of grants.[33]

T. Parrish simplifies this by suggesting that it is a "nongovernmental institution which makes grants."[34]

Foundations are distinguished from other charitable organizations in that they receive funds from a single person or small group, their major function being to provide grants rather than to engage in other activities.[34] Thus, they perform a service as well as a research function.

A guide to existing foundations and their research and grant orientations is *The Foundation Directory*.[33] According to the Foundation Center, there are some 23,000 foundations that distribute funds in a variety of ways and at different time periods.

Many foundations focus on health promotion and are interested in nutrition-related activities. The following discussion briefly reviews certain foundations of particular interest to nutrition advocates.

Nutrition Foundation

The Nutrition Foundation was founded in 1941 to promote education and research in nutritional science. The stated mission of the foundation is "to take an active role in the stimulation of public education programs, in focusing objective scientific attention on current issues in food safety and nutrition and in hammering out research priorities."[35] Priority research topics include infant and pregnancy nutrition considerations and food safety considerations. In addition to sponsoring research, the foundation also sponsors various seminars and conferences.

Another prominent activity of the Foundation is the publication of the monthly *Nutrition Reviews,* a journal which contains authoritative reviews of current nutrition literature. The Foundation also publishes *Present Knowledge in Nutrition* and a monograph series.

American Dietetic Association Foundation

This foundation administers funds for awards, scholarships, research, and educational activities. The purpose is to advance "education and science in the fields of nutrition and dietetics . . . for the benefit of the public welfare and the improvement of the nutrition of human beings."[36]

American Home Economics Association Foundation

The foundation administers funds for scholarships and sponsors workshops, seminars, research, and the development of educational materials.[37]

Kellogg Foundation

This foundation offers aid for education and training programs, and has a primary interest in health promotion.[33] The particular concern of the Kellogg Foundation is the utilization of knowledge in areas of health, agriculture, and education. Current foundation-aided programs emphasize the preparation of nutrition professional education and human nutrition education to maintain or improve health. In 1972 the Foundation funded a Study Commission on Dietetics, which advocated a blending of the art and the science of nutrition in the education of health professionals.

Rockefeller Foundation

This is another foundation dedicated to promoting health and eliminating malnutrition and its consequences. A program of the Rockefeller Foundation, "Conquest of Hunger," is involved in trying to increase food production and in distributing this food to needy populations. Grants have been provided to a variety of fields including medical education, public health, medical and biological research, agricultural, and social sciences.[33]

Ford Foundation

The mission of the Ford Foundation is to advance public welfare through contributing to the solution of national and international problems. Grants, made principally to institutions, are for experimental, demonstration, and development efforts that show the potential of yielding significant advances.

Interests of the Ford Foundation include improving education in schools, colleges, and universities; training teachers and administrators; educational research; increasing educational opportunity; research in the environment and ecology; and international research and development assistance.[33]

Juvenile Diabetes Foundation

This foundation is a nationally accredited voluntary health agency founded to raise money for research on diabetes. Grants are provided for direct research and as postdoctoral fellowships. The foundation also provides services intended to help the diabetic, such as counseling, education, and group meetings.

VOLUNTARY AGENCIES

Many nongovernmental, voluntary organizations include nutrition-related activities in their programs and operations. Such organizations may be health agencies, professional organizations, business and industry organizations, or private foundations.

The nutritionist should be familiar with these agencies and with the nutrition component of their programs. The nutrition professional may be influential in strengthening nutritional activities. The nutritionist may frequently obtain valuable assistance or resources from these agencies. Another reason for the importance of close working relationships between agencies and nutritionists is the opportunity for the referral of clients to the resources provided through many voluntary agencies. Finally, the nutrition community may have the opportunity to join forces with strong agency groups to achieve political support and to gain influence into the nutrition policy-making process. It is to the mutual advantage of the various agencies and the nutrition community to combine their efforts and to work for common goals.

A voluntary health agency has been defined as a

> private nonprofit organization, chartered and licensed by an appropriate government agency, conducting activities designed to mitigate a specific health problem, and funded by contributions from individual citizens or private organizations. Most voluntary agencies have national organizations with state affiliates and local branches.[31]

The National Health Council has established operational standards and guidelines that national voluntary agencies must meet. Such standards require the agency to be directed by a board of volunteers drawn from a wide geographical area. The agencies are to obtain technical guidance for specific activities from professionals with related expertise so that the public good may be best served.[31]

D. Wilner et al. suggest that voluntary health agencies have three basic orientations: concern for the effects of a specific disease (such as heart, cancer, diabetes), concern for a particular part of the body (heart, stomach), or concern for a vulnerable population group (such as pregnant women, the elderly, the retarded individual).[31,38] The activities of different health agencies may often be indirectly related to nutrition through the education and promotion of health and the prevention of disease. Some agencies are more directly concerned with nutrition. Activities of agencies whose activities are widespread and relate especially to nutrition are summarized in Appendix IV.

STATE-LEVEL NUTRITION AGENCIES

Health in the United States is primarily a state-administered function. Nowhere in the U.S. Constitution is there any authorization for federal involvement in either health or nutrition. Thus, the state has great responsibility for health matters.

At the state level, the State Health Planning and Development agencies (mandated by the National Health Planning and Resources Development Act of 1974, see pages 35-38) assume much responsibility for nutrition programs and services.

Much of the nutrition-related activity at the state level emanates from the state health department. There are 50 state health departments or organizations with different titles that have responsibility for public health. This responsibility involves some of the following activities.[39]

Examination of state health problems and responses to such problems.

Provision of financial support to local health departments.

Collection of health statistics.

Establishment of health personnel qualifications and health facility standards.

Coordination and supervision of local health-related activities.

Collection and dissemination of information for health promotion and the prevention of disease.

Formulation of plans to meet state health needs.

State-level public health programs concerned with health promotion include those programs that prevent communicable disease in addition to maternal and child health programs, environmental health activities, alcohol and drug abuse programs, and rehabilitation at the community level through cooperation with neighborhood health centers and other primary, secondary, or tertiary care facilities.[31]

State health departments vary tremendously in power; the majority of them formulate state health codes and regulations, but some have the duty to conduct health studies or have supervisory power over local health boards.

Various state health agencies function differently in response to varying regional needs. The health programs operated at each state level also vary according to needs, demands, and available resources.

In general, state health departments are responsible, not for direct nutritional services, but for the provision of plans, development of policies, program planning, implementation and evaluation, legislation, and setting of quality criteria and standards. They are also responsible for providing technical support, consultation, and financial support; conducting research related to various needs and problems; enforcing state regulations; and coordinating various local and community level programs and the basic health and nutrition-related activities, such as assessment, surveillance, and education. In addition, state health departments provide linkages between the federal government, national programs, and local communities.[31]

Nutritional activities may be found in various state administrative agency units. For example, the nutrition component for the elderly may be found in the State Office of Aging, and the nutrition component for the School Lunch Program may be found in the State Department of Education. The state health departments typically employ nutrition specialists who work with local health departments to foster nutrition programs and to improve the provision of nutrition services.

Most state-level nutrition units have public health nutrition directors. These directors have formed an Association of State and Territorial Public Health Nutrition Directors (ASTPHND).[31,37]

ASTPHND, founded in 1953, is affiliated with the Association of State and Territorial Health Officers (ASTHO). Its activities include those of communication, legislation, and public policy.

A recent study commissioned by the Office of Planning, Evaluation, and Legislation of the Health Resources Administration (HRA) was conducted to provide insights on the impact of specific federal health programs upon the health goals and activities at the state levels.[40]

Specific questions researched by the study were the following:

How supportive are federal health programs of the goals of individual states?

Do federal programs force individual states to go in directions to which they are opposed?

How do states use federal program assistance in reaching their goals?

The study found that state goals related to health were extremely varied, ranging from total absence of a stated goal, to goals precipitated by federal efforts, to well-formulated goals already established by the state.

The conclusion of the study noted that:

> states do not always have formulated goals; that the federal government does not always support one goal position to the exclusion of another; that federal impact is most successful in terms of agenda-setting — for beyond placing a goal on a state's agenda, federal influence is limited; that states are rarely "withering" under federal activity, for states tend to use the programs to support their own needs; and finally, that as PHS (Public Health Service) programs are formulated and implemented, recognition should be made of both the policy environment into which they will fit and the reactions and perceptions of elected state officials to administrative issues.[40]

This points up the importance of nutrition advocates' taking an active role in helping to formulate state goals and plans that are supportive of nutritional concerns. Nutrition professionals must assume the responsibility for the direction that the state public health nutrition department takes. Informed leadership and active participation in state-level activities can foster a strong nutrition component.

One example of the fruits borne by the efforts and input of dietetic professionals is the establishment of the Board of Nutrition for the state of Massachusetts. Responsibilities of the board include monitoring nutritional status of state residents, planning long-range nutrition programs, and reviewing, evaluating, and coordinating statewide nutrition programs. Members of the Massachusetts Dietetic Association were "credited with the major input in the 'tortuous legislative process' that brought the bill (five years in the drafting process) to fruition."[41]

There is also potential in states' joining together to advance common nutritional goals. Six northeastern states (Maine, Vermont, New Hampshire, Massachusetts, Rhode Island, and Connecticut) joined together to form the New England Nutrition Committee, the first regionwide food advocacy coalition in the United States. Early activities of the committee included the publication of a regionwide needs assessment, the channeling of training and technical assistance funds for the New England area, and the sponsoring of workshops on school breakfasts in member states.[42]

LOCAL AGENCIES

More than 16,000 full-time local health departments serve 25,000 counties and more than 300 cities in the nation. These departments differ greatly in their responsibilities and activities, in those to whom they are responsible, in the resources they command, and in the personnel and manpower who serve them. Many local health departments are concerned, at least indirectly, with the provision of nutritional care as they conduct assessments, control and prevent disease, educate the public on important health matters, and protect the health of the infants, mothers, and other particularly vulnerable groups.[39]

Local health departments are also involved in regional planning and in liaison with state health departments, as well as with other private and voluntary health agencies. Local health agencies include those of county and city agencies and those developed by the health systems agency for a given region.

In most cases, states delegate to local or county levels the authority to establish health agencies to serve the population within the area. Formal organization of these agencies and their relationships to the state vary. In some instances, the county agencies function as branches of the state government; in others they are autonomous agencies.

Although services provided by local health departments vary, they usually include preventing and controlling of communicable diseases or other preventable disease; rehabilitation; protecting the health of vulnerable groups, such as pregnant and lactating mothers, infants, and children; monitoring the quality of care provided in institutions such as hospitals and nursing homes; maintaining current vital statistics and records; and sponsoring other health programs.[31]

Local programs are often funded primarily by private means, frequently by churches. Because the resources of local programs tend to be limited, the coverage they provide is often narrow.

Nutrition councils are an example of local nutrition agencies. They are composed of nutrition professionals and exist in many local communities. The functions of nutrition councils include providing educational programs, sponsoring public seminars and awareness campaigns, and working to influence nutrition policies and education for the public, schools, and other health professionals.[43]

CONCLUSION

Numerous agencies, both public and private, are engaged in advancing nutrition goals and objectives. The federal agencies receive their program mandates from legislation passed by the Congress. Thus, their activities and programs are largely matters of general public social and health policy. The legislative process and ways to influence it are discussed in Chapter 15; Chapter 17 discusses federal food and nutrition programs, their administration, operation, and effectiveness.

USDA ADDRESSES

For more information on the U.S. Department of Agriculture, the address is:

U.S. Department of Agriculture
Independence Street (btw 12th and 14th Streets), SW
Washington, D.C.

Other USDA addresses include

U.S. Department of Agriculture (USDA)
Food and Nutrition Service
500 12th Street, SW
Washington, D.C.

National Agricultural Library
Baltimore Blvd.
Beltsville, Maryland

Consumer and Food Economics Institute
Hyattsville, Maryland

Animal and Plant Health Inspection Service
14th and Independence Street, SW
Washington, D.C.

Agricultural Research
Beltsville, Maryland

Community Services Administration (CSA)
1200 19th Street, NW
Washington, D.C.

THE FOOD AND NUTRITION SERVICE (FNS) REGIONAL OFFICES

To learn more about the Food and Nutrition Service Programs and activities in your state or region, contact the regional office in the region in which you reside.

New England Region, Food and Nutrition Service, USDA, 34 Third Avenue, Burlington, MA 01803: Connecticut, Maine, Massachusetts, New Hampshire, Rhode Island, Vermont.

Mid-Atlantic Region, Food and Nutrition Service, USDA, 1 Vahlsing Way, Robbinsville, NJ 08691: Delaware, District of Columbia, Maryland, New Jersey, New York, Pennsylvania, Puerto Rico, Virginia, Virgin Isl., W. Virginia.

Southeast Region, Food and Nutrition Service, USDA, 1100 Spring Street, N.W., Atlanta, GA 30309: Alabama, Florida, Georgia, Kentucky, Mississippi, North Carolina, South Carolina, Tennessee.

Midwest Region, Food and Nutrition Service, USDA, 536 South Clark Street, Chicago, IL 60605: Illinois, Indiana, Michigan, Minnesota, Ohio, Wisconsin.

Southwest Region, Food and Nutrition Service, USDA, 1100 Commerce Street, Room 5-C-30, Dallas, TX 75202: Arkansas, Louisiana, New Mexico, Okalahoma, Texas.

Mountain Plains Region, Food and Nutrition Service, USDA, Post Office Building, 1823 Stout Street, Denver, CO 80202: Colorado, Iowa, Kansas, Missouri, Montana, Nebraska, North Dakota, South Dakota, Utah, Wyoming.

Western Region, Food and Nutrition Service, USDA, 550 Kearney Street, Room 400, San Francisco, CA 94108: Alaska, American Somoa, Arizona, California, Guam, Hawaii, Idaho, Nevada, Oregon, Trust Territory, Washington.

DHEW ADDRESSES

For more specific information on the Office of the Assistant Secretary for Health or the Public Health Service, in general, write to the

Office of Public Affairs
Public Health Service
Room 17–22
5600 Fishers Lane
Rockville, Maryland 20852

Similarly, should you wish to take a closer look at the activities and responsibilities of any of the six PHS agencies, you may address inquiries directly to the agencies in which you are interested, at the addresses given:

Table 16–4
Public Health Service Regional Offices

Region	States	Address
I	Connecticut, Maine, Massachusetts New Hampshire, Rhode Island, Vermont	Regional Health Administrator John F. Kennedy Federal Bldg. Boston, Massachusetts 02203
II	New Jersey, New York, Puerto Rico, Virgin Islands	Regional Health Administrator 26 Federal Plaza New York, New York 10007
III	Delaware, District of Columbia, Maryland, Pennsylvania, Virginia, West Virginia	Regional Health Administrator P.O. Box 13716 Philadelphia, Pennsylvania 19101
IV	Alabama, Florida, Georgia, Kentucky, Mississippi, North Carolina, South Carolina	Regional Health Administrator 50 Seventh Street, N.E. Atlanta, Georgia 30323
V	Illinois, Indiana, Michigan, Minnesota, Ohio, Wisconsin	Regional Health Administrator 300 South Wacker Drive Chicago, Illinois 60606
VI	Arkansas, Louisiana, New Mexico, Oklahoma, Texas	Regional Health Administrator 1114 Commerce Street Dallas, Texas 75202
VII	Iowa, Kansas, Missouri, Nebraska	Regional Health Administrator 601 East 12th Street Kansas City, Missouri 64106
VIII	Colorado, Montana, North Dakota, South Dakota, Utah, Wyoming	Regional Health Administrator 19th & Stout Streets Denver, Colorado 80202
IX	American Samoa, Arizona, California, Guam, Hawaii, Nevada, Trust Territory of the Pacific Islands	Regional Health Administrator 50 Fulton Street San Francisco, California 94102
X	Alaska, Idaho, Oregon, Washington	Regional Health Administrator 1321 Second Avenue Seattle, Washington 98101

ADAMHA
Office of Communications and Public Affairs
Alcohol, Drug Abuse, and Mental Health Administration
Room 16-95
5600 Fishers Lane
Rockville, Maryland 20852

CDC
Office of Information
Center for Disease Control
Atlanta, Georgia 30333

FDA
Food and Drug Administration
HFI-10
5600 Fishers Lane
Rockville, Maryland 20852

HRA
Office of Communications
Health Resources Administration
Room 10A-31
5600 Fishers Lane
Rockville, Maryland 20852

HSA
Office of Communications and Public Affairs
Health Services Administration
Room 14A-55
5600 Fishers Lane
Rockville, Maryland 20852

NIH
Division of Public Information
National Institutes of Health
Building #1, Room 307
Bethesda, Maryland 20014

REFERENCES

1. *U.S. Government Manual.* Washington, D.C.: Government Printing Office, 1978.
2. U.S. Department of Agriculture. *USDA: Your United States Department of Agriculture,* Rept. No. PA-824. Washington, D.C., October 1977.
3. Food and Agriculture Act of 1977, P.L. 95-113, September 1977.
4. U.S. Department of Agriculture. The organization of S.E.A. (internal communication). Washington, D.C., December 15, 1977.
5. Bergland, R. *Statement in Observance of National Nutrition Week, March 4-10, 1979,* Rept. No. USDA 505-79. Washington, D.C.: U.S. Department of Agriculture, March 1979.
6. U.S. House Committee on Appropriations. *Agriculture and Related Agen-*

cies' Appropriations for 1976. Part 2. Agricultural Program. Washington, D.C.: Government Printing Office, 1975, p. 269.

7. Mertz, W. In U.S. Senate Select Committee on Nutrition and Human Needs, *Nutrition and Diseases, 1973. Part 2. Sugar in Diet, Diabetes, and Heart Diseases.* Washington, D.C.: Government Printing Office, 1973, p. 148.

8. Consumer and Food Economics Institute. *Organization and Program.* Hyattsville, Md.: U.S. Department of Agriculture, Agricultural Research Service, May 1977.

9. U.S. House Committee on Appropriations. *Agriculture and Related Agencies' Appropriations for 1976, op. cit.*, p. 468.

10. Nielson, J. Testimony before U.S. House Subcommittee on Domestic Marketing, Consumer Relations, and Nutrition. Washington, D.C.: Government Printing Office, October 1977.

11. Leidenfrost, N. B. Testimony before the U.S. House Subcommittee on Nutrition, Committee on Agriculture, Nutrition, and Forestry. Washington, D.C.: Government Printing Office, March 1977.

12. USDA's economics, statistics, and cooperatives agencies merged. *Nat'l Food Rev.* 5 (April 1978): 35.

13. Foreman, C. Quoted in *CNI Week. Rep.* 8 (1978): 4.

14. Comptroller General, Report to the Congress. *Informing the Public about Nutrition: Federal Agencies Should Do Better.* Washington, D.C.: General Accounting Office, March 22, 1978.

15. U.S. Department of Health, Education, and Welfare. *This Is HEW*, Rept. No. 0-256-465. Washington, D.C.: Government Printing Office, 1978.

16. Barclay, W. Legislative highlights. *J. Am. Diet. Assoc.* 71 (1977): 55.

17. U.S. Department of Health, Education, and Welfare. *Forward Plan for Health, FY 1978-82.* Washington, D.C.: Government Printing Office, 1976.

18. Lashof, J. C. Testimony before U.S. House Subcommittee on Domestic Marketing, Consumer Relations, and Nutrition, *op. cit.*, October 6, 1977.

19. Cooper, T. Testimony before the U.S. Senate Select Committee on Nutrition and Human Needs, *Diet Related to Killer Diseases.* Washington, D.C.: Government Printing Office, July 27, 1976.

20. Grant, J. D. Food and Drug Administration, in J. Mayer, ed., *U.S. Nutrition Policies in the Seventies.* San Francisco: W. H. Freeman, 1973, p. 208.

21. Kennedy, D. *U.S. Food and Nutrition Policy: Food and Drug Administration*, American Public Health Association Annual Meeting, Washington, D.C. 1977.

22. Labuza, T. P. *Food and Your Well-being.* St. Paul. West Publishing, 1977, pp. 337-351.

23. Relic, P. D. Testimony before U.S. House Subcommittee on Domestic Marketing, Consumer Relations, and Nutrition, *op. cit.*, October 6, 1977, p. 529.

24. Hunt, H. K. Advertising in the public interest: FTC influences. *Human Ecol. Forum* 4 (1974): 23-25.

25. Stone, A. *Economic Regulation and the Public Interest.* Ithaca, N.Y.: Cornell University, 1977.

26. Wehr, E. House/Senate committees propose changes in FTC. *Cong. Quar.* 23 (1977): 1156.

27. Hobson, L. B. Quoted in U.S. Senate Select Committee on Nutrition and Human Needs. *The Role of the Federal Government in Human*

Nutrition Research. Washington, D.C.: Government Printing Office, March 1976.

28. Langworthy, C. F., and R. D. Milner. *Investigations on the Nutrition of Man in the United States.* Washington, D.C.: Government Printing Office, 1904, p. 5.
29. U.S. Congress, Community Services Act, Sec. 222 (a) (5), 1974.
30. Ashley, I. R. Communication with U.S. House Subcommittee on Domestic Marketing, Consumer Relations, and Nutrition, November 15, 1977.
31. Obert, J. *Community Nutrition.* New York: John Wiley, 1977.
32. National Academy of Sciences. Food and Nutrition Board (pamphlet). Washington, D.C., January 1979.
33. Foundation Center. *The Foundation Directory,* 5th ed. New York: Columbia University Press, 1975.
34. Parrish, T. Cited in J. Obert, *op. cit.*
35. Nutrition Foundation announces new goals and new leadership. *Nutr. Rev.* 30 (1972): 1.
36. American Dietetic Association. *All about the A.D.A.* Chicago, undated.
37. National Organizations of the U.S. *Encyclopedia of Associations,* 9th ed. Detroit: Gale Research, 1975.
38. Wilner, D. M., R. P. Walkley, and L. S. Goerke. *Introduction to Public Health.* New York: Macmillan, 1973.
39. Gray, S. E. *Community Health Today.* New York: Macmillan, 1978.
40. Miller and Byrne, Inc. *Final Report: Evaluations of the Impact of the PHS Programs on State Health Goals and Activities,* Publ. No. (HRA) 77-604. Washington, D.C.: U.S. Department of Health, Education, and Welfare, 1977.
41. Board of Nutrition established in Massachusetts. *J. Am. Diet. Assoc.* 66 (1975): 241.
42. Community Nutrition Institute. CFNP Rept. No. 1, January 5, 1978, p. 3.
43. Nutrition Council as a tool for change: a workshop in effective action. *J. Nutr. Educ.* 6 (1974): i–iv.

17

Federal food and nutrition programs

Reader Objectives

After completing this chapter, the reader should be able to
1. State the target group and purpose for the following nutrition programs: WIC, School Breakfast and School Lunch programs, Food Stamp Program, and National Nutrition Program for the Elderly.
2. Evaluate the effectiveness of federal nutrition programs in terms of general expenditures, participation, and nutritional benefits.
3. Describe five general problems with federal food programs.

Today's nutrition programs are a great source of pride to me and, I hope, to the entire nation. They are our real national defense. I thought many, many times that we need a new definition of national defense. I read in the Washington Post *this morning that the administration had decided to go ahead with another new generation of missiles, the so-called MX system, the one that will be operated on long, 20-mile segments of railroads buried underground. It's going to cost us $30 to $32 billion to erect that new system.*

Now, recognizing that we live in a dangerous world and we have to have an adequate national defense, I couldn't help but think what we could do with that $32 billion over the next few years, if it could be invested in the nutrition, the health, the education, the housing, energy sources for the American people. It might very well turn out that, invested in programs of that kind to strengthen the domestic fiber of this country, we would be a stronger force in the world than adding to the nuclear stockpile.

— Senator George McGovern

INTRODUCTION — HISTORICAL PERSPECTIVE

Although feeding and nutrition programs in the United States date back to the early 1900s, most federal nutrition programs as they are known today have been largely the result of attacks on poverty and malnutrition that were made in the 1960s. Many events of this time and of the following years helped to shape current programs. Significant among these events were:

— Examination into the extent of poverty and malnutrition by the Citizen's Board of Inquiry.

— Establishment and work of the U.S. Senate Select Committee on Nutrition and Human Needs.

— Work of the White House Conference on Food, Nutrition, and Health.

A brief historical perspective on these events will serve as an introduction into a more specific examination of certain federal food and nutrition programs.

In April 1967 the Subcommittee on Employment, Manpower, and Poverty of the Senate Committee on Labor and Public Welfare, as a section of its analysis of the war on poverty, held public hearings and conducted a field inspection trip in Mississippi to hear and see, firsthand, the extent and severity of malnutrition and hunger in the Delta counties.[1,2] As a result, the subcommittee noted conditions "that can only be described as shocking and which we believe constitute an emergency."[1]

The subcommittee requested that the secretary of the USDA send a department inspection team to make a personal field study of the situation. The findings were summarized as follows.[1]

1. There is clear evidence of acute malnutrition and hunger among many families in the Mississippi Delta.

2. Many families subsist without discernible income and cannot afford to meet the minimum purchase requirements for food stamps.

3. Many low-income families also have serious difficulty in meeting the purchase requirements for food stamps.

To support these findings, the subcommittee cited a specific example of a family with 13 children who ". . . told us that they had had grits and molasses for breakfast, no lunch, and would have beans for supper." Some of the children were unable to attend school because they did not have shoes, they had enlarged stomachs (the result of protein-calorie malnutrition) and chronic sores around the mouth, and they were very apathetic and lethargic — "all of which are the tragic evidence of serious malnutrition."[1]

A team of medical doctors reported their findings and recommendations, which resulted from their personal observations and medical examinations of rural families and children in six Mississippi counties. Their conclusions were stated as follows:

> In sum we saw children who are hungry and who are sick — children for whom hunger is a daily fact of life and sickness in many forms, an inevitability. We do not want to quibble over words, but "malnutrition" is not quite what we found; the boys and girls we saw were hungry — weak, in pain, sick; their lives are being shortened; they are, in fact, visibly and predictably losing their health, their energy, their spirits. They are suffering from hunger and disease and directly or indirectly they are dying from them — which is exactly what "starvation" means. . . . It is unbelievable to us that a nation as rich as ours, with all its technological and scientific resources has to permit thousands and thousands of children to go hungry.[2]

In April 1968 the Citizens Board of Inquiry published *Hunger, U.S.A.* The report noted that the investigation had revealed:

> Substantial numbers of new-born, who survive the hazards of birth and live through the first month, die between the second month and their second birthday from causes which can be traced directly and primarily to malnutrition;
>
> Protein deprivation between the ages of 6 months and a year and one-half causes permanent and irreversible brain damage to some young infants;
>
> Nutritional anemia, stemming primarily from protein deficiency and iron defi-

ciency, was commonly found in percentages ranging from 30 to 70 per cent among children from poverty backgrounds;

Teachers report children who come to school without breakfast, who are too hungry to learn, and in such pain that they must be taken home or sent to the school nurse;

Mother after mother in region after region reported that the cupboard was bare . . .

Doctors personally testified to seeing case after case of premature death, infant deaths, and vulnerability to secondary infection, all of which were attributable to or indicative of malnutrition;

In some communities people band together to share the little foods that provide inadequate sustenance.[3]

The report went on to charge that there was a "shocking absence of exact knowledge in this country about the extent and severity of malnutrition", that federal food programs were not successfully reaching the poor, and finally that ". . . hunger and malnutrition in a country of abundance must be seen as consequences of a political and economic system that spends billions to remove food from the market, to limit production, to retire land from production, to guarantee and sustain profits for large producers of basic crops."[3] The report was an impassioned plea for action against hunger and malnutrition in the United States. Response to the report was generally that of incredulity, anger, and denial.

The airing of the CBS documentary "Hunger in America" and the publication by the Committee on School Lunch Participation of a booklet entitled *Their Daily Bread* added fuel to the fire and provoked a broad variety of responses from politicians, health and medical professionals, and farm leaders.[4,5]

The Senate recognized a need for congressional response to such a national situation, and, as a result, 39 senators from both parties cosponsored a Senate resolution (S. Res. 281) introduced by Senator George McGovern asking that the executive branch establish a select committee to report back to the Senate "legislation necessary to establish a coordinated program or programs which will assure every U.S. resident adequate food, medical assistance, and other basic necessities of life and health."[6]

On July 30, 1968, the resolution was amended and agreed to, and the Select Committee on Nutrition and Human Needs was thus established. The committee was charged with the mandate for determining

1. The extent and causes of hunger and malnutrition in the United States, including educational, health, welfare, and other matters related to malnutrition.

2. The effectiveness of food programs designed to reach citizens who lack adequate quantity or quality of food.

3. The means by which this nation can bring an adequate supply of nutritious food and other related necessities to every American.

4. The divisions of responsibility and authority within Congress and the executive branch to assure that every resident of the United States

has adequate food, medical assistance, and the other basic related necessities of life and health.

5. The degree of additional federal action desirable in these areas.

The U.S. Senate Select Committee on Nutrition and Human Needs focused attention on the extent and effect of hunger and malnutrition, the effectiveness and the need for reform of federal food assistance programs, the development of a national nutrition policy, basic nutrition research, preventive health care, and the relationship of U.S. food and nutrition to the world food crisis. Hearings, staff studies, legislative activities, and committee recommendations resulted from the committee work. The Select Committee went out of existence in 1977.

Another part of the federal response to the identification of large-scale nutritional problems in the United States was the convening of the White House Conference of Food, Nutrition, and Health on December 2–4, 1969, in Washington, D.C. The conference was called by President Nixon to advise the president, the Congress, and the North American people on the formulation of national policy designed to eliminate poverty and malnutrition resulting from economic deprivation, and also to improve the nutritional status of the North American people.[7,8]

Membership of the conference, numbering nearly 5,000, was as broad as possible. University professors and students, medical professionals and their patients, labor leaders, factory workers, businessmen, women's rights representatives, and over 400 of the very poor themselves were included.

Jean Mayer was appointed to head and organize the conference, and Robert Choate was also greatly involved in the organization and activity of the conference. These two men were of dissimilar backgrounds and general objectives. Mayer, a Frenchman and Harvard professor, was well known for his research into the problems of obesity; his interest was in the relationship between nutrition and health. Choate, an engineer by profession, was very interested in the politics of hunger and in the elimination of poverty.[8]

During the summer of 1969 much preliminary work was done by 26 panels, working in 6 different sections and 8 different task forces. The concerns of the panels are summarized in Table 17–1. The panels were headed by academic and professional people — medical, industry, and university experts in nutrition and food. These panels were asked to draft recommendations for improving the nutritional status of the North American population. Panelists were appointed by conference leaders, primarily by Mayer. The recommendations of the panels were reviewed by the task forces that represented clergy, farmers, the poor themselves, and various social action and community groups.

From the outset there was an indecisiveness about the conference — it was unclear whether the mission of the conference was to improve the nutritional status of the North American people, in general, or to eliminate poverty-related hunger and malnutrition. Mayer and the academicians on the panels focused their attention on the first, and Choate invited and encouraged the participation of social action people, those who composed the task forces; their emphasis was on hunger and poverty.

Table 17-1

Sections and Work of the White House Conference on Food, Nutrition, and Health

Section	Concerns and Recommendations
The surveillance and evaluation of the North American people	Recommended that prime responsibility for identification of malnutrition in the United States be placed in the USDHEW.
Vulnerable groups	Considered programs for children, pregnant women, the elderly, and the sick. Emphasized that special programs could operate only with provision of free food stamps for very poor, or reasonable family allowance. Stressed importance of nutrition education in all programs.
Provision of food as it affects the consumer	Directed recommendations to simplify legislation, allow greater innovation in industry, and ensure greater consumer protection through establishment of standards.
Nutrition education	Stressed need for improved quality of education. Suggested more effective use of media and of community aides.
Food delivery and distribution systems	Suggested that the federal government provide managerial assistance for food distributors in poor rural and city areas to facilitate distribution of good food at low prices. Made recommendations concerning federal food distribution and assistance programs.
Voluntary action to help the poor	Various subgroups considered farmers, industry social action groups, health, agriculture, and labor organizations. Emphasized the need for urgent measures to combat poverty-related hunger and malnutrition. Stressed the need for improved outreach to poor, and the need to increase the purchasing power of the very poor.

Source: White House Conference on Food, Nutrition, and Health. *Final Report.* Washington, D.C.: Government Printing Office, 1970.

The conference thus attempted to deal with virtually all nutrition-related issues from food safety, health, and consumerism, to problems of the poor and disadvantaged and the solution of these problems.

In trying to be all things to all participants, the conference was not able to please any of the factions. The political debate and passionate public interest in the topic of hunger, which stimulated the conference in the first place, acted to further fuel the controversy and debate at the conference. Political controversies plagued the participants throughout the conference, and conference leaders felt that they were not given the support to carry out the job expected of them. Funds came from various sources but often from funds already allocated to other programs. The money from the USDHEW, for instance, came from funds previously allocated to the National Nutrition Survey. Needless to say, this caused great resentment from individuals who might otherwise have been very supportive of the conference. In addition, the issue of defining nutrition in terms of scope and depth had far-reaching political implications —

should the focus be on hunger and the poor, or on overnutrition and the average American citizen? The issue was never really resolved.

The final panel recommendations were reviewed by the largely lay, nonprofessional, nonscientific task forces. The social side of nutrition, the hunger issue, seemed to be predominant in the final recommendations.

The combined task force action/priority action program included five major points:

1. Declaration of a national emergency on hunger and malnutrition.

2. A guaranteed adequate income with a floor of $5,500 annually for a family of four.

3. Interim food programs.

4. Universal free school food programs, including breakfasts and lunches for all children.

5. Administrative responsibility for nutrition programs to be shifted from the USDA to the USDHEW.

On the last day of the conference all participants were presented with the statement of the task forces. The presentation was done in a rather confused and hasty manner. Most delegates had never had a chance to discuss the various proposals in their panels. A vote was called for the statement amid a loud cheer from the task force groups and the proposal was declared unanimously endorsed. There was no opportunity for debate.[8]

Mayer returned to Harvard after the conference, and responsibility for implementing the conference recommendations then fell to the President's Council for Urban Affairs. The recommendations were assigned to a subcommittee on food and nutrition made up of the secretaries of Agriculture, Health, Education, and Welfare, and Commerce — none of whom had strongly supported the conference.[8]

Panel Recommendations

At the request of Dr. Mayer, William D. Carey, chairman of the panel on Federal and State Administrative Structures of Monitoring Organizations, read the following statement at the plenary session.

I shall be brief.

I am not here to sum up what went on in all the workshops. It would take a greater talent than mine to do that.

But I believe that my co-chairmen would want me to make these points:

1. Hunger is not a statistical abstraction. It is real, and it is a disgrace.
2. This nation *can* afford — now — to erase that disgrace. And it must.
3. Hunger is the dark side of poverty. It will end when we escalate and finish the war we started against poverty.
4. We can, and inevitably will, argue over *means*. But this Conference is in no doubt whatsoever concerning *ends*.
5. We must be clear about our priorities. The paramount priority is action now: *Action* to cut red tape and get food to the poor on an emergency basis.

Action to make *realistic* income payments to the poor.

Action to convince an apathetic society that its big successes are matched by equally big failures.

6. Balancing the Federal budget is a hollow achievement while people go hungry, live in shacks, and cannot obtain health care.

7. Food programs for the poor, and especially poor children, must be fully funded; and then we can get on with the rest of our unfinished business in food, nutrition, and health — emphasizing education and prevention, monitoring of diets and remedial programs, and manpower training.

8. The job before us is not Government's alone but is shared with industry, the health professions, the mass media, advertisers, schools and universities, churches, voluntary groups and organizations of poor people.

9. Control of policy and program delivery is not reserved to the high and mighty but is equally the right of the low and the weak.

If we got this much through our heads in two days, the Conference accomplished something. There has been plenty of plain talk in the workshops. I got my comeuppance more than once. The procedures were wide open and I think that everybody had his say. Most of us were struck by the presence of so many responsible members and leaders of the local Community Action groups. They held our feet to the fire. The panel recommendations were taken apart mercilessly. They won't look so placid when they're put back together.

We found that words and phrases and meanings don't always come through clearly on paper. They can be frigid and lifeless. So the workshops did what a report can never do — bring out in the open the hurt and the urgency and the anger that go with hunger.

The President brought us here. And we will leave here changed and less sure that we know it all than when we arrived. And we leave knowing one other thing: you can have a conference like this once but if it doesn't produce results not many of us will answer the phone next time.

Some of the frustrations as well as the joys of the conference are evident in the Panel Recommendation Statement read at the plenary session and presented here. For many, the conference did not achieve what its supporters had expected. The political climate surrounding the conference and the failure of the conference to carefully define its mission and the scope of its focus were largely responsible.

However, the effects of the conference as well as of these other activities on current food and nutrition programs have been significant. The federal government has revised and extended the Food Stamp Program; expanded many child nutrition programs; developed new programs to meet the special needs of women, infants and young children, and the elderly; and developed a nutrition label. But nutrition advocates and many critics are not yet satisfied that current nutrition programs reach their stated goals or that they are really effective in attempts to alleviate hunger and malnutrition in the United States. The following sections review some of these programs and problems.

MATERNAL AND CHILD HEALTH PROGRAMS

The original legislative authority for maternal and child health programs was the Social Security Act of 1935, which provided for federal assistance to the states to improve the health services for mothers and their children.

Probably the most successful and well-known projects are the Maternity and Infant Care (M&I, or MIC) and the Children and Youth (C&Y) projects. The purpose of the MIC project is to reduce the complications and poor outcomes of pregnancy that frequently result in mental retardation, physical handicaps, and infant and maternal mortality. Special care is provided for high-risk mothers and their infants. High-risk, nutrition-related factors include anemia, malnutrition, hypertension, diabetes, pregnancy under the age of 16 or over the age of 36, a history of premature birth, or other similar circumstance.[9]

The project objectives are to provide prenatal care including dietary and nutritional supports, education, and counseling. Nutritional screening, assessment, monitoring, and referrals where necessary are provided. The emphasis is on multidisciplinary provision of care, with professionals from a variety of fields collaborating to maximize the quality of services provided. Other services include family planning, dental care for expectant mothers, classes for expectant parents, well-baby clinics, pediatric clinics, hospital care of premature infants, school health examinations, and mental retardation clinics.

The C&Y projects are designed to provide comprehensive health care to the preschool and school child in low-income areas. Services include medical, dental, and mental health services, which provide assessment, screening, monitoring, diagnosis, intervention, and treatment. C&Y projects are to be integrated into existing service delivery systems. For example, the C&Y project might be coordinated with local school or social programs. Program activities are planned according to individual needs. Staffs include physicians, nurses, nutritionists, social workers, and health aides. In many urban areas, MIC and C&Y projects are the only places in which poor mothers and children are able to obtain the nutritional services they need.

In addition to these programs are the Special Crippled Children Services (CC) in each state. These programs are designed to locate children with crippling conditions and to see that these children are provided with needed social, health, and welfare services. The state unit responsible for administering these various programs is the Maternal and Child Health Program Unit.

Family planning projects, which are also provided for under the Social Security Act, aim to give families the freedom of choice in determining the number and spacing of children through access to information and medical support services. These projects are employing nutritionists in increasing numbers.

Another important program intended for pregnant women, lactating women, infants, and children is the Special Supplemental Program for Women, Infants, and Children (WIC).

WIC PROGRAM

Sometimes I have the feeling that WIC isn't a program . . . it really is a course in survival . . . survival for those of you who have tried so hard to bring the benefits of WIC to our urban and rural poor, survival for those of us in Congress who wondered if the law would ever be fully implemented, and, most importantly, survival for millions of women, infants and children that WIC really serves.[10]

Introduction

The Special Supplemental Food Program for Women, Infants, and Children was established as a pilot program in 1972. However, WIC projects were not funded until 1974 when the U.S. Department of Agriculture issued regulations in the wake of pressure from Congress, community groups, and a lawsuit.

In 1975, the WIC program was extended for three years and funding for the program was increased. Significant in the 1975 legislation was language stating that WIC was to be a preventive health program. The legislation provided for the inclusion of nutrition education programs. The Child Nutrition Bill of 1978 authorized continuation of the WIC program through 1982.

Definition of the WIC Program

The WIC program is designed to provide supplemental foods to pregnant women up to 6 months postpartum, nursing mothers up to 1 year postpartum, infants up to 1 year of age, and children up to 5 years of age. The program goals are twofold: to provide nutrition education and supplemental food to low-income participants and to provide clinical and administrative data for program evaluation. The program is thus both research and service oriented.

Eligibility of the program is based on the following[11,12]

1. Residence: Local participants must live in a specific geographical area.

2. Income: National income standards specify economic eligibility criteria.

3. Nutritional risk: Participants must be determined at nutritional risk by a health professional. Definitions of nutritional risk are presented in Table 17-2.

Participants in the program receive supplemental foods to help them meet their nutritional needs. Supplemental foods are those that contain nutrients known to be limited in the diets of populations who are at nu-

Table 17-2
WIC Regulations Defining Nutritional Risk

For Pregnant and Lactating Women	*For Infants and Children*
1. Known inadequate nutritional patterns	1. Deficient patterns of growth
2. High incidence of anemia	2. High incidence of nutritional anemia
3. High rates of prematurity or miscarriage	3. Known inadequate nutritional patterns
4. Inadequate patterns of growth (underweight, obesity, or stunting)	

Source: Committee on School Lunch Participation, *Their Daily Bread.* 1969.

tritional risk. The foods contain high-quality protein, iron, calcium, vitamin C, and vitamin A. Commercially fortified products that are designed specifically for infants are also included. Thus, only specific food selections are allowed. These foods are listed in Figure 17-1.[12] Although various counties must conform to the federal regulations for the food package, within these regulations there is freedom of choice. For example, Montgomery County, Maryland (whose food package is listed here),

Figure 17-1. Acceptable WIC foods list from Montgomery County, Maryland.

SPECIAL FORMULA

13 oz. Concentrated with Iron

SMA Iron-Fortified Infant Formula	Soyalac	Nutramigen	Isomil
Similac with Iron	1-Soyalac	Pregestimil	Nursoy
Enfamil with Iron	Neo-Mull-Soy	Lofenalac	Prosbce
	Portagen	Meat Base Formula	Prosobee

TYPES: Concentrated/Powdered/Ready to Feed

INFANT JUICE	INFANT CEREAL	
Gerber — All Varieties	Barley	Oatmeal
Beechnut — All Varieties	Hi Protein	Rice
Heinz — All Varieties	Mixed	
	NO CEREAL WITH FRUIT OR SUGAR ADDED	

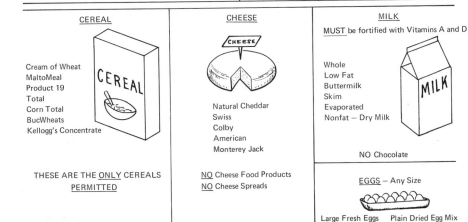

CEREAL	CHEESE	MILK
		MUST be fortified with Vitamins A and D
Cream of Wheat		Whole
MaltoMeal		Low Fat
Product 19		Buttermilk
Total		Skim
Corn Total	Natural Cheddar	Evaporated
BucWheats	Swiss	Nonfat — Dry Milk
Kellogg's Concentrate	Colby	
	American	
	Monterey Jack	NO Chocolate
THESE ARE THE ONLY CEREALS PERMITTED	NO Cheese Food Products NO Cheese Spreads	EGGS — Any Size
		Large Fresh Eggs Plain Dried Egg Mix

JUICES

THE LABEL SHOULD READ:

JUICE and NOT "Drink"

"NO SUGAR ADDED" OR "UNSWEETENED"
Supply 90% of the USRDA for
Vitamin C in six ounces

ORANGE — Any Brand
GRAPEFRUIT — Any Brand

PINEAPPLE	APPLE	TOMATO	GRAPE JUICE
Dole	Seneca (Frozen)	Delmonte	*Welch's (bottle)
Delmonte			
Grand Union			
Aunt Nellie			
Town House			
Co-op			

*On the Pink and Yellow vouchers clients can substitute 2 — 40 oz. bottles of
Welch's Grape Juice in place of the 2 — 46 oz. cans of Fruit Juice.
(Frozen Welch's Juice not allowed)

chose not to allow presweetened cereals such as Kaboom and King Vitamin in its food package. The WIC food package is currently being re-evaluated and revisions in the allowed foods may result.

Participants receive the food at no charge. Direct distribution, voucher system, and central distribution are the three methods of distribution. In direct distribution, the foods are delivered monthly to the participant's home. In central distribution, foods are distributed from a central location. In the voucher system, the participant receives a monthly coupon booklet. The participant then presents coupons to the grocer or supermarket when the food is purchased and pays only for the cost above the amount allowed.

Program Organization and Operation

WIC is funded by the USDA, administered by a state agency, and sponsored by a local agency. The USDA Food and Nutrition Service (FNS) is responsible for the administration and overall evaluation of the program.

The state agency must be a health department or equivalent agency of each state, Indian tribe, or group recognized by the Department of the Interior or the Indian Health Service of the USDHEW. The state agencies are responsible for the food delivery system design, and they recommend local agencies for funding, and monitor approved local agencies. Local agencies must be nonprofit, private agencies or public health or welfare agencies that provide continuous health services to residents of a largely low-income area, and must serve women, infants, and children at nutritional risk. Staffing must include professionals who are able to meet the health needs of the WIC participants.

Local WIC agencies are responsible for the examination and certification of individuals; distribution of the WIC food package; and collection and computation of clinical, administrative, and fiscal data required by the FNS. The local agency must ensure the integration of a nutrition education program, and it is also responsible for ensuring that grocers authorized to accept WIC food vouchers in exchange for foods allow only those items approved by the WIC Program for this exchange.

Nutrition Education

WIC Programs are provided with funds to be used specifically for nutrition education.[13] The 1978 Child Nutrition legislation strengthened nutrition education as a benefit of the WIC program.

Each state agency is required to prepare an annual, detailed plan specifying operation of the education program. The nutrition education must be provided to all WIC program participants and to parents or guardians of infants and children in the program.

The overall goal of nutrition education in the WIC program is that, through the utilization of the supplemental and other nutritious foods, individuals will improve food habits and hence their nutritional status, while preventing nutrition-related problems. Thus, participants are taught to recognize the relationships between proper nutrition and good health; emphasis is on the nutritional needs of the pregnant, postpartum and breast-feeding woman and on the infant and child under the age of 5 years. PL-95-627 mandated that the state agency provide training to persons providing the nutrition education.[14]

Subject matter to be included in the WIC program to meet stated program goals includes:[14,15]

1. Explanation of recipient's nutritional need and the importance of the supplemental foods being consumed by the recipient rather than by other members of the family.

2. Reference to the special nutritional needs of the recipient and ways to meet these needs.

3. An explanation of the program as a supplemental rather than a total food program; focus on the need for using the foods provided by the WIC program with other nutritious foods to achieve a balanced diet.

4. Information on ways to use supplemental foods and the nutritional value of these foods.

5. Participants at high nutritional risk should receive individual care plans that will aid them in meeting their nutritional needs.

Program Effectiveness

There is increasing evidence that the WIC program is one of the most effective health and nutrition programs operated by the federal government. Data collected by various state WIC programs (e.g., Arizona, Oregon, and Louisiana) indicate that WIC participants evidenced a significant decrease in anemia and in the prevalence of low-birth-weight infants, as well as an improvement in attaining improved weight levels among participants who were underweight when they began to participate in the WIC Program.[16]

Arizona reported that anemia was reduced by 81 per cent among children. Eighty-two per cent of surveyed children improved their underweight status, and 64 per cent of the children improved their height measurements. Arizona also reported a significant reduction in the incidence of low-birth-weight infants born to mothers enrolled in the program. Oregon reported similar findings; 94 per cent of the children initially at high risk because of anemia were no longer at risk after one year in the program. The condition of obesity was corrected among 56 per cent of those initially obese, and 49 per cent of those initially under height for age achieved normal heights after a year. The results in Louisiana were similar.

The Center for Disease Control has data from the nutrition surveillance program that include WIC program records from 13 states. The CDC has reported that of those children with low hemoglobin/hematocrit levels, 94 per cent had acceptable levels by their second WIC follow-up visit. The greatest improvement was noted among those children who were most severely anemic. CDC data also document the considerably decreased incidence of low birth-weight infants among WIC program participants.[16]

The Urban Institute conducted an extensive evaluation of the WIC program. The report, *Toward Efficiency and Effectiveness in the WIC Delivery System*, describes the survey. The WIC program was found to be popular with participants. In addition, the program was found to be significant in increasing the use of medical services by WIC participants. WIC programs were responsible for a 77 per cent increase in clinic attendance by children, a 27 per cent increase for infants, and a 14 per cent increase for pregnant women.[17]

However, many negative findings were reported. For instance, more than 10 per cent of WIC households were found to have incomes that were 200 per cent above the poverty line, and 3 per cent had incomes more than 250 per cent above the cutoff line. This was identified to be a grave problem in view of the very limited enrollment that is possible in the program and the numerous women and children who are not able to participate in WIC.

The study also reported that many clinics did not operate at capacity, whereas other clinics had long waiting lists. More than half the clinics surveyed had waiting lists — the average number on the list was 94 persons. This contrasts sharply with the tens of thousands of unused WIC slots in other clinics. Principal reasons identified for nonparticipation included the lack of transportation or the feeling that transportation to the clinic would entail too much time, effort, or money; the lack of child care during a visit to the clinic; and the inconvenient clinic operating hours. The study noted that "these impediments to participation hit hardest and most frequently among the poorest, and therefore presumably the most needy."[17]

Approximately two thirds of the clinics studied had made some efforts at outreach. Techniques included public service announcements, newspaper advertisements, posters, displays, and speakers at meetings. Only about 5 per cent of the participants studied had been informed of the WIC program through these outreach efforts.

Nutrition education efforts were found to be, for the most part, worthless. There was a good deal of nutrition education activity — an average of 11 per cent of the administrative budget went to nutrition education, and almost 70 per cent of the clinics offered individual counseling to participants. However, only 12 per cent of the 75 per cent who recalled receiving nutrition education felt that they had profited from it. Nutrition education was found to be most effective when the educators had an idea of what the participants ate, the money available for food, and the cultural and ethnic values of the participants relating to food. The most effective nutrition education messages were simple, concrete, and well illustrated. Education offerings were more successful when they were integrated into other program services, when desired changes in food habits were minimal, and when individuals were provided with personal follow-up. More than half the clinics were viewed as ineffective in nutrition education efforts by more than 90 per cent of the participants.

The study also considered WIC administrative costs. Approximately 20 per cent of the costs went to the administration of the program. More than 92 per cent of the WIC participants studied said that they would purchase some of the WIC foods without WIC vouchers. Thus, the WIC program actually operated as a form of supplemental income; 81 per cent of the participants used WIC foods to feed other family members. This illustrates the issue of more general policy goals. The WIC program, as well as other food assistance programs, must be considered not only as food programs but also as a form of income supplementation. At the high level of administrative cost (approximately double the administrative costs involved in many other welfare programs) federal dollars may be spent unwisely — monies that could go to benefit the poor, and ultimately improve their nutritional status, may be used up in program administration.[17]

The medical evaluation of the WIC program conducted by the University of North Carolina at Chapel Hill was designed to evaluate the impact of the WIC program on the health and nutritional status of its participants. Data were collected from 19 projects in 14 states; 100 individual clinics were represented. Women were examined at the time of enrollment, approximately every 3 months until delivery, and 4 to 8 weeks postpartum. Infants and children were examined at enrollment and after receiving the food package for 6 and 11 months.[18]

The findings included the following.[18]

1. Ninety-one per cent of the participants lived in urban locations and were predominantly from very low-income households. Average household size was 4.6 persons.

2. For infants and children, participation in the WIC program was associated with a statistically significant increase in the rate of growth. After participation, 6- to 12-month-old infants had increased their daily intakes of iron, vitamin A, thiamine, and ascorbic acid. Participating children showed increased intakes of all nutrients except energy. Six-month participation reduced the incidence of anemia to 40 per cent in all age groups. After 11 months, there was a significant decrease in the anemia rate in the 12- to 24-month-old group.

3. Pregnant women participants increased their consumption of protein, calcium, phosphorous, iron, vitamin A, thiamine, folacin, riboflavin, niacin, and ascorbic acid, but not energy. After participation, women gained more weight during pregnancy than women in the initial population.

4. There was an association between WIC program participation and increased infant birth weight.

5. The WIC program was associated with a reduced prevalence of anemia among pregnant women in the third trimester and in postpartum mothers.

Recommendations

Many aspects of the WIC program are clearly in need of improvement. The National Advisory Council on Maternal, Infant, and Fetal Nutrition made a number of recommendations for legislative and operating changes in the WIC program. Such recommendations were thought to improve the WIC program and include the following:[19]

1. Increased emphasis on preventive aspects of the WIC program — The WIC program should be used to promote health and not merely

to treat disease. Eligibility requirements for program participation should give priority to the most vulnerable relative to nutritional risks and benefits from intervention. These groups should include (in this order) pregnant teenagers up to age 16, other pregnant women, infants up to 18 months of age, and children, with reduced priority for each year of life.

2. Coordination of benefits provided by federal assistance programs — Legislation should provide for a coordination of programs and integration of programs into existing efforts at federal, state, and local levels. Such coordination and integration should be mandated by federal program regulations.

3. Future funding level based on need — Funding should be determined according to those vulnerable groups in great need of intervention. Funding levels should be determined according to the priorities identified in recommendation 1.

4. Alternative formulas for allocating funds to state agencies — Formula should make sure that funds are distributed on an equitable basis and guarantee state agencies a minimum amount of funds for program operation.

5. Alternative methods for determining administrative costs — Funds should be authorized in needed amounts for WIC program operations. Methods should provide adequate funds for the operation of high-quality WIC programs and should encourage cost management practices, advanced planning, and the reduction of administrative costs through efficient program management.

6. Funds for demonstration projects and for program evaluation — Funds should be authorized for demonstration projects that might improve program operation and the success and effectiveness of the WIC program. Program evaluation should be required and funds should be allocated for this activity.

7. Targeting nutrition education — The nutritional status of WIC participants should be assessed, and this assessment should serve as the basis for nutrition education efforts. Funds should be available for the development of model nutrition education programs; such models should then be used by other WIC programs.

8. Changes in food packages — Because program participants have varying nutritional needs, different food packages should be offered. In particular, foods for infants and children should be consistent with their nutritional needs, which may be vastly different from the needs of pregnant mothers.

9. Providing WIC program benefits to migrants — A system to provide continuity in WIC program benefits to migrants as they travel through the migrant stream should be developed and implemented. Special consideration should be given to areas with a heavy migrant population.

HEAD START PROGRAM

The goal of the Head Start program is to

Bring about a greater degree of social competence in children of low-income families. By social competence is meant the child's everyday effectiveness in dealing with both present environment and later responsibilities in school and life. Social competence takes into account the interrelatedness of cognitive and intellectual development, physical and mental health, nutritional needs, and other factors that enable a developmental approach to helping children achieve social competence.[20]

Introduction

Head Start was originally created to provide low-income children with the individualized and specialized services they require to "overcome the physical, social, and emotional deprivation of poverty in order that they may achieve social competence." Basic parts of the Head Start program include nutritional, medical, dental, and mental health services, education, and social services.[21]

Current Program Administration and Operation

Head Start is administered by AOCYF and ten regional U.S. Department of Health, Education, and Welfare offices. The regional offices allocate funds, enforce standards, and coordinate training for Head Start programs.[20]

Most regional offices have nutritionists available on a part-time consulting basis for training and coordination of nutrition activities. At the national office level there is a senior nutrition specialist. The national office also publishes several guides for local nutrition programs. These include the *Rainbow Series* and six booklets covering different aspects of the nutrition component, as well as a *Handbook for Local Head Start Nutrition Specialists* and the *Leadership Development and Training for Head Start Coordinators of Nutrition and Cook Managers*.[21-28]

The Head Start Program is administered locally by community-based organizations or other nonprofit organizations. Head Start is federally funded, but local programs must provide matching funds. This can be in noncash or in volunteer help forms. Head Start programs may also participate in the Child Care Food Program, which reimburses each program for the cost of the food service.

Eligibility for Head Start programs is determined from family income and the age of the child. Yearly family income guidelines are established by the federal government; no more than 10 per cent of children in the program are to be from nonpoverty families. The age of the participants ranges from 3 to 5 years. Another eligibility requirement is that at least 10 per cent of Head Start enrollment be handicapped children.

Goals of the Program

The basic concept of the Head Start program is that all children have certain needs; for low-income children whose needs are often unmet, a comprehensive, interdisciplinary program offering various services is needed.

Further, the philosophy of the Head Start program is to involve both family and community in the program. The general goal of the program is to overcome the deprivation of poverty to enable low-income children to reach a greater level of social competence. Objectives designed to reach this goal are summarized as follows: [29]

1. Improve the child's health and physical abilities.
2. Encourage self-confidence, spontaneity, curiosity, and self-discipline.
3. Enhance the child's mental skills.
4. Establish patterns and expectations of success.
5. Improve the communication between the child and family.
6. Enhance the child's and his or her family's sense of dignity and self-worth.

Components of the Program

There are four major components in the Head Start program. Each program must submit a detailed plan each year stating how the goals of each component will be achieved. The components are as follows:

Education

The education component is to provide each child with experiences that will aid his or her intellectual, physical, social, and emotional development. The children are individually assessed and evaluated. Teachers and aides plan activities that emphasize basic developmental concepts such as self-concept, interaction with others, problem solving, language development, and large and small motor coordination. Activities are designed to involve parents in the educational process.

Social Services

This component is responsible for outreach, recruiting and enrolling children, and for helping the families of Head Start children to improve the quality and condition of family life. [30]

Parent Involvement

All components stress parent involvement, considered to be one of the most important aspects of Head Start. The program must provide experiences and activities that support the parents as significant influences in their child's life and encourage their involvement in all aspects of Head Start.

Health

The health component is designed to provide each child with comprehensive medical, dental, mental health, and nutrition services. Emphasis is on assessment, early intervention, and prevention of health problems. Nutrition and services to handicapped children (required to be 10 per cent of total enrollment) are included in the health component. Each child receives many health-screening services early in the year. Identified problems are followed up by parents and Head Start staff. The health coordinator works closely with those involved in other aspects of Head Start to provide health education and services to families.

Nutrition in Head Start

"For children to gain maximum benefits from the Head Start educational program they must bring healthy bodies and minds sustained by nutritious foods to the learning process."[21] Thus, nutrition can be envisioned as a part of almost every aspect of Head Start. The primary objectives of the nutritional component are:

1. To provide the children with a stimulating physical and emotional environment so that they will be able to develop positive food habits and fulfill their socialization needs.

2. To provide well-balanced and nutritious meals and snacks for the children.

3. To help the families of Head Start youngsters and the local Head Start staff to learn about the importance of food and nutrition in promoting health, physical, mental, emotional, and social well-being and to help the families to provide nourishing food to meet the child's nutritional needs.

4. To establish linkages with other food and nutrition programs at all levels so that the totality of family nutritional needs can be met.

5. To involve parents, staff, and community in the nutritional care of the children so that the Head Start center's efforts will complement those of the home and community.

Head Start is required to serve meals and snacks to meet one third of the RDA for children in part-day programs and two thirds of the RDA for children in full-day programs. Children attending the part-day program receive lunch or supper and a snack or breakfast. Children attending for the full-day have a lunch or supper plus two snacks, or one snack and breakfast. Lunch and supper patterns are similar to the type A school lunch (meat or meat substitute, two fruits or vegetables, bread, butter, and milk) but with smaller portions. A snack consists of bread and milk, fruit, or juice, and breakfast supplies juice or fruit, cereal or protein-rich food, bread, and milk. Breakfast must be offered to any children who arrive in the morning without it. An effort is made to include some unfamiliar foods, finger foods, and ethnic foods. (See Figure 17-2.)

If the goal for the nutrition component is to attain and maintain the best possible nutritional status for the children, the staff must work closely with each child and with the family. Each child is assessed for health and diet-related problems early in the school year; problems are followed up by the health, social services, or nutrition staff with the parents. Information about food, menus, and nutrition activities is shared with parents through newsletters and home visits. Parents are involved in the centers as volunteers in the kitchen, classroom, and lunchroom, and as members of a policy council that approves yearly nutrition plans and menus. Par-

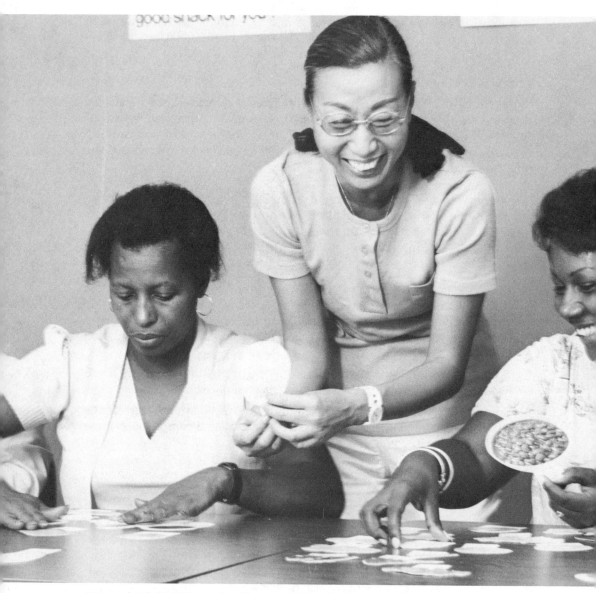

Figure 17-2. Nutrition education program at a community center. (American Dietetic Association/Doyle Pharmaceutical Company)

ents are encouraged to attend parent activities involving food, nutrition, or cooking and to use all available community resources and programs.

Effectiveness of the Program

Numerous studies have attempted to determine program effectiveness in accomplishing stated goals.[31-39] Many of these studies have noted that Head Start has had a positive effect on the participating children, making them better prepared to enter school than nonparticipants from low-income families.[34,36] However, other studies have concluded that these educational benefits decline after the children leave the Head Start program, and, by the end of the third grade, the early gains from the program are often lost.[34,35] The type of Head Start program, the appropriateness of learning experiences provided, and the the degree of parental involvement have all been found to affect the later ability of the child to maintain the gains experienced from the program.[35,36]

The Head Start program has also had a positive effect on child health in terms of lower school absenteeism, fewer cases of anemia, more immunizations, and improved nutritional practices.[36] An examination of the nutritional impact of Head Start was conducted by R. Cook et al.[39,40] These researchers found that the dietary intake of the children who regularly attended the program improved, particularly with respect to calcium and ascorbic acid intakes. However, the dietary patterns in the home appeared unchanged. Thus, upon completion of the Head Start program, the children may resume their previous poor food intakes. This finding further emphasizes the need for a strong nutrition education program that involves the parents and community as well as the children.

CHILD NUTRITION PROGRAMS

Historical Perspective [41]

The first recorded organized school-feeding program in the United States was implemented by the Children's Aid Society in New York City in 1853. The program served meals to the children attending a New York City vocational school.

Figure 17-3. Day care center. (United Nations/B. Weinbaum)

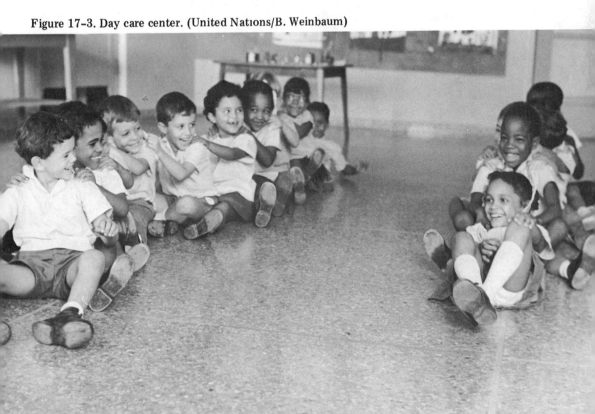

In 1910 an experimental lunch program was started by a group of volunteer social organizations in selected New York City schools. The meal was provided at a cost of $.03 for the student. By 1912 the New York City Board of Education authorized the expansion of the program to other city schools and subsidized the cost of equipment and space.

In 1916 the U.S. Department of Agriculture reviewed the importance of eating an adequate lunch and recommended some simple recipes for meals that could be served in a lunch program. The bulletin suggested that the lunch program provide food from various food groups, including protein-rich foods, fruit and vegetables, cereals or starches, fats, and simple sweets.

During the 1920s and 1930s, various state and local legislative mandates authorized local school districts to offer meals for schoolchildren. However, it soon became clear that local school districts were unable to financially support these programs. By 1935, federal funds, through programs such as the Civil Works Administration, the Emergency Relief Administration, and the Works Progress Administration (WPA) provided assistance for foods and lunch programs in the nation's schools.

The 74th Congress, on August 24, 1935, approved legislation that mandated making available federal funds in the amount of 30 per cent of the gross receipts from duties collected under custom laws for the purchase of surplus foods from the domestic market. The aim was to remove such foods that would depress farm prices. This food was to be used as export foods and to be offered to provide domestic food assistance to needy individuals. Part of these purchased foods were distributed to the schools, thus initiating the Commodity Distribution Program.

A milk program was authorized in 1940, and, in 1944 and 1945, specific amounts of money were set aside for school lunch and milk programs. The National School Lunch Act, passed on June 4, 1946, mandated a National School Lunch Program whose primary mission was to "safeguard the health and well-being of the Nation's children." The law provided assistance to individual states to establish, maintain, operate, and expand nonprofit school lunch programs. Another purpose of this legislation was to encourage the domestic consumption of nutritious agricultural commodities.

The Child Nutrition Act of 1966 strengthened and expanded the School Lunch Program. In addition, federal appropriations were provided for a special milk program, a breakfast program, nonfood assistance program, and for technical support and assistance. Following a brief description of these and additional child nutrition programs, this section focuses on the School Lunch Program.

CURRENT CHILD NUTRITION PROGRAMS[42]

Direct Food Assistance

This program helps schools to provide nutritious lunches to students at low or no cost. Most of these schools are those in the National School Lunch Program; however, public and nonprofit schools not in the National

School Lunch Program may also receive donated foods, provided they serve nutritious meals that contain foods from the basic four food groups.

Foods purchased especially for the National School Lunch Program are selected according to the nutritional needs of the children, recommendations of state school lunch officials, and market supplies and prices. The variety and quantity of donated foods vary according to market conditions that affect purchases.

The School Breakfast Program

This children's nutrition program provides cash assistance to state educational agencies to help schools to operate nonprofit breakfast programs that meet established nutritional standards. The program is important in improving the diets of needy children who may receive breakfast free or at reduced prices. (See Figure 17–4.)

The Special Milk Program for Children

This program is designed to improve child nutrition by paying a share of the cost of increased servings of fluid milk made to children. Food assistance is given to the states to reimburse eligible schools and child-care institutions that provide this milk to children. Funds for this program are provided by direct appropriation. (See Figure 17–5.)

The Summer Feeding Program for Children

This program helps to provide nutritious meals to needy preschool children and school-aged children in recreation centers and summer camps or during vacations in areas operating under a continuous school calendar. Through grants-in-aid and other means, states can initiate, maintain, and expand nonprofit food service programs for children in such institutions.

Any nonresidential public or private nonprofit institution or residential public or private nonprofit summer camp is eligible if it develops a summer food program for children from low-income areas. All meals are served free.

The Special Food Service Program

Legislative authority in 1968 enables this program to help provide nutritious food to children (mainly of low-income families) who do not participate in the School Lunch Program. Institutions participating in the program may provide breakfast, lunch, supper, two snacks, or some modification of this schedule. If USDA standards are met, schools can be reimbursed for meals served.

Child Care Food Program

The U.S. Department of Agriculture, under this program, provides cash reimbursement or commodities to nonprofit, licensed, and qualified child-care agencies to facilitate the provision of nutritious meals to needy preschool children.

Reimbursement is provided to the institution for food service and related costs, based on the income of the children's parents and the meals served.

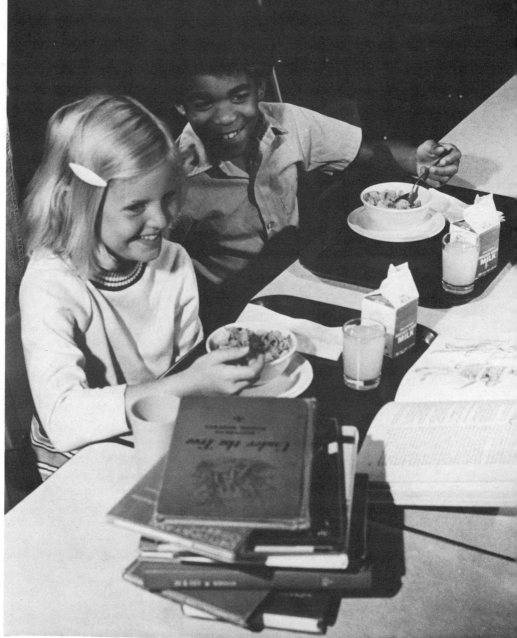

Figure 17-4. Project Head Start aims to improve child health by creating an environment to bring children to their full potential. Nutrition is an integral component of the program. (UDS USDA Food and Nutrition Service)

NATIONAL SCHOOL LUNCH PROGRAM

Introduction

The federally subsidized National School Lunch Program picks up the world's largest restaurant tab and serves more than 26 million elementary students at over 90,000 locations. The program is a grant-in-aid program providing federal assistance to the states, which are then to provide,

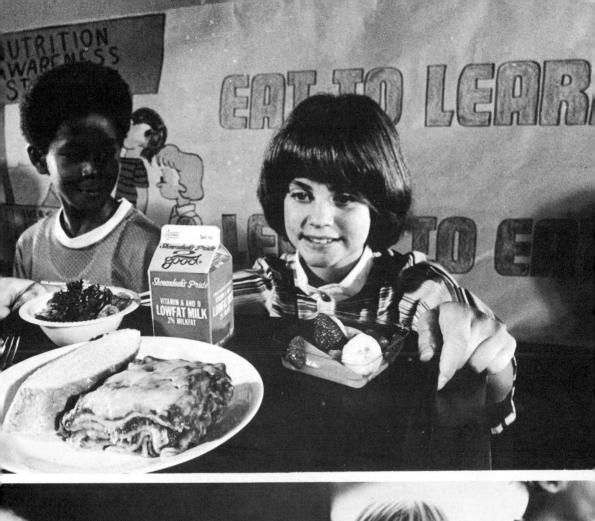
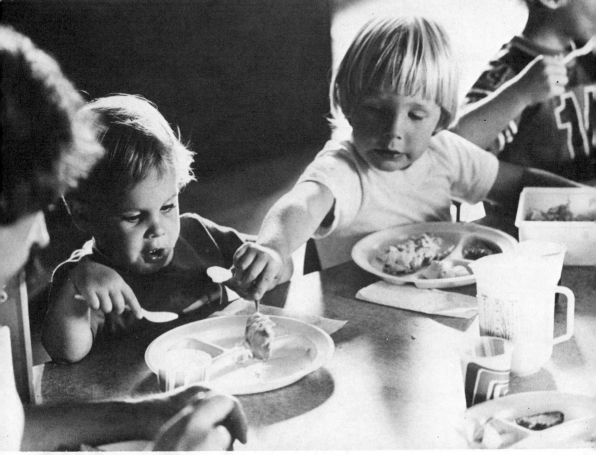

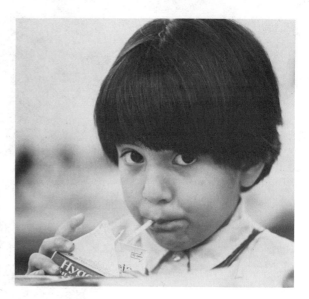

Figure 17-5. The Special Milk Program is designed to encourage milk consumption by children in a variety of settings. (U.S. Department of Agriculture, Food and Nutrition Service)

through cash reimbursement and donated foods, nominally priced, wholesome, and appetizing lunches to the nation's schoolchildren.

Program Administration

The U.S. Department of Agriculture, through the Food and Nutrition Service headquarters and regional offices, has the primary responsibility for program administration. At the state level, the state educational agency administers the program in public and private schools where permitted. The state agency is responsible for supervising, assisting, and monitoring local program operation.

At the local level, the schools or school districts carry out the program and determine those students who are eligible for free or reduced-price lunches. To participate in the program, each school and district must enter into a written agreement with the state and must keep appropriate records to support reimbursement claims.

Eligibility

All public and nonprofit elementary and secondary schools (such as parochial, sectarian, and denominational schools) are eligible. To obtain federal aid, schools must agree to:

— Operate the program on a nonprofit basis for all children regardless of race, color, or national origin.

— Provide free or reduced-price lunches to children unable to pay the full price of the lunch. Children receiving free or reduced-price lunches must not be so identified or otherwise discriminated against.

— Serve nutritious lunches that meet the meal requirements established by the USDA.

Children are considered to be eligible for free lunches according to economic criteria established annually by the USDA and for reduced-price lunches according to criteria developed by individual states or school districts.

Meal Pattern

The original School Lunch Program recognized three approved meal patterns. Type A was intended to provide one third or more of the RDAs; type B offered a supplemental lunch in schools where facilities were not available to prepare a type A lunch; and type C consisted of one half pint of whole milk. In subsequent years, types B and C were dropped and some modifications were made in the type A lunch.

The type A lunch included the following:

— 2 ounces of meat and/or alternate,

— ¾ cup of two or more vegetables and/or fruit,

— one slice of enriched or whole-grain bread or equivalent, and

— ½ pint of milk.

This pattern was based on the 1968 RDAs for children aged 10 to 12. New USDA regulations drop the term "Type A Lunch" and modify the meal pattern.

Regulations require local schools to expand the bread alternatives to include rice and pasta; to serve low fat milk rather than whole milk; and to involve parents and students in the planning, development, and service of the lunch program. The meals are to include only a moderate level of sugar, fat, and salt, and adequate amounts of iron, vitamin A, and vitamin C.[43,44]

Nutrition Education

The National School Lunch Act and Child Nutrition Amendments of 1977 added a new section to the National School Lunch Act, "Nutrition Education and Training," which authorized a system of grants through the USDA to state educational agencies. The program was funded in FY 1978 and 1979 through an entitlement of $.50 per child. No state was to receive less than $75,000 a year. The program was authorized for FY 1980, but was subject to regular nonentitlement appropriations processes in that year.

The legislation included four mandates:[45]

1. Instruction in nutrition for students.

2. Training for school food service employees.

3. Teacher instruction in food and nutrition.

4. Development of resources and curriculum.

The legislation also provided for the development of a state plan to consider, with other agencies, an initial needs assessment and a program evaluation. An education coordinator was to be appointed in each state to direct the expansion of nutrition education and training.

Problems in the School Lunch Program

Many problems in the program have been identified. Nonparticipation of eligible schools and children is a major difficulty. Lack of cooking and storage equipment are primary reasons for nonparticipation. Although free or reduced-price lunches are available to many needy students, numerous obstacles to participation have been identified:

1. Schools adopt practices that are not in compliance with FNS requirements.

2. Needy families refuse to have their children accept free or reduced-price lunches because of pride.

3. Inadequate monitoring by FNS regional offices and state agency reviewers of schools' implementation of the program hinders compliance with regulations.

4. Some schools choose not to participate.

5. Some schools lack food service facilities and equipment and the funds to acquire them.

6. Some schools participate with limited facilities and are not able to see all who need meals.

Another major criticism of the program relates to food wastage. Studies have suggested that neary $600 million worth of food goes untouched and that as much as 15 per cent of the menu is wasted.[46]

The effectiveness of the program and the quality of food served to the children who participate have been a subject of investigation and have gained considerable publicity. A study conducted by the *Chicago Tribune* monitored the effectiveness of Chicago's programs. The study consisted of samples from 12 lunches at 6 different schools. Lunches were evaluated for proximate composition of carbohydrate, fat, protein, fiber, water, and ash, as well as for content of vitamins A and C, thiamin, riboflavin, niacin, calcium, and iron. A variety of different types of food service were represented by the schools: commercially prepared prefrozen meals, nonselective menu prepared on site, catered cold lunches, and lunches made at a central site and delivered to decentralized school sites were included.

Nutrients were compared with the standard, set at one third of the RDA for children aged 11–14. The researchers found that protein, riboflavin, and calcium consumption were greater than the standard, whereas vitamin A, vitamin C, and iron intakes were less than the standard.

Plate waste was used to evaluate the students' acceptance of the meals. The most plate waste was found in the school serving cold lunches, whereas food acceptance was highest in the school in which hot lunches were served in a setting where teachers ate with the children and provisions for nutrition education were made.[47]

Innovative Programs

Various programs have initiated innovative efforts to combat food wastage in the School Lunch Program. In Clark County, Nevada, school lunch is patterned after the fast-food offerings: "Our lunches look like junk food, taste like junk food but are actually health food" according to the food service director. Food is merchandised to appeal to the children. Snappy posters promote the school lunchroom as "a fun place to eat." The children are able to order from colorful menus describing such items as "taco combo," "big Nevad'n," "big Tex'n," "mile-long cheese dog," and "super shake."

The foods available are imitations of fare that is available at various fast-food franchises, but are intended to be "healthy." Foods are cooked in liquid vegetable oil and fortified with vitamins. Wheat germ, whole-wheat flour, and low-fat ingredients including kelp are used. In 1972, before the start of these innovations, the Clark County school food program was losing about $200,000 annually. Today the program has doubled the number of meals served and has a huge cash surplus.[48] However, the program is severely criticized on the grounds that children are not being educated to make wise food choices outside of the school lunchroom.

A successful program in Milwaukee enjoys a 70–75 per cent student participation in the school lunch program, compared with a 40–50 per cent national average participation rate. Meals are prepared from scratch; students participate in the planning of program and menus and in evaluating program results. Nutrition education is an integral part of the program and is intended to provide the students with techniques to keep nutritionally fit for the rest of their lives. Other innovations in school lunch include a salad bar in lunchrooms, picnics and small dining settings, smorgasbords, and family-style food service.[49]

Another school lunch director's innovations include the use of cartoon characters, such as "Nutritious Nellie" (a cow), to teach about dairy products, especially yogurt, and "Vita-Man." Active student involvement is emphasized. Another successful school lunch manager in Huron, South Dakota, with a 94 per cent participation rate, uses a formula that includes menu planning by a student committee chosen from children in K–12. San Antonio's method is primarily through parent feedback. Parents eat in the school cafeterias, participate in lunchroom committees, and make monthly reports. Youth councils are used in Florida to promote lunch programs by planning special cafeteria events. These examples of successful programs demonstrate that one important ingredient of any effective program is student involvement.

Future Recommendations

Foundations for future programs were laid in Vail, Colorado, in September 1976. Principles on which an effective program should be based, according to the Vail conference, include the following:[50]

1. The feeding program should be an important part of the total school curriculum.

2. The feeding program should be a learning experience for the children.

3. School food centers should be a focal point for the attack on chronic diseases.

4. School food service must change to accommodate new societal demands.

5. School lunch must become community oriented, serving people of all ages, all day, all year.

6. Accountability is necessary for the resources used in providing food service.

7. Establishing a national nutrition policy that is comprehensive in planning and realistic in implementation is important to the success of the program.

8. Service is the ultimate yardstick of success.

9. Sound nutrition education for all age groups is sound preventive medicine.

In the fifth annual report to the president and Congress, the National Advisory Council on Child Nutrition recommended that continued emphasis be placed on children's nutrition education. To combat plate waste, the council encouraged schools to offer a variety of foods, involve secondary school students in menu planning, and allow adequate time for the lunch period. The council also suggested that the USDA redirect the bulk of its extra efforts away from nonprogram schools and toward increased participation and minimizing food waste in those schools already having school lunch programs.[51]

FOOD STAMP PROGRAM

The Food Stamp Program began in the 1930s when agricultural economists became interested in food stamp plans as instruments to expand the market demand for agricultural products. The objectives of the early programs were to aid in the disposal of surplus agricultural commodities and hence to indirectly subsidize the income of farm families and to subsidize an improved nutrition program for low-income families. The program enabled relief clientele and a small number of low-income people not on relief to receive stamps to obtain foods on a special surplus list. The program grew to reach over 3 million people a month.[52]

In 1943, at the height of World War II, the program was terminated because of the war effort. To feed the poor, many local governments began surplus commodity distribution programs, in which the participants received free foods (such as flour, beans, and potatoes).

The present Food Stamp Program was initiated in 1961 as a pilot program in eight areas under the authority of an executive order issued by President Kennedy.[53] By August 1964, this pilot program operated in 43 areas in 22 states. The pilot program was extended and instituted on a permanent basis with the Food Stamp Act of 1964.[54] The primary purpose was to alleviate hunger and malnutrition among the poorest individuals in the country, while at the same time assisting the agricultural economy. The program enables households with incomes below the poverty line to receive, or purchase at a discount, food stamps whose face value is, in theory, adequate to allow them to purchase a nutritional diet. Retail food stores redeem the stamps at face value.

The program is designed to provide assistance to eligible households in purchasing food through normal marketing channels. There are few restrictions on the foods that the recipients may purchase. (Some gourmet items for example are not permitted.) However, nonfood items, such as pet food, alcoholic beverages, paper products, tobacco, soap, or other cleaning products may not be purchased with the stamps.

Current Program

The current Food Stamp Program has changed from that initiated by the Food Stamp Act of 1964. As the food supply and demand conditions altered over the years, and, as Congress has gained experience with the program in light of changing priorities, the program has been amended and the emphasis of the program has shifted. More emphasis has been placed on program participation. The primary purpose of the program now is to improve the nutritional status of low-income households whose limited food purchasing power contributes to hunger and malnutrition among members. Changes made in the program include several features that were directed toward increasing the benefits to recipients and encouraging participation. These changes included organized efforts by states to inform the public of the availability and benefits of the program.

Further amendments broadened the program by making it mandatory nationwide. When the Commodity Distribution Program* for families coexisted with the Food Stamp Program, each county had to make the decision about which program it wished to use. For many, the economics of the situation was a disincentive to having the Food Stamp Program. But in 1974, with the amendment to the Food Stamp Act, the Commodity Distribution Program to individual families was disallowed.

In 1974, Congress authorized a 50 per cent reimbursement of state administrative expenses. In 1975 a full-time state outreach coordinator and additional personnel to effectively perform outreach activities were required.[53]

The Food and Agriculture Act of 1977, signed into law in September 1977, included the Food Stamp Act of 1977. One of the major reforms of this legislation was the elimination of the purchase requirement (EPR).[55] Previously, recipients had been required to purchase stamps on a monthly basis. The value of the food stamps was greater than the purchase price, the difference being termed the food stamp "bonus." Because many food stamp recipients were too poor to pay for the stamps, they could not purchase them on the specified day each month.

The new law eliminates the purchase requirement. Those who are eligible for food stamps can now receive them in the amount of their bonus with no money transfer. For example, a family previously required to pay $150 for stamps worth $200 can now receive $50 in stamps without a money transaction. This system, in addition to increasing the participa-

---

*The Commodity Distribution Program allowed eligible families to receive bulk commodities such as peanut butter, rolled oats, canned meat, and nonfat dry milk.

tion of the very poor, will reduce the total number of stamps in circulation and will eliminate much cash exchange.[56]

Other changes in the program included an increase in the material assets that a family can own and continue to be eligible for food stamps; and a change in some of the deductions used in figuring food stamp allowances.[57]

Native American tribes are to have the choice of food stamps or a commodity food program. If the food stamp option is selected, Indian tribes will be allowed to administer the program on reservations if the states do not administer the program adequately.

Eligibility

Any household that meets eligibility standards and complies with work registration requirements can participate in the Food Stamp Program. Eligibility is determined by national standards, and is primarily based on income and material resources.[57]

To obtain food stamps, the head of the household must complete an application, supply a detailed account of finances, and be interviewed. This information is used by the local food stamp office to determine eligibility. The approved applicant is then able to receive food stamps for a stated period of time (the certification period).

Program Administration

Program administration is the responsibility of the Food and Nutrition Service of the USDA. This agency writes program regulations and sets uniform national standards. Certain program operations, such as outreach, certification, and issuance of stamps, are administered by a state agency (usually the welfare or social services office).

Effectiveness of the Food Stamp Program

The program has increased both in participation and in cost over the years.[58,59] But how effective is the Food Stamp Program in improving the nutritional status of participants? Studies in Pennsylvania have found that participation in the program can increase total food expenditures. These studies also found that some nutritional benefits can result from participation in the program. The impacts of the program were most significant immediately after the stamps had been purchased and after time had passed from receiving the last income. The intakes of iron, thiamine, protein, and riboflavin were higher among food stamp recipients than among nonrecipients of comparable income levels.[60]

Lane, in a comparison of food consumption and nutritional quality of diet between participants and nonparticipants in food assistance programs, found that food stamp recipients spent a lower percentage of their income on food, but appeared to have a better nutritional status relative to certain nutrients. These nutrients included calories, protein, calcium, iron, vitamin A, thiamine, and riboflavin.[61]

The Community Services Administration funded a recent study to examine the ability of federal food assistance programs to improve the nutritional status of low-income households.[62] The study found that the ability of the program to meet family nutritional needs varied greatly. For example, because the food stamp allotments are based on household size rather than on household composition, the cost of adequately feeding older children would be greater than that of feeding toddlers. Thus, the family with adolescent boys would experience a greater hardship than the family with preschool children.

The study also reported that the Food Stamp Program could not adequately supply dietary assistance without overlapping benefits from other food assistance programs, such as the WIC Program and the School Lunch and School Breakfast Programs.

Economic Program Benefits

The Food Stamp Program has a dual purpose: to improve nutrition and to strengthen the agricultural economy. The Food Stamp Act of 1964 clearly stated the legislative intent:

> The Congress hereby finds that the limited food purchasing power of low-income households contributes to hunger and malnutrition among members of such households. The Congress further finds that increased utilization of food in establishing and maintaining adequate levels of nutrition will promote the distribution in a beneficial manner of our agricultural abundances and will strengthen our agricultural economy, as well as result in more orderly marketing and distribution of food.[54]

The federal food programs have a significant effect, not only on the nutritional status of program participants but on the general U.S. economy. Programs affect local food purchases and, hence, food demand, food prices, food production, marketing and processing, employment, and income. These effects are especially significant in low-income areas, where a larger proportion of the population are eligible to participate in the programs. Food stamps have even been referred to as a "grass roots form of revenue sharing."[63]

It has been estimated that up to 65 per cent of the bonus food stamp money buys food that would not have been purchased otherwise. Thus, one of the primary effects of the program is the expansion of food demand.[64] If this estimate is correct, in 1976 an expanded demand for food resulted in approximately $2.5–3.5 billion extra for food at the retail level.[63] An estimated $1.10–1.45 billion of these dollars were received by farmers in 1976.

Indirect economic benefits from the Food Stamp Program are not limited to food producers and retailers. Additional money they receive must be used to purchase needed farm inputs, such as equipment, seeds, and fertilizer or to pay for other supplies, goods, and services. Persons who supply goods and services to retailers must buy replacements from the sectors that produced them, and these, in turn, must buy raw material and labor to produce the replacement items.

The "multiplier effect" refers to the level of business stimulated by such an expanded economy. The multiplier effect for the Food Stamp Program has been estimated to be 3.64. In other words, $1.00 of food stamp bonus spent will result in $3.64 of new business transactions.

This, in turn, generates new jobs and the cycle of economic improvement continues.[65]

Research studies confirm these ideas. A USDA report summarized the impact of the Food Stamp Program on three rural economies. In Haywood County, Tennessee, the program cost the government an estimated $1.2 million, but resulted in an additional business value of $1.5 million and the creation of 60 additional jobs. The other counties studied experienced similar benefits. According to the Economic Research Service, business receipts in the United States were more than $1.2 billion higher in 1974 than they would have been without the program.[65] In 1974, an estimated 76,500 new jobs resulted from the program, primarily in agriculture, forestry, fisheries, food processing, and retailing.

Problems of the Food Stamp Program

One of the most significant problems is that of nonparticipation. According to a Bureau of the Census report, only 40 per cent of eligible households participate. Particularly problematic is nonparticipation among the elderly and among migrant workers.

Why is the rate of nonparticipation so high? Factors include inconvenient food stamp office locations, inconvenient office hours, long waits for interview appointments, lack of understanding by non-English speaking persons, the long time involved in certification and issuance procedures, the personal pride that keeps many from accepting "handouts," and the lack of outreach resulting in lack of knowledge or understanding about the program and its benefits.[58]

The regulations promulgated as a result of the Food Stamp Act of 1977 may help to alleviate some of these problems. Participation in the program is expected to increase in cases where those working poor who did not have the needed itemized deductions are now eligible because of the standard deduction and the increase in allowed asset values. Further, participation may increase with the elimination of the purchase requirement. In general, the revisions are expected to increase participation by 10–15 per cent.[44]

A variety of other problems, common to the Food Stamp Program and to other federal food programs, are discussed on pages 601–608.

NATIONAL NUTRITION PROGRAM FOR THE ELDERLY

In an effort to meet the multifaceted needs of the elderly, the Administration on Aging, established under the U.S. Department of Health, Education, and Welfare by the Older Americans Act of 1965 (Title IV), conducted research and demonstration projects to improve the nutrition and diets of the elderly.

The specific objectives were to demonstrate methods of providing appetizing and nutritionally adequate meals in settings that were conducive to eating and to social interactions with peers for the elderly. Other objectives included improving the diet and nutritional status of the participants, evaluating various settings for the program, determining the impact of education on changing the dietary habits of the participants, and analyzing the needs of subgroups of older Americans and determining appropriate meals to meet these needs.

Thirty-two nutrition programs were funded. Each project provided meals in group settings, nutrition education and information, systematic evaluation, supportive services, and outreach services.[66]

Results of the projects suggested that the programs include five components:[67]

1. An outreach plan to reach those who were most in need of the program.

2. Service of meals in a socially stimulating environment.

3. Nutrition education.

4. Related and ancillary services.

5. Ongoing, objective, and systematic evaluation.

Current Program Activities

As a result of the Title IV demonstration projects, Congress in 1972 enacted the Title VII Nutrition Program. In October 1978, Congress changed the AOA titles and the National Nutrition Program for the Elderly is now funded under Title III of the Older Americans Act.

The main goals of the program are summarized in Table 17-3.[68] The mission of the program is to provide inexpensive, nutritionally balanced

Table 17-3
Goals of the National Nutrition Program for the Elderly

1. Improve the health of the elderly with the provision of regularly available low-cost nutritious meals served largely in congregate settings and when feasible, to the homebound.

2. Increase the incentive of elderly persons to maintain social well-being by providing opportunities for social interaction and the satisfying use of leisure time.

3. Improve the capability of the elderly to prepare meals at home by providing auxiliary services including nutrition and homemaker education, shopping assistance, and transportation to markets.

4. Increase the incentive of the elderly to maintain good health and independent living by providing counseling and information and referral to other social and rehabilitation services.

5. Assure that those elderly most in need, primarily the low-income, minorities, and the isolated, can and do participate in nutrition services by providing an extensive and personalized outreach program and transportation service.

6. Stimulate minority elderly interest in nutrition services by assuring that operation of the projects reflects cultural pluralism in both the meal and supportive service components.

7. Assure that program participants have access to a comprehensive and coordinated system of services by encouraging administration coordination between nutrition projects and area agencies on aging.

Source: U.S. Department of Health, Education, and Welfare, Committee on Research and Development, Gerontological Society. *Evaluative Research on Social Programs for the Elderly*. Washington, D.C.: Government Printing Office, 1973, p. 142.

meals for the elderly. The program aims to help the elderly who participate to be motivated to maintain their social well-being through the provision of opportunities for social interaction.

Meals are provided in congregate meal settings at specified, centralized
locations. They are designed to provide at least one-third of the basic nutrient requirements. Although volunteer contributions for meals are accepted, the elderly are not required to pay for their food.

A variety of supportive services are to be provided to encourage and
facilitate participation in the program: transportation to the meal site
and back home, information and referral services, health or welfare
counseling, ongoing nutrition education, assistance in food shopping,
recreation activities, and outreach.

Eligibility and Participation

Individuals aged 60 or older and their spouses (who may not necessarily
be 60) are eligible if they have difficulty meeting their nutritional needs
because they

1. Cannot afford to do so.
2. Lack the skills to select and prepare nutritionally sound meals.
3. Are restricted in mobility, which may impair their ability to shop and
   cook for themselves.
4. Are lonely, isolated, and in need of social activities to stimulate the
   motivation to eat a well-balanced meal.

The U.S. Senate Select Committee on Nutrition and Human Needs conducted surveys on the Title VII and the Meals on Wheels projects and
found that 97 per cent of the private meal delivery programs were located in metropolitan areas where Title VII programs were located. But
40 per cent of the Title VII programs were located in rural areas where
the home-delivered meals are not available.[69]

Administration

The meal program provides formula grants to individual states, based on
the ratio of a state's eligible population (those aged 60 and over) to the
national population of those aged 60 or over. The states then award funds
to designated projects established to provide meals for the target population. In addition, the U.S. Department of Agriculture provides surplus
commodities to the program.

State and local governments also offer funds for the operation of the
meal programs. States must provide matching funds to the federal funds.
Program participants also contribute income to the program as their
abilities permit.

The primary responsibility for supervision, administration, and program administration rests with the individual states, and the District of
Columbia, Puerto Rico, Guam, American Samoa, the Virgin Islands, and
the trust territories of the Pacific Islands.

HOW EFFECTIVE ARE FOOD AND NUTRITION ASSISTANCE PROGRAMS IN COMBATING MALNUTRITION?

Today, the United States finds the cost of a sound diet and of nutrition education for all its children to be too expensive. Yet a truly adequate program of nutrition and nutrition education for our children would require approximately the same expenditure that we make each year to feed our dogs and cats. It would require a billion dollars a year less than we spend each year on horse racing; only one-half of what we spend each year on tobacco; less than one-third of what we spend each year on alcoholic beverages. If we seriously consider our priorities, surely we will decide that a nation that can afford to spend 30 million dollars on candy for its children on one Halloween night can afford to feed the same children a balanced diet throughout the year. We talk too much about the cost of good nutrition and too little about the cost of bad nutrition. The cost of illness in the United States has increased 400 per cent in the past ten years and continues to skyrocket. A strong program of nutrition and nutrition education for our youth would cut billions from the medical costs of our nation.[70]

We do not hesitate to outlaw murder when it is quick but when it comes in the form of a slow decline due to hunger and malnutrition even we equivocate and refuse to take a stand.

We search our souls when a soldier is killing civilians, but we would rather look the other way when civilians — in and out of government — condemn people to slow starvation by refusing to implement programs.[71]

Federal food and nutrition programs have many outspoken critics who contend that the North American public and the federal government, in particular, have no real desire to alleviate hunger and malnutrition but, instead, toss out token aid to the deprived, like crumbs to a starving man. Can these criticisms be substantiated? The following section assesses some of the successes as well as some of the weaknesses of federal food assistance programs.

Expenditures and Participation

Public food and nutrition programs have been greatly expanded since 1969. Federal expenditures for these programs have greatly increased. Further, the WIC Program, the Child Care Feeding Program, and various nutrition education programs have been implemented since 1969. Tables 17-4 and 17-5 illustrate the growth in federal food and nutrition programs.

A very important issue relative to the increase in federal involvement in these food and nutrition programs is whether the effort has significantly reduced nutrition problems. There are really two parts to the answer to this question. First, if the programs are successful in achieving their objective of reducing hunger and malnutrition, the food assistance must reach those in need of such aid. Second, even if food assistance dollars reach the poor, these programs must have influenced changes in food consumption and improved the nutritional status of vulnerable assistance recipients if they are successful.

Early studies provided little evidence that federal food assistance was able to significantly improve nutritional status. Research in five counties

Table 17–4

Federal Cost of USDA Food Programs

			1977		1978			
	1975	*1976*	*1977*	*IV*	*I*	*II*	*III*	*IV*[1]
Item				*Million Dollars*				
Food stamps								
Total issued	7,680	7,818	7,425	1,784	1,925	1,861	1,878	1,893
Bonus stamps[2]	4,602	4,657	4,373	1,037	1,183	1,133	1,146	1,137
Food distribution[3]								
Needy families	11	8	11	2	2	2	2	2
Schools[4]	364	448	528	136	193	109	85	152
Other[5]	33	33	49	11	28	17	31	20
Child nutrition[6]								
School lunch	1,340	1,505	1,645	525	565	471	226	576
School breakfast	94	118	147	49	52	49	22	51
Special food[7]	116	240	236	32	36	55	128	35
Special milk	134	147	152	46	39	35	20	43
WIC[8]	106	182	281	81	89	99	106	113
Total[9]	6,800	7,337	7,422	1,921	2,190	1,969	1,766	2,129

[1] Preliminary.
[2] Includes Food Certificate Program.
[3] Cost of food delivered to state distribution centers.
[4] Includes special food services.
[5] Includes supplemental food, institutions, elderly persons.
[6] Money donated for local purchase of food. Excludes nonfood assistance.
[7] Includes child care and summer food programs.
[8] Special Supplemental Food Program for Women, Infants, and Children begun January 1974.
[9] Excludes those food stamps paid for by the recipient. Do not add due to rounding.
Source: Bunting, F.: Food spending and income. *National Food Review*, Winter 1979, p. 10.

in Pennsylvania noted that the provision of commodity foods to low-income households did not actually improve dietary quality but did free up money to be used for other purposes, such as clothes and housing. A later study of the Food Stamp Program also indicated that the primary benefit of the program was an income maintenance one.[60]

The WIC Program has been found to be important in improving the nutritional status of the participants. Other programs providing meals, such as the Title III and school feeding programs, may free up income that would otherwise have been used for food, but they may also improve nutritional status.[72]

In fiscal 1969, per capita food assistance program expenditures for those in identified "hunger counties" (counties chosen according to the percentage of population below the poverty line and the rate of postneonatal mortality) with the highest postneonatal mortality rates (PMR, an indicator of the existence of malnutrition) were an estimated $26. In fiscal 1976, this figure rose to over $127. Thus, in absolute dollars, the per capita expenditures for food assistance in these areas of nutritional vulnerability rose by more than $100. In the total United States, per person expenditures for the same programs increased by only $44.[73]

Table 17-5.

Participation Growth in Federal Food Assistance Programs, Fiscal Years 1969-77, in thousands

	1969	1970	1971	1972	1973	1974	1975	1976	Transition Quarter	1977
Family food assistance programs (monthly average)										
1. Food stamp program	2,878	4,340	9,368	11,103	12,129	12,896	17,063	18,557	17,315	17,054
2. Commodity distribution program (needy families)	3,611	3,812	3,756	3,438	2,660	1,982	330	80	72	82
Child feeding programs (peak):										
1. National school lunch program:										
(a) Total (sec. 4)	22,079[1]	23,127	24,640	24,941	25,164	25,019	25,289	25,857	25,104	26,812
(b) Free (sec. 11)	3,334[1]	4,787[1]	5,421	7,612	8,586	9,007	9,595	10,280	10,020	10,598
(c) Reduced price (sec. 11)			899	499	199	300	599	897	993	1,292
2. School breakfast program	330	573	960	1,142	1,313	1,534	1,993	2,334	2,141	2,561
3. Child care food program	40	93	176	216	225	377	457	463		552
4. Summer food service program for children	99	227	569	1,205	1,437	1,403	1,785	2,454	3,467	2,666
5. Special milk program (half-pints)	2,944,423	2,901,931	2,569,975	2,498,215	2,560,711	1,425,923	2,138,993	2,305,143	313,429	2,253,274
6. Special supplemental food program for women, infants, and children (WIC):	[2]	[2]	[2]	[2]	[2]	206	498	592	656	994
(a) Women						38	77	98	118	199
(b) Infants						62	151	146	162	257
(c) Children						105	270	348	376	538
Nutrition program for the elderly	[2]	[2]	[2]	[2]	41	195	1,277	1,723	667	2,392[3]

[1] This figure represents a combined total for free and reduced-price meals, separate data are not available.

[2] Program not in existence.

[3] First three quarters in 1977 data only.

Source: U.S. Senate Select Committee on Nutrition and Human Needs, *Final Report*. Washington, D.C.: U.S. Government Printing Office, December 1977.

These figures suggest that food assistance funds are reaching those areas where hunger and malnutrition are likely to be most severe. Figure 17-6 illustrates federal per person expenditures for food assistance in counties with the highest and the lowest postneonatal mortality rates.

Food Sales[73]

If federal food assistance in the form of food stamp expenditures is actually reducing nutritional problems, then it is to be expected that this influence could be observed through increased local per capita retail sales of food in areas of poverty and deprivation. The results of a recent study show that increases in federal expenditures for food stamps actually did exert a statistically significant influence on per capita retail food sales in the counties with the highest PMR, but not in counties with the lowest PMR.

These data suggest that funds have been channeled to those areas of particular nutritional vulnerability, but they do not indicate that hunger or malnutrition has been eliminated in the United States. The data from the USDA Nationwide Food Consumption Survey (1977-1978) will aid in defining the incidence of dietary problems in the population at large. It is clear, however, that we lack evidence to suggest that nutritional problems have been alleviated, and, as noted in Section II, substantial research indicates the continued existence of hunger and malnutrition in the United States, despite tremendous federal expenditures for food assistance and nutrition programs.

Nutritional Benefits

Programs designed to combat malnutrition have often met with success as demonstrated by improved nutritional status. As examples, two nutri-

Figure 17-6. Federal expenditures per person for domestic food assistance in U.S. counties with the highest and lowest post-neonatal mortality rates.

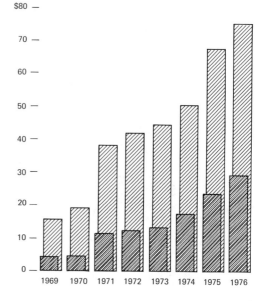

HIGHEST▨ AND LOWEST▨ POST NEONATAL MORTALITY RATES

tion program evaluations are now reviewed. P. Zee et al. reported a nutrition and health survey of black preschool children in a low-income area in Memphis, Tennessee. Median family income was $1,838 and household size was 6.8 individuals. A random sample of 300 children was studied; 50 per cent of the children were below the twenty-fifth percentile for height and weight standards. Anemia was widespread — 28 per cent of the children under the age of 3 years presented hemoglobin values less than 10 gm/100 ml, and 25 per cent of children over the age of 3 had values less than 11 gm/100 ml. Forty-four per cent of the sample presented low serum vitamin A values.[74]

Following this initial survey, coordinated efforts of county health departments, model cities programs, and local medical and health personnel initiated a supplementary feeding program. Participants in the program were low-income children under the age of 6, pregnant women, and mothers up to 1 year postpartum.

In 1972 a resurvey of 250 children randomly selected from the same population studied in 1969 showed significant improvement in many of the nutritional status indicators, such as hemoglobin, height, and weight as a result of the program.[75]

In another study, nutritional intervention in the form of iron-enriched milk formula was provided to a group of about 100 Baltimore, Maryland, infants for the first 9 months of life. A control group received no enriched supplement. The prevalence of low hemoglobin levels (below 10 mg/100 ml) was 2.5 per cent for the experimental versus 55 per cent in the control group.[76]

Another Baltimore study monitored 5,284 inner-city schoolchildren over a four-year period during which time free school meal programs were implemented. Significant nutritional improvements were evidenced in the reduction of low hemoglobin, serum albumin, and vitamin A levels and in the number of children falling below the third percentile in skinfold thickness measurements.[76]

Problems with Federal Food Programs

The Citizens Board of Inquiry, in a follow-up to their 1968 report, cited many reasons for the inefficient functioning of federal food programs. One factor limiting the passage of effective food assistance legislation centers on *political considerations* and *"bureaucratic sensitivity."*

Although the right of individuals to adequate food is verbally honored by policymakers, the attack on hunger and malnutrition is often conducted to advance political gains. For example, in early 1969, President Nixon was quoted as stating, "You can say that this administration will have the first complete, far-reaching attack on the problems of hunger in history. Use all the rhetoric, so long as it doesn't cost any money."[77] Thus, the charge was made by the Citizens Board of Inquiry that the position of the executive, as well as of the legislative branch, was one of "rhetoric, but not resolve."

The passage of legislation that is beneficial to solving hunger problems is often contingent on political factors. To illustrate this, the Citizens Board cites the following:

The original Food Stamp Act was successfully enacted in 1964 in large part because Congresswoman Leonor Sullivan . . . was astute enough to sense that the bill which she sponsored on behalf of the hungry could be used in trade by the urban House members in exchange for farm legislation desired by the farm bloc. She took skillful advantage of her bargaining position to exchange a wheat-cotton subsidy program for food stamps. In 1967 and in 1968 she repeated her strategy of linking urban support for farm programs with rural and farm support for food programs and was thus able to extend and expand the Act and its authorization level.[78]

Although this view of the passage of "antihunger" legislation is no doubt simplistic, as well as controversial, there is little doubt that the political arena is the setting for progress in combating malnutrition and that politics is a strong influence on the way food programs and legislation are handled.

As Congresswomen Shirley Chisholm noted, many politicians and lawmakers see federal humanism to be a form of "erosion of American ideal." Thus, they tend to be "overprotective and overdefensive" "about the federal programs; when there is a budgetary constraint, an administration difficulty or a service delivery difficulty, these politicians respond by trying to show that such programs should be eliminated, cut back, that they can't be workable, efficient or effective, that they are a waste of federal tax dollars."[79]

There are many angles to the story of politics and food. One interesting one that illustrates vividly the behind-the-scene actions is told by J. Kramer when he was special counsel for the House Committee on Agriculture:

In 1970 we had the major school lunch bill scheduled on Washington's Birthday, thanks to Senator Mansfield who had no interest in the bill. We had a major vote about just how many children could get school lunch for free. . . . We lost 36 to 35 . . . Senator Javits, who was one of the major spokesmen in *Esquire, Playboy* and elsewhere for anti-hunger programs, stayed in Acapulco to finish off his weekend and help finish off the children. Senator Hollings was skiing. . . . And Senator Percy — this is the best of all — . . . delivered a speech in Chicago . . . saying it is time we turned our priorities around and put more money into feeding children . . .[80]

Many problems inherent in the food programs are the result of those who participate in the legislative and regulatory process, for example, congressmen who do not keep up with the events and do not know what is happening and, consequently, are not able to help the nutrition cause.

Another problem involves the time taken to develop regulations. It is not unheard of for three years to pass between the passage of legislation and the publication of regulations specifying how the law is to be made into reality. Problems of this nature were discussed in Chapter 15.

Program administration is another major problem. No single committee or department has the responsibility for the effects of the whole system; each deals with legislation that directly affects only a few programs. This is part of the broader problem that Congress lacks an effective mechanism for setting priorities. Thus, although there are hundreds of programs, most with promising legislative preambles, the funds are insufficient to extend the benefits of the programs to all who are eligible under the law.[81] Table 17-6 illustrates the jurisdiction of Congress over various nutrition education programs revealed in a Congressional Research Service study in 1977. The problem of lack of universal goals and overall coordination is clear. Figure 17-7 illustrates the maze of administrative flows for major federal food and nutrition programs.

When federal feeding programs are examined for their *bureaucratic*

Table 17-6

Committee Jurisdiction over Nutrition Education Related Programs

Program	Committee Jurisdiction	
	House	Senate
A. EXTENSION SERVICE Extension Food and Nutrition Program (other than EFNEP)	Subcommittee on Domestic Marketing, Consumer Relations and Nutrition, Committees on Agriculture	Subcommittee on Agricultural Research and General Legislation, Committee on Agriculture and Forestry
Expanded Food and Nutrition Education Program (EFNEP)	Subcommittee on Domestic Marketing, Consumer Relations and Nutrition, Committee on Agriculture	Subcommittee on Agricultural Research and General Legislation, Committee on Agriculture and Forestry
B. AGRICULTURAL RESEARCH SERVICE Food and Nutrition Research Program	Subcommittee on Departmental Operations and Investigations, Committee on Agriculture	Subcommittee on Agricultural Research and General Legislation, Committee on Agriculture and Forestry
C. FOOD AND NUTRITION SERVICE Food Stamp Program	Subcommittee on Domestic Marketing, Consumer Relations and Nutrition, Committee on Agriculture	Subcommittee on Agricultural Research and General Legislation, Committee on Agriculture and Forestry
Child Nutrition Program	Subcommittee on Elementary and Secondary Education, Committee on Education and Labor	Subcommittee on Agricultural Research and General Legislation, Committee on Agriculture and Forestry
Special Supplemental Food Program for Women, Infants, and Children (WIC)	Subcommittee on Elementary and Secondary Education, Committee on Education and Labor	Subcommittee on Agricultural Research and General Legislation, Committee on Agriculture and Forestry Select Committee on Nutrition and Human Needs
D. COOPERATIVE STATE RESEARCH SERVICE	Subcommittee on Departmental Operations and Investigations, Committee on Agriculture	Subcommittee on Agricultural Research and General Legislation, Committee on Agriculture and Forestry

Committee Jurisdiction over Nutrition Education Related Programs *(continued)*

Program	Committee Jurisdiction House	Senate
Department of Health, Education, and Welfare (HEW)		

A. ADMINISTRATION ON AGING

Program	House	Senate
Nutrition Program Aging Nutrition Program for the Elderly	Subcommittee on Select Education, Committee on Education and Labor	Subcommittee on Aging, Committee on Labor and Public Welfare

B. OFFICE OF CHILD DEVELOPMENT

Program	House	Senate
Head Start Program	Subcommittee on Equal Opportunities, Committee on Education and Labor	Subcommittee on Employment, Poverty, and Migratory Labor, Committee on Labor and Public Welfare

C. OFFICE OF CONSUMER AFFAIRS

Program	House	Senate
Food, Nutrition, and Affairs Food, Nutrition, and Health Campaign	Subcommittee on HUD and Independent Agencies, Committee on Appropriations	Subcommittee on HUD and Independent Agencies, Committee on Appropriations

D. OFFICE OF EDUCATION

Program	House	Senate
Consumer and Home-making Education, Part F	Subcommittee on Elementary and Secondary Education, Committee on Education and Labor	Subcommittee on Education, Committee on Labor and Public Welfare
Follow Through	Subcommittee on Elementary and Secondary Education, Committee on Education and Labor	Subcommittee on Education, Committee on Labor and Public Welfare
The Library and Services Construction Act	Subcommittee on Select Education, Committee on Education and Labor	Subcommittee on Education, Committee on Labor and Public Welfare
Part B, Basic Grants, State Vocational Education Programs, Occupational Home Economics Education	Subcommittee on Elementary and Secondary Education, Committee on Education and Labor	Subcommittee on Education, Committee on Labor and Public Welfare
Consumers' Education	Subcommittee on Elementary and Secondary Education, Committee on Education and Labor	Subcommittee on Education, Committee on Labor and Public Welfare
Adult Education Program	Subcommittee on Elementary and Secondary Education, Committee on Education and Labor	Subcommittee on Education, Committee on Labor and Public Welfare
School Health and Nutrition Services for Low-income Families	Subcommittee on Elementary and Secondary Education, Committee on Education and Labor	Subcommittee on Education, Committee on Labor and Public Welfare

Committee Jurisdiction over Nutrition Education Related Programs *(continued)*

	Committee Jurisdiction	
Program	*House*	*Senate*
Centers and Services for Deaf-Blind Children	Subcommittee on Select Education, Committee on Education and Labor	Subcommittee on Education, Committee on Labor and Public Welfare
Severely Handicapped Children and Youth	Subcommittee on Select Education, Committee on Education and Labor	Subcommittee on Education, Committee on Labor and Public Welfare
Handicapped Children's Early Education Program	Subcommittee on Select Education, Committee on Education and Labor	Subcommittee on Education, Committee on Labor and Public Welfare
E. HEALTH SERVICES ADMINISTRATION		
Bureau of Community Health Services	Subcommittee on Public Health and Environment, Committee on Interstate and Foreign Commerce	Subcommittee on Health, Committee on Labor and Public Welfare
Service	Subcommittee on Indian Affairs, Committee on Interior and Insular Affairs	Subcommittee on Indian Affairs, Committee on Interior and Insular Affairs
Bureau of Quality Assurance	Subcommittee on Public Health and Environment, Committee on Interstate and Foreign Commerce	Subcommittee on Health, Committee on Labor and Public Welfare
Bureau of Medical Services	Subcommittee on Public Health and Environment, Committee on Interstate and Foreign Commerce	Subcommittee on Health, Committee on Labor and Public Welfare

Source: Congressional Research Service, Subcommittee on Domestic Marketing, Consumer Relations, and Nutrition. *The Role of the Federal Government in Nutrition Education.* Washington, D.C.: Government Printing Office, March 1977, pp. 5–7.

limitations, we see many specific examples of these larger problems: lack of coordination between various programs designed to increase the nutritional status of individuals and families, lack of funds to adequately administrate these programs, lack of sufficient supervision to prevent abuse within programs, and failure of programs to be offered to those who are eligible to participate.

"Jurisdictional rights" have also been suggested as severely handicapping food programs by the "reluctance of various governmental arms to cross jurisdictional boundaries." The reluctance of federal administrators to supervise and regulate programs at the state and local levels has often impaired the success of food programs. Lack of uniform and universal eligibility standards, program authorization standards, and financial authorization for various programs has resulted in an inequity, geographically as well as economically, socially, and culturally, in available benefits from the federal food programs.[78]

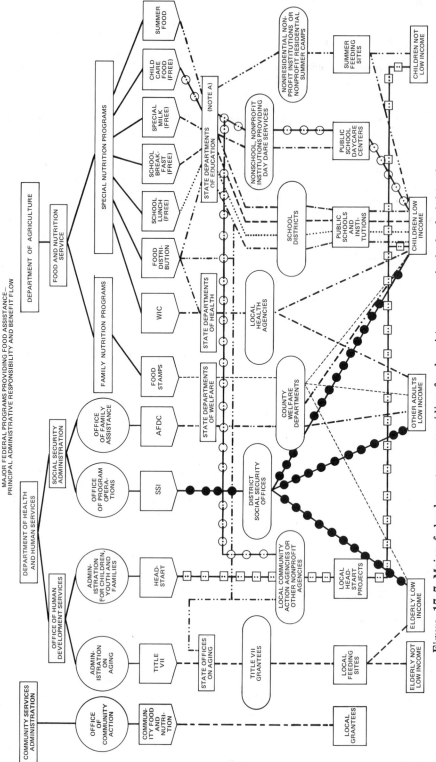

Figure 17-7. Major federal programs providing food assistance — principal administrative responsibility and benefit flow. (Office of Management and Budget)

As the Citizens Board charged:

> The hungry poor remain a federal problem if you are a county commissioner or welfare official and a state or local problem if you are the Department of Agriculture. Local failures to deliver are supported by federal failures to intervene. No jurisdiction is willing to accept the full responsibility for seeing that the benefits Congress intended to bestow upon the hungry poor ever reach them.[78]

Another charge made concerning the federal response to nutritional problems is that the *discipline of the budget,* rather than efficient and effective reimbursement of funds authorized for programs, characterizes efforts to administer food programs. The Citizens Board made its case for these various charges by citing specific instances of lack of appropriate funding in family food programs, school programs, and programs for pregnant women, nursing mothers, and their children. The burden of problems in the programs is felt by participants. What this actually means in terms of inhuman treatment that may result is illustrated by the following excerpt taken from a case study of a blue-collar family living in the Washington, D.C. area.[82]

> Bobbi, however, still received the AFDC check for Bubba and still qualified for food stamps. On the morning of April 7, I accompanied her to the welfare department to be recertified. When I picked her up at six-thirty in the morning, Bobbi was waiting for me and said that she had been up since five. When we arrived at seven, a half-dozen people were ahead of us. By seven-thirty there were sixteen; by eight there were thirty; and by eight-thirty, when the receptionist arrived, there were well over fifty people, mostly white, mostly women, with a scattering of blacks and a scattering of older males. Also there were at least a half-dozen long-haired young people.
>
> While we were waiting, Bobbi and the black woman sitting next to her agreed that they knew exactly what was going to happen. Bobbi said: "Listen, I can tell you. I've been here enough times, I know exactly what the routine is going to be. About eight-thirty, when they are supposed to open up, the caseworkers will come wandering in. Some of them will have coffee, some of them won't. They won't say a word; they'll just breeze past the line of people, sort of turn their noses up, and go into the back room. Then a little after eight-thirty the receptionist will sort of mosey on out. She might look around and then go back in and get a cup of coffee. Take her first coffee break for about fifteen minutes. Then about eight forty-five they will be ready to start the line. They'll call out the names of the people who were there yesterday but who weren't seen. Then everybody will rush to the front and sort of jam around and try to get in front of the line. Then they'll take names of people today who are supposed to get certified. She'll see a few people, then take another coffee break, smoke a cigarette, sort of take it easy. By nine-fifteen or nine-thirty, if we're lucky and in the first of the line, we'll get seen. That's what will happen. You mark my words."
>
> Bobbi was exactly right. The receptionist came out about eight forty-five with a cup of coffee. She said, "Two lines will be formed. One for food stamps and one for public assistance."
>
> "Which line is which?" someone asked.
>
> "I don't know," said Bobbi.
>
> "Well, which line am I in?" asked the person next to us.
>
> "I guess you're in the food stamp line," said Bobbi.

People shifted lines. Two crude lines were formed. Though there was some shoving and pushing, most of the people were content to keep their original place in line. We should have been third, but some people hung around the reception desk and managed to get ahead of us.

The receptionist said, "I'm sorry, but only four people will be seen today for food stamps." The person who was fifth in line said, "Only four people? I've been here since six in the morning. The person who is first, he didn't get here until much later."

"I'm sorry, I wasn't here. I don't know," replied the receptionist condescendingly.

"But other people know. . ." Several people voiced agreement.

"I'm sorry. I wasn't here, and I don't know who was first."

"But I came over here from way over the other side of the county. I can prove it. You can call my house. I can prove it. I can't come back tomorrow."

"I'm sorry."

"But that's not fair. There are two people who got ahead of me who weren't here. . .".

Bobbi said, "Ain't that some shit. We ain't going to get seen today. I knew it. I always have to come back."

There were several women standing in line with small children, who were crying. By this time the hallway was filled with smoke, and everyone seemed as discomforted as I felt. Bobbi commented to the receptionist, "Look, I was here before he was," pointing to the person ahead of us.

"I'm sorry. You'll have to wait your place in line."

"Listen, we were here at seven and he didn't come in until later." The receptionist took the gentleman's name anyway and said that he should go into room number three. When our turn came, being so far down the list, Bobbi was told to come back tomorrow. She later commented that it would take probably at least until eleven or eleven-thirty tomorrow to get re-certified for food stamps.

Bobbi went through this every single month. Every month she arrived between the hours of five and seven in the morning and stood in line for two or three hours.

Conclusion — Problems of U.S. Food Assistance Programs

There are, without doubt, numerous problems inherent in the structure and operation of food assistance programs in the United States. Perhaps the fundamental problem is the assumption on which the programs are founded. Historically, federal approaches to nutritional problems have been categorical; most programs have focused on individual groups with specific problems or with special vulnerability to developing such problems. Traditional benefactors of nutrition programs have included the school-aged child, the poor, and more recently, pregnant/lactating mothers, infants, children, and the elderly.

However, this approach may have to be re-evaluated, especially in light of the increasing recognition that nutrition is essential for preventive health care.

Implementation of a more effective federal initiative will require closer linkages between local, state, and federal activities, those undertaken by consumer and advocate groups, and those supported by industry, foundations, or other funding sources.

Some states have developed mechanisms to provide nutritional services to residents through the delivery of services at the county or multicounty level. Even with federal, state, and regional cooperation, successful nutrition program efforts appear to be dependent on the active participation of the local community, including the public, health professionals, and organizations.

REFERENCES

1. U.S. Senate Subcommittee on Employment, Manpower, and Poverty. *Letter to President Johnson.* Washington, D.C., April 27, 1967.
2. Brenner, J., R. Coles, A. Mermann, M. Senn, C. Walwyn, and R. Wheeler. *Children in Mississippi: A Report to the Field Foundation.* Washington, D.C., June 1967.
3. Citizens Board of Inquiry. *Hunger, U.S.A.: A Report by the Citizens Board of Inquiry into Hunger and Malnutrition in the United States.* Washington, D.C.: New Community Press, 1968.
4. Columbia Broadcasting System. "Hunger in America." New York, 1969.
5. Committee on School Lunch Participation. *Their Daily Bread,* 1969.
6. U.S. Senate Select Committee on Nutrition and Human Needs. *National Nutrition Policy Study.* Washington, D.C.: Government Printing Office, 1974.
7. White House Conference on Food, Nutrition, and Health. *Final Report.* Washington, D.C.: Government Printing Office, 1970.
8. Enloe, C. Hitched to everything in the universe. *Nutr. Today* 4 (Winter 1969-1970): 2-17.
9. U.S. Department of Health, Education, and Welfare, Maternal and Child Health Services. *Program of Projects: Guidelines.* Rockville, Md.: U.S. Public Health Service, September 1976.
10. Percy, C. In *Overcoming Malnutrition: Putting Federal Programs to Work.* Washington, D.C.: The Children's Foundation, May 1977.
11. U.S. Department of Agriculture, Food and Nutrition Service. WIC program on regulations, Sect. 246.2(p). 39 *Fed. Reg.* 44731.
12. Goodwin, M. T., and R. Bohdan. *A Guide to Food Programs in Montgomery County, Maryland.* Rockville, Md.: Montgomery County Health Department, Nutrition Services, June 1978.
13. National School Lunch Act and Child Nutrition Act of 1966, PL-94-105, 1975 amendments, October 1975.
14. Child Nutrition Act of 1966, PL-95-627, 1978 amendments, November 10, 1978.
15. U.S. Department of Agriculture, Food and Nutrition Service. *Nutrition Education Guidelines.* Washington, D.C.: Government Printing Office, 1976.
16. Foreman, C. T. Testimony before U.S. Senate Subcommittee on Agriculture, Nutrition, and Forestry. Washington, D.C.: Government Printing Office, April 12, 1978.
17. Benedick, M., I. H. Campbell, D. L. Bawden, and M. Jones. *Towards Efficiency and Effectiveness in the WIC Delivery Service.* Washington, D.C.: The Urban Institute, 1976.
18. U.S. Senate Select Committee on Nutrition and Human Needs. *Evaluation of the Special Supplemental Food Program for Women, Infants, and Children.* Washington, D.C.: Government Printing Office, 1976. See, also, Edozein, J. C., B. R. Switzer, and R. B. Bryan. Medical evaluation of the

special supplemental food program for women, infants, and children. *Am. J. Clin. Nutr.* 32 (1974): 677–692.

19. National Advisory Council on Maternal, Infant, and Fetal Nutrition. *1977 Annual Report*. Washington, D.C.: U.S. Department of Agriculture, 1977.

20. U.S. Department of Health, Education, and Welfare, Office of Child Development. *Head Start Program Performance Standards*. Washington, D.C.: U.S. Department of Health, Education, and Welfare, 1975.

21. U.S. Department of Health, Education, and Welfare, Office of Child Development. *Handbook for Local Head Start Nutrition Specialists*. Washington, D.C.: U.S. Department of Health, Education, and Welfare, 1975.

22. U.S. Department of Agriculture; U.S. Department of Health, Education, and Welfare. *Head Start Food Buying Guide and Recipes*. Washington, D.C.: U.S. Department of Health, Education, and Welfare, 1969.

23. U.S. Department of Health, Education, and Welfare, Office of Child Development. *Head Start Nutrition Instructor's Guide for Training Leaders — Parent Education in Nutrition and Food*. Washington, D.C.: U.S. Department of Health, Education, and Welfare, 1969.

24. U.S. Department of Health, Education, and Welfare, Office of Child Development. *Head Start Nutrition Staff Training Program*. Washington, D.C.: U.S. Department of Health, Education, and Welfare, 1969.

25. U.S. Office of Economic Opportunity. *Head Start Leader's Handbook for a Nutrition and Food Course*. Washington, D.C.: U.S. Department of Health, Education, and Welfare, 1967.

26. U.S. Department of Health, Education, and Welfare, Office of Child Development. *Head Start Nutrition Film — "Jenny Is a Good Thing" Leader's Discussion Guide*. Washington, D.C.: U.S. Department of Health, Education, and Welfare, 1969.

27. U.S. Department of Health, Education, and Welfare, Office of Child Development. *Head Start Nutrition Education for Young Children*. Washington, D.C.: U.S. Department of Health, Education, and Welfare, 1969.

28. U.S. Department of Health, Education, and Welfare, Office of Child Development. *Leadership Development and Training for Head Start Coordinators of Nutrition and Cook Managers*. Washington, D.C.: U.S. Department of Health, Education, and Welfare, 1975.

29. U.S. Department of Health, Education, and Welfare, Office of Child Development. *Head Start: A Child Development Program*. Washington, D.C.: U.S. Department of Health, Education, and Welfare, 1977.

30. *Head Start Newsletter* 9 (May–June 1977): 8.

31. General Accounting Office. *Federal Domestic Food Assistance Programs — A Time for Assessment and Change*, Rept. No. CED 78–113. Washington, D.C., June 13, 1978.

32. Office of the Comptroller General of the United States. *Project Head Start: Achievements and Problems*. Washington, D.C.: General Accounting Office, May 20, 1975.

33. Stearns, M. S. *Report on Preschool Programs: The Effects of Preschool Programs on Disadvantaged Children and Their Families*. Washington, D.C.: U.S. Department of Health, Education, and Welfare, Office of Child Development, 1971.

34. Grotberg, E. *Review of Research, 1965 to 1969, of Project Head Start*. Washington, D.C.: U.S. Department of Health, Education, and Welfare, Office of Child Development, 1969.

35. Datta, L., C. McHale, and S. Mitchell. *The Effects of the Head Start Classroom Experience on Some Aspects of Child Development: A Summary Report of National Evaluations, 1966 to 1969*. Washington, D.C.:

U.S. Department of Health, Education, and Welfare, Office of Child Development, 1976.

36. Mann, A. J. *A Review of Head Start Research since 1969 and an Annotated Bibliography.* Washington, D.C.: U.S. Department of Health, Education, and Welfare, Office of Child Development, 1977.

37. Kirschner Associates, Inc. *A National Survey of the Impacts of Head Start Centers on Community Institutions: Summary Report.* Albuquerque, N.M., 1970.

38. Datta, L. *A Report on Evaluation Studies of Project Head Start.* Washington, D.C.: U.S. Department of Health, Education, and Welfare, Office of Child Development, 1969.

39. Cook, R. A., S. B. Davis, F. H. Radke, and M. E. Thornbury. Nutritional status of Head Start and nursery school children. I. Food intake and anthropometric measurements. *J. Am. Diet. Assoc.* 68 (1976): 120-126.

40. Cook, R. A., S. B. Davis, F. H. Radke, and M. E. Thornbury. Nutritional status of Head Start and nursery school children. II. Biochemical measurements. *J. Am. Diet. Assoc.* 68 (1976): 127-132.

Child Nutrition Programs

41. The University of the State of New York. *Nutrition Programs for Children in New York State.* Albany, N.Y.: State Education Department, July 1975.

42. Federal programs dealing with domestic hunger. *Hunger* (January 1978).

43. FNS implements initial changes in meal standards. *CNI Weekly Rep.* 34 (1979): 1.

44. USDA food programs. *Nat'l Food Rev.* 5 (January 1978): 10. *Fed. Reg.* 43 (22 August 1978): 163.

45. National School Lunch Act and Child Nutrition Act, P.L. 95-166, 1977 amendments, sec. 19, 1977.

46. *Newsweek*, March 21, 1977, p. 52.

47. Voichick, J. School lunch in Chicago. *J. Nutr. Educ.* 9 (1977): 102.

48. School lunches that kids really love. *Parade*, January 15, 1978, p. 13.

49. Benezra, N. Would you eat your child's school lunch? *Fam. Health* 9 (1977): 40.

50. Schaefer, A. Nutrition 1986 — Vision of Vail: School food service in 1986. *School Food Serv. J.* 31 (1977): 56.

51. National Advisory Council on Child Nutrition. *1976 Annual Report.* Washington, D.C.: U.S. Department of Agriculture, August 1977.

Food Stamp Programs

52. U.S. House of Representatives. *Food Stamp Act of 1977. Appendix III. A History of the Origins of the Food Stamp Program*, Rept. No. 95-464. Washington, D.C.: Government Printing Office, 1977.

53. U.S. Department of Agriculture, Food and Nutrition Service. In U.S. Senate Committee on Agriculture and Forestry, *Food Stamp Program.* Washington, D.C.: Government Printing Office, July 21, 1975.

54. Food Stamp Act of 1964, P.L. 88-525, August 31, 1964.

55. Food and Agriculture Act of 1977, P.L. 95-113, September 1977.

56. U.S. Department of Agriculture, Food and Nutrition Service. *Summary of the Food Stamp Act of 1977.* Washington, D.C.: Government Printing Office, 1977.

57. Food Research Action Center. *FRAC's Guide to the Food Stamp Program.* Washington, D.C., 1978.

58. U.S. Senate Select Committee on Nutrition and Human Needs. *Final Report.* Washington, D.C.: Government Printing Office, December 1977.
59. U.S. Department of Agriculture, Food and Nutrition Service. *Characteristics of Food Stamp Households.* Washington, D.C.: Government Printing Office, 1977.
60. Madden, J. P., and M. D. Yoder. *Program Evaluation: Food Stamps and Commodity Distribution in Rural Areas of Central Pennsylvania,* Bull. No. 780. University Park, Pennsylvania State University Agricultural Experiment Station, June 1972.
61. Lane, S. Food distribution and food stamp program effects on food consumption and nutritional "achievement" of low-income persons in Kern County, California. *Am. J. of Ag. Econ.* 60 (1978): 108–116.
62. Temple-West, P., and C. Mueller. *Preliminary Evaluation of the Contribution of Federal Food Assistance Programs to Low-income Households.* Philadelphia: Nutritional Development Services, 1978.
63. Oklahoma Nutrition Council. *Food Stamps and the Oklahoma Economy.* Oklahoma City, September 1976.
64. U.S. Department of Agriculture. Food stamp report to the Senate, in U.S. Senate Select Committee on Nutrition and Human Needs, *The Food Stamp Controversy of 1975: Background Materials.* Washington, D.C.: Government Printing Office, October 1975, chaps. 7 and 8.
65. U.S. Department of Agriculture, Economic Research Service. *Economic Effects of the U.S. Food Stamp Program.* Washington, D.C.: Government Printing Office, 1976.

Nutrition Programs for the Elderly

66. Dechill, W. G., and I. Wolganot. In U.S. Department of Health, Education, and Welfare, Social and Rehabilitation Service, *Nutrition for the Elderly.* Washington, D.C.: Government Printing Office, 1973, pp. 5–6.
67. Pelcovits, J. Nutrition for older Americans. *J. Am. Diet. Assoc.* 58 (1971): 17.
68. U.S. Department of Health, Education, and Welfare, Committee on Research and Development, Gerontological Society. *Evaluative Research on Social Programs for the Elderly.* Washington, D.C.: Government Printing Office, 1973, p. 142.
69. Federal programs dealing with domestic hunger. *Hunger* (January 1978).

Effectiveness of Programs

70. Perryman, J. School lunch programs, in J. Mayer, ed., *U.S. Nutrition Policies in the Seventies.* San Francisco: W. H. Freeman, 1973, p. 221.
71. Young, J. H. and National Executive Committee of United Presbyterian Women. Testimony before the U.S. Senate Select Committee on Nutrition and Human Needs. Washington, D.C.: Government Printing Office, May 4, 1971.
72. U.S. Senate Select Committee on Nutrition and Human Needs. *Testimony on the WIC Program* (North Carolina State University Project). Washington, D.C.: Government Printing Office, August 1976.
73. Boehm, W. T., and A. E. Gallo. Has food assistance helped? *Nat'l Food Rev.* 5 (December 1978): 23–25.
74. Zee, P., T. Walters, and C. Mitchell. Nutrition and poverty in preschool children: A nutritional survey of preschool children from impoverished black families, Memphis. *J.A.M.A.* 213 (1970): 739.

75. Zee, P., and A. G. Kafatos. Nutrition and federal food assistance programs: A survey of impoverished preschool blacks in Memphis, Tennessee. *Fed. Proc.* 32 (1973): 926 (abstr. 3980).
76. Schaefer, A. F. Nutrition in the United States of America, in D. S. McLaren, ed., *Nutrition in the Community.* London: John Wiley, 1976, p. 382.
77. Kotz, N. *Let Them Eat Promises.* Englewood Cliffs, N.J.: Prentice-Hall, 1969, p. 210.
78. Citizens Board of Inquiry. *Hunger, U.S.A. Revisited.* Washington, D.C.: New Community Press, 1972.
79. Chisholm, S. Quoted in J. Kramer, *Overcoming Malnutrition: Putting Federal Programs to Work.* Speech presented at the First National WIC Symposium. Washington, D.C.: The Children's Foundation, May 1977.
80. Kramer, J. *Overcoming Malnutrition: Putting Federal Programs to Work.* Washington, D.C.: The Children's Foundation, May 1977.
81. Griffiths, M. W. Of government and welfare. *Human Ecol. Forum* 6 (Summer 1975).
82. Howell, J. T. *Hard Living on Clay Street.* Garden City, N.Y.: Anchor Books, 1973, pp. 123–125.

18

Toward a national nutrition policy

Reader Objectives

After completing this chapter, the reader should be able to
1. Define a food and nutrition policy.
2. Describe general policy issues related to the development of a national nutrition policy.
3. State the controversy over the need for a national nutrition policy.
4. List five goals to be addressed by a national nutrition policy.
5. State how the goals might be implemented.
6. Describe the controversy regarding the *Dietary Goals.*

Food policy, which is now in the adolescent stage, is in the painful process of growing up. Let us hope that the youth grows to become a happy productive adult.

— D. Paarlberg[1]

Public policy involves all activities that impact on the lives of individuals or affect groups within a given community. These activities may include individual actions, community activities, public laws, programs, institutions, and the like. Food and nutrition policy is a very important component of public policy.

E. Peterson has defined food and nutrition policy as "a framework for issues of concern to users of food, or consumers." Thus, food policy includes considerations ranging from the Recommended Dietary Allowances, to world food developments and supplies, to the use of energy in food production, to government price supports, to nutrition education.[2]

In its broadest sense, a food and nutrition policy would include tax rates levied, air pollution control laws, regulations affecting land availability, and numerous other similar issues. But, for the present purpose, food and nutrition policy is interpreted more narrowly to include food and nutrition programs, nutrition education programs, and other elements directly related to improving the nutritional status of the American public.

POLICY ISSUES

A policy is simply a blueprint for a specified plan of action; it is a course— of action selected from among many alternatives and is oriented to achieve a particular goal. In short, it is a map detailing how to get to the desired point.

Thus, before a policy can be formulated, policymakers must be clear about the directions in which they want to go. When goals and objectives have been clearly formulated and agreed upon, goal-directed activities can be determined.

Where do we want to go with nutrition? What is the goal of a nutrition policy? Should nutrition be viewed as an individual responsibility, a matter of life-style, personal preference, and affordability, or should nutrition be regarded as a matter of public concern? If the latter question deserves a "yes" answer, then can it be agreed that social action is warranted to achieve a high level of national nutrition?

It is clear that there is no consensus about answers to these difficult questions. Perhaps the basic question to be posed and answered, is, Is access to an adequate and nutritious diet a right or a privilege for the American public?

If adequate nutrition is to be regarded as a privilege, its attainment may be reserved for specially favored individuals. This privilege is an inherently private matter, and there is no public responsibility implicated in assuring adequate nutrition for all.

But, if proper diets are to be a basic human right in the United States, the right is something to which all are entitled. The protection of this right then becomes a matter of public concern and government regulation. If nutrition is declared as a basic human right, then access to this right must be assured and protected, just as the fundamental freedoms guaranteed by the Constitution are protected. These are some of the many complex issues involved in the determination of national nutrition policy.[3]

"A nation needs to look to its food farm policies from a nutritional viewpoint."[4] This statement, made in December 1977, seems innocuous enough to the consumer; the notion has been bandied around in nutrition circles for years. But coming from Lauren Soth, the dean of American farm journalists, the statement implied that no longer could farm policy be formulated in isolation from the nutritional needs of consumers. The statement illustrated the point that the time had come for a broader consideration of nutrition policy.

In November 1977, USDHEW Secretary Joseph Califano contended that "nutrition policy must reflect the health needs of consumers and patients, not the market needs of producers." He argued that the health needs of the American public would be better served if nutrition programs were transferred from the USDA to the USDHEW. His proposal had been made years earlier by the White House Conference, but it had been largely ignored. These and other developments, such as the excitement as well as furor stimulated by the 1977 publication of the *Dietary Goals*, brought the nutrition policy issue to the forefront.[4,5]

IS THERE NEED FOR A NATIONAL NUTRITION POLICY?

The need for a national nutrition policy has been voiced by many nutrition and health experts. As the National Nutrition Consortium noted, a stated national nutrition policy is needed to ensure that food will be available to provide an adequate diet at a reasonable cost to every person within the United States.[6]

Most nutritionists, dietitians, and nutrition educators and many consumer advocates agree that the United States needs to have a national nutrition policy. Other individuals from health and education-related professions who share this view believe that such a policy should ultimately aim to provide all Americans the opportunity to consume a diet that will promote optimum health. Beyond this general premise, it is difficult to get consensus on what should be contained in a national nutrition policy.

Suggested components for such a policy include nutrition and food assistance programs, nutrition education and counseling, assurances to provide a safe and wholesome food supply, nutrition research, manpower training, and institutional arrangements responsible for enforcing policy implementation. Because nutrition is "a web of many strands" and is intertwined with other policies and programs, it is difficult to work with nutrition-related concerns in isolation from other federal activities. Nutrition is a concern of those responsible for export policy, national economic and financial planning, environmental and energy policy, interstate commerce, education, and the welfare of vulnerable population groups, such as infants, children, pregnant women and lactating mothers, and the elderly. For example, the high cost of energy causes the price of fertilizer to rise, which in turn influence the availability of fertilizer and food production and, ultimately, food prices and food availability.

The development of a national nutrition policy is a very complex process. Many who believe that the time is not ripe for this process suggest that, if much time, effort, and energy were expended to develop a policy and the policy ultimately failed to "make it," future efforts would necessarily be shelved for many years. Few people, especially nutrition professionals, can really comprehend the total picture. Legislators seem to be better able to grasp the larger policy issues rather than the individual pieces. D. M. Hegsted's statement that "no one has yet been able to grasp all of the essential components or describe an organizational structure that would be adequate to administer or enforce a national policy" is equally, if not more, true today.[3]

The development of a policy in food and nutrition is probably a more difficult task than in other areas of human welfare because it will eventually come to bear on very personal and intimate individual practices, behaviors, and needs.

Policy development usually follows the recognition of a public need. Policy typically responds to specific situations, circumstances, or personalities. Thus, the initial step in developing a policy requires a general assessment of needs to identify the needs and problems to be addressed by the policy. Examples of policy that have been developed to follow identified needs include the WIC Program, the Food Stamp Program, price supports for agricultural production, PL 480, Food for Peace to provide food assistance overseas, the FDA mandate to regulate the safety of the food supply, and the federal initiative in nutrition education and research.

From this brief list of nutrition-related policy activities, it is clear that there is not so much a lack of nutrition policy directions as there is a lack of coordination, long-term objectives, and integration of nutrition policy into broader policy schemes. The Panel on Nutrition and Government summarized the current status of nutrition program and policy coordination at the federal level by noting that:[7]

1. No one in the executive office of the President is in charge of the nutrition policy questions.
2. No single focus exists anywhere in the executive branch of the government to assess and advocate nutrition policies.
3. No overall coordinating machinery exists at either the executive office level or the interdepartmental level for nutrition planning, program management, or research and development.

TOWARD A NATIONAL NUTRITION POLICY

The National Nutrition Consortium developed five general goals to be addressed by a national nutrition policy:

1. Assure an adequate wholesome food supply at reasonable cost to meet the needs of all segments of the population. This supply is to be available at a level consistent with the affordable life-style of the era.
2. Maintain food resources sufficient to meet emergency needs, and to fulfill a responsible role as a nation in meeting world food needs.
3. Develop a level of sound public knowledge and responsible understanding of nutrition and foods that will promote maximal nutritional knowledge.
4. Maintain a system of quality and safety control that justifies public confidence in its food supply.
5. Support research and education in foods and nutrition with adequate resources and reasoned priorities to solve important current problems and to permit exploratory basic research.[6]

As these goals are broadly stated, they seem to be abstract and even ambiguous. They must be translated into behaviorally oriented objectives, and specific, measurable criteria should be developed to facilitate the evaluation of goal attainment. Programs and efforts recommended to meet these goals are presented in Table 18–1.

Table 18–1
Guidelines for a National Nutrition Policy

The National Nutrition Consortium recommended a variety of programs and efforts needed to meet the objectives for a national nutrition policy:

1. A plan for national nutritional surveillance to monitor the nutritional status of the population. Ongoing reporting should include information on:

   a. The prevalence of specific nutritional problems.
   b. The effects of nutrition intervention and nutrition promotion programs on nutritional status.
   c. Food consumption of different population subgroups.

2. Nutritional programs in the health care system should be implemented to address the following considerations:

   a. (1) Promotion of good nutrition should occur throughout all of the population.

Guidelines for a National Nutrition Policy *(continued)*

      (2) Attention should be given to those vulnerable to nutritional problems.

      (3) Nutrition should be promoted in health care centers where assessment and counseling should be offered.

      (4) Nutrition should also be a component of hospitals, long-term care facilities, prisons, day-care centers, and the like.

  b. A significant effort should be made to eliminate malnutrition among groups vulnerable to nutrition problems. These groups include infants, pregnant and lactating women, the elderly, migrant workers, Indians, and other minority groups. Programs should include Food Stamps and other programs designed to improve nutritional status.

  c. Health promotion through positive nutrition should be the responsibility of public health programs and personnel. Problems include anemia, poor growth and development, nutrient deficiencies, and nutritional problems related to disease states (e.g., coronary heart disease, dental caries, and cancer), malabsorption states, inborn metabolic defects, allergies, diabetes, and renal disorders.

  d. Programs should provide a nutritional component in all health care centers throughout the nation. Nutritional services should be provided under the guidance of a trained nutritional professional; support for such programs should be provided by national health insurance.

  e. Nutritional centers of excellence for assessment, diagnostic treatment, education, and research should be established in various regions in the United States.

3. Nutrition education should be integrated into all strata of formal education:

  a. In schools, nutrition should be part of the basic curriculum in secondary and elementary schools; teachers should be provided with training in nutrition; the School Lunch Program should become a vehicle for nutrition education. In addition, colleges and universities should offer courses in nutrition.

  b. Training of nutrition and other health professionals and paraprofessionals, including physicians, nurses, dentists, veterinarians, social workers, physical education teachers, and health educators should be given high priority. College undergraduate, graduate, and postgraduate education and continuing education in nutrition should be provided.

     Medical schools should develop resources for nutrition education, and nutrition training and services should be promoted in all programs of primary, secondary, and tertiary health care.

  c. The media at all levels, including federal, state, and local education departments, Cooperative State Extension Services, community agencies, industry, and mass media should promote dissemination of sound nutrition information.

     Nutrition education components should be established in federal food assistance programs, such as the Food Stamp and WIC Programs.

4. Nutritional research should be supported; basic and applied research should be ongoing and expanded.

  a. Colleges, universities, nutrition centers, health care facilities, industry, and federal agencies should support nutrition research.

  b. Support should be provided to research in food production, processing, and use.

  c. Federal agencies involved in nutrition research (including the FDA, NIH, DOD, VA, DOC, and EPA) should have their activities coordinated.

5. Food production and distribution should be considered from the vantage point of nutritional objectives. Global food concerns should be considered and planned for, as should domestic food needs. Increased food production, improved distribution, food reserves, and international trade policies should be planned with nutritional objectives in mind.

Guidelines for a National Nutrition Policy *(continued)*

6. Nutrient composition, quality, and food safety should be studied and assessed.

   a. Encouragement should be given for the development of wholesome foods.
   b. Food labeling should be used as a tool for nutrition education.
   c. Food regulation should assess quality and safety; review of regulatory agencies should also be conducted.

7. National nutrition policy should consider the responsibilities of the United States to other nations. Issues of concern related to global malnutrition that should be addressed include population and family planning, food production, food science and technology, economic development, and applied nutrition education and sociocultural factors related to nutrition.

POLICY IMPLEMENTATION

Successful implementation of a nutrition policy demands that the measure designed to influence food consumption be undertaken in conjunction with the cooperation and collaboration of the public sector, the relevant agencies, organizations and individuals in the private sector, and the individual consumers themselves.

If nutritional goals are to be realized, institutions should exist that are responsible for the future coordination and development of food and nutrition policy. Specific institutions should be available to:

— Assess and evaluate food and nutritional status of the population; such assessment should form an integral part of a long-term surveillance plan; its purpose would be to determine developments in food and nutrition habits relative to the formulated nutrition goals.

— Determine, based on the nutritional surveillance, problems that must be solved.

— Specify methods to attach the identified problems, define projects, and develop plans for the ongoing implementation of the food and nutrition policy.

— Oversee the implementation of specified plans within stated time limits.

— Coordinate the activities of various agencies responsible for implementing food and nutrition policy.

— Evaluate the effectiveness of policy and planning implementation.

— Contribute to professional development in nutrition and health, education, and related disciplines.

— Provide ongoing advice and counsel for future public policy.

WHAT HAS BEEN DONE TO IMPLEMENT THESE GOALS AND ACTIVITIES?[7,8]

Much of the work toward developing a national nutrition policy was done by the U.S. Senate Select Committee on Nutrition and Human Needs. The

Committee advocated the development of a comprehensive national nutrition plan to ensure accountability. The suggested format was a written document, prepared and submitted annually to the Congress. Specific characteristics of the plan were to include

- A formal analysis of national nutritional status.
- A set of specific goals, such as promoting good health, meeting adequate food production for domestic as well as international needs, ensuring adequate food safety and quality, facilitating the equitable distribution of food supplies, and allowing the consumer the chance to make an informed choice of diet from available food supplies.
- Statement of specific actions needed to implement the goals — these should be stated in such a way as to be compatible with evaluation.
- Provision for cooperation among institutions and between federal, state, and local levels for communication, interaction, implementation, and evaluation of the plan.

The Select Committee envisioned this plan not as an ideal plan but as what is currently being done. Agencies involved in nutrition-related activities would submit parts of the plan, based on what they were doing; these pieces would then be assembled into a national nutrition plan.

The formal nutrition plan would be almost worthless without an agency charged with implementing it. The Select Committee suggested the need for an agency to judge the appropriateness of the plan as well as the total picture of the national nutrition status and to determine how closely the reality approached what was identified as the idea.

A Federal Nutrition Office as envisioned by the Select Committee would be responsible for coordinating the nutritional activities of other agencies. The office would not administer or supervise nutrition programs, but it would monitor activities in terms of how they met the goals of the plan. The office would also describe and interpret these activities for the President and for the Congress, and would be responsible for reviewing ideas, program recommendations, and legislative proposals before they were implemented. The office would not, however, have the power to veto proposed changes. It was hoped that the knowledge that their proposals would be reviewed by the Federal Nutrition Office would stimulate individual agencies to carefully consider all the aspects and impacts of their programs before they were implemented.

In addition to this Federal Nutrition Office, the Select Committee endorsed the idea of a need for a National Nutrition Center, established within the U.S. Department of Health, Education, and Welfare, to administer expanded nutrition programs. The Select Committee believed that nutrition activity should be centralized in the U.S. Department of Health, Education, and Welfare. The proposed Nutrition Center would administer the nutrition education programs, supervise nutritional surveillance activities, coordinate federally supported nutrition research, and administer nutrition manpower programs. The level of operations and functions of the two proposed offices are summarized in Table 18-2.

Additional proposals included the establishment of a position, the

Presidential Assistant for Nutrition, and of a National Nutrition Policy Board to serve as a national forum for the discussion of nutrition policy concerns.

Other needs discussed by the Select Committee paralleled those outlined by the National Nutrition Consortium:[8]

1. The need to improve nutrition surveillance. Such an effort should consider the changing dietary pattern of the U.S. public as well as the changing nature of the food supply. An effort aimed at improving nutritional surveillance should include food consumption surveys, a national consumer panel, composition of food (including nutrient content), monitoring of food additives, and evaluation of nutritional status.

2. The need to improve nutrition education.

3. The need to improve nutrition research.

These proposals have not advanced very much beyond the discussion stage. What are the possibilities for consensus, agreement, and legislative authority for, and final implementation of this, or perhaps a similar national nutrition policy? There is no easy answer to this question. A consideration of *Dietary Goals for the United States* may provide insight into the possibilities for development and implementation of a broader national nutrition policy.

DIETARY GOALS

The essence of knowledge is, having acquired it, to apply it.

— *Confucius*

In February 1977, the U.S. Senate Select Committee on Nutrition and Human Needs proposed dietary goals for the United States. These goals, revised in December 1977, are the following:[5]

1. To avoid overweight, consume only as much energy as is expended; if overweight, decrease energy intake and increase energy expenditure.

2. Increase the consumption of complex carbohydrates and "naturally occurring" sugars from about 28 per cent of energy intake to about 48 per cent of energy intake.

3. Reduce the consumption of refined and processed sugars by about 45 per cent to account for about 10 per cent of total energy intake.

4. Reduce overall fat consumption from approximately 40 per cent to about 30 per cent of energy intake.

5. Reduce saturated fat consumption to account for about 10 per cent of total energy intake, and balance that with polyunsaturated and

Table 18-2

Functions and Operations of the Proposed Institutional Structures to Guide National Nutrition Plans

	Level of Operation	*Functions*
Federal Nutrition Office	Cabinet level: Director would report to the President; director would participate in cabinet meetings related to nutrition policy or in other meetings dealing with food and nutrition issues.	Responsible for coordination and overview of nutritional activities of various agencies; responsible for overall guidance in national nutritional plan.
National Nutrition Center	Subcabinet level within USDHEW: Director would report to Secretary of USDHEW.	Formulate USDHEW's input into National Nutrition Plan; responsible for monitoring programs; administers and monitors nutrition manpower programs.

monounsaturated fats, which should account for about 10 per cent of energy intake each.

6. Reduce cholesterol consumption to about 300 mg/day.

7. Limit the intake of sodium by reducing the intake of salt to about 5 gm/day.

The goals are to be achieved by an increased consumption of fruits, vegetables, whole grains, poultry, fish, skim milk, and vegetable oils and a reduced consumption of whole milk, meat, and eggs by the population (with the possible exception of children, premenopausal women, and the elderly who should obtain needed nutritional benefits of needed animal products) and of foods rich in sugar, salt, and fat. Recommendations to further implement the practices advocated in the *Dietary Goals* are summarized in Table 18-3.[5]

The stimuli for the development of the *Dietary Goals* were, according to the introductory statement of the report and the comments made in support of the goals at the time of their publication:[5]

1. "Killer diseases," "epidemic in our population" include heart disease, stroke, cancer, and various other chronic diseases.

2. "Six of the ten leading causes of death in the United States have been linked to our diet."

3. The "epidemic" of "killer diseases" is related to changes in the U.S. diet that pose a significant "threat to public health."

The *Dietary Goals* has been endorsed by a number of prominent nutrition and health authorities (such as J. Mayer, D. M. Hegsted, J. Gussow, J. Dwyer, and M. Latham) and interest groups (including the Center for Science in the Public Interest and the Council for Responsible Nutrition, a trade association of food supplement manufacturers). Despite these

Table 18-3
Recommendations Prompted by Dietary Goals

1. Congress should provide increased funds for a public nutrition education campaign to reach five general areas:

   a. health and nutrition education in the classrooms and lunchrooms of schools.
   b. nutrition and health education for school food service personnel.
   c. nutrition education component in all federally funded food and nutrition programs.
   d. nutrition education sponsored by Extension in USDA.
   e. increased use of mass media for the purposes of public nutrition education.

2. Food labeling should be required for all foods; information to be contained should help the consumer to make comparisons on the basis of percentage and type of fats, per cent of sugar, milligrams of cholesterol and salt, calories, and food activities.

3. Increased funds should be allocated to the USDA and the USDHEW to conduct joint studies and demonstration or pilot projects to develop new methods of food preparation and product development to decrease dietary risk factors in the population.

4. Increased funding should be available for human nutrition research.

5. The USDA and the USDHEW should form a joint committee to consider, on an ongoing and periodic basis, the implications of nutritional and health issues of agricultural concerns and policies.

endorsements, considerable controversy and criticism surrounded the publication of the *Dietary Goals*. Notable among the issues that surfaced are the following:[9-11]

1. How would adoption of the goals really influence the nutrition-related "killer diseases" in the United States?

Many suggest that the dietary changes indicated in the goals would produce hoped-for results in terms of improved health. For example, the relationship between dietary fat intake and atherosclerotic heart disease suggests that a reduction in saturated fat and cholesterol intake would influence the prevalence of heart disease. (See Chapter 7.) Recognizing the fact that all data relative to these issues are not totally clear, many suggest that:

> At some point between complete adoption and outright rejection of the Goals, there is evidence that Americans, in general, would do well to look closely at present eating practices. While data are incomplete . . . it is sufficient to expect that many people . . . would certainly benefit.[10]

Others are less certain and believe that scientific evidence on these issues is so incomplete and controversial that recommendations to the public are not yet indicated. They suggest that widespread promotion of the goals, without a significant improvement in health, would ultimately be detrimental. Erosion of public confidence in nutritional science would result, and later dietary and nutrition advice would be ignored. As L. A. Barness suggested: "I hope that the statement . . . might make many investigators so angry that they will take up the cudgels to find out what a good diet is. Until such time, I do not think that we have the information to make universal changes."[11] D.M. Hegsted responded to this position by noting that:

> The diet we eat today was not planned or developed for any particular purpose. It is a happenstance related to our affluence, the productivity of our farmers and the activities of our food industry. The risks associated with eating this diet are demonstrably large. The question to be asked, therefore, is not why should we change our diet, but why not? What are the risks associated with less salt, and more fruits, vegetables, unsaturated fat and cereal products — especially whole grain cereals? There are none that can be identified and important benefits can be expected.[5]

Some experts agree with the general pattern of the goals, but disagree with the specific recommendations. Still others suggest that the adoption of the goals might even be nutritionally harmful for particularly vulnerable subgroups. For example, a reduction in meat intake, in an effort to reduce dietary saturated fat and cholesterol, may also reduce iron intake in the face of a significant prevalence of anemia in certain pockets throughout the United States.

2. How should the goals be implemented? What organizational structures would be necessary?

The issue of implementation is clearly crucial to the success of the goals. If the government believes in the importance of the goals, should it consider itself responsible for setting general policy directives for the implementation of the goals? The goals as published did not link dietary goals to national policy objectives to aid in attaining them. The *Dietary Goals* suggests only a weak link to the policy and planning processes. "The logical process whereby necessity for *diet change* leads to the formation of policy to *change the food system* is not addressed. The creation of institutions . . . is effectively ignored in *Dietary Goals* in favor of recommendations for food labeling, research, and education."[12] The notion persists that individual change, rather than societal change, is needed to implement the goals.

The *Dietary Goals* also effectively ignores the fact that what the government actively does, as well as what it does not do, largely determine the nature of the environment. For example, agriculture and food supplies are greatly influenced by government price supports, product subsidies, loans, regulations, grading, and the like. There is a disinclination to obviously interfere with the "free market" forces that produce the supply of food available. However, more subtle interventions into factors that affect the food supply, as well as the price of food, such as price supports, the use of a commodity food supply to reduce domestic food surplus, and land use policies, are rarely criticized.

3. What possible side effects might result from the widespread adoption of the goals?

It is clear that there could be drastic economic repercussions. If the demand for food shifts from animal and dairy products to more fresh produce and whole-grain products, there could be severe economic problems for the dairy and meat industries. National economic difficulties could result as employees lost jobs, enterprises went out of business, production was cut back, and prices rose. How could these results be prevented so that an orderly transition in food consumption patterns could take place? As the demand for certain food increased, the laws of supply and demand would probably result in higher prices for these food items. What programs and policies could be used to ensure that consumers, especially those in the low-income strata, could afford these items?

Agricultural policies formerly operated to provide price supports to improve the income of food producers. Will these policies have to be modified to switch support from the producers of meat, egg, and dairy products to those who grow grain, fruits, and vegetables? Could agricultural research aid adjustments in food consumption? What is the appropriate role for the government in this process?

Although none of the specific recommendations promoted in the *Dietary Goals* has yet been formally implemented by the government, there has been an increased evidence of a recognition of the importance of nutrition at the national level:[13]

1. In December 1977, the executive office of the President published a report entitled "New Directions in Federally Supported Human Nutrition Research." The report recommends the formation of an interagency working group chaired by the Assistant Secretary for Health, Education, and Welfare to evaluate the recommendations contained in *Dietary Goals.* The report also recommends that the USDA, USDHEW, USDOD, and AID support the formation of nutrition goals and habits that are conducive to positive health.

2. The USDA approved a mission-oriented basic research grant program and is funding proposals dealing with human nutrient requirements and factors related to the formation of food habits.

3. The USDA is implementing a mass media education experiment designed to determine the most effective way of providing children with nutrition education.

4. Two appointments have been made in the USDA and the USDHEW for positions to assume *responsibility for* coordinating efforts between the two departments in terms of nutrition.

CONCLUSIONS

What can we conclude relative to a national food and nutrition policy? A couple of facts stand out:

1. There is a lack of consensus, not only among health professionals, scientists, policymakers, and administrators but also among nutritionists

themselves, as to what constitutes appropriate dietary goals for the U.S. population.

2. Given this lack of consensus over the relationship between dietary status and health, and recommendations for changes in dietary patterns, there is little likelihood that significant consensus and goal implementation and broad policy development could be reached in the near future.

If a national food and nutrition policy seems a very remote goal, where should nutrition activity center, relative to the broad policy-making process? Should nutrition advocates push for a national policy? The following fable was narrated in answer to this question:

"The fox knows many things, but the hedgehog knows one big thing."

Imagine a President who promises a sweeping national welfare policy that will sculpt the divergent programs which the 40-plus years of Federal concern for the needy have accreted into one coherent reform. Suppose that he uses his coordinating authority to pressure one department that would offer only cash to ally with another department that would supply only jobs. Assume that he persuades his legislative leaders to create a super subcommittee to overcome jurisdictional barriers that might otherwise inhibit adequate consideration of a plan that, at once, touches the tax, welfare, food program, and manpower systems. Finally, speculate on the end product of all this endeavor: a miscalculated monster with a price tag of between \$20 and \$25 billion that turns most politicians to stone, pits agency against agency, committee against committee, and is prematurely laid to rest, perhaps jeopardizing any hope for progress, however modest. At the same time, the monster, by focusing attention exclusively upon itself, manages to divert notice from efforts to curtail existing benefits that may, therefore, succeed.[14]

J. Kramer related this fable to point up the moral "to think small like the fox and survive. Do not blunder like the hedgehog into an intellectual trap of your own devising. Hesitate to relate everything to a single, central vision or organizing principle that operates to unite rather than divide the enemies of your objectives and partial, minor victories that yield meaningful change, however incremental." The wisdom of focusing great energy on national policy development is questionable.[14]

Kramer and others argue that the time is not right to push for a national nutrition policy. Their advice to those eager for a national policy is to take one step at a time, to clearly understand and gain a consensus on what such a policy should include. Work should proceed within the system: "You have to live with and learn the Congressional jurisdiction rules, not expect to change them . . . at the same time you have to be constantly alert for sneak attacks from the rear." The job should involve recognizing and then using to the full extent all available "pressure points" to advance the appropriate nutritional goal. Efforts should involve developing pronutrition attitudes among influential congressmen on relevant authorizing committees, as well as the other activities designed to influence specific policy and program considerations. (See Chapter 15.)

The moral, in sum, is to "fight little skirmishes effectively, after thorough preparation, not big wars, when your supply lines are exhausted before you start."[14]

REFERENCES

1. Paarlberg, D. Food and economics. *J. Am. Diet. Assoc.* 71 (1977): 107.
2. Petersen, E. *Statement* before Technology Assessment Board, Office of Technological Assessment, February 4, 1976. Washington, D.C.: Government Printing Office, 1976.
3. Hegsted, D. M. Food and nutrition policy — Now and in the future. *J. Am. Diet. Assoc.* 64 (1974): 367.
4. Nutrition policy has come of age. *CNI Week. Rep.* 8 (1978): 4.
5. U.S. Senate Select Committee on Nutrition and Human Needs. *Dietary Goals for the United States*, rev. Washington, D.C.: Government Printing Office, December 1977.
6. National Nutrition Consortium, Inc. In U.S. Senate Select Committee on Nutrition and Human Needs, *Guidelines for a National Nutrition Policy*. Washington, D.C.: Government Printing Office, May 1974.
7. U.S. Senate Select Committee on Nutrition and Human Needs, Panel on Nutrition and Government. *National Nutrition Policy Study Hearings*. Washington, D.C.: Government Printing Office, June 21, 1974, vol. 7–A.
8. U.S. Senate Select Committee on Nutrition and Human Needs. *Toward a National Nutrition Policy*. Washington, D.C.: Government Printing Office, May 1975.
9. U.S. Senate Select Committee on Nutrition and Human Needs. *Dietary Goals for the United States — Supplemental Views*. Washington, D.C.: Government Printing Office, November 1977.
10. American Dietetic Association. Statement: Dietary goals. *J. Am. Diet. Assoc.* 71 (1977): 227.
11. Barnes, L. A. In Twenty commentaries. *Nutr. Today* 12 (1977): 12.
12. Winikoff, B. Nutrition and food policy: The approaches of Norway and the United States. *Am. J. Publ. Health* 67 (1977): 552.
13. LeBovit, C. U.S. dietary goals — An update. *Nat'l Food Rev.* 3 (June 1978): 33.
14. Kramer, J. *Better a Live Fox than a Dead Hedgehog*, speech delivered to Conference on Nutrition and American Food System. Washington, D.C.: Community Nutrition Institute, May 1978.

section five
END OF SECTION ACTIVITIES

1. Choose a nutrition issue of current concern to the Congress. Investigate the issue and then write a letter to your congressman in support of a particular position.

2. The following figure (page 630) illustrates the interactions between agencies formed to aid in the development of a rural health care delivery

system. Contact the sponsors of a local community nutrition program to determine the problems involved in the planning and implementation of the program. What communication lines were formed with other agencies? Develop a similar model to illustrate this.

3. Design a model program to meet the specifically identified nutritional needs of a target population. Discuss your program idea with others, obtain their reactions, and, where appropriate, modify program design. Write up a description of the program to include:

— background, need, justification.

— program long-term goals and short-range objectives.

— program administration; what agencies and individuals will be responsible? Your operation may be integrated into existing programs, but all levels of administration should be clearly identified.

— program activities; what specifically will the program do?

— needed resources.

Community and extracommunity relationships. G. J. Cummings. Rural response to a physician shortage. Family and Community Health 1(1978): 74–76 See explanation for the figure on facing page.

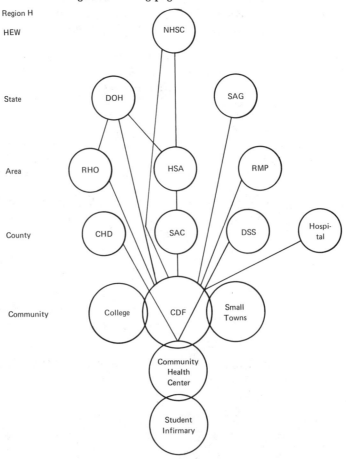

— source of resources.

— barriers to program and ways in which to address these barriers.

— method for evaluation of program operation.

Present this description to others, and try to gain their support for your program. Form a small coalition of supportive individuals and meet with them to work out a strategy to promote your program. Identify the following:

— What are the program strengths? Try to define these strengths in measurable terms.

— What specific benefits will result?

---

1. NHSC — The agency within HEW that supplies physicians for two or three years to under-served areas for partial financial reimbursement with the expectation that the community will develop a program for recruiting medical providers from the private sector.
2. DOH (Department of Health) — The state agency that is authorized to issue a certificate to operate diagnostic and treatment centers and establishes Medicaid rate.
3. SAG (The State Attorney General) — The office that approves applications to establish not-for-profit corporations for stated public purposes such as providing health services.
4. RHO (The Regional Health Office) of the State Health Department makes on-site inspections to determine adequacy of a facility to provide intended health services.
5. RMP — A source of federal development monies for assisting communities to obtain needed health services. This agency's functions were taken over by area Health Systems Agencies (HSA), established by Congress in 1974.
6. HSA — An area agency legally responsible in conjunction with the states for planning and development of all health facilities and services financed from federal sources. It has recommendatory responsibilities regarding the need for services in a community.
7. DSS (The Department of Social Services) — Responsible for the local administration of Medicaid and certain other health service funds.
8. SAC (The Subarea Council) — A subsidiary of HSAs usually organized on a one-county or two-county basis to assist in initial screening of applications for facilities, programs, and services.
9. CHD (The County Health Department) — Responsible for operating various public health clinics and nursing services as well as enforcing sanitary and environmental safety codes and regulations.
10. Hospital — Provides inpatient and emergency care of patients; determines, through medical committees, who shall be allowed certain staff privileges within the hospital.
11. College — A small women's private college.
12. Small Towns — The five towns or townships making up the primary catchment area for health services.
13. CDF (The Community Development Federation) — A legally created organization to sponsor the medical center.
14. Community Health Center — The facility that houses the staff who provide primary health care services to the area and college students.
15. Student Infirmary — A college-owned building that provides nurse services to its students and houses the medical center.

— What are the drawbacks? On what points do individual members of your group disagree? Try to work out these differences to obtain solid group support.

— What sources of support can you identify (these might be industry, in public sector, health or educational professionals, and the like)?

— What individuals of local, state, or national importance might you get to support your program?

Develop a broad strategy to obtain support for your program and to obtain needed legislation to institutionalize your program. List all the steps you would need to go through to the possible final passage of a bill authorizing your program and a bill appropriating needed funds to support the program.

4. Investigate the WIC program in your area. What type of outreach activities are included? What percentage of eligible individuals participate? What type of nutrition education is included in the program activities? Is nutritional assessment an important part of the program? How is information from nutritional assessments used to aid program participants? Is there a program for ongoing monitoring and follow-up of individuals' nutritional status? If not, discuss the reasons for the lack of these components with the WIC program personnel. What might be done to include these elements in the program?

5. You have been approached by a citizen's action group that desires your help in "improving" the quality of the lunches served in the local school lunch program. The group is very disturbed over the limited menu offered to the children. Menus revolve around hamburgers, pizza, meat loaf, spaghetti, and hot dogs. Fresh fruits and vegetables are rarely served, white bread is standard for sandwiches, and fried, high-fat foods seem to be the rule, rather than the exception. The group feels that children will not learn to like and accept a wide variety of foods if such foods are not offered in the lunch program. The group approached the director of the lunch program who said that the program must pay for itself and that a balanced budget must be achieved. Serving new foods, such as the vegetarian dishes requested by the citizen's group, said the director, would result in fewer children participating in the program and would result in increased plate waste. In addition, these foods are more expensive than currently used foods. What suggestions would you make to resolve the conflict?

6. You are the director of a Title III meal program for the elderly. You are aware of the lack of nutrition education in such programs and have scheduled a meeting with the director of the state office on aging to ask for more funds to include a nutrition education component in your program. However, you are aware that funds are extremely limited and you know that the director would rather use the limited funds to feed more people rather than for nutrition education. How would you justify your request for money for nutrition education? State your case convincingly.

7. Survey your local health department to learn of nutrition-related

activities. What nutrition programs come under the purview of the local health department?

8. Mr. and Mrs. Bradley live in Springfield. Mr. Bradley works in a metal factory; he makes $110 a week before payroll deductions are taken out. He takes home $90 weekly.

Mrs. Bradley does not work, but receives $30 monthly from a previous husband. In addition the Bradley's son Billy, a teenager, works a few hours after school and earns $14 weekly.

The Bradley's pay $20 a month for hospitalization insurance and $15 a month for prescription medicine. Mr. Bradley has also been previously married and must pay his first wife a monthly sum of $25. Mrs. Bradley frequently feels the need to "get away" for a few hours and, to do this, hires a sitter for 3-year-old Amy. The family pays $150 monthly for rental of an apartment. Other expenses, such as telephone, heat, utilities, etc., total $70 a month.

What is the monthly net food stamp income? What is their monthly food stamp allowance? What is the maximum cost of these stamps?

Refer to the table and instructions below to determine the Bradley's monthly food stamp allowance and maximum cost.

Number in Family	Net Monthly Income Limit*	Monthly Food Stamp Allotment	Maximum Cost
1	$ 277	$ 54	$ 44
2	363	100	80
3	480	144	126
4	607	182	158
5	720	216	188
6	867	260	228
7	953	286	250
8	1,093	328	288

*To find the net monthly income limit for households of over eight people, add $140 for each additional person.

How to Figure Income for Food Stamps

a. Determine total monthly family income (including income of all family members).

b. Subtract the following:

1. Paycheck deductions such as taxes, retirement, union dues, and and Social Security.

2. Medical bills, if they are greater than $10 per month.

3. Education expenses, including tuition and mandatory fees.

4. Work expense (10 per cent of pay, but only up to $30 per month).

5. Unusual expenses such as those resulting from funerals or fire, theft, or flood.

6. Court-ordered child support or alimony payments.

7. Payments to support care for household dependent (of any age) to allow a household member to work, attend school, or participate in a training program.

8. Payments for rent or mortgage and utilities costs. Subtract only those payments in excess of 30 per cent of income after all the other deductions.

This determines net food stamp income.

9. Food and nutrition policies are also important at the state level. The following state food policy was developed by the Center for Science in the Public Interest. What is your response to this program? Would you modify it in any way? Have any of the provisions been implemented in your state? What premise do you feel needs to have top priority in terms of implementation? What strategies might you take to further its implementation?

A State Food Policy*

1. Every American should have a guaranteed income adequate to insure access to a nutritionally adequate diet. Until this is a reality, all state (or city) agencies, including the legislature, executive, and departments of health, welfare, and education, should make a major effort to see that all federal food assistance programs — including food stamps, school lunch, school breakfast, food for day care centers, and meals for the elderly — are *fully* and fairly implemented. This means that all the poor and near poor should be informed of their eligibility, and that administrative procedures should be made as efficient and humane as possible, so that all those in need may be served.

2. High prices, low quality, and reduced variety are due in part to monopoly and oligopoly in the food industry. Antitrust actions should be taken by the State Attorney General to end existing monopolies in the food industry. State (or city) officials should lobby for Federal actions to the same end.

3. In recent years, states have seen many thousands of acres of prime agricultural land lost to urbanization, resort development, highways, energy siting, and other uses. The state (or county) should assess its current and future patterns of land uses and ownership, and develop a strong program to protect its agricultural land, utilizing agricultural districts, acquisition or transfer of development rights, use-value assessment of agricultural land, and other means at its disposal.

4. The family farmer should be protected by the enactment and strong enforcement of state laws restricting involvement in farming by corporations other than "family farm" or other relatively small and closely-held corporations.

5. Nourishing food should be easily accessible, whether in a country grocery store, a city supermarket, a fast-food restaurant, or a vending machine.

6. The state should undertake a major nutrition education effort, making full use of schools, TV, radio, and other media, to encourage the public (a) to eat a balanced diet based to a large extent on whole grains, vegetables, nuts, low-fat dairy products, poultry, grass-fed beef, seafood and fruit; and (b) to reduce their intake of fat, sugar, and cholesterol.

7. Consumer interests should be equitably represented on state market order boards that help determine production levels, quality standards, and prices of certain foods.

*prepared by CSPI

8. Individual, school, and community gardens yield learning, recreation, community spirit, and high-quality, low-cost foods. The state should encourage its citizens to garden, and should assist municipalities and groups in setting up community garden projects by coordinating information and resources and making vacant public land available for gardens.

9. Agricultural research and extension, through the state's land grant college, should orient its efforts to assist small-scale farmers, and to breed more nutritious and less energy-intensive crops and livestock.

10. Direct farmer-to-consumer marketing, as well as other "alternative" marketing structures, can provide great benefits for both consumers and small farmers. The state's Department of Agriculture should develop specific programs to encourage and assist farmers to market through farmers markets, "U-Pick" operations, roadside markets, and other direct marketing enterprises, and to assist municipalities wishing to organize farmers' markets. The state (or city) should also identify, promote, and provide technical assistance to consumer food buying clubs and cooperatives, and help facilitate their purchase of farm goods directly from producers. The state should develop a revolving credit fund to help establish food production, distribution, and retailing cooperatives.

11. The potential for conflicts of interest in state agencies that regulate food should be minimized by (a) forbidding employees to join a regulated industry after leaving the agency until substantial time has elapsed; and (b) balancing former industry people in government agencies with persons who have worked with pro-consumer groups.

12. State sales taxes on food clearly impose a special burden on those least able to afford an adequate diet. If the state has a sales tax on food items, it should be repealed, and replaced by more equitable revenue sources.

13. The State Department of Agriculture should issue guidelines defining "organically grown" food to prevent consumer fraud and to facilitate an ecologically sound way of farming. The Department should encourage all farmers to be judicious and frugal in their use of fertilizers, pesticides, and fuel.

10. The concepts of a national food and nutrition policy have been reviewed. Develop your own ideas for a national nutrition policy. What are the basic premises to be included? What means do you suggest for implementation? How would you evaluate such a policy? Would your policy be acceptable to nutrition professionals? To legislators and public planners? Critique the policy developed by another student. Compare your policy to the Citizen's Food Policy outlined below. This policy was developed and endorsed by the Consumer Federation of America, the Children's Foundation, the Food Research and Action Center, the National Consumer Congress, and the National Consumer League. Do you agree with the premises of the Citizen's Food Policy? Would you modify it in any way? How would administrators in the USDA and HEW respond to the Citizens Food Policy?

Citizen's Food Policy

The Citizen's Food Policy places human need before corporate profit and recognizes that an adequate diet is a basic right of every individual.

American food policy reflects disparate political pressures more than careful thought and planning. These pressures are usually wielded by multibillion dollar global corporations. Our current "food policy" consists of such elements as inadequate government control over giant food companies, a poorly publicized food stamp program, uncontrolled TV advertising that induces small children to buy foods that are bad for their health, and no nutrition education whatever. The Federal government must articulate a comprehensive national food policy, covering agricultural production, nutrition education, and aid to needy nations.

1. Every American should have a guaranteed adequate income to insure access to a nutritionally adequate diet. Until this is a reality, all Federal food assistance programs — such as food stamps, school lunch, school breakfast, food for day care centers, and meals for the elderly — should be fully funded and implemented.

2. High prices, low quality, and reduced variety are due in part to monopoly and oligopoly in the food industry. Immediate antitrust actions should be taken by the Justice Department and Federal Trade Commission to end existing monopolies in the food industry. Future problems should be avoided by laws limiting the size of corporations and the percentage of the market that they control.

3. The family farmer should be protected by laws restricting corporate involvement in farming and by price support programs progressively structured to assure adequate income for small farmers, but not to allow undue benefits to large farmers.

4. A major nutrition education effort, making full use of TV, radio, and other media, should encourage the public to eat a balanced diet based to a large extent on whole grains, vegetables, nuts, low-fat dairy products, poultry, grass-fed beef, and fruit, and to reduce their intake of fat, sugar, and cholesterol.

5. Nourishing food should be easily accessible, whether in a country grocery store, a city supermarket, a fast-food restaurant, or a vending machine.

6. The potential for conflicts of interest in the FDA, USDA, and other agencies that regulate food should be minimized by (1) forbidding employees to join a regulated industry after leaving the agency until a substantial period of time has elapsed, and (2) balancing former industry people in government agencies with persons who have worked with pro-consumer groups.

7. Agricultural research, particularly at land-grant colleges, should develop technology to assist small-scale farmers and to breed more nutritious crops and livestock. The agricultural extension services should focus their efforts on disseminating the results of this research.

8. Energy conservation measures should be promoted throughout the food industry. Farmers should be judicious and frugal in their use of pesticides, herbicides, fertilizer, and fuel. Regional markets should be emphasized to save on transportation costs.

9. Consumer interests should be equitably represented on state and Federal boards that help determine levels, quality standards, and prices of certain foods.

10. The medical community should focus its efforts on implementing the findings of current nutrition research, which show strong connections between diet and obesity, heart disease, dental caries, and other health problems.

11. Federal and state governments should have revolving credit funds earmarked for setting up food production, processing, distributing, and retailing cooperatives.

Appendices

Appendix I ASSESSMENT OF NUTRITIONAL STATUS

Table I-A
Information Needed for the Assessment of Nutritional Status

Sources of Information	Nature of Information Obtained	Nutritional Implications
1. Agricultural data; food balance sheets	Gross estimates of agricultural production; agricultural methods	Approximate availability of food supplies to a population
	Soil fertility, predominance of cash crops; overproduction of staples; food imports and exports	
2. Socioeconomic data; information on marketing, distribution, and storage	Purchasing power; distribution and storage of foodstuffs	Unequal distribution of available foods between the socioeconomic groups in the community and within the family
3. Food consumption patterns; cultural-anthropological data	Lack of knowledge, erroneous beliefs and prejudices; indifference	
4. Dietary surveys	Food consumption	Low, excessive, or unbalanced nutrient intake
5. Special studies on foods	Biological value of diets; presence of interfering factors (e.g., goitrogens); effects of food processing	Special problems related to nutrient utilization
6. Vital and health statistics	Morbidity and mortality data	Extent of risk to community; identification of high-risk groups
7. Anthropometric studies	Physical development	Effect of nutrition on physical development
8. Clinical nutritional surveys	Physical signs	Deviation from health because of malnutrition
9. Biochemical studies	Levels of nutrients, metabolites and other components of body tissues and fluids	Nutrient supplies in the body; impairment of biochemical function
10. Additional medical information	Prevalent disease patterns, including infections and infestations	Interrelationships of state of nutrition and disease

Table I–B
Household Record of Food Used for One Week

Record No. _____			Date Record Started _____	
		MEALS EATEN THIS WEEK		
Person	*Sex*	*Age*	*Number of Meals Eaten at Home or Lunches Carried*	*Number of Meals Eaten Out, not Using Home Food Supply*

ON THE FOLLOWING PAGES, WE WOULD LIKE A RECORD OF THE FOODS AND
DRINKS USED IN YOUR HOME FOR ONE WEEK.

1. When you start the record, write down the amounts of the foods *on hand* which you may
   use during the week.
2. As food is brought into the house from store, farm, or elsewhere during the week, write
   it down.
3. At the end of the week, write down the amounts of food left from those you have put
   on your record.

HOW TO KEEP THE RECORD:

Under *amount*, put down the numbers, weights, measure, or sizes.
Under *kind* of food, write the exact name of the food, for example, "cornflakes," not
   "cereal." Write whether foods are fresh, canned, dried, or frozen.
Under *price for amount bought*, put down price.
Under *source*, write whether foods are from store, own farm, bought from farm, dairy, bak-
   ery, gift, etc. If food is home-canned or home-frozen, record this, and tell the original
   source of the fresh food.

Amount	*Kind of Food*	*Price for Amount Bought*	*Source*

End of Week:
   Amounts of food left over from those listed above:

Amount	*Kind of Food*

Table I–C
Household Dietary Questionnaire

Name	Address	Date

1. Persons fed: (Give sex and age for each)

2. Grade of school completed
    by homemaker

3. Occupation of
    head of household

4. Income level $ Sources of Income

5. Where do you usually get your food supplies?
    If purchased:
       Kind of store?   Cash or credit?
       Distance to store?   Transportation?
       How often shop for food?   Why?
    If home produced, what?

    Do you home preserve?   What? How much?

    Other sources?

    Are food stamps available?   Do you purchase?
       How much do you pay? $ Value get?
    Are donated or surplus foods available?   Do you use?

6. How much did you spend for food last week?
    Is this the usual amount?
7. Do you feel you have adequate storage facilities for food?
8. Do you feel you have adequate cooking facilities?
    Kind?   Working Oven?
9. Do you feel you have adequate refrigeration?
    Kind?

Adapted from National Nutrition Survey, Nutrition Program; Division of Chronic
Disease Program, DHHS, Atlanta, Georgia

Table I-D
24-Hour Recall Form

Name

Date and time of interview

Length of interview

Date of recall

Day of the week of recall

1-M   2-T   3-W   4-Th   5-F   6-Sat   7-Sun

"I would like you to tell me everything you (your child) ate and drank from the time you (he/she) got up in the morning until you (he/she) went to bed at night and what you (he/she) ate during the night. Be sure to mention everything you (he/she) ate or drank at home, at work (school), and away from home. Include snacks and drinks of all kinds and everything else you (he/she) put in your (his/her) mouth and swallowed. I also need to know where you (he/she) ate the food, and now let us begin."

What time did you (he/she) get up yesterday?

Was it the usual time?

What was the first time you (he/she) ate or had anything to drink yesterday morning? (list on the form that follows)

Where did you (he/she) eat? (list on form that follows)

Now tell me what you (he/she) had to eat and how much?

(Occasionally the interviewer will need to ask:)
  When did you (he/she) eat again? Or, is there anything else?
  Did you (he/she) have anything to eat or drink during the night?

Was intake unusual in any way? Yes   No

(If answer is yes)   Why?

                  In what way?

What time did you (he/she) go to bed last night?

Do(es) you (he/she) take vitamin or mineral supplements?

                  Yes   No

(If answer is yes) How many per day?

                  Per week?

What kind? (Insert brand name if known)

Multivitamins

Ascorbic Acid

Vitamins A and D

Iron

Other

Table I-E
Dietary Questionnaire for Children

Name

Date

1. Does the child eat at regular times each day?

2. How many days a week does he/she eat —
    a morning meal?
    a lunch or mid-day meal?
    an evening meal?
    during the night

3. How many days a week does he/she have snacks —
    in mid-morning?
    in mid-afternoon?
    in the evening?
    during the night

4. Which meals does he usually eat with your family?
    None Breakfast Noon meal Evening meal

5. How many times per week does he/she eat at school, child care center, or day camp?
    Breakfast Lunch Between meals

6. Would you describe his/her appetite as Good? Fair? Poor?

7. At what time of day is he/she most hungry?
    Morning Noon Evening

8. What foods does he/she dislike?

9. Is he/she on a special diet now? Yes No
    If Yes, why is he/she on a diet? (Check)
       for weight reduction (own prescription)
       for weight reduction (doctor's prescription)
       for gaining weight
       for allergy, specify
       for other reason, specify
    If No, has he/she been on a special diet within the past year? Yes No

10. Does he/she eat anything which is not usually considered food? Yes No
    If Yes, what?   How often?

11. Can he/she feed himself? Yes No
    If Yes, with his/her fingers? with a spoon?

12. Can he/she use a cup or glass by himself/herself? Yes No

13. Does he/she drink from a bottle with a nipple? Yes No
    If yes, how often?   At what time of day or night?

14. How many times per week does he eat the following foods (at any meal or between meals)? Circle the appropriate number:

Bacon	0 1 2 3 4 5 6 7	>7, specify
Tongue	0 1 2 3 4 5 6 7	>7, specify
Sausage	0 1 2 3 4 5 6 7	>7, specify
Luncheon meat	0 1 2 3 4 5 6 7	>7, specify
Hot dogs	0 1 2 3 4 5 6 7	>7, specify

Dietary Questionnaire for Children *(continued)*

Liver — chicken	0 1 2 3 4 5 6 7 >7, specify
Liver — other	0 1 2 3 4 5 6 7 >7, specify
Poultry	0 1 2 3 4 5 6 7 >7, specify
Salt pork	0 1 2 3 4 5 6 7 >7, specify
Pork or ham	0 1 2 3 4 5 6 7 >7, specify
Meat in mixtures (stew, tamales, casserole, etc.)	0 1 2 3 4 5 6 7 >7, specify
Beef or veal	0 1 2 3 4 5 6 7 >7, specify
Other meat	0 1 2 3 4 5 6 7 >7, specify
Fish	0 1 2 3 4 5 6 7 >7, specify

15. How many times per week does he eat the following foods (at any meal or between meals)? Circle the appropriate number:

Fruit juice	0 1 2 3 4 5 6 7 >7, specify
Fruit	0 1 2 3 4 5 6 7 >7, specify
Cereal — dry	0 1 2 3 4 5 6 7 >7, specify
Cereal — cooked or instant	0 1 2 3 4 5 6 7 >7, specify
Cereal — infant	0 1 2 3 4 5 6 7 >7, specify
Eggs	0 1 2 3 4 5 6 7 >7, specify
Pancakes or waffles	0 1 2 3 4 5 6 7 >7, specify
Cheese	0 1 2 3 4 5 6 7 >7, specify
Potato	0 1 2 3 4 5 6 7 >7, specify
Other cooked vegetables	0 1 2 3 4 5 6 7 >7, specify
Raw vegetables	0 1 2 3 4 5 6 7 >7, specify
Dried beans or peas	0 1 2 3 4 5 6 7 >7, specify
Macaroni, spaghetti, rice, or noodles	0 1 2 3 4 5 6 7 >7, specify
Ice cream, milk pudding, custard, or cream soup	0 1 2 3 4 5 6 7 >7, specify
Peanut butter or nuts	0 1 2 3 4 5 6 7 >7, specify
Sweet rolls or doughnuts	0 1 2 3 4 5 6 7 >7, specify
Crackers or pretzels	0 1 2 3 4 5 6 7 >7, specify
Cookies	0 1 2 3 4 5 6 7 >7, specify
Pie, cake, or brownies	0 1 2 3 4 5 6 7 >7, specify
Potato chips or corn chips	0 1 2 3 4 5 6 7 >7, specify
Candy	0 1 2 3 4 5 6 7 >7, specify
Soft drinks, popsicles, or Koolaid	0 1 2 3 4 5 6 7 >7, specify
Instant breakfast	0 1 2 3 4 5 6 7 >7, specify

16. How many servings per day does he/she eat of the following foods? Circle the appropriate number:

Bread (including sandwich), toast, rolls, or muffins (1 slice or 1 piece is 1 serving)	0 1 2 3 4 5 6 7 >7, specify
Milk (including on cereal and other foods) (8 ounces is 1 serving)	0 1 2 3 4 5 6 7 >7, specify
Sugar, jam, jelly, syrup (1 tsp. is 1 serving)	0 1 2 3 4 5 6 7 >7, specify

17. What specific kinds of the following foods does he eat most often?
    Fruit juices
    Fruit
    Vegetables
    Cheese
    Cooked or instant cereal
    Dry cereal
    Milk

Taken from Screening Children for Nutritional Status: Suggestions for Child Health Programs. Washington DC: U.S. Government Printing Office, 1971.

Table I-F
Dietary Questionnaire for Adults and Adolescents

Name   Sex   Date of birth

Address   Marital status   Date

1. Grade of school   2. Still in   3. Occupation
   completed?   school?

4. Are you employed?   Full time?   Part time?

5. Income level $ Sources of income

Where appropriate:

6. Are you pregnant?   Stage?   Lactating?

If pregnant have you changed the way you eat or drink? How?

On whose advice?

8. Where do you usually get your food supplies?

If home produced, what?

Do you home preserve? What? How much?

If purchased:

Kind of store?   Cash or credit?
Distance to store?   Transportation?
How often shop for food?   Why?

Are food stamps available?   Do you purchase?

How much do you pay? $ Value get? $

Are donated or surplus foods available?   Do you use?

9. Do you feel you have adequate storage facilities for food in your home?

10. Do you feel you have adequate cooking facilities?

Kind?   Working oven?

11. Do you feel you have adequate refrigeration?   Kind?

12. Do you eat at regular times each day?

13. How many days a week do you eat:

a morning meal?
a lunch or mid-day meal?
an evening meal?
during the evening or night?

14. How many days a week do you have snacks, and what do you have then?

in mid-morning
in mid-afternoon
in the evening
during the night

15. Where do you usually eat your meal?
Morning   Mid-day   Evening

16. With whom do you usually eat?
Morning   Mid-day   Evening

Dietary Questionnaire for Adults and Adolescents *(continued)*

17. How many times a week do you usually eat away from home?

18. Would you say your appetite is Good?   Fair?   Poor?

19. What foods do you particularly dislike?

20. Are you on a special diet?   If yes, what kind?   Who prescribed?

21. Are there foods you don't eat for other reasons?

22. Do you eat anything not usually considered food (e.g. clay, dirt, starch, other)?

    If yes, what?   when?   how much?

23. Do you add salt to your food at the table?

24. Do you have any difficulty chewing?

25. How many times per week do you eat the following foods (at any meal or between meals)? Circle the appropriate number:

Bacon	0 1 2 3 4 5 6 7 >7, specify
Tongue	0 1 2 3 4 5 6 7 >7, specify
Sausage	0 1 2 3 4 5 6 7 >7, specify
Luncheon meat	0 1 2 3 4 5 6 7 >7, specify
Hot dogs	0 1 2 3 4 5 6 7 >7, specify
Liver — chicken	0 1 2 3 4 5 6 7 >7, specify
Liver — other	0 1 2 3 4 5 6 7 >7, specify
Poultry	0 1 2 3 4 5 6 7 >7, specify
Salt pork	0 1 2 3 4 5 6 7 >7, specify
Pork or ham	0 1 2 3 4 5 6 7 >7, specify
Bones (neck or other)	0 1 2 3 4 5 6 7 >7, specify
Meat in mixtures (stew, tamales, casseroles, etc.)	0 1 2 3 4 5 6 7 >7, specify
Beef or veal	0 1 2 3 4 5 6 7 >7, specify
Other meat	0 1 2 3 4 5 6 7 >7, specify
Fish	0 1 2 3 4 5 6 7 >7, specify
Cheese and cheese dishes	0 1 2 3 4 5 6 7 >7, specify
Eggs	0 1 2 3 4 5 6 7 >7, specify
Dried beans or pea dishes	0 1 2 3 4 5 6 7 >7, specify
Peanut butter or nuts	0 1 2 3 4 5 6 7 >7, specify

26. How many servings per day do you eat of the following foods? Circle the appropriate number:

Bread (including sandwich), toast, rolls, muffins (1 slice or 1 piece is 1 serving)	0 1 2 3 4 5 6 7 >7, specify
Milk (including on cereal or other foods) (6 ounces is 1 serving)	0 1 2 3 4 5 6 7 >7, specify
Sugar, jam, jelly, syrup (1 tsp. is 1 serving)	0 1 2 3 4 5 6 7 >7, specify
Butter or margarine (1 tsp. is 1 serving)	0 1 2 3 4 5 6 7 >7, specify

27. How many times per week do you eat the following foods (at any meal or between meals)? Circle the appropriate number:

Fruit juice	0 1 2 3 4 5 6 7 >7, specify
Fruit	0 1 2 3 4 5 6 7 >7, specify
Cereal — dry	0 1 2 3 4 5 6 7 >7, specify
Cereal — cooked or instant	0 1 2 3 4 5 6 7 >7, specify
Pancakes or waffles	0 1 2 3 4 5 6 7 >7, specify
Potato	0 1 2 3 4 5 6 7 >7, specify
Other cooked vegetables	0 1 2 3 4 5 6 7 >7, specify

Dietary Questionnaire for Adults and Adolescents *(continued)*

Raw vegetables	0 1 2 3 4 5 6 7 >7, specify
Macaroni, spaghetti, rice, or noodles	0 1 2 3 4 5 6 7 >7, specify
Ice cream, milk pudding, custard, or cream soup	0 1 2 3 4 5 6 7 >7, specify
Sweet rolls or doughnuts	0 1 2 3 4 5 6 7 >7, specify
Crackers or pretzels	0 1 2 3 4 5 6 7 >7, specify
Cookies	0 1 2 3 4 5 6 7 >7, specify
Pie, cake, or brownies	0 1 2 3 4 5 6 7 >7, specify
Potato chips or corn chips	0 1 2 3 4 5 6 7 >7, specify
Candy	0 1 2 3 4 5 6 7 >7, specify
Soft drinks, popsicles, or Koolaid; sherbets	0 1 2 3 4 5 6 7 >7, specify
Instant breakfast	0 1 2 3 4 5 6 7 >7, specify
Artificially sweetened beverage	0 1 2 3 4 5 6 7 >7, specify
Coffee or tea	0 1 2 3 4 5 6 7 >7, specify
Beer	0 1 2 3 4 5 6 7 >7, specify
Wine	0 1 2 3 4 5 6 7 >7, specify
Whiskey, vodka, rum, scotch, gin	0 1 2 3 4 5 6 7 >7, specify

28. What specific kinds of the following foods do you eat most often?
    Fruit juices
    Fruit
    Vegetables
    Cheese
    Cooked or instant cereal
    Dry cereal
    Milk
    Cream or cream substitute
    Butter or margarine
    Salad dressings

Adapted from Screening Children for Nutritional Status: Suggestions for Child Health Programs. Washington, D.C.: U.S. Government Printing Office, 1971.

Table I-G
Physical Signs Indicative or Suggestive of Malnutrition

Body Area	*Normal Appearance*	*Signs Associated with Malnutrition*
Hair	Shiny; firm; not easily plucked	Lack of natural shine; hair dull and dry; thin and sparse; hair fine, silky and straight; color changes (flag sign); can be easily plucked
Face	Skin color uniform; smooth, pink, healthy appearance; not swollen	Skin color loss (depigmentation); skin dark over cheeks and under eyes (malar and supra-orbital pigmentation); lumpiness or flakiness of skin of nose and mouth; swollen face; enlarged parotid glands; scaling of skin around nostrils (nasolabial seborrhea)
Eyes	Bright, clear, shiny; no sores at corners of eyelids; membranes a healthy pink and are moist. No prominent blood vessels or mound of tissue or sclera	Eye membranes are pale (pale conjunctivae); redness of membranes (conjunctival injection); Bitot's spots; redness and fissuring of eyelid corners (angular palpebritis); dryness of eye membranes (conjunctival xerosis); cornea has dull appearance (corneal xerosis); cornea is soft (keratomalacia); scar on cornea; ring of fine blood vessels around corner (circumcorneal injection)
Lips	Smooth, not chapped or swollen	Redness and swelling of mouth or lips (cheilosis); especially at corners of mouth (angular fissures and scars)
Tongue	Deep red in appearance; not swollen or smooth	Swelling; scarlet and raw tongue; magenta (purplish color) of tongue; smooth tongue; swollen sores; hyperemic and hypertrophic papillae; and atrophic papillae
Teeth	No cavities; no pain; bright	May be missing or erupting abnormally; gray or black spots (fluorosis); cavities (caries)
Gums	Healthy; red; do not bleed; not swollen	"Spongy" and bleed easily; recession of gums
Glands	Face not swollen	Thyroid enlargement (front of neck); parotid enlargement (cheeks become swollen)
Skin	No signs of rashes, swellings, dark or light spots	Dryness of skin (xerosis); sandpaper feel of skin (follicular hyperkeratosis); flakiness of skin; skin swollen and dark; red swollen pigmentation of exposed areas (pellagrous dermatosis); excessive lightness or darkness of skin (dyspigmentation); black and blue marks due to skin bleeding (petechiae); lack of fat under skin

Physical Signs Indicative or Suggestive of Malnutrition *(continued)*

Body Area	Normal Appearance	Signs Associated with Malnutrition
Nails	Firm, pink	Nails are spoon-shape (koilonychia); brittle, ridged nails
Muscular and skeletal systems	Good muscle tone; some fat under skin; can walk or run without pain	Muscles have "wasted" appearance; baby's skull bones are thin and soft (craniotabes); round swelling of front and side of head (frontal and parietal bossing); swelling of ends of bones (epiphyseal enlargement); small bumps on both sides of chest wall (on ribs) — beading of ribs; baby's soft spot on head does not harden at proper time (persistently open anterior fontanelle); knock-knees or bow-legs; bleeding into muscle (musculoskeletal hemorrhages); person cannot get up or walk properly
Internal Systems:		
Cardiovascular	Normal heart rate and rhythm; no murmurs or abnormal rhythms; normal blood pressure for age	Rapid heart rate (above 100 tachycardia); enlarged heart; abnormal rhythm; elevated blood pressure
Gastrointestinal	No palpable organs or masses (in children, however, liver edge may be palpable)	Liver enlargement; enlargement of spleen (usually indicates other associated diseases)
Nervous	Psychological stability; normal reflexes	Mental irritability and confusion; burning and tingling of hands and feet (paresthesia); loss of position and vibratory sense; weakness and tenderness of muscles (may result in inability to walk); decrease and loss of ankle and knee reflexes

Source: G. Christakis, editor. *Nutritional Assessment in Health Programs.* Am. J. Public Health 63, Suppl. (1973):1.

Table I–H
Physical Signs and Nutritional Terms Associated with Malnutrition

---

1. General Appearance

Apathy: Unreactive, unresponsive, disinterested, and inattentive to surroundings.

Clinical Marasmus: Evidence of pronounced wasting of subcutaneous fat without edema. Significant apathy may be present. Frequently the face and eyes of the child may appear unusually bright due to the combination of wasting and prominance of the eyes. The child is usually considerably underdeveloped in relation to age and there may or may not be associated hair changes such as dyspigmentation, thinness, easily pluckable, or signs of avitaminosis.

Irritability: Hyperresponsive, excessive or overreaction to minor stimuli, particularly manifest through crying or unusual indication of fear as a result of minor or relatively insignificant happenings.

Kwashiorkor: Pitting edema at least on the pretibial region, underweight, undersize, underdeveloped for age. Muscular wasting may be present but masked by edema. Apathy of some degree is present. Changes in the hair are usually noted, such as thinning, easily pluckable with dyspigmentation or flag sign, and change in texture to silken, sparse hair. Dermatosis with desquamation of the so-called flaky-paint type, with or without hyperpigmentation. In severe cases the dermatosis may resemble a relatively severe burn but lacks erythema.

Pallor: Paleness and loss of color of skin, nail beds, mucosa and lips.

Prekwashiorkor: An underweight, undersized, underdeveloped child, without the evident pronounced wasting present in marasmus. Child is thin and undersized, but has relatively normal body proportions, has rather poor muscle tone, and hair changes may be present. Not apathetic, though would not be described as alert.

---

2. Hair

Dry staring: Dry, wirelike, unkempt stiff hair, often brittle; sometimes may exhibit some bleaching of the normal color.

Dyspigmentation: Definite change from normal pigment of the hair, most usually evident distally and best seen by carefully combing hair strands upward and viewing the orderly array of hair in good light. Dyspigmentation includes both change of pigment (usually lightening of color) and depigmentation. Not to be confused with dyed or tinted hair. Dyspigmentation is often bandlike in character and usually is associated with some change in texture of hair in the depigmented band. In some groups, particularly among Negroid people, the pigment may be slightly reddish in color. In others, especially peoples with straight black hair, the bandlike depigmentation ("flag sign") is common.

Easily pluckable: Easily pluckable hair is that in which the shafts are readily removed with minimum tug when a few strands are grasped between the finger and thumb and gently pulled. In such cases there is a lack of reaction of the child, indicating a lack of pain associated with removing of the hair.

---

3. Skin

Crackled skin: Definite scales larger in size than those seen in xerosis. It is often congenital and is most prominent in cool weather. It is non-nutritional in origin.

Dependent edema: The presence of abnormally large amounts of fluid in the intercellular tissue spaces of the body; usually applied to demonstrable accumulation of excessive fluid in the subcutaneous tissues which are dependent upon position and gravity.

Dermatitis, with desquamation, or crazy-pavement type: Under this heading should be recorded those desquamating changes of the skin, usually with increased pigmentation,

Physical Signs and Nutritional Terms Associated with Malnutrition *(continued)*

which occur on the extremities, especially legs, thighs and buttocks, but may occur over the trunk in association with kwashiorkor. (These have been termed "flaky-paint" dermatoses.) Small circumscribed bleblike lesions sometimes seen in association with kwashiorkor and which on occasion may precede the desquamation. In addition, any "crazy-pavement" type of lesions observed should be noted. These are characterized by a thin-appearing epithelium marked by striations usually resembling in outline the microscopic picture of epithelial cells. Not to be confused, however, with ichthyosis (scaly skin).

Follicular hyperkeratosis: This lesion has been likened to "gooseflesh" which is seen on chilling, but it is not generalized and does not disappear with brisk rubbing of the skin. Readily felt, as it presents a "nutmeg grater" feel. Follicular hyperkeratosis is more readily detected by the sense of touch than by the eye. The skin is rough, with papillae formed by keratotic plugs which project from the hair follicles. The surrounding skin is dry and lacks the usual amount of moisture or oiliness. Differentiation from adolescent folliculosis can usually be made through recognition of the normal skin between the follicles in the adolescent disorder. It is distinguished from perifolliculosis by the ring of capillary congestion which occurs about each follicle in scorbutic perifolliculosis.

Pellagrous dermatitis: Symmetrical lesions typical of acute or chronic, mild or severe pellagra are observed; lesions are usually red, often swollen or blistered like sunburn, pigmented, scaly over exposed areas; clearly demarcated from normal skin.

Purpura or petechia: Small localized extravasations of blood, red or purplish in color, depending on the time elapsed since formation. Usually distributed at sites of pressure and may be perifollicular.

Xerosis: Xerosis is a clinical term used to describe a dry and crinkled skin which is accentuated by pushing the skin parallel to its surface. In more pronounced cases it is often mottled and pigmented, and may appear as scaly or alligator-like pseudo-plaques, usually not greater than 0.5 cm in diameter. Nutritional significance is not established. Differential diagnosis must be made from changes due to dirt and exposure and ichthyosis.

4. Skeletal

Bowleg: An outward curve of one or both legs at or below the knee (genu varum).

Costochondral beading: Palpable and visible enlargement of the costochondral junctions.

Cranial bossing: Abnormal prominence or protusion of frontal of parietal areas.

Enlarged joints: When the more obvious ends of long bones are enlarged; i.e., the wrist, ankles, knees.

Winged scapula: A scapula having a prominent vertebral border.

5. Muscle

Muscle wasting: When appearance indicates abnormal loss of muscle substance, as exhibited by unusual prominence of bony skeleton, undue degree of folding of the skin of the buttocks, or the abnormal flabby feel (sometimes described as jelly-like) of the child with poor muscle tone.

6. Eyes

Bitot's spots: Bitot's spots are small circumscribed grayish or yellowish gray, dull, dry, foamy superficial lesions of the conjunctiva. They most often occur on the lateral aspect of the bulbar conjunctiva in the interpalpebral area. Do not confuse with pterygium.

Blepharitis: Inflammation of eyelids.

Keratomalacia: Softening of the cornea.

Physical Signs and Nutritional Terms Associated with Malnutrition *(continued)*

Thickened opaque bulbar conjunctivae: All degrees of thickening may occur. The blueness of the sclera may disappear and the bulbar conjunctivae develop a wrinkled appearance with increase in vascularity. The thickened conjunctivae may result in a glazed, procelain-like appearance, obscuring the vascularity.

Xerosis conjunctivae: The conjunctivae, upon exposure by holding the lids open and having the subject rotate the eyes, appear dull, lusterless, and exhibit a striated or roughened surface.

7. *Face*

Angular lesions: Present bilaterally when mouth is held half open. May appear as pink or moist whitish macerated angular lesions which blur the mucocutaneous junction. Angular fissures are recorded when there is definite break in continuity of epithelium at the angles of the mouth.

Angular scars: Scars at the angles, which, if recent, may be pink; if old, may appear blanched.

Cheilosis: Condition in which the lips are swollen, tense, or puffy; where it appears, the buccal mucosa extends out onto the lips. These lesions are also denuded. This category may be used to record vertical fissuring of the lips, but not for lesions of the angles of the mouth only.

Nasolabial seborrhea: Definite greasy yellowish scaling or filiform excrescences in the nasolabial area which become more pronounced on slight scratching with the fingernail or a tongue blade.

8. *Mouth*

Filiform papillary atrophy: Filiform papillae exceedingly low or absent, giving the tongue a smooth appearance which remains after scraping slightly with an applicator stick. "Mild" involves less than ¼ of the tongue (tip and lateral margins only); "moderate" involves ¼ to ¾ of the tongue; "severe" involves over ¾.

Glossitis: Glossitis is any increase in redness, fissuring or swelling with color change (break in lingual mucosa) or diffuse involvement of mucosa. Geographic tongue has the typical irregularly shaped and distributed areas of atrophy with irregular white patches resembling leukoplakia. Glossitis is usually associated with some sensation of pain or burning, particularly upon eating.

Magenta colored: The color of alkaline phenolphthalein.

Swollen gums: Swollen red interdental papillae, with more than one papilla involved.

9. *Teeth*

Carious teeth: Molecular decay of a tooth in which it becomes friable, thinned, and dark, and gradually breaks down with the formation of pus.

Fluorosis: Opaque paper-white areas in the enamel of the tooth, ranging in size from a few flecks to entire enamel surface. In the latter case brown stain is a frequent accompaniment as is attrition of opposing surfaces. The most severe forms of fluorosis include discrete or confluent pitting, with widespread brown staining and a general, corroded appearance.

10. *Glands*

Parotid enlargement: Because of various types of facial configuration, parotid enlargement may be easily missed in certain populations. Check by palpation, moving the gland with fingers upward and backward toward the ear. Check if bilateral.

Physical Signs and Nutritional Terms Associated with Malnutrition *(continued)*

Thyroid enlargement: Thyroid enlargement is a condition in which a visually perceptible enlargement definitely palpable with or without swallowing is noted. It is preferable to examine the subject with his head slightly extended in order to detect thyroid enlargement.

11. Organs

Hepatomegaly: Liver edges more than 2 cm below the costal margin. (In children, the liver edge may be normal palpable.)

Splenomegaly: Spleen is palpable.

Source: G. Christakis, editor. *Nutritional Assessment in Health Programs.* Am. J. Public Health 63, Suppl. (1973):1.

Physical Signs of Malnutrition

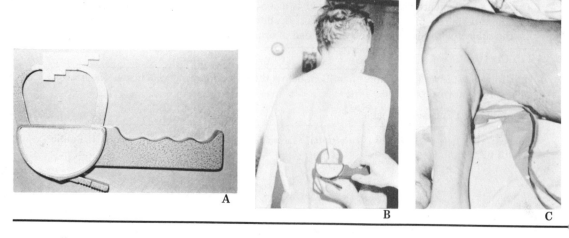

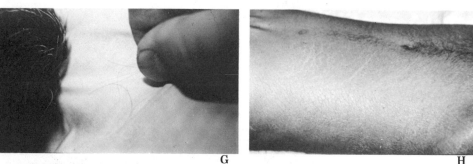

Fig. A Lange skinfold calipers with standardization device, manufactured by Cambridge Scientific Industries, Inc., Cambridge, Maryland.   Fig. B Lange skinfold calipers in use for measurement of subscapular skinfold thickness.   Fig. C Resorption of gastrocnemius muscle in an obese subject who had lost 60 pounds of body weight in 60 days (from 320 to 260 pounds) during a complicated postoperative period following cholecystectomy. There had been marked limitation of nutrient intake. Total serum protein was 5.4, albumin 2.4 g/dl along with numerous other abnormal laboratory findings. The general appearance and abundant subcutaneous fat tended to obscure extensive loss of lean body mass. Nutritional assessment was: protein-calorie malnutrition; severe, acute visceral attrition superimposed on chronic perietal muscle depletion (marasmic-kwashiorkor-like syndrome).   Fig. D Nail changes during PCM. A 36-year-old man developed an enterocutaneous fistula following an injury, lost approximately 40 per cent of his body weight and developed multiple nutritional deficiencies. This illustration shows abnormal nail, characterized by brittleness and lack of luster, being displaced by normal nail that has grown during a period of total parenteral nutrition.   Figs. E, F Cheilosis, glossitis, scorbutic gums, and periodontal disease in a patient with multiple deficiencies of vitamins and iron due to inadequate intake. She had eaten nothing but canned soup for four months and had pulled several of her own teeth when they became loose. Hospitalization was brought on by acute urinary tract infection, probably facilitated by impaired immune mechanisms. The clinical diagnosis of scurvy was confirmed by a plasma ascorbate value in the deficient range. Other features of malnutrition included: iron deficiency anemia (low serum iron and low transferrin saturation); hypoproteinemia; hypoalbuminemia; hypoprothrombinemia; and subnormal levels of thiamin in blood and urine. Despite cheilosis, the riboflavin levels in blood and urine were in the acceptable range. There was rapid and dramatic improvement

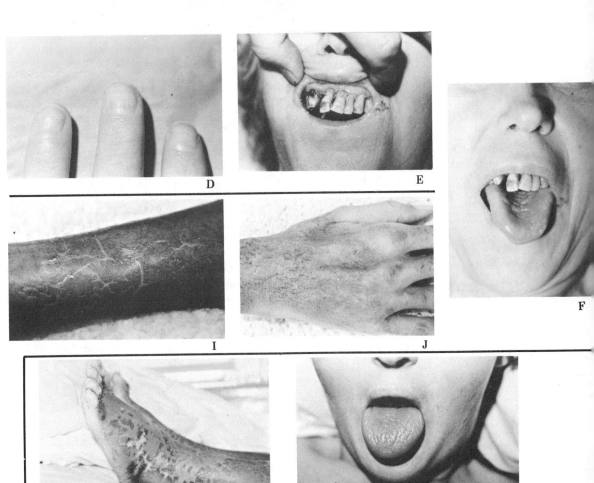

D

E

F

I

J

K

L

in her general state following replacement therapy with multiple vitamins and iron, along with treatment of infection. Dental extractions were carried out successfully after correction of nutritional deficiencies. However, she would have run a considerable risk of post-operative complications if dental surgery (or any other surgery) had been attempted without adequate prior preparation. She illustrates the value of early assessment of nutritional status.   Fig. G Easily pluckable hair. Gentle traction on hair between thumb and fore-finger, sliding toward the tip, normally yields no hairs or at most one or two. In cases of PCM larger numbers are released and with greater ease. Although this is difficult to quantify, it becomes possible with experience to distinguish between "easily pluckable" and "firmly attached" hair, making this simple procedure a useful adjunct to the bedside evaluation of a patient's status. Valuable information can sometimes be gained by inspection of the comb or brush at the bedside for evidence of excessive shedding of hair.   Figs. H, I Flaky paint dermatosis of protein-calorie malnutrition. This pattern has been described in young children suffering from kwashiorkor, but may also be seen in adults. Like hair changes, it seems to be associated with hypoalbuminemia and is probably related to deficiencies of essential amino acids.   Figs. J, K Symptoms of pellagra. Note erythema, hyperpigmentation, desquamation, and sharp margination.   Fig. L The tongue of a 25-year-old woman with multiple nutritional deficiencies 7 months after ileal by-pass surgery for obesity has been performed. The patient complained of a sore, dry tongue and lack of taste. She was subsequently found to have abnormally low levels of serum zinc and folate.

Table I–I

Table of Current Guidelines for Criteria of Nutritional Status for Laboratory Evaluation

Nutrient and Units	Age of Subject (years)	Criteria of Status		
		Deficient	Marginal	Acceptable
*Hemoglobin	6–23 mos.	Up to 9.0	9.0– 9.9	10.0+
(gm/100ml)	2–5	Up to 10.0	10.0–10.9	11.0+
	6–12	Up to 10.0	10.0–11.4	11.5+
	13–16M	Up to 12.0	12.0–12.9	13.0+
	13–16F	Up to 10.0	10.0–11.4	11.5+
	16+M	Up to 12.0	12.0–13.9	14.0+
	16+F	Up to 10.0	10.0–11.9	12.0+
	Pregnant (after 6+ mos.)	Up to 9.5	9.5–10.9	11.0+
*Hematocrit	Up to 2	Up to 28	28–30	31+
(Packed cell volume)	2–5	Up to 30	30–33	34+
in percent)	6–12	Up to 30	30–35	36+
	13–16M	Up to 37	37–39	40+
	13–16F	Up to 31	31–35	36+
	16+M	Up to 37	37–43	44+
	16+F	Up to 31	31–37	33+
	Pregnant	Up to 30	30–32	33+
*Serum albumin	Up to 1	—	Up to 2.5	2.5+
(gm/100ml)	1–5	—	Up to 3.0	3.0+
	6–16	—	Up to 3.5	3.5+
	16+	Up to 2.8	2.8–3.4	3.5+
	Pregnant	Up to 3.0	3.0–3.4	3.5+
*Serum protein	Up to 1	—	Up to 5.0	5.0+
(gm/100ml)	1–5	—	Up to 5.5	5.5+
	6–16		Up to 6.0	6.0+
	16+	Up to 6.0	6.0–6.4	6.5+
	Pregnant	Up to 5.5	5.5–5.9	6.0+
*Serum ascorbic acid (mg/100ml)	All ages	Up to 0.1	0.1–0.19	0.2+
*Plasma vitamin A (mcg/100 ml)	All ages	Up to 10	10–19	20+
*Plasma carotene (mcg/100ml)	All ages	Up to 20	20–39	40+
	Pregnant	—	40–79	80+
*Serum iron (mcg/100ml)	Up to 2	Up to 30	—	30+
	2–5	Up to 40	—	40+
	6–12	Up to 50	—	50+
	12+M	Up to 60	—	60+
	12+F	Up to 40	—	40+
*Transferrin saturation (%)	Up to 2	Up to 15.0	—	15.0
	2–12	Up to 20.0	—	20.0+
	12+M	Up to 20.0	—	20.0+
	12+F	Up to 15.0	—	15.0+
**Serum folacin (%)	All ages	Up to 2.0	2.1–5.9	6.0+
**Serum vitamin B$_{12}$ (pg/ml)	All ages	Up to 1.0	—	100+

Table of Current Guidelines for Criteria of Nutritional Status for Laboratory Evaluation
(continued)

Nutrient and Units	Age of Subject (years)	Criteria of Status		
		Deficient	*Marginal*	*Acceptable*
*Thiamine in urine	1–3	Up to 120	120–175	175+
(mcg/g creatinine)	4–5	Up to 85	85–120	120+
	6–9	Up to 70	70–180	180+
	10–15	Up to 55	55–150	150+
	16+	Up to 27	27– 65	65+
	Pregnant	Up to 21	21– 49	50+
*Riboflavin in urine	1–3	Up to 150	150–499	500+
(mcg/g creatinine)	4–5	Up to 100	100–299	300+
	6–9	Up to 85	85–269	270+
	10–16	Up to 70	70–199	200+
	16+	Up to 27	27– 79	80+
	Pregnant	Up to 30	30– 89	90+
**RBC transketolase-TPP-effect (ratio)	All ages	25+	15– 25	Up to 15
**RBC glutathione reductase-FAD-effect (ratio)	All ages	1.2+	—	Up to 1.2
**Tryptophan load (mg xanthurenic acid excreted)	Adults (Dose: 100mg/kg body weight)	25+(6 hrs.) 75+(24 hrs.)	— —	Up to 25 Up to 75
**Urinary pyridoxine	1–3	Up to 90	—	90+
(mcg/g creatinine)	4–6	Up to 80	—	80+
	7–9	Up to 60	—	60+
	10–12	Up to 40	—	40+
	13–15	Up to 30	—	30+
	16+	Up to 20	—	20+
*Urinary n'methyl nicotinamide (mg/g creatinine)	All ages Pregnant	Up to 0.2 Up to 0.8	0.2–5.59 0.8–2.49	0.6+ 2.5+
**Urinary pantothenic acid (mcg)	All ages	Up to 200	—	200+
**Plasma vitamin E (mg/100ml)	All ages	Up to 0.2	0.2–0.6	0.6+
**Transaminase Index (ratio)				
†EGOT	Adult	2.0+	—	Up to 2.0
‡EGPT	Adult	1.25+	—	Up to 1.25

*Adapted from the Ten State Nutrition Survey
**Criteria may vary with different methodology
†Erythrocyte Glutamic Oxalacetic Transaminase
‡Erythrocyte Glutamic Pyruvic Transaminase
Source: G. Christakis, editor. *Nutritional Assessment in Health Programs.* Am. J. Public Health 63, Suppl. (1973):1.

Table I–J

Desirable Weights for Men and Women According to Height and Frame
Ages 25 and Over

Height (in shoes)*	Weight in Pounds (in indoor clothing) Men		
	Small Frame	Medium Frame	Large Frame
5 ft 2 in	112–120	118–129	126–141
5 ft 3 in	115–123	121–133	129–144
5 ft 4 in	118–126	124–136	132–148
5 ft 5 in	121–129	127–139	135–152
5 ft 6 in	124–133	130–143	138–156
5 ft 7 in	128–137	134–147	142–161
5 ft 8 in	132–141	138–152	147–166
5 ft 9 in	136–145	142–156	151–170
5 ft 10 in	140–150	146–160	155–174
5 ft 11 in	144–154	150–165	159–179
6 ft 0 in	148–158	154–170	164–184
6 ft 1 in	152–162	158–175	168–189
6 ft 2 in	156–167	162–180	173–194
6 ft 3 in	160–171	167–185	178–199
6 ft 4 in	164–175	172–190	182–204
	Women		
	Small Frame	Medium Frame	Large Frame
4 ft 10 in	92– 98	96–107	104–119
4 ft 11 in	94–101	98–110	106–122
5 ft 0 in	96–104	101–113	109–125
5 ft 1 in	99–107	104–116	112–128
5 ft 2 in	102–110	107–119	115–131
5 ft 3 in	105–113	110–122	118–134
5 ft 4 in	108–116	113–126	121–138
5 ft 5 in	111–119	116–130	125–142
5 ft 6 in	114–123	120–135	129–146
5 ft 7 in	118–127	124–139	133–150
5 ft 8 in	122–131	128–143	137–154
5 ft 9 in	126–135	132–147	141–158
5 ft 10 in	130–140	136–151	145–163
5 ft 11 in	134–144	140–155	149–168
6 ft 0 in	138–148	144–159	153–174

*1-inch heels for men and 2-inch heels for women
Source: Prepared by the Metropolitan Life Insurance Company (1960). Derived primarily from data of the *Build and Blood Pressure Study*, 1959.

Table I-K
Growth Standards for Boys from Birth to Age 18*

Age	Height (inches) Percentiles			Weight (pounds) Percentiles			Height (centimeters) Percentiles			Weight (kilograms) Percentiles		
	5th	50th	95th	5th	50th	95th	5th	50th	95th	5th	50th	95th
Birth	18.4	19.8	21.1	5.9	7.5	9.1	47	50	54	2.7	3.4	4.1
1 mo.	19.9	21.4	22.9	7.3	9.4	11.1	51	54	58	3.3	4.3	5.0
3 mo.	22.6	24.0	25.4	9.8	13.4	16.0	57	61	65	4.4	6.1	7.3
6 mo.	25.1	26.7	28.3	14.7	18.0	21.3	63	68	72	6.7	8.2	9.7
9 mo.	27.2	28.7	30.2	16.8	21.4	25.1	69	73	77	7.6	9.7	11.4
1 yr.	28.4	30.2	32.0	18.7	23.3	27.8	72	77	81	8.5	10.6	12.4
2 yr.	32.1	34.6	37.1	28.3	28.3	33.3	82	88	94	10.6	12.8	15.1
3 yr.	35.3	37.8	40.3	27.1	32.5	37.9	90	95	102	12.3	14.8	17.1
4 yr.	38.3	40.8	43.3	30.0	36.1	42.4	97	104	110	13.6	16.4	19.2
5 yr.	40.3	43.4	46.4	33.0	40.3	47.6	102	110	118	15.0	18.3	21.6
6 yr.	42.8	45.9	49.0	36.0	44.7	53.4	109	117	124	16.3	20.3	24.2
7 yr.	44.8	48.1	51.4	40.3	50.9	61.5	114	122	131	18.3	23.1	27.9
8 yr.	46.9	50.5	54.1	44.4	57.4	70.4	119	129	137	20.2	26.1	32.0
9 yr.	48.8	52.8	56.8	48.0	64.4	80.4	124	134	144	21.8	29.2	36.5
10 yr.	50.6	54.9	59.2	51.4	71.4	91.4	129	139	150	23.3	32.4	41.5
11 yr.	51.9	56.4	60.9	53.3	78.9	102.5	132	143	155	24.2	35.8	46.5
12 yr.	53.5	58.6	63.7	60.0	86.0	113.5	136	149	162	27.2	39.0	51.5
13 yr.	55.2	61.3	67.4	65.3	98.6	131.9	140	156	171	29.6	44.8	59.9
14 yr.	57.5	64.1	70.7	75.5	111.8	148.1	146	163	180	34.3	50.8	67.2
15 yr.	61.0	66.9	72.8	88.0	124.3	160.6	155	170	185	40.0	56.4	72.9
16 yr.	63.8	68.9	74.0	97.8	133.8	169.8	162	175	188	44.4	60.7	77.1
17 yr.	65.2	69.8	74.4	106.5	139.8	174.0	166.	177	189	48.3	63.5	79.0
18 yr.	65.9	70.2	74.5	110.3	144.8	179.3	167	178	189	50.0	65.7	81.4

*Height in inches and weight in pounds from: *Obesity and Health*, Pub. 1485, Public Health Service. U.S. Department of Health, Education, and Welfare, 1966; height in centimeters and weight in kilograms calculated from these data.

Table I-K continued
Growth Standards for Girls from Birth to Age 18*

Age	Height (inches) Percentiles			Weight (pounds) Percentiles			Height (centimeters) Percentiles			Weight (kilograms) Percentiles		
	5th	50th	95th	5th	50th	95th	5th	50th	95th	5th	50th	95th
Birth	18.3	19.5	20.7	5.3	7.3	8.8	47	50	53	2.4	3.3	4.0
1 mo.	19.5	21.0	22.5	6.6	8.3	9.8	50	53	57	3.0	3.8	4.4
3 mo.	22.2	23.6	25.0	10.2	12.4	14.4	56	60	64	4.6	5.6	6.5
6 mo.	24.6	26.1	27.6	13.4	16.7	19.8	63	66	70	6.1	7.6	9.0
9 mo.	26.3	27.9	29.5	15.3	19.8	24.1	67	71	77	6.9	9.0	10.9
1 yr.	27.6	29.4	31.2	17.4	21.7	26.0	70	75	79	7.9	9.9	11.8
2 yr.	31.6	33.8	36.0	22.3	27.1	31.9	80	86	91	10.1	12.3	14.5
3 yr.	35.3	37.5	39.7	26.3	32.3	38.3	90	95	101	11.9	14.7	17.4
4 yr.	38.1	40.7	43.3	28.8	36.1	43.4	97	103	110	13.1	16.4	19.7
5 yr.	40.6	43.4	46.2	32.2	40.9	49.6	103	110	117	14.6	18.6	22.5
6 yr.	42.8	45.9	49.0	35.5	45.7	55.9	109	117	124	16.1	20.7	25.4
7 yr.	44.5	47.8	51.1	38.3	51.0	63.7	113	121	130	17.4	23.2	28.9
8 yr.	46.4	50.0	53.6	42.0	57.2	72.4	118	127	136	19.1	26.0	32.9
9 yr.	48.2	52.2	56.2	45.1	63.6	82.1	122	133	143	20.5	28.9	37.3
10 yr.	49.9	54.5	59.1	48.2	71.0	95.0	128	138	150	21.9	32.2	43.1
11 yr.	51.9	57.0	62.1	55.4	82.0	108.6	132	145	158	25.1	37.2	49.3
12 yr.	54.1	59.5	64.9	63.9	94.4	124.9	137	151	165	29.0	42.9	56.7
13 yr.	57.1	62.2	66.8	72.8	105.5	138.2	145	158	170	33.1	47.9	62.7
14 yr.	58.5	63.1	67.7	83.0	113.0	144.0	149	160	172	37.7	51.3	65.4
15 yr.	59.5	63.8	68.1	89.5	120.0	150.5	151	162	173	40.6	54.5	68.3
16 yr.	59.8	64.1	68.4	95.1	123.0	150.1	152	163	174	43.2	55.9	68.1
17 yr.	60.1	64.2	68.3	97.9	125.8	153.7	153	163	174	44.4	57.1	69.8
18 yr.	60.1	64.4	68.7	96.0	126.2	156.4	153	164	174	43.6	57.3	71.0

*Height in inches and weight in pounds from: *Obesity and Health*, Pub. 1485, Public Health Service. U.S. Department of Health, Education, and Welfare, 1966; height in centimeters and weight in kilograms calculated from these data.

Table I–L
Triceps Skin-fold Measurements

Triceps Skin-fold, Birth to 60 Months, Sexes Separate
Triceps Skin-fold (mm)

Age (months)	Standard		90% Standard		80% Standard		70% Standard		60% Standard	
	M	F	M	F	M	F	M	F	M	F
Birth	6.0	6.5	5.4	5.9	4.8	5.2	4.2	4.6	3.6	3.9
6	10.0	10.0	9.0	9.0	8.0	8.0	7.0	7.0	6.0	6.0
12	10.3	10.2	9.3	9.2	8.2	8.2	7.2	7.1	6.2	6.1
18	10.3	10.2	9.3	9.2	8.2	8.2	7.2	7.1	6.2	6.1
24	10.0	10.1	9.0	9.1	8.0	8.1	7.0	7.1	6.0	6.1
36	9.3	9.7	8.4	8.7	7.5	7.8	6.5	6.8	5.6	5.8
48	9.3	10.2	8.4	9.2	7.5	8.2	6.5	7.2	5.6	6.1
60	9.1	9.4	8.2	8.5	7.3	7.5	6.4	6.6	5.5	5.7

Triceps Skin-fold, 5–15 Years, Sexes Separate
Triceps Skin-fold (mm)

Age (years)	Standard		90% Standard		80% Standard		70% Standard		60% Standard	
	M	F	M	F	M	F	M	F	M	F
5	9.1	9.4	8.2	8.5	7.3	7.5	6.4	6.6	5.5	5.7
6	8.2	9.6	7.4	8.6	6.6	7.7	5.8	6.7	4.9	5.8
7	7.9	9.4	7.1	8.5	6.3	7.5	5.5	6.6	4.7	5.7
8	7.6	10.1	6.8	9.1	6.1	8.1	5.3	7.1	4.5	6.1
9	8.2	10.3	7.4	9.2	6.6	8.2	5.8	7.2	4.9	6.2
10	8.2	10.4	7.4	9.3	6.6	8.3	5.7	7.3	4.9	6.2
11	8.9	10.6	8.1	9.6	7.2	8.5	6.3	7.5	5.4	6.4
12	8.5	10.1	7.6	9.1	6.8	8.1	5.9	7.0	5.1	6.0
13	8.1	10.4	7.3	9.4	6.5	8.3	5.7	7.3	4.9	6.2
14	7.9	11.3	7.1	10.1	6.3	9.0	5.5	7.9	4.8	6.8
15	6.3	11.4	5.7	10.2	5.0	9.1	4.4	8.0	3.8	6.8

Triceps Skin-fold, Adults, Sexes Separate
Triceps Skin-fold (mm)

Sex	Standard	90% Standard	80% Standard	70% Standard	60% Standard
Male	12.5	11.3	10.0	8.8	7.5
Female	16.5	14.9	13.2	11.6	9.9

Appendix II REFERRALS

Sample Nutrition Referral Form

CLIENT'S NAME (Last)	(First)	REASON FOR REFERRAL

ADDRESS	CITY	STATE	ZIP	PHONE NUMBER

DATE OF BIRTH	AGE	SEX	HEIGHT	WEIGHT	PHYSICIAN

DIAGNOSIS

MODIFIED DIET

SUMMARY OF PERTINENT MEDICAL HISTORY (Laboratory, physical findings)

SUMMARY OF PERSONAL BACKGROUND AS IT RELATES TO REFERRAL (Such as economic status, educational background, food stamps, and WIC)

OTHER PROBLEMS RELATED TO THE PRACTICE OF GOOD FOOD HABITS

PLANS FOR FOLLOW-UP

REFERRED TO:		REFERRED FROM:		
Person	Title	Person	Title	Date

661

Appendix III GRANTSMANSHIP

Table III-A

Basic Components of a Grant Proposal

I. Introduction
   A. Overview
   B. Statement of the problem
   C. Justification and significance of proposed study
   D. Research questions or hypothesis
   E. Objectives
II. Review of Relevant Literature: Summary of Related Research and/or Work in the Field; References; Methodology
III. Procedure or Plan of the Project
   A. Populations to be served or samples to be studied
   B. Design or plan of project operation
   C. Location of project
   D. Personnel required for project and specified responsibilities
   E. Duration (timeline) of project
   F. Evaluation of project operation
IV. Budget
   A. Personnel (including base pay, fringe benefits, and the like)
   B. Operating expenses
   C. Consultants
   D. Supplies, materials, and equipment
   E. Travel
   F. Other expenses
   G. Overhead
   H. Other sources of funds for proposed project

Table III-B

Common Reasons for Lack of Funding of Proposals

I. The Problem
   A. Statement about the purpose of the project is not clear.
   B. Unlikely that any new or useful information would result from project.
   C. Limited significance of problem.
   D. Research questions not properly formulated.
   E. Objectives broad and general, rather than specific.
   F. Literature review incomplete.
II. Plan or Approach of Project
   A. Description of procedures or plan of operation is not clear.
   B. Objectives and procedures are not properly coordinated.
   C. Methodological errors: inadequate selection of subjects, statistical errors, and inadequate evaluation.
   D. Proposed methods are not likely to result in valid or reliable data.
   E. Budget too high or too low for proposed project.
III. Ability and Competence of Investigators
   A. Limited training and/or experience for proposed area of project.
   B. Lack of familiarity with relevant literature and appropriate procedures.
   C. Poor record of achievement in previous grant attempts.
   D. Inexperienced or inadequate support staff, or insufficient description of personnel and their responsibilities.

Table III–C

Suggestions for More Effective Proposal Writing

The following is a list of questions that those who review proposals *may* ask when reading them.

1. Is the proposal relevant to priority areas as stated and/or implied in legislation, guidelines, and/or rules and regulations?
2. Is the proposed activity needed in the area to be served by the program? Or is the applicant merely looking for money?
3. Is the need documented and substantiated?
4. Has a need analysis been made? Is it convincing?
5. Are the resources set out by the agency sufficient to do the task?
6. Are goals and objectives sharply defined and clearly stated? Goals and objectives should state and/or clearly imply (a) What will be done? (b) How will it be done? (c) How will it be measured?
7. Remember: Do not be too grandiose. Reviewers will be sure to ask (a) Can the goals be attained by the proposed procedures? (b) Can the program be measured?
8. Is the proposed plan of operation sound? Is the project based on theory and practice?
9. Do the people involved in the project have adequate qualifications? What is their relevant background and related experience? Have they demonstrated the ability to do the task?
10. Is the organizational structure conducive to project attainment? If the project has merit, will it become institutionalized or will the program die when the supply of money ends?
11. Is the proposed evaluation plan sound? Is it based on theory and practice? (Here you may want to note that some objectives cannot be measured. Acknowledge this and do not state them as primary objectives.)
12. Are the evaluation practices and procedures appropriate for measuring progress and are they appropriate to the objectives?
13. Is some attention given to latent effects? Are they taken into account?

(From *Pedagogy*, 1 (3). Feb. 24, 1977)

Appendix IV AGENCIES WITH NUTRITION-RELATED ACTIVITIES

Agency/Address	Type of Organization	Primary Objectives of Organization	Key Activities
Al-Anon Al-Anon Family Group Headquarters, Inc. P.O. Box 182 Madison Square Sta. New York, N.Y. 10010	Nonprofit, voluntary	To focus attention on the recognition of alcoholism as a problem of the total family group, to provide help and information for the total family.	Public service spot announcements. Labor-management program. Literature, books, monthly publication, *Forum*, newsletter, and other educational materials. Nutrition is a concern in its effect on the alcoholic and his or her family.
Alcoholics Anonymous World Service, Inc. (AA) Box 459 Grand Central Sta. New York, N.Y. 10017	Nonprofit, voluntary fellowship	To provide aid to willing alcoholics.	Group meetings, speakers, and publications. Nutrition is a concern as it becomes a problem for those seeking help.
Action for Children's TV 46 Austin St. Newtonville, Mass. 01260	Nonprofit, voluntary	To encourage and support quality programming for children; to eliminate commercialism and require a reasonable amount of weekly programming for children of various ages.	Involved in legislation and work with the FTC to improve broadcast practices. Develop resource materials in children's programming. Conducts national symposiums on children and media. Supports research on children's television. Maintains resource library and offers award achievements in children's TV.
American Academy of Pediatrics (AAP) 1801 Hinman Avenue Evanston, Ill. 60204	Nonprofit, professional	To help children attain their full potential by setting standards for child health care and by acting as an advocate for child health needs and providing education to providers of child health care.	Programs public service television announcements, television educational programs, publications on various facets of child health including nutrition and nutrition-related diseases. Committee on Nutrition is involved in education and technical assistance in nutrition-related issues.
American Cancer Society (ACS) 777 3rd Ave. New York, N.Y. 10017	Nonprofit, voluntary health agency	To eliminate cancer, to prvent cancer and to save lives of cancer victims, and enhance the quality of life for those suffering from cancer.	Health education program stresses prevention, early diagnosis, and treatment. Stresses preventive habits, such as adequate and proper diet. Publishes wide variety of educational materials such as films, posters, displays, booklets, and pamphlets.
American Dental Association (ADA) 211 E. Chicago Ave. Chicago, Ill. 60611	Professional membership	To encourage improved public health and promote dentistry.	Dental health education program including teaching materials. Development of materials and programs for public awareness campaigns about dental health. Training for professionals and educators. Wide variety of education materials cover various health topics, including nutrition.

Organization	Type	Purpose	Programs and Activities
American Diabetes Association (ADA) 600 Fifth Ave. New York, N.Y. 10020	Nonprofit, voluntary	To develop educational materials to promote better understanding of diabetes for the public, patients, and professionals. To promote research related to diabetes mellitus.	Wide variety of educational materials for the professional and the public. Publishes *Diabetes Forecast*, bimonthly magazine; programmed instruction, cookbook, and exchange lists for diabetic meal planning. Provides speakers, public detection programs, and technical assistance and training for professionals and laymen. Sponsors research into causes, prevention, and treatment of diabetes.
American Dietetic Association (ADA) 430 North Michigan Ave. Chicago, Ill. 60611	Educational and professional membership	To advance the science and art of dietetics. To improve nutritional status of mankind and improve nutrition education and public awareness of good nutrition.	Programs include annual national nutrition week, speakers bureaus, technical assistance, and a number of materials for public and professional use. Monthly *Journal of the American Dietetic Association*. Maintains Washington staff to keep abreast of national nutrition-related activities. Participates in legislative process and inform members of current events and developments.
American Heart Association (AHA) 7320 Greenville Ave. Dallas, Tex. 75231	Nonprofit, voluntary	To reduce premature death and disability from cardiovascular diseases. To sponsor research, education, and community service programs aimed at the prevention and treatment of heart disease.	Provides public awareness and information through national media, printed literature, and publications. Local chapters address specific local needs; examples of local chapter activities include dietary counseling, screening, and modification of risk factors related to coronary heart disease, and speakers bureau. Training programs for health education of the young, training in cardiopulmonary resuscitation (CPR), and emergency cardiac care. Materials, including publications and audiovisuals, cover topics including nutrition, diet, and heart disease. Publications include monthly: *Circulation, Circulation Research, Modern Concepts of Cardiovascular Disease*; bimonthly: *Stroke — Journal of Cerebral Circulation*; quarterly: *American Heart and Heart Research Newsletter*.

Agency/Address	Type of Organization	Primary Objectives of Organization	Key Activities
American Home Economics Association (AHEA) 2010 Massachusetts Ave., N.W. Washington, D.C. 20036	Professional and educational	To improve individual and family quality of life.	Programs include family management, economics, child care, nutrition, and consumer education. Publishes a monthly *Journal of Home Economics*, a quarterly *Home Economics Research Journal*, and an *AHEA Action* newspaper. Publishes The *Home Economics Research Abstracts*, which summarizes master's theses and doctoral dissertations related to home economics.
American Hospital Association (AHA) 840 North Lake Shore Dr. Chicago, Ill. 60611	Nonprofit, membership	To promote general welfare and to assist health care providers in improving health care.	Engaged in training hospital personnel and others to develop health education programs. Materials include printed literature and audiovisuals; a film library is maintained and provides materials to members.
American Institute of Baking 400 E. Ontario St. Chicago, Ill. 60611	Nonprofit, industry sponsored	To advance public welfare through research, education and promotion of food, and nutrition: special emphasis on baked products	Provides placement service and maintains library. Conducts basic research and educational projects; publications include bimonthly *Institute's News, Library Quarterly Index,* and research bulletins.
American Institute of Nutrition 9650 Rockville Pike Bethesda, Md. 20014	Professional membership	To advance scientific nutrition knowledge and to facilitate personal contact between professionals in nutrition and related fields.	Sponsors and conducts nutrition research. Publishes research. Publishes *American Journal of Clinical Nutrition* and the *Journal of Nutrition*.
American Medical Association (AMA) 535 North Dearborn St. Chicago, Ill. 60610	Professional membership	To enable individuals to understand and appreciate the relationship between health behavior and their health status.	Provides the public with health information through the media, public service announcements, and publications; nutrition is an important topic of concern, as are nutrition-related diseases such as diabetes and atherosclerosis. Workshops, lectures, and meetings are sponsored for public and professional education. Acts as a clearinghouse for a vast amount of health-related topics. Provides technical assistance and a wide variety of materials on various health topics; included topics are nutrition, education, cancer, alcohol, child care, ecology, fitness sports, and kidney disease.

Organization	Membership	Purpose	Programs/Activities
American Nurse's Association (ANA) 2420 Pershing Rd. Kansas City, Mo. 64108	Professional membership	To foster nursing practice legislation, implement standards of nursing research, and encourage the development of advanced and continuing education programs.	Programs in community health, geriatrics, maternal and child health, nutrition, and other public health areas. Sponsors national conferences and congresses. Represents nursing profession in federal and legislative areas, and implements ethical standards and quality assurance standards.
American Osteopathic Association (AOA) 212 East Ohio St. Chicago, Ill. 60611	Professional membership	To promote public health, stimulate scientific research, and maintain high standards of medication education for the osteopathic profession.	Provides training and materials on such topics as prenatal care, nutrition, and cancer. Conducts an annual campaign to increase public awareness of the problems inherent in hypertension.
American Public Health Association (APHA) 1015 18th St., N.W. Washington, D.C. 20036	Professional membership	To protect and promote public, personal, and environmental health.	Engages in community health education projects, develops guidelines and models for health education programs, and sponsors the Prevention Practitioner Project to stimulate awareness for the health practitioner and to promote positive health and prevention. Publishes the *Nation's Health*, a monthly *American Journal of Public Health*, and newsletters for members of the 23 special interest sections, one of which is foods and nutrition. Involved in developing guidelines and standards for nutritional assessment of the community and of individuals. Involved in health-related research.
American School Food Service Association (ASFSA) 4101 E. Iliff Ave. Denver, Col. 80222	Membership composed of those involved in school food programs	To improve quality of school food service.	Publications include *The School Food-service Journal*, *ASFS Action*, and film catalog. Sponsors National School Lunch Week. Sponsors workshops and other formal and informal education programs on nutrition.
American School Health Association (ASHA) 7263 SR 43 ASHA Building Kent, Ohio 44240	Professional membership	To promote comprehensive and constructive school health programs, health services, and education and environment. To establish guidelines for school health education and to cooperate with local, state, and national organizations. To advance improvement of school health education.	Programs include an annual convention, publications, the publication of a directory of National Organizations concerned with School Health, and teaching guides and position papers on school health education issues; publication of reports on current status of various school health programs.

Agency/Address	Type of Organization	Primary Objectives of Organization	Key Activities
Center for Science in the Public Interest CSPI) 1755 S. St., N.W. Washington, D.C. 20009	Private public interest and consumer protection	To help science to be responsive to human problems and needs. To provide the public with reliable information about food, the food industry, and government food regulations. Its goal is to improve the quality of the American diet through research and education at the national and local levels.	Provides technical assistance and training for activities aimed to improve public awareness on a number of health-related topics; serves as a clearinghouse for requests for such information. Publishes variety of reports on subjects including nutrition and a popular publication, *Nutrition Scoreboard: Your Guide to Better Eating*, which rates the nutritional value of about 200 various foodstuffs. Publishes *Nutrition Action*, monthly publication. Organizes and publicizes annual "Food Day" to increase public nutrition awareness.
Cereal Institute 135 S. LaSalle St. Chicago, Ill. 60603	Nonprofit, industry sponsored	To increase public awareness of importance of good nutrition and the role of cereal products in diet.	Conducts nutrition-oriented research and education projects on the role of cereals in human diet. Provides filmstrips, literature, teaching aids on nutrition, and consumer education.
Children's Foundation (CF) 1420 New York Ave., N.W. Room 800 Washington, D.C. 20005	Nonprofit, public interest and advocacy	To assist low-income poor to be better able to use food assistance programs.	Provides technical assistance to community groups desiring to organize activities around federal food and nutrition programs, in particular the USDA school lunch and breakfast programs, Head Start, WIC, and Food Stamp Program.
Community Nutrition Institute (CNI) 1146 19th Street, N.W. Washington, D.C. 20006	Private, nonprofit	To develop effective and successful nutrition services at the community level; special target groups are the poor and minority groups.	Major activity is to publish the *CNI Weekly Report* on nutrition policy, programs, and developments. Publishes other materials on food stamp outreach, volunteer activities, and community worker education. Contracts in states provide training workshops for community organization, outreach, planning, and education efforts. Provides nutrition and technical assistance to individuals, groups and programs.
Concern, Inc. 2233 Wisconsin Ave., N.W. Washington, D.C. 2007	Nonprofit, tax-exempt	To develop public awareness of environmental issues and recommend appropriate citizen action.	Studies on energy conservation, drinking water, food additives, and toxic substances; findings are published in environmental guides, called Eco-Tips. Arranges conferences, provides advisory and consulting services, testifies before Congress, and appears on radio and television programs.

Organization	Type	Purpose	Activities
Consumer Federation of America (CFA) 1012 14th St., N.W. Suite 901 Washington, D.C. 20005	Network of national, state, regional, and community organizations involved in protecting the rights of consumers through education and legislation	To promote rights of consumers.	Provides assistance and direct consultation to those involved in community consumer-related issues. Publications include material on advertising, food, drugs, and organizing for consumer action.
Consumers Union (CU) 256 Washington St. Mount Vernon, N.Y. 10550	Nonprofit	To provide consumers with education and information on consumer goods and services. To provide assistance on family-income related matters. To cooperate with efforts designed to improve standard of living.	Publishes monthly *Consumer Reports* that contains buying information; also publishes buying guides and a book, *The Medicine Show*, a practical guide to common health problems.
Food Research and Action Center (FRAC) 2011 I St., N.W. Washington, D.C. 20006	Private, nonprofit public interest law firm and advocacy center	To end hunger and malnutrition in the United States. To influence federal policies toward the expansion and improvement of effective nutrition programs to aid the poor.	Provides legal aid, organizing assistance, training, and information to the poor and their groups working to improve federal food programs. Publishes pamphlets, booklets, guides, and newsletters on current developments concerning nutrition issues and programs.
Health Research Group 2000 P St., N.W. Suite 708 Washington, D.C. 20036	Action group supported by Public Citizen.	To influence legislation, make government more responsive to public needs, and make public and private organizations more accessible and responsive to public needs.	Efforts include research, education, community organization, litigation, and advocacy to advance public interest concerns; activities include consumer health care delivery, food and nutrition, and product safety.
La Leche League International, Inc. (LLLI) 9616 Minneapolis Ave. Franklin Park, Ill. 60131	Nonprofit, voluntary service	To provide information and encouragement through personal contact with mothers who desire to nurse their infants.	Sponsors local meetings, provides speakers. Publishes a variety of pamphlets and books for public and professional use; nutritional concerns of the infant and the mother are prominent topics of focus.
Maternity Center Association (MCA) 48 East 92nd St. New York, N.Y. 10028	Nonprofit, voluntary	To assure high standards of health care for mothers and infants.	Maintains Childbearing Center for families desiring normal, natural childbirth. Sponsors childbearing classes that include nutrition education. Provides technical assistance and training for universities, hospitals, and health-related groups. Conducts workshops on expectant parent education. Distributes a variety of educational materials on topics including nutrition.

Agency/Address	Type of Organization	Primary Objectives of Organization	Key Activities
National Child Nutrition Project 303 George St. New Brunswick, N.J. 08901	Nonprofit, voluntary	To improve nutritional well-being of American children.	Works with individuals, state, and local groups to improve delivery of nutrition services. Initiates *Hunger Task Forces* to extend food assistance benefits to those in need. Education and training programs, provision of technical assistance. Supports food stamp outreach campaigns. Provides speakers, workshops, television spots, and other public awareness resources. Publishes *Food Action* a bimonthly journal of New Jersey food program descriptions.
National Dairy Council 111 North Canal St. Chicago, Ill. 60606	Nonprofit research and educational organization supported by the dairy industry	To promote optimum health and welfare through the use of milk products in accord with scientific recommendations and ultimately to contribute to American agriculture and national welfare.	Wide variety of educational resources including films, pamphlets, brochures, posters, slides, and other materials. Development of nutrition education curriculum for use in schools. Public service information bulletins, media spots. Sponsors research on dairy foods. Publishes *Dairy Council Digest*.
National Foundation — March of Dimes (NFMOD) 1275 Mamaroneck Ave. White Plains, N.Y. 10605	Nonprofit, voluntary	To prevent birth defects and to improve the outcome of pregnancy.	The national office focuses on genetic, personal, and environmental conditions affecting the outcome of pregnancy; subjects of particular interest include proper nutrition, prenatal care, and sound health habits. Provides health education materials for the public and for professionals. Nutrition projects and programs are carried out with the aim of improving public and professional education. Conferences, institutes, and a number of youth programs are made available. Publishes materials for public and professional education. Provides speakers bureau for nutrition topics. Supports relevant research on the effects of proper nutrition and pregnancy outcome.

Organization	Membership	Purpose	Activities
National Livestock and Meat Board (NLSMB) 444 N. Michigan Ave. Chicago, Ill. 60611	Livestock and meat industry representatives	To promote health through the use of meat and livestock products. To serve as the service organization for the livestock and meat industry.	Conducts extension programs of promotion, education, and information about meat products. Sponsors research on meat products and their relation to health. Sponsors projects such as recipe testing and development, food demonstrations, food photography, educational offerings for colleges, experimental meat-cutting methods, and preparation of educational materials for dissemination in the mass media.
National Nutrition Consortium, Inc. 2121 P St., N.W. Washington, D.C. 20037	Composed of numerous professional societies: American Dietetic Association, American Institute of Nutrition, American Society for Clinical Nutrition, Institute of Food Technologists, Society for Nutrition Education, American Academy of Pediatrics, Food and Nutrition Board, and American Home Economics Association	To provide leadership in the development and coordination of food nutrition policies. To aid in providing the American public with sound nutrition information. To provide coordination and communication among member organizations.	Works to provide government and the public with accurate nutrition information. Developed national nutrition policy. Publications include material on nutrition labeling and interpretations of complicated nutrition information for public understanding.
National Retired Teachers Association/American Association of Retired Persons (NRTA/AARP) 1909 K St., N.W. Washing, D.C. 20049	Nonprofit membership organization	To help older individuals to improve the quality of life.	Programs include health education on such topics as foods, facts, and frauds; diet, nutrition, and health; and health quackery.
Nutrition Today Society 101 Ridgely Ave. P.O. Box 773 Annapolis, Md. 21404	Professional, nonprofit	To increase public awareness of new developments in nutrition. To increase nutritional knowledge of all professionals engaged in nutrition-related concerns.	Produces audiovisual learning materials and other nutrition resources. Publishes *Nutrition Today*.
Society for Nutrition Education (SNE) 2140 Shattuck Ave. Berkeley, Calif. 94704	Professional membership	To promote good nutrition for the public by making sound nutrition education more available and effective. To improve the effectiveness of nutrition education, communication, and research.	Provides technical assistance and consultation for interested groups. Maintains the National Nutrition Education Clearing House (NNECH) to serve as a source of published nutrition education materials and information relevant to sound nutrition education. Develops extensive bibliographies with evaluated annotations of content. Publishes *Journal of Nutrition Education*. Makes available Nutrition Education Resource Series of reference lists on subjects such as nutrition and aging, food additives, and the like.

Agency/Address	Type of Organization	Primary Objectives of Organization	Key Activities
			Publishes monographs in the area of curriculum guide evaluations and mass media. Committees are involved in legislation, liaison with industry, and local groups.
Society for Public Health Education, Inc. (SOPHE) 655 Sutter St. San Francisco, Calif. 94102	Professional membership.	To promote and advance public health through methods of improved public health education.	Provides technical assistance to community health education programs. Publishes *Health Education Monographs.*
SOURCE, Inc. P.O. Box 21066 Washington, D.C. 20009	Group of six people who do research and publish for community organizers.	To provide a resource agency for those involved in community organizations.	Activities include the publication of catalogs that serve as working tools for those attempting to improve health care. A recent catalog, *Source III: Organizing for Health Care,* describes models of groups who have organized around issues including nutrition, health, and environmental health. The catalog also lists films, tapes, periodicals, pamphlets, and books of use to community organizers.

672

Appendix V ABBREVIATIONS

Abbreviations

AA		Alcoholics Anonymous
AAP		American Academy of Pediatrics
ACS		American Cancer Society
ADA		American Dietetic Association
	or	American Dental Association
	or	American Diabetic Association
ADAMHA		Alcohol, Drug Abuse, and Mental Health Administration (DHHS)
AFDC		Aid to Families with Dependent Children
AHA		American Hospital Association
	or	American Heart Association
AHEA		American Home Economics Association
AHP		Appalachian Health Program (USDHHS)
AIB		American Institute of Baking
AID		Agency for International Development
AIN		American Institute of Nutrition
AMA		American Medical Association
AMS		Agricultural Marketing Service (USDA)
AOA		Administration on Aging (USDHHS)
AOCYF		Administration on Children, Youth, and Families (USDHHS)
APA		Assistance Payments Administration (USDHHS)
APHA		American Public Health Association
ARC		American Red Cross
ARS		Agricultural Research Service (USDA) (replaced by Agricultural Research)
ASCN		American Society of Clinical Nutrition
ASFSA		American School Food Service Association
ASTPHND		Association of State and Territorial Public Health Nutrition Directors
BATF		Bureau of Alcohol, Tobacco, and Firearms (Treasury)
BCHS		Bureau of Community Health Services (USDHHS)
BHI		Bureau of Health Insurance (USDHHS)
BMS		Bureau of Migrant Services (USDHHS)
BQA		Bureau of Quality Assurance (USDHHS)
CAA		Community Action Agency
C & Y		Children and Youth
CAP		Community Action Program
CBO		Congressional Budget Office
CC		Crippled Children's Services (USDHHS)
CCFP		Child Care Feeding Program
CDC		Community Development Corporation
	or	Center for Disease Control (USDHHS)
CF		Children's Foundation
CFA		Consumer Federation of America

CFNP		Community Food and Nutrition Program
CHAP		Child Health Assessment Program
CHC		Community Health Center
	or	Comprehensive Health Center
CIHP		Coalition of Independent Health Professions
CMHC		Comprehensive Mental Health Centers
CNI		Community Nutrition Institute
CPSC		Consumer Product Safety Commission (USDA)
CRIS		Current Research Information System (USDA)
CRS		Congressional Research Service
CSA		Community Services Administration
CSPI		Center for Science in the Public Interest
CU		Consumers Union
DHHS		Department of Health and Human Services
DISPAC		Domestic and International Scientific Planning, Analysis, and Cooperative Science and Technology Subcommittee (House of Representatives)
DOD		Department of Defense
ESCS		Economics, Statistics and Cooperative Services (USDA)
EFNEP		Expanded Food and Nutrition Education Program (USDA)
EMS		Emergency Medical Services
EPA		Environmental Protection Agency
EPR		Elimination of Purchase Requirement (Food Stamp Program)
EPSDT		Early Periodic Screening, Detection, and Treatment
ERDA		Energy Research and Development Administration
FAO		Food and Agriculture Organization (United Nations)
FCS		Farmer's Cooperative Service (USDA)
FDA		Food and Drug Administration
FHA		Farmer's Home Administration (USDA)
FHS		Family Health Service (USDHHS)
FIC		Federal Information Center
FICIN		Federal Intercommunications in Nutrition Group
FNIERC		Food and Nutrition Information and Education Resources Center (USDA)
FNB		Food and Nutrition Board (NAS–NRC)
FNS		Food and Nutrition Service (USDA)
FPP		Family Planning Program (USDHHS)
FRAC		Food Research and Action Center
FSQS		Food Safety and Quality Service (USDA)
FTC		Federal Trade Commission
GAO		General Accounting Office
HANES		Health and Nutrition Examination Survey
HCFA		Health Care Financing Administration (USDHHS)

HHS		Home Health Service (USDHHS)
HMO		Health Maintenance Organization (USDHHS)
HRA		Health Resources Administration (USDHHS)
HRF		Health Related Facility
HSA		Health Systems Agency
	or	Health Services Administration (USDHHS)
HURA		Health to Underserved Rural Areas (USDHHS)
ICC		Interstate Commerce Commission
ICF		Intermediate Care Facility
ICNND		Interdepartmental Committee on Nutrition and National Defense
IFT		Institute of Food Technologists
IHS		Indian Health Service
JCAH		Joint Commission on Accreditation of Hospitals
JNRPB		Joint Nutrition Research Planning Board (DOD)
LLLI		La Leché League International
LRC		Lipid Research Clinics (USDHHS)
MCH		Maternal and Child Health (USDHHS)
MCS		Marketing and Consumer Service (USDA)
	or	Medical Care Standards (USDHHS)
MCE		Medical Care Evaluation
MHP		Migrant Health Program (USDHHS)
MOW		Meals on Wheels
MRFIT		Multiple Risk Factor Intervention Trials (USDHHS)
MSA		Medical Services Administration (USDHHS)
NAL		National Agricultural Library (USDA)
NAS–NRC		National Academy of Sciences — National Research Council
NCHS		National Center for Health Statistics (USDHHS)
NCI		National Cancer Institute
NDC		National Dairy Council
NDRC		Nutrient Data Research Center
NFCS		National Food Consumption Survey (USDA)
NFMOD		National Foundation, March of Dimes
NHLBI		National Heart, Lung, and Blood Institute (USDHHS)
NHSC		National Health Service Corporation (USDHHS)
NIAAA		National Institute on Alcohol Abuse and Alcoholism (USDHHS)
NIDA		National Institute on Drug Abuse (USDHHS)
NIE		National Institute of Education (USDHHS)
NIH		National Institutes of Health (USDHHS)
NIMH		National Institute of Mental Health (USDHHS)
NLSMB		National Livestock and Meat Board
NMRP		National Migrant Referral Project (USDHHS)
NNC		National Nutrition Consortium, Inc.

NNDB	National Nutrient Data Bank (USDA)
NSF	National Science Foundation
NSMS	Nutritional Status Monitoring System
OCA	Office of Consumer Affairs
OCD	Office of Child Development (USDHHS)
OE	Office of Education
OEO	Office of Economic Opportunity
OHD	Office of Human Development (USDHHS)
OHIHP	Office of Health Information and Health Promotion (USDHHS) (this title is now changed to the Office of Health Information, Health Promotion and Physical Fitness and Sports Medicine.)
OLTCSE	Office of Long-term Care Standards Enforcement
OMB	Office of Management and Budget
ONAP	Office of Native American Programs (USDHHS)
ORD	Office of Rural Development (USDHHS)
OSFS	Office of School Food Service
OSTP	(White House) Office of Science and Technology Policy
OTA	Office of Technology Assessment
OYD	Office of Youth Development (USDHHS)
PCM	Protein Calorie Malnutrition
PEP	Performance Evaluation Procedure
PHS	Public Health Service (USDHHS)
POMR	Problem Oriented Medical Record
PSRO	Professional Standards Review Organization
QAP	Quality Assurance Program
R & D	Research and Development
RDA	Recommended Dietary Allowances
RHI	Rural Health Initiative
RDS	Rural Development Service (USDA)
RPA	Research Problem Areas
RSA	Rehabilitation Service Administration (USDHHS)
SA	State Health Planning and Development Agency
SBP	School Breakfast Program
SCOR	Specialized Centers for Research
SAES	State Agricultural Experiment Stations (USDA)
SEA	Science and Education Administration (USDA)
SFP	Summer Feeding Program
SIDS	Sudden Infant Death Syndrome
SLP	School Lunch Program
SNE	Society for Nutrition Education
SNF	Skilled Nursing Facility
SRS	Social and Rehabilitation Services (USDHHS)
SSA	Social Security Administration (USDHHS)

UR	Utilization Review
USAMRNL	U.S. Army Medical Research and Nutrition Laboratory (DOD)
USC	U.S. Congress
USDA	U.S. Department of Agriculture
USRDA	U.S. Recommended Dietary Allowances
VA	Veterans Administration
WHO	World Health Organization
WIC	Women, Infants, and Children (USDA)
WIN	Work Incentive Program (DOL)

Glossary

Absolute Poverty — Type of economic poverty characterized by a quality of life so deprived that basic needs are left unfulfilled.

Acquired Pellicle — Initial process in development of dental decay — a protein film, derived from glycoproteins in saliva, that is adsorbed onto the surface of tooth enamel.

Allowances — A general term for the daily amounts of food or nutrients recommended per person (Allowances are usually expressed in practical terms with a margin of safety about physiologically determined requirements. They may be stated in terms of quantities of food, specific foods, or allowances for specific nutrients such as the recommendations of the Food and Nutrition Board of the National Research Council of the National Academy of Sciences).*

Ambulatory Care Center — An organization providing health care services to meet the needs of noninstitutionalized or nonhousebound clients.

Amino Acids, Limiting — The essential amino acid of a protein that shows the greatest percentage deficit relative to the amino acids contained in the same quantity of a standard protein.*

Amino Acid Reference Pattern — A theoretical and ideal combination of amino acids in proportion and amount to meet known physiological requirements; designed to serve as basis for determination of minimum nitrogen and amino acid requirements.*

Amino Acid Sequences — The order or sequence of amino acids in the chains of a specific protein.*

Amino Acids, Essential — Those amino acids that cannot be synthesized by the animal organism, out of the materials ordinarily available, at a speed commensurate with the demands for normal growth; they must be provided preformed in the diet.*

Anthropometric Assessment — Evaluation of physical aspects and gross composition of body at varying age levels and degrees of health and nutrition.

Assay — Determination of the quantity, relative to some standard of reference, of a nutrient present in a foodstuff or biological material.*

Atherogenic Diets — Diets designed to produce atheromas in the arteries of a given species.*

At-risk Concept — A major, identifiable biological or environmental circumstance that increases the risk of severe illness, especially malnutrition, and thus suggests the need for prevention and special intervention measures.

Availability (physiological) — The extent to which a nutrient is present in a form that can be absorbed and utilized in metabolic processes. (Some

Entries marked with * adapted from E. N. Todhunter. *A Guide to Nutrition Terminology for Indexing and Retrieval*, USDHEW/PHS/NIH publ. Supt. of Documents, Washington, D.C.: Government Printing Office, July 1970.
Entries marked with † adapted from R. Frankle, and A. Yanochik-Owen. *Nutrition in the Community: The Art of Delivering Services*. St. Louis, Mo.: C. V. Mosby, 1978.

nutrients may be bound to a compound, be insoluble, or combine in the intestinal tract with some other compound to form an insoluble substance, so that they cannot be absorbed and hence are not available for nutritional processes).*

Balance (Metabolic) — The comparison of the intake and excretion of a specific nutrient; the "balance" may be negative (excess of excretion), or positive (retention in the body), or in equilibrium.

Biotin — The designated term for the compound also known as "coenzyme II."*

Blood Volume — The total number of liters of whole blood in the body.*

Body Balance Method — A nonrespiratory method for the determination of heat production and overall accumulation of substances in small animals maintained in metabolism cages for several weeks. Analysis of total food intake, excreta, and carcass for nitrogen and other elements and calorie value by bomb calorimeter determination are the basis of computation.

Body Cell Mass — The totality of cellular components of skeletal, cardiac, and smooth muscles, the parenchymatous viscera, the intestinal tract, blood, glands of the body, and cellular components of the brain. It is a basic reference entity used for the consideration of energy conversion of foodstuffs, oxygen requirement, carbon dioxide production, or work performance.

Calcium — A metallic divalent element that is a major mineral constituent of the body, making up approximately 1.5-2.0 per cent of the body weight of the mature human; 99 per cent of body calcium is present in bones and teeth.*

Calculated Nutrient Content — The nutrient content of a diet or a food recipe calculated from food composition tables; it is not determined directly by analysis of that specific food, or dietary composite.*

Caloric Excess — Intakes of calories in excess of calories required for growth and metabolic processes, or for adult maintenance of desirable weight for age.*

Cariostatic Foods — Foods exerting protective effects on the teeth.

Child Care Food Program — Federal program providing financial support to organized licensed child care programs to aid them in improving the nutritional status of children up the age of 19 years.

Child Health Assessment Program (CHAP) — *See* Early Periodic Screening, Detection, and Treatment.

Choline — An essential dietary constituent for the guinea pig and fowl and, under usual experimental conditions, for the growing rat, mouse, pig, dog, cat, and rabbit; choline deficiency has not been demonstrated in man, and whether or not it is an essential dietary nutrient for man is unknown.*

Community Assessment — Broad, general evaluation of food and nutritional status of a given community; it entails reliance on existing sources of information, such as hospital records, statistics, and the like.

Community Nutrition — Aspect of nutritional science that deals with the assessment of public health problems and strategies to solve public health, nutrition-related problems.

Consumption Units — Units expressing the amount of food, types of food, or of nutrients present in foods consumed per person or per household, or in terms of money spent, or some other selected basis.*

Convenience Foods — Foods in which one or more steps in preparation have been completed before the product is offered for retail sale, for example, semiprepared foods, such as frozen vegetables and mixes, or finished foods such as ready-to-eat, ready-to-bake, or heat-and-serve foods.*

Critical Periods — Time periods in which an individual is especially vulnerable to a particular condition.

Cross-sectional Data — Data collected over a short time period describing given parameters in groups of various ages.*

Crude Fiber — The residue of plant food that remains after sequential extraction with solvent, dilute acid, and alkali.

Cyanocobalamin — The designated form to use for the compound α- (5, 6-dimethylbenzimidazolyl) cobamine cyanide; also known as vitamin B_{12} or cyanocobalamine.*

Decennial — Occurring every ten years, as *decennial census.**

Deficiency Diseases — Disorders or disease conditions with characteristic clinical signs caused by a dietary deficiency of nutrients. They can be cured or prevented by supplying the nutrients that are lacking.*

Demographic Data — Quantitative data on characteristics of human populations such as size, growth, density, distribution, and vital statistics.*

Demonstration Area — An area or region selected for the purpose of demonstrating methods (such as agricultural food production or food processing) or the effectiveness of following some procedure such as a particular nutrition program.*

Dental Caries — Cavities produced by certain microorganisms that live on the teeth and produce acids from ingested sugar and starches.

Dental Plaque — White, gray, or yellow gelatinous adherent material that covers the teeth as a result of contact with food and neglect of oral hygiene habits.

Determinants of Change — Factors that can be identified by study and research as responsible for change in the attitudes, beliefs, or behavior of individuals or groups, especially relative to the acceptance of new food products and new methods for food preparation.*

Deviance — Behavior that differs from the normal or average accepted for a specific age or cultural group.*

Dietary Assessment — Evaluation of food intake of an individual or of a group of individuals.

Dietary Counseling — Providing individualized professional guidance to aid an individual in adjusting the diet to meet health needs; it entails interviewing, counseling, and consulting.

Dietary Fiber — Material in foods that includes undigested storage polysaccharides present within cellular contents, as well as undigested poly-saccharides and lignin present in the cell wall.

Dietary History — A detailed account of the kind, estimated amount, and preparation methods of the usual daily food intake and variations for an individual, obtained in interview by a professional worker.*

Dietary Survey — Assessment of the dietary (food) intake of a group of individuals. It is used to determine the adequacy or inadequacy of diets, or to collect information about food habits and dietary patterns, and factors influencing them. Methodology may include estimation by recall, food record, dietary history, or weighed intake of food consumed.

Dietetics — A profession concerned with the science and art of human nutritional care, an essential component of health science. It includes the extending and imparting of knowledge concerning foods that will provide nutrients sufficient to health and during disease throughout the life cycle, and the management of group feeding (American Dietetic Association).

Digestibility — The extent to which the nutrients present in food are chemically changed within the digestive tract and absorbed into the body system.*

DMF Index — The total number of decayed, missing, and filled teeth; sometimes used in nutritional status surveys.*

Early Periodic Screening, Detection, and Treatment Program (EPSDT) — Sometimes referred to as Child Health Assessment Program (CHAP), under an amendment to the Social Security Act, it is designed to make comprehensive health services available to Medicaid-eligible individuals under the age of 21 years.

"Empty Calorie" Food — A term used to refer to snack-type foods and beverages that in large measure provide only "empty calories," for example, fat and carbohydrate but little or no protein, minerals, vitamins, or other micronutrients.*

Enrichment — Addition of nutrients to foods to replace those nutrients lost in processing.

Epidemiological Triad — A triad of factors considered to be responsible for the development of disease conditions.

> **Agent** — the immediate cause of the disease.
>
> **Host** — factors related to the individual, such as previous and present nutritional status.
>
> **Environment** — other factors such as the availability of food.

Estimated Intake — Food intake estimated by the individual or by the observer, usually in terms of household measures rather than by weight or extract measurement.*

Expanded Food and Nutrition Education Program (EFNEP) — Federal program designed to aid low-income families to learn skills needed to achieve adequate dietary intakes.

Experimental Diets — Diets of known composition (preferably by direct analysis) fed to animals or humans during experimental periods.*

External Poverty — Generally a transitory type of poverty, as for example, that occurring when a middle-class family head temporarily loses a job.

Family Composition — The number of persons in the household or family group, including the age, sex and kinship of the group.*

Family Eating Patterns — Food habits of the family, such as the order of serving food to family members, who eats with the men of the family, and when and with whom the children and women eat.*

Family Food Distribution — How food is given and consumed within the family, particularly what kind and amount of food is given the father or men in the family and what foods are given to the women and children.*

Fetal Alcohol Syndrome — The typical pattern resulting from excessive alcohol intake by a pregnant woman; it is characterized by a delay in development and in psychomotor responses, growth retardation, retarded intellectual performance, and abnormalities in various physiological systems of the newborn.

Fluoridation — Addition of fluoride to food or drink, such as fluoridation of water.

Fluorine — A chemical and a nutrient important for development of bones and teeth.

Fluorosis — Mottling of enamel resulting from excessive fluoride intake.

Folacin — The generic descriptor used for folic acid and related compounds exhibiting qualitatively the biological activity of folic acid.*

Folic Acid — The designated term used for the compound monopteroylglutamic acid.*

Food Additives — Substances other than a basic foodstuff, which are present in a food as a result of any aspect of production, processing, storage, or packaging. The term does not include chance contaminants.*

Food Balance Sheets — Annual total national food production and imports minus exports gives the food supply available for the year; divided by the population number, gives the food available per person for consumption.*

Food Checklist — A list of foods that an individual may be requested to check in some way, for those foods he or she usually or regularly eats; may also be used to determine likes and dislikes or other specific reactions to a given list of foods.*

Food and Nutrition Board (NAS/NRC) — This board, established in 1940 under the Division of Biology and Agriculture of the National Academy of Sciences/National Research Council, serves as an advisory body in the field of food and preparation. A well-known activity of the Food and Nutrition Board is the preparation of Recommended Dietary Allowances (RDAs), which are revised periodically.*

Food Exchanges — Foods grouped according to similarities in composition so that foods within a group may be used interchangeably in diet planning. (Exchange lists, prepared jointly by the American Diabetes Association and the American Dietetic Association, are used by diabetics as a guide to their food selection. Similar food exchange lists have been prepared for reducing diets and other therapeutic diet plans).*

Food Patterns — The types of foods customarily used by people in a given area, region, or ethnicity, and the way those foods are prepared and served.*

Food Record — A listing of foods eaten for a specific length of time.

Food Restrictions — Foods to be avoided or limited for cultural or clinical reasons. For example, for children and for women in pregnancy and other conditions, there may be cultural restrictions on the kind of foods that may be eaten; this differs with different cultures.*

Food Stamp Program — Federal program designed to provide adequate level of nutrition to low-income households. Food stamps or food coupons issued through the USDA are used to purchase food.

Formula Diets — Liquid preparations with a balanced composition of nutrients. (Early examples were infant formulas. Formulas in dry form are available for reconstitution for use of adults on special diets. These diets are used in tube feedings or orally in research studies in which constant composition is necessary).*

Fortification Agents — Nutrients such as minerals, vitamins, and amino acids added to foods to increase the specific nutrient content.*

Frequency of Eating — Number of times a day an individual consumes food or nutrient-containing beverages.*

Grant — Award of financial or direct support under programs providing for such assistance on the basis of the review and approval of an application outlining proposed need for assistance, objectives, and methods for use and support.†

Head Start — Program designed to aid the disadvantage preschool children from low-income areas reach their growth and physical and mental potential before entering school. Nutrition is an integral component of the project.

Health — A state of complete physical, mental, and social well-being and not merely the absence of disease or infirmity (World Health Organization).

Health and Nutrition Examination Survey (HANES) — Nutritional status survey conducted by the National Center for Health Statistics (USDHEW) of the U.S. population to determine nutritional status.

Health Care — Provision of services to maintain health; its focus is on environment, nutrition, and the like.

Health Care Evaluation — Program designed to measure the quality of health care provided by an institution; it is concerned with two dimensions of quality.†

> **Health care (medical) audit** — a retrospective evaluation of the application of health care as indicated by a review of medical records.

> **Utilization review** — study of efficiency of care based on appropriateness of admissions to an institution, ordered and provided services, length of stay, and discharge plans.

Health Care Team — A group of health care professionals who provide coordinated services to achieve optimal health care of the client.†

Health Field Concept — Broad approach to health developed by the National Health and Welfare Department of Canada; it suggests that matters related to health can be divided into four principal elements; human biology, environment, life-style, and health care organization.

> **Human biology** — aspects of health developed within the human body as a result of the basic biology of man and the organic makeup of the individual.
>
> **Environment** — those matters related to health that are external to the human body and over which the individual has little control.
>
> **Life-style** — the decisions made by individuals that affect their health and over which they have no control.
>
> **Health care organization** — the quantity, quality, arrangement, nature, and relationships of people and resources in the provision of health care.

Health Maintenance — Preventive, diagnostic, curative, and restorative health services available to a client, group, or community.†

Health Maintenance Organization (HMO) — An organization that integrates the provider elements necessary to deliver a comprehensive range of services for organized health care.

Health Promotion and Disease Prevention Act (P.L. 94–317) — Established an office for the coordination of all health education and health promotion efforts nationwide. It provides authority for activities of health promotion and health prevention (June 1976).

Health Promotion Organizations (HPO) — Proposed voluntary, community-based organizations that would reward healthy life-styles and provide incentives for the promotion of health by supporting a close collaborative relationship among government, private industry, labor, the health care system, the community, and individuals.

Health Systems Agency (HSA) — The governing body for each health service area provided for under the National Health Planning and Resources Development Act (P.L. 93–641) of 1974. Responsible for planning and developing health services, manpower, and facilities and for preventing inefficiencies in the delivery of health care.

Hyperplasia — Increased number of cells.

Hypertrophy — Increased size of cells.

Incidence — Number of new cases of a disease or condition occurring during a specified period of time and for a specified population.*

Infant — Age period of 29 days through 12 months.*

Infant Feeding Practices — Methods of feeding (breast or bottle), the kind and amount of supplements given, weaning age, method and kind of foods given at weaning, and similar information.*

Internal Poverty — Represents the culture of poverty into which an individual is born and is rarely able to escape; it is characterized by lack of power, helplessness, lack of self-worth, inability to provide for needs of self and family, and disregard for traditional values of middle and upper class.

Iodine — A nonmetallic chemical that is part of thyroid hormones and is an essential nutrient for man.*

Iron — A nutrient and metallic element occurring in the hemoglobin of red blood cells, stored in tissues in the form of ferritin; it is an essential part of important respiratory enzymes.*

Kwashiorkor — A severe clinical condition occurring most frequently in children 1 to 3 years of age resulting from a deficiency of protein (and other nutrients) in the face of a relative excess of calories; it is characterized by growth failure, edema, and muscle wasting. It is usually preceded by or associated with infection (e.g., diarrhea, respiratory infection, measles, and the like). Frequently associated symptoms include dyspigmentation and easy pluckability of the hair, liver enlargement, dermatosis, and mental apathy, some or all of which may be present.*

Lean Body Mass —Totality of the skeleton, tendon, fascia, collagen, elastin, dermis components of the body, and the structural lipids.*

Legumes — Edible seeds of leguminous plants (e.g., beans, peas, peanuts, and soybeans) used primarily for human consumption.*

Life-style — An individual's mode of living as affected by physiologic, psychosocial, environmental, economic, and religious influences.†

Longitudinal Studies — Continuous or repeated experimental observations and measurements carried on for a number of years with the same group of human subjects or through one or more generations of animals.*

Magnesium — A mineral element important as a constituent of soft tissue and bone; this trace mineral is an enzyme activator. The adult human body contains approximately 20–25 gm of magnesium; about one half is located in the skeleton.*

Malformation — A deformity of a given body part or parts.*

Malnutrition — A state of poor health with symptoms clinically identified as the result of inadequate intake of one or more essential nutrients over a sustained period.*

Marasmus — A condition occurring most frequently in infants (3–18 months) as a result of gross deficiency of calories, protein, and other nutrients over a period of time; it is frequently accompanied by diarrhea. Characteristics of marasmus are low body weight, loss of subcutaneous fat, and wasting of muscle tissue (some cases of marasmus show edema and are best described as kwashiorkor rather than marasmic kwashiorkor).*

Meal Patterns — Pattern of the types and amounts of food eaten at the various meals of the day.*

Meals on Wheels — Federal program providing nutritionally adequate meals for the elderly, handicapped, or convalescent homebound.

Medicaid — Federal program providing for payment of medical care services to recipients of categorical public assistance.

Medical Care — The care provided under the control of the physician. It is usually crisis oriented and in response to illness or symptoms of a health disorder.

Medical Care Evaluation Studies — Retrospective health care evaluation involving detailed assessments of the quality or utilization of health care services.

Medicare — Provides federal health insurance to individuals over the age of 65.

National Health Planning and Resources Development Act (P.L. 93-641) of 1974 — Legislation designed to provide a national health planning system and to coordinate state health plans, health facilities expenditures, the development of new institutional health services, and the ongoing review of existing health services.

National Nutrition Survey (also called the Ten-State Survey) — USDHEW survey of malnutrition and related health problems in ten states (Kentucky, Louisiana, South Carolina, Texas, West Virginia, California, Massachusetts, Michigan, New York, and Washington).

National Poverty Line — The income level in cash or cash equivalent, determined as the amount below which poverty exists.*

National School Breakfast Program (SBP) — Federal program aimed at schools serving needy children, or children who must travel long distances and who come to school without adequate breakfasts. The program provides for breakfasts in accordance with USDA regulations.

National School Lunch Program (SLP) — Program of federal financial support to schools to enable students to receive a free, a reduced-price, or a paid nutritious meal at lunchtime.

Neonate — A baby during the period from birth through 28 days.*

Niacin — The generic descriptor for pyridine-3-carboxylic acid and derivatives exhibiting qualitatively the biological activity of nicotinic acid.*

Nicotinamide — The designated term used to refer to the compound known as niacinamide or nicotinic acid amide.*

Nonfood Assistance Program — Federal program providing financial support for eligible schools and child care institutions to allow them to acquire needed equipment for school food service.

Nursing Bottle Syndrome — Also referred to as the baby-bottle caries or bottle-mouth syndrome, it refers to enhanced caries development as a result of a child's taking a bottle of sugar-sweetened liquid at bedtime and falling asleep sucking.

Nutrient Toxicity — Toxicity due to an excessive intake of certain nutrients; for example, vitamin A and vitamin D, in excessive amounts, are toxic to man.*

Nutrients — Components of food: protein, fat, carbohydrate, minerals, vitamins, and water.*

Nutrition — Nutrition is the science of food, the nutrients, and other substances therein; their action, interaction, and balance in relation to health and disease; and the processes by which the organism ingests, digests, absorbs, transports, utilizes, and excretes food substances. In addition, nutrition must be concerned with social, economic, cultural, and psychologic implications of food and eating (Council on Foods and Nutrition, American Medical Association, 1963).

Nutrition Education — Planned use of any educational processes to modify food and nutrition behavior in pursuit of improved health.

Nutrition Policy — Framework for issues of concern to users of food.

Nutrition Program for the Elderly — Federal program providing a hot nutritious noontime meal to individuals over the age of 60 and their spouses, usually in congregate settings.

Nutrition Units — The recognized units of weight (gm, mg, μg) or other designations such as IU (international units) used to quantitatively record the various nutrients, also kcal, for the energy value of foods.*

Nutritional Care — The application of nutrition science to the health care of people, used in reference to individual or community care; it encompasses the following essential elements:

> **Assessment of nutritional status** — collecting information on the availability and acceptability of food, biochemical measurement of nutrients in body fluid or tissues, clinical and anthropometric measurements.
>
> Planning and implementing nutritional counseling and education to meet normal and therapeutic needs.
>
> **Referral** -- appropriating resources for aid in attaining optimal nutrition.
>
> Program planning, implementation, monitoring, and evaluation to determine the effectiveness of nutritional care and to modify care as appropriate.

Nutritional Status — The health condition of an individual as influenced by his or her intake and utilization of nutrients, determined from the correlation of information obtained from physical, biochemical, clinical, and dietary studies.*

Nutritional Status Assessment — Evaluation of nutritional status accomplished by the use of one or more of the following methods:

> **Dietary assessment** — to identify inadequate diet.
>
> **Medical and clinical examination** — to detect conditioning elements leading to poor nutritional status.
>
> **Biochemical tests** — to detect tissue, blood, or urine levels of nutrients.
>
> **Anthropometric tests** — to detect physical and anatomical changes resulting from faulty diets.

Nutritional Stress — Stress on the organism because of deficiency and/or imbalance of one or more nutrients and/or calories, or caloric or nutrient excess.*

Nutritional Survey — A study of the nutritional status of a community of individuals. A survey usually implies an assessment on a one-time basis.

Nutritional Surveillance — Ongoing monitoring of nutritional status. It implies continuity, a frequent and continuous "watching over."

Nutriture — The state of nutrition of an individual or animal relative to a specific nutrient, for example, calcium nutriture or riboflavin nutriture. Nutriture differs from nutritional status, which is a general term for the overall state of nutrition.*

Obesity — A body condition characterized by an excessive amount of stored fat.

Overweight — Weight in excess of the average for a given sex, age, and height in a given population. (Excessive weight may be the result of muscle tissue or related body fluid, not fat tissue. Thus, overweight may not be synonymous with obesity).

Pantothenic Acid — The designated term used for the compound also known as pantoyl-β-alanine.*

Patient Care Audit — Evaluation of health care using objective criteria developed by professionals with the aim of improving the quality of health care.

Peer Review — Formal evaluation of quality and efficiency of health care by health care practitioners.†

Per Capita Consumption — The amount of food or nutrients consumed per person in a given period.*

Periodontal Disease — The breakdown and decay of structures supporting the teeth.

Phosphorus — A nonmetallic chemical element that is a major inorganic component in bones, teeth, blood, and cells.*

Plate Waste — Uneaten food remaining on the subject's plate after a meal. (Weight, kind, and nutrient composition of plate waste should be determined in metabolic studies and at least estimated, or calculated, in food consumption studies.)*

Poverty — A situation in which the income level of an individual, family, or group is below the standard of living of the community either in terms of subsistence or in contrast to normal standards of income required for at least modest participation in community life.*

Poverty Line — Income level determined as the amount below which poverty exists; in the United States, it is based on calculations made on the cost of the thrifty USDA food plan.

Precursors of Disease — Factors that precede a health disorder.

Prekwashiorkor — A condition found most commonly in infants and young children; characterized by growth retardation for both height and weight, skin pallor, and dyspigmentation and easy pluckability of the hair.*

Premature — Born before full gestation term (37 weeks); sometimes applied to infants of low birth weight (below 2.5 kilograms) regardless of gestational age.*

Preschool Child — Age period of 1 year through 5 years.*

Presymptomatic Disease — The condition of an individual who has a disease but is not yet experiencing symptoms. For example, an individual may have slightly elevated blood sugar levels, but not be experiencing overt symptoms of diabetes. Detection may involve screening procedures or complete physical and diagnostic workups.

Prevalence — The number of cases of a disease or a particular condition occurring in a given group or area and at a specified time or during a given period of time. (No distinction is made between new or old cases; it is the total of all cases evident at the time the count is made.)*

Prevention — Avoidance of a disease; may involve four distinct levels of health care.

Primary prevention — the fostering of health and prevention of disease before it begins; involves the removal of the underlying cause of the disorder or health problem.

Secondary prevention — early intervention into existing illness; includes early detection of disease and speedy action and intervention to relieve discomfort and prevent disability and death.

Tertiary prevention — encouraging recovery from episodes of sickness; includes attempts to relieve discomfort, help people live acceptable lives while suffering from a chronic dysfunction, and improve health status through various rehabilitative techniques.

Rehabilitation — prevention to the extent of retarding development of further sequelae of disease condition.

Primary care — Medical care coordinated to patient needs and health status, possessing the following characteristics:

It includes "first-contact" care, the patient's entry point into the health care system.

It assumes outreach and follow-up responsibility for patient and community.

It is comprehensive and multidisciplinary.

It assumes ongoing responsibility for patient in terms of both health and sickness.

It assumes the responsibility for coordinating the care of all the patient's health problems.

It is "personal care in the broadest sense."

Profession — A career requiring specialized knowledge and intensive preparation, including instruction in skills and methods as well as in scientific, historical, or scholarly principles underlying such skills and methods; maintaining by force of organization or concerted opinion high standards of achievement and conduct; and committing its members to continued study and to a kind of work that has for its primary purpose the rendering of a public service (*Webster's Third International Dictionary*).

Professional Standards Review Organization (PSRO) — Under P.L. 92-603, mandated to monitor health care paid for under Title V, XVIII, and XIX of the Social Security Act.

Protein, Biological Value (BV) — The proportion of absorbed nitrogen retained in the body for maintenance and growth when a given protein is fed. If the correction for metabolic and endogenous losses is not made, the value is termed "apparent biological value."*

Protein-Calorie Malnutrition (PCM) — Malnutrition in persons (usually infants and young children) whose diets are deficient in proteins and calories; the disease condition is frequently precipitated by other factors such as infections (parasitic, bacterial, and viral). PCM may be classified clinically as marasmus, prekwashiorkor, or kwashiorkor.* It is sometimes referred to as protein-energy malnutrition, PEM.

Pyridoxine — The designated term to use for the compound 3 hydroxy-4, 5-bis (hydroxymethyl)-2-methylpyridine; also known as vitamin B_6, adermin, or pyridoxol.*

Recall — A method used in dietary surveys in which the subject is asked to recall everything he or she has eaten for the past 24 hours or other specific period; the reliability of this procedure is highly variable.*

Recommended Dietary Allowances (RDAs) — The specific term used by the Food and Nutrition Board of the National Research Council of the National Academy of Sciences (NAS/NRC) for recommendations for daily intake of specific nutrients, for groups of healthy individuals according to age and sex. The recommended dietary allowances, designed to be adequate for practically all the population of the United States, allow a margin of safety for individual variations.*

Reliability — The degree to which a given result can be reproduced in a second assessment.

Riboflavin — The designated term to be used for the compound also known as vitamin B_2, lactoflavin, or riboflavin.*

Skin-fold Thickness — Measurement, with calibrated calipers, of thickness of a fold of skin at a selected body site. Commonly selected sites for measurement, particularly in nutrition surveys, are the upper arm or triceps, subscapular region (just below the shoulder blade), and upper abdomen.*

Snacks — Any food or beverage consumed other than at a regular meal period.*

Special Milk Program — Federal program designed to allow schools, child care institutions, and camps to receive financial reimbursement for milk served to children.

Special Supplemental Food Program for Women, Infants, and Children (WIC) — Federal program for pregnant women, lactating mothers, and young children who cannot afford an adequate diet. The program provides extra food needed to promote growth, prevent malnutrition, and reduce other factors that may contribute to complications during pregnancy.

Standards — Professionally developed statements specifying level of health care performance in given areas.

Standards of Practice — Models or criteria designated to provide effective dietetic service to clients.

State Health Planning and Development Agency (SA) — The vehicle for operationalizing the mandate of the Health Systems Agency in each state.

Summer Feeding Program — Federal program designed to improve nutritional status of children under the age of 19 years through initiation, maintenance, or expansion of nonprofit food service programs where school food programs do not exist.

Susceptibility to Specific Disease — Understood in terms of a healthy person in danger of contracting disease upon exposure unless he or she is protected or immunized.

Ten-State Survey — See National Nutrition Survey.

Thiamin — The designated term to be used for vitamin B_1, or thiamin.*

Tocopherols — The designated term to use as the generic descriptor for all methyl tocols. Thus, the term is not synonymous with the term "vitamin E."*

Undernutrition — Inadequate intake of one or more nutrients and/or of calories. (The converse term "overnutrition" is not a recommended term.)*

USDA Food Plans — Dietary plans at four different cost levels — thrifty, low-cost, moderate-cost, and liberal. Provides estimates of the cost of an adequate diet on a monthly basis for 12 different age–sex combinations and for pregnant women and lactating mothers, according to one of these four cost levels.

Validity — Degree to which information actually measures what is intended to be assessed.

Vegans — Individuals who eat only food and food products from plant sources; all animal foods including meat, fish, poultry, milk, eggs, cheese, and seafoods in any form are avoided.*

Vegetarians — (1) Those who refrain from eating meat of any kind but use milk, milk products, and eggs — more specifically described as ovolactovegetarians; (2) those who refrain from eating meat and eggs — specifically called lactovegetarians; (3) those who eat only foods from plant sources — sometimes called pure (true) vegetarians.*

Vitamin A — The generic descriptor to use for all β-ionone derivatives, except pro-vitamin A carotenoids, exhibiting qualitatively the biological activity of retinol.*

Vitamin B_6 — The generic descriptor to use for all 2-methylpyridine derivatives exhibiting qualitatively the biological activity of pyridoxine.*

Vitamin B_{12} — The generic descriptor to use for all corrinoids exhibiting qualitatively the biological activity of cyanocobalamin.*

Vitamin C — The generic descriptor to use for all compounds exhibiting qualitatively the biological activity of ascorbic acid.*

Vitamin D — The generic descriptor to use for all steroids exhibiting qualitatively the biological activity of cholecalciferol.*

Vitamin E — The generic descriptor to use for all tocol derivatives exhibiting qualitatively the biological activity of α-tocopherol.*

Vitamin K — The generic descriptor to use for 2-methyl-1, 4-napthoquinone and all derivatives exhibiting qualitatively the biological activity of phylloquinone.*

Weaning — The period from the first consistent addition of a food supplement until breast- or bottle-feeding ends.*

Weanling — (1) A child in the course of being weaned. (2) An animal that can survive without suckling and is able to consume an experimental diet.*

Women, Infants, and Children (WIC) — *See* Special Supplemental Food Program.

Index

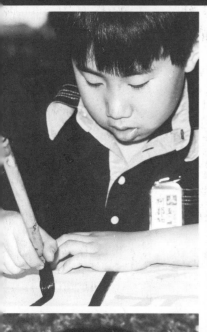
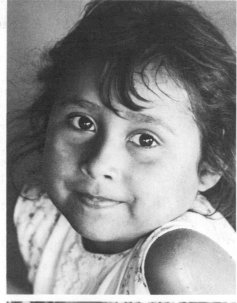
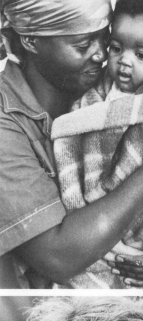
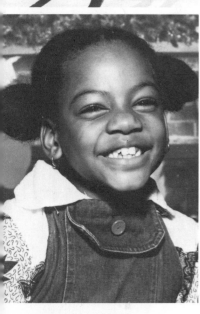
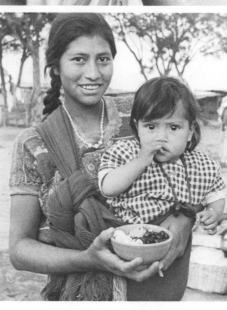
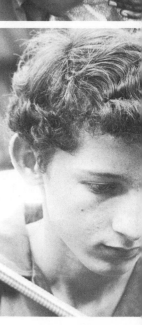
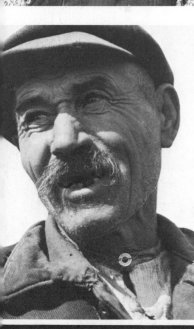
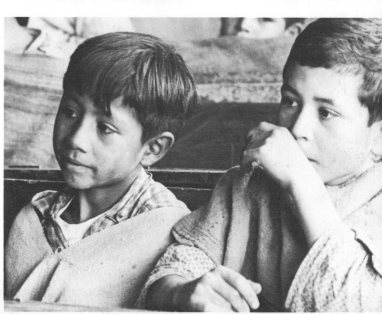